CRC Handbook of Lethality Guides for Low-Acid Canned Foods

Volume I Conduction-Heating

Authors

C. R. Stumbo
K. S. Purohit
T. V. Ramakrishnan
D. A. Evans
F. J. Francis

Department of Food Science
and Nutrition
University of Massachusetts
Amherst, Massachusetts

CRC Press, Inc.
Boca Raton, Florida

Library of Congress Cataloging in Publication Data
Main entry under title:

Handbook of lethality guides for low-acid
canned foods.

Includes bibliographies.

Contents: v. 1. Conduction-heating --
v. 2. Convection-heating.
1. Food, Canned--Sterilization--Tables.
2. Food--Bacteriology--Tables. I. Stumbo,
C. R. (Charles Raymond), 1914-
TP371.35. H36 1982 664'.0282 82-12900
ISBN 0-8493-2961-2 (v. 1)
ISBN 0-8493-2962-0 (v. 2)

Direct all inquiries to CRC Press, Inc., 2000 Corporate Blvd., N.W., Boca Raton, Florida, 33431.

International Standard Book Number 0-8493-2961-2 (Volume I)
International Standard Book Number 0-8493-2962-0 (Volume II)

Library of Congress Card Number 82-12900
Printed in the United States

FOREWORD

The thermal processing of food in sealed containers, or canning as it is known to the consumer, is a very old industry. It had its beginnings in France when Napoleon was concerned about the quantity and quality of food for his army. He offered a prize of 12,000 francs, a large sum in those days, to anyone who could develop a practical method of extending the shelf life of food. Nicolas Appert, an obscure Parisian confectioner, entered the contest and was awarded the prize in 1809. He published the first treatise on canning in 1810. His method was simply to place the food in a sealed container and subject the container to heat in boiling water. The reason why his method worked was unknown until a half century later from the researches of another Frenchman, Louis Pasteur. Regardless of his understanding, Appert was a capable experimenter, and he described canning procedures for more than 50 foods. Later food packers, without Appert's zeal for sanitation and adherence to processing details, had numerous failures primarily because of underprocessing, as many military personnel could testify. Nevertheless, the process succeeded and soon spread to many other countries.

The canning industry in America is believed to have been started by William Underwood who founded a company in Boston in 1819. In 1820, Underwood in Boston and Thomas Kensett in New York were producing canned foods. These early beginnings led to the very large industry we know today.

The microbiological basis of a successful canning industry in the U.S. was initiated by the work of Samuel C. Prescott and William L. Underwood in 1895 on the spoilage of corn. Progress was accelerated by the development of a chemical laboratory by the American Can Co. in 1906 and by the founding of the National Canners Association (now the National Food Processors Association) in 1907. The mathematical basis of assuring food safety in canning was first established in the era 1923 to 1928. The years between 1925 and 1945 saw much research effort culminating in a number of publications which established the safety of canned foods.

In the early 1950s, the canning industry was considered to be mature and research interest in thermal process calculation decreased considerably. Even the universities, which were training food scientists, decreased the time devoted to thermal process calculation. There were considered to be no problems since cases of botulism attributed to commercially processed food were rare indeed. A whole generation of food scientists grew up with minimal awareness of potential problems in thermally processed food.

This state of affairs came to an abrupt end in June 1971 with the infamous vichyssoise incident in which an underprocessed soup resulted in a death due to botulism. It became obvious that proper processing controls in this case were not being followed. Further, it is not difficult to imagine that a process schedule might not meet the minimum standards, since the scientific principles of thermal processing and the mathematics involved in process evaluations are relatively complex. The FDA was concerned about the potential public health aspects in an industry as large as this one. This resulted in more surveillance, the development of "Good Manufacturing Practices", and the requirement that all companies have a certified retort operator present at all times in which food was being processed.

The surveillance aspect of thermal processing from a public health point of view is not easy. The calculation of an adequate process is tedious and requires special training. The mere time involved in one calculation would ensure that food inspectors were not likely to calculate very many processes even if they did have the appropriate background. It was with this scenario that the idea of designing the process lethality guide tables was conceived. The complex mathematical steps involved in the process calculations were computerized and applied to a broad range of practical processing situations. Over 250,000 evaluations were done and the guide tables, which were originally developed under the auspices of a grant from the FDA to C. R. Stumbo, would enable anyone to assess the status of his process schedule for a given set of process parameters. This provides a quick check on the adequacy of a process for most practical situations designed for the sterilization of low-acid canned foods. The decision to publish these tables was based on the assumption that food processors would also welcome this type of information.

C. R. Stumbo
K. S. Purohit
T. V. Ramakrishnan
D. A. Evans
F. J. Francis

THE AUTHORS

Dr. Charles R. Stumbo, a native of Kansas, received a B.S., M.S., and Ph.D. in Bacteriology from Kansas State University with minors in physical and biological chemistry. He has held faculty positions at Kansas State University, South Dakota State College, Michigan State University, Washington State College, and the University of Massachusetts.

Dr. Stumbo has held a number of industry positions, including the John Morell Co., Owens-Illinois Glass Co., Food Machinery Corp., H. J. Heinz Co., and the Producers Creamery Co. He has also held two government positions with the Division of Soil Microbiology, U.S.D.A. and the Michigan State Department of Health. In all of these positions, his major responsibilities were in the microbiological aspects of food processing. The quality and public health safety aspects of processed food were paramount in his entire professional career.

His extensive industrial experience made him exceptionally well qualified for an academic appointment as Professor at the University of Massachusetts in Food Science and Technology. His research support came from the Food and Drug Administration of HEW and the Glass Container Manufacturers Institute. Dr. Stumbo is the author of 35 research papers and 3 books. One entitled *Thermobacteriology in Food Processing* is considered to be a classic in this professional discipline. Dr. Stumbo is retired.

Kailash S. Purohit,* a native of India, received his Ph.D. (Food Engineering) in 1972 from the University of Massachusetts, Amherst. For the next 2 years, he taught a course in Sterilization Process Engineering and worked at the Heat Sterilization Process Evaluation Center in Amherst.

He joined the General Foods Technical Center in 1974 and was involved in alternate energy sources and Decaffeination R&D. Since 1977 he has been employed by Travenol Laboratories, and has worked in their Corporate Sterilization Department developing processes for drugs, devices, and parenteral solutions. He is presently a Group Manager for Heat and Aseptic Process Development.

His professional interests include biochemistry, biophysics, and microbiology, as they relate to the industrial production, preservation processing, and handling of biological materials.

Dr. T. V. Ramakrishnan received a Ph.D. in Food Science from the University of Massachusetts in 1973. He received a B.S. in Chemistry and a M.S. in Biochemistry from the University of Bombay, India. He is currently with the Department of Food Science and Nutrition at the University of Massachusetts doing research on various aspects of thermal processing and chemistry of foods. He was with Heinz for a year in 1975 and prior to that spent a year as a Postdoctoral Research Associate at the Process Evaluation Center for FDA, Department of Food Science and Nutrition at the University of Massachusetts. He was with Bhabha Atomic Research Center in Bombay for 5 years and conducted research on food pigments, proteins, and radiation preservation of foods. He has published several papers on chemistry and processing aspects of foods. He has also participated in several technical symposia.

* Present address — Baxter Travenol Laboratories, Chicago, Ill.

Dr. David A. Evans received the Ph.D. degree in Food Science from the University of Massachusetts. He has been in his present position as Associate Professor since 1972. His teaching and research interests include thermobacteriology and food processing, food microbiology, and food fermentations. He has held positions in the commercial food industry in Pennsylvania and Arizona. He has also served on several industry and government task force committees over the years, including the FDA Advisory Committee on Thermal Process Evaluation and the NFPA Ad Hoc Committee for Reveiw and Development of Processes for Low-Acid Foods in Glass Containers. Dr. Evans has authored or co-authored more than 30 technical and/or research papers relating to the microbiological quality and thermobacteriology of foods.

Dr. F. J. Francis, a native of Ottawa, Canada, received a B.A. in Biochemistry and a M.A. in Food Chemistry from the University of Toronto. He received a Ph.D. in Food Technology from the University of Massachusetts. He has held faculty positions at the University of Toronto, the University of Guelph, and since 1954, the University of Massachusetts.

Dr. Francis has held his current position as Professor since 1977, and prior to that was Department Head, Food Science and Nutrition from 1971 to 1977, and Nicolas Appert Professor from 1964 to 1971 at the University of Massachusetts. His research interests include food pigments, food colorimetry, food composition, thermal processing, and post-harvest physiology of fruits and vegetables. In recent years, his interests have also included technical methods for increasing food supply and food safety.

He has been very active in the Institute of Food Technologists and served as President in 1980 to 1981. He has served on the Board of Directors of both Food Update, sponsored by the Food Drug and Law Institute and the Research and Development Associates for Military Food and Packaging Systems. He is a Fellow of both the Institute of Food Technologists and the American Association for the Advancement of Science, as well as being a member of ten other professional societies. His honors include Distinguished Scientist of the Year, New York Section of IFT; Nicolas Appert Medal, Institute of Food Technologists; and the International Award, Institute of Food Technologists.

Dr. Francis is the author of over 260 technical papers and co-author of 3 books: *Food Colorimetry: Theory and Applications* (AVI, 1975), *Food, Nutrition and You* (Prentice-Hall, 1976), and *Human Ecological Issues: A Reader* (Kendall/Hunt, 1980).

CRC HANDBOOK OF LETHALITY GUIDES FOR LOW-ACID CANNED FOODS

Authors

C. R. Stumbo, K. S. Purohit, T. V. Ramakrishnan, D. A. Evans, and F. J. Francis

Volume I
CONDUCTION-HEATING
Basic Considerations
Thermal Process Lethality Guides for Conduction-Heating Low-Acid Canned Foods
References
Appendix

Volume II
CONVECTION-HEATING
Basic Considerations
Thermal Process Lethality Guides for Convection-Heating Low-Acid Canned Foods
References
Appendix

TABLE OF CONTENTS

Volume I

BASIC CONSIDERATIONS
Introduction to Thermal Processing of Low-Acid Foods 3
Thermobacteriology and Process Variables 3
Methods of Process Evaluation and Their Complexity 5
Thermal Process Evaluation Procedures 6
Order of Death of Bacteria and Target Process Value 6
Thermobacteriological and Heat Penetration Data 6
Mathematical Methods of Evaluation 9
Process Evaluation for Conduction-Heating Products 10
Development of Computer Programs for Thermal Process Evaluations and the Establishment of Process Lethality Guides 18
Microbiological Basis for Thermal Process Lethality Guides 20
Safe Thermal Processes 20
Commercial Sterility 22
Application of the Tables to Practical Processing Schedules 23

THERMAL PROCESS LETHALITY GUIDES FOR CONDUCTION-HEATING LOW-ACID CANNED FOODS
Heat Penetration and Processing Parameters 27
Use of the Tables for Conduction-Heating Products 28
Section I: Safe Thermal Processes with z Values from 12 to 18; Tables 1 to 164 31
Section II: Safe Thermal Processes with z Values from 18 to 24; Tables 165 to 328 197
Section III: Commercial Sterility with z Values from 16 to 22; Tables 329 to 498 363

REFERENCES 531

APPENDIX
Symbols and Definitions 535
Can Volume and Process Values for 41 Can Sizes 537
An Example of Using the Process Lethality Guide Tables for Conduction-Heating Products 539

Basic Considerations

INTRODUCTION TO THERMAL PROCESSING OF LOW-ACID FOODS

In order to understand the fundamentals of thermal processing of foods in sealed containers, it is essential to classify the food products on the basis of pH. A widely recognized classification is as follows:

- Low-acid foods: pH above 4.5
- Acid foods: pH 4.0 to 4.5
- High-acid foods: pH below 4.0

Preservation of foods by thermal processing is based on reducing the probability of survival of a vegetative organism or a bacterial spore that is of concern either because of possible toxin formation in the food, or because of possible economic spoilage of the food. Those organisms which are of most concern to the acid and high-acid foods are normally less heat resistant than those organisms or spores that are of concern to low-acid foods. Consequently, the low-acid foods require more severe thermal processing than do the acid and high-acid foods. From the public health standpoint, microbiological safety aspects require that the thermal process must be adequate to insure the inactivation of spores of *Clostridium botulinum*. Also, the industrial sterilization processes for low-acid foods are designed for commercial sterility in order to reduce the economic loss due to spoilage. However, processing for commercial sterility is secondary in importance to processing for a high degree of safety. In most cases, a process designed to insure commercial sterility with a high degree of assurance, for a given set of variables, is more severe than a process, with the same variables, designed to provide a high degree of public health safety.

The concepts and the mathematical steps involved in the process evaluations are relatively complex, and the calculations tend to be tedious and time consuming. So far, there has not been any attempt made to develop comprehensive process lethality guides so that a food processor could quickly check, at least approximately, the adequacy of a process schedule. We undertook a serious effort in this direction by first developing elaborate computer programs for all the mathematical routines needed for effective and accurate process calculations. The potential of these programs was utilized to establish the process lethality guides for low-acid canned foods. An accurate evaluation of the critical thermal resistance and process variables on the lethality requirements for safe thermal processes and commercial sterility was made. Approximately 250,000 evaluations were required for both conduction- and convection- heating products. A broad range of processing criteria were covered by considering low-acid foods of different heat transfer properties for the standard 41 can sizes under widely varying processing conditions. The process variables associated with a particular industrial process most probably will not match exactly with the value of the corresponding variables listed in the appropriate process lethality guide tables. However, with proper use of the tables, it is possible, in most cases, to check the adequacy of an industrial sterilization process, at least in approximate terms.

Volume I includes detailed discussions on thermobacteriological considerations, process evaluation methods, and lethality guide tables for conduction-heating products. Volume II deals with the evaluation methods and the tables for convection-heating products.

Thermobacteriology and Process Variables

In the sterilization of foods which have a pH above 4.5, special attention should be given to several microorganisms of concern. The most important bacteria from the standpoint of safety is the neuroparalytic toxin-forming bacterium *C. botulinum*. Under the anaerobic conditions of hermetically sealed cans, the surviving spores of *C. botulinum* could germinate to vegetative cells that might produce a toxin in the medium of low-acid foods. Because of this, the safety aspects of sterilization of low-acid foods are based on achieving a considerable reduction of the probability of survival of spores of *C. botulinum* in processed foods.

In the canning industry, the public health safety aspects of low-acid foods must be given the highest possible considerations. Also, from a commercial standpoint, the storage stability of the canned product is an extremely important aspect. Thermal processing of low-acid foods in the industry is generally directed towards achieving commercial sterility which would assure different degrees of freedom from economic spoilage. The entities of concern in this respect are bacterial spores of some of the thermophilic and mesophilic anaerobes and facultative anaerobes. For the most part, spores of these bacteria have a greater resistance to heat than do *C. botulinum* spores. Consequently, thermal processes for commercial sterility are in most cases more severe than those required for public health safety.

The amount of processing to be given to a low-acid food would depend on the following basic considerations.

1. Thermobacteriological aspects
2. Size of the container and the heat transfer characteristics of the food per se
3. The actual processing conditions

The primary aspect of the thermobacteriological criterion is to select the degree of processing, whether it should merely be safe from a public health point of view or whether it should also assure commercial sterility. The organism of concern should be defined along with its initial population, heat resistant characteristics, and the extent of reduction needed. From these data, a target value for the process is derived that is generally expressed in terms of minutes of processing time at a specified temperature, usually 250°F.

The next step in thermal process evaluation is to determine the actual process time from the target process value. The heat penetration data corresponding to a specific food in a particular container size are plotted and the necessary related data are deduced for use in the subsequent calculation by a suitable method. Even though two different products may have the same target process value, the process time needed to achieve safety or commercial sterility would differ considerably because of the influence of the heat transfer characteristics of the food in a particular can size and the variability of parameters associated with the actual processing conditions. The size of the can could easily vary from a small size such as 202 × 204 to a large size such as 603 × 700. The dimensions and the volume of the container are major factors that influence the calculation of the process time. Under similar conditions, the larger the size of the can, the greater will be the process time needed. The heat transfer properties of the food itself are important factors. In thermal process evaluation of low-acid foods these are generally expressed in terms of thermal diffusivity values. In practice, the size of the can and the thermal diffusivity are treated together and the resultant function is derived from the plot of the heat penetration data.

The actual processing conditions in industrial plants generally vary widely from one situation to another. The retort temperature has a very significant influence on the final process time necessary to achieve the target process value. The higher the retort temperature, the shorter will be the process time needed. The temperature of the food at the beginning of processing can also modify the process time. The higher the initial food temperature, the shorter will be the process time. The rate of cooling can also indirectly affect the evaluation of the process time although to a lesser degree compared to the other variables. When the cooling rate is slow the process time will be shortened slightly. Different processing equipment such as still retorts, agitating retorts, or continuous processors affect the rate of transfer of heat within the food itself. In the evaluation of the process time the heat transfer properties of a specific food in a particular container should be determined under the normal operating conditions of the equipment, and the corresponding functions derived should be used in the calculation. The heat transfer function would include in itself any variability that may arise due to the design of the processing equipment.

Methods of Process Evaluation and Their Complexity

It should be clear from the discussion on the thermobacteriology of food processing and related process variables that determination of the process time from the target-process value for a low-acid food packed in a container of particular size and to be processed under certain conditions involves several variables. The first scientific approach to the problem of applying bacteriological and physical data to evaluation of thermal processes for foods was the general method described by Bigelow et al.[3] This method is essentially a graphical procedure for integrating the lethal effects of various time-temperature relationships existent at some given point in a confined body of food during heat processing. Notable improvements in the general method were made by Schultz and Olson.[12] These improvements greatly increased the applicability of the general method, however, the method is still laborious and is ordinarily used only for the calculation of processes which cannot be readily evaluated by the simpler mathematical procedures developed by Ball.[1,2] This method mathematically accomplishes the integration of the lethal effects produced by the time-temperature relationships existent at the point of greatest temperature lag in a container of food during the process. The equations developed can be applied to any case in which the major portion of the heating curve on a semilogarithmic paper approximates a straight line or two straight lines, and also, where the thermal death time curve on semilogarithmic paper is, or can be assumed to be, a straight line. Provisions were made in the method for applying the given heat penetration data to all can sizes and retort temperatures. In Ball's method it was assumed that the point of greatest temperature lag was the primary point of concern with respect to calculating a process time to accomplish sterilization. The other points in the container generally receive more severe heat treatments and their consideration may be valuable in assessing the overall reduction of bacterial load per container particularly for conduction-heating products. Stumbo[19] developed and refined a mathematical procedure for integrating the lethal effects of time-temperature combinations existent throughout a container of a conduction-heating food during the process. This procedure is reasonably accurate, but it is complex and tedious.

The mathematical method of Ball and the subsequent modification by Stumbo for conduction-heating products are basically versatile. The actual evaluation involves many repeated calculations and several references to tables of values. The evaluations are not only complex but also demand a sound understanding of thermobacteriology of food processing. The complexity involved has limited the application of these methods. In order to make the evaluations simpler and more easily applicable to practical processing situations, elaborate computer programs were developed, which would automatically perform the detailed operations involved. The speed and accuracy were greatly improved and the versatility of the programs enabled us to undertake a rather difficult task of making an extensive study in the thermal processing of low-acid foods. Thousands of calculations were performed to obtain safe thermal processes and processes for commercial sterility at comparable processing situations. The purpose of this effort is to present the process evaluations in the form of tables, and it is hoped these values will be helpful to the food processors as a guide in establishing the process time and also to determine the adequacy of processes.

THERMAL PROCESS EVALUATION PROCEDURES

The process evaluations for the establishment of thermal process lethality guides are based on the mathematical methods of Ball[1,2] and the further refinements made by Stumbo.[19] The mathematical methods are described here along with typical examples of process calculations explaining most of the steps involved. Also a brief account of the thermobacteriological aspects and the heat penetration data are given. For a full understanding of these basic considerations and the various symbols, the reader is referred to the book *Thermobacteriology in Food Processing.*[20]

Order of Death of Bacteria and Target Process Value

The order of death of bacteria is considered to be essentially logarithmic and a general equation defining the survivor curve may be written as follows:

$$t = D(\log a - \log b)$$

t = time, in minutes, of heating at a constant lethal temperature
D = time, in minutes, to kill 90% of the population
a = initial number of viable cells in the population
b = number of viable cells in the population after time t (1)

The bacterial population considered here is per unit volume. The unit volume may be 1 mℓ, or the volume of food in a container of given size.

For the purpose of comparing the relative sterilizing capacities of different heat processes, it is necessary to consider a unit of lethality. For convenience, 1 min of heating at 250°F is defined as the unit of lethality. In sterilization processes, the total process lethality is designated by the symbol F. Equation 1 may be modified and written as:

$$F = D(\log a - \log b) \qquad (2)$$

Without any subscript the symbol F is a general term. It may refer to the sum of all the effects at any one point in a container or to the sum of all the effects at an infinite number of points throughout a container of food. If F corresponds to the lethal effects at the geometrical center of the container, which is considered to be the slowest heating point, it is designated as F_c. In conduction-heating evaluations, an infinite number of points in the whole container is considered and the total lethal effects would be referred as F_s.

Thermobacteriological and Heat Penetration Data

In order to establish the process time for low-acid foods, an understanding of the heat resistant characteristics of the spores of the bacteria of concern is essential. The two factors which define the heat resistance of spores are D_r and z values. When bacteria are subjected to moist heat, death expressed in terms of reduction of individual organisms is quite orderly. The number of viable cells is generally reduced exponentially with time of exposure to a lethal temperature. The D_r value is defined as the time required at any designated reference temperature to destroy 90% of the spores or vegetative cells of a given organism.

During thermal processing, the food is subjected to different temperatures. The resistance of a bacterial spore at different temperatures varies widely. Thermal destruction curves (TD) reflect the relative resistance of bacteria to different lethal temperatures. They are most conveniently constructed by plotting the logarithm of D against the corresponding temperatures of exposure. The TD curves are essentially straight lines over the range of temperatures of chief concern in food sterilization. The term z is numerically equal to the number of fahrenheit degrees required for the TD curve to traverse one log cycle. Thus, the z value employed in the process calculations accounts for the relative resistance of microorganisms to different lethal temperatures.

There are several methods of determining the D and z values of bacterial spores.[20] The D value is evaluated by studying the reduction in population at a constant temperature and the z value is calculated from the data on D values at different temperatures. For the public health significance, the organisms of concern in the sterilization of low-acid foods are *C. botulinum* types A and B. They are characterized by D_{250} values of the order of 0.10 to 0.20. The types A and B of *C. botulinum* are considerably less resistant than the mesophilic organisms of the *C. sporogenes* group which are of significance in the economic spoilage of low-acid foods. A good example of this is the organism Putrefactive Anaerobe 3679 (P.A. 3679) which is characterized by D_{250} values ranging from 0.50 to 1.50. Because of its heat resistance, nontoxicity, and other practical advantages, P.A. 3679 frequently is used as a test organism to establish the adequacy of canning processes. The spores of a thermophilic spoilage organism such as the facultatively anaerobic *Bacillus stearothermophilus* are extremely heat resistant and D_{250} values as high as 5.0 min may be encountered. The z values of most of the spores important to the sterilization of low-acid foods range usually from 12 to 22 F°.

There are a number of food factors that may influence the bacterial resistance to heat and growth of bacteria. One of the most important of these is acidity, generally expressed in terms of pH. For this reason, in a discussion of bacterial spoilage, foods are generally classified as low-acid (above 4.5), acid (pH 4.0), and high-acid (below pH 4.0).[20]

Inherent resistance of bacterial spores varies not only with species but also with different strains of the same species. Environmental factors active during the growth of bacteria have been observed to exert widely variable influences on the resistance of different species and strains of bacteria. The resistance of a bacterial spore when the heat is being applied is also affected by the nature of the food in which it is suspended. Because of these reasons, in process evaluations for a particular low-acid food, the D and z values used should be based on their practical determination in the chosen food itself under the normal operating conditions to be employed.

In order to evaluate the process time from the target process value for the sterilization of low-acid foods, it is important to obtain experimental data on the heat transfer characteristics of the chosen food in the specified container under actual processing conditions. The temperature of the food at different stages of processing is determined at the point of slowest heating in the container using thermocouples. The experimental data recorded should be transformed into proper form for further use in the calculation of process time by mathematical methods. The time-temperature data are plotted on a semilogarithmic paper. To construct the heating curve, the difference between retort temperature and food temperature is plotted on a logarithmic scale against time on a linear scale. This can be conveniently accomplished by rotating the semi-log paper through 180° and labeling the top line 1° below retort temperature and plotting the temperature of food directly (Figure 1). For the cooling curve, the semilogarithmic paper is kept in its normal position and the food temperature is used directly after labeling the bottom line 1° above the cooling water temperature.

There are several parameters associated with the processing conditions and the heat transfer properties of the food (see Figure 1) in a particular can size. They are as follows:

Initial temperature (T_{ih}) — This is the temperature of the food at zero time of heating or cooling.

Retort temperature (T_r) — The retort temperature is the controlled temperature of the heating medium, in the retort, in processing a product.

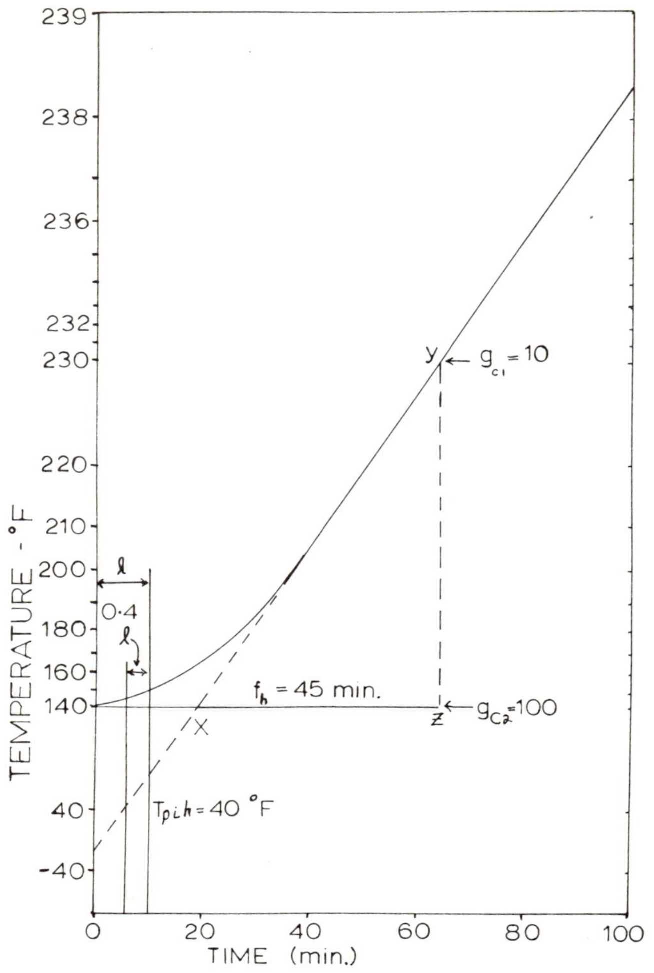

FIGURE 1. Semilogarithmic heat penetration plot.

Process time (B) — This refers to the time elapsing from the instant the retort is up to a desired processing temperature until the instant the steam is turned off plus 0.4 of the time (ℓ) required to bring the retort to the processing temperature.

$$B = P_t + 0.4\,\ell$$

P_t is the operators process time and corresponds to the time elapsing from the instant the retort is up to processing temperature until the steam is turned off.

$$P_t = B - 0.4\,\ell$$

The function (I_h) — This function is defined as the difference between the retort temperature and initial food temperature.

$$I_h = T_r - T_{ih}$$

Pseudo-initial temperature (T_{pih}) — This is the temperature represented by the intersection of the extension of the straight line portion of the semi-log heating curve and a verticle line corresponding to the beginning of the process (Figure 1).

The heating lag factor (j_{ch}) — This factor on being multiplied by I_h locates the intersection of the extension of the straight line portion of the heat penetration curve and a verticle line representing the beginning of the process. Mathematically, it is defined as follows:

$$j_{ch} = \frac{T_r - T_{pih}}{T_r - T_{ih}}$$

The cooling lag factor (j_{cc}) — This factor corresponds to the cooling curve and is similar to j_{ch} and is mathematically defined as follows:

$$j_{cc} = \frac{T_w - T_{pic}}{T_w - T_{ic}}$$

T_w = cooling water temperature, T_{pic} = pseudo-initial cooling temperature, and T_{ic} = initial cooling temperature.

The function (f_h) — This function expresses the combined effects of the heat transfer properties of the food per se, the thermal diffusivity (k), and the size of the container on the rate of increase in temperature at the geometrical center of the food during processing. The f_h is defined as the time in minutes required for the straight line portion of the semi-log heat penetration curve to traverse one log cycle (Figure 1). It is numerically equal to the reciprocal of the slope of the curve.

Mathematical Methods of Evaluation

The mathematical methods of evaluating the process time were originally developed by Ball.[1,2] These methods are based on the integration of lethal effects produced by time-temperature relationships existent at the point of greatest temperature lag in a container of food during thermal processing. The mathematical steps involved can be applied to most processing situations in which the products exhibit a straight line semi-log heating curve after the initial lag. The equation developed by Ball may be written as follows:

$$B = f_h \log \frac{j_{ch} I_h}{g_c} \tag{3}$$

g_c is the difference, in degrees Farenheit, between the retort temperature and the maximum temperature reached by the food at the geometrical center which is considered to be the point of greatest temperature lag. An analysis of Figure 1 would indicate the basis for Equation 3. From the triangle XYZ and the heat penetration curve

$$\text{Slope} = \frac{\log g_{c2} - \log g_{c1}}{f_h}$$

$$\log g_{c2} - \log g_{c1} = 1$$

since this corresponds to a difference of one log cycle. Therefore,

$$\text{Slope} = 1/f_h$$

If the process time (B) is the x-coordinate, the corresponding y-coordinate is $\log j_{ch} I_h - \log g_c$. Also

$$\text{Slope} = \frac{\log j_{ch} I_h - \log g_c}{B}$$

Therefore,

$$\frac{\log j_{ch} I_h - \log g_c}{B} = 1/f_h$$

$$B = f_h(\log j_{ch} I_h - \log g_c) \qquad (4)$$

This equation is a modified form of Equation 3.

During the cooling process there is also some heat left in the product. Even though it is not obvious, Equations 3 and 4 do take into account the lethal effects of heat available during cooling. This is done through the relationship of g to the ratio f_h/U, where U is the time required at retort temperature to accomplish the same amount of bacterial destruction equivalent to the F value of the process. This can be explained by constructing a hypothetical TD curve passing through 1 min at 250°F.[20] Here,

$$U = F F_i$$

also

$$F_i = \log^{-1} \frac{250 - T_r}{z}$$

where F_i is the time at the given retort temperature (T) equivalent to 1 min at 250°F.

It is important to note that the variations in the values of z significantly affects f_h/U:g relationships. It has also been found that these relationships are virtually independent of the process parameters such as the retort temperature, container dimensions, initial food temperature, cooling water temperature, and the j value of the heating curve. However, they are greatly influenced by the j value of cooling curves. Stumbo and Longley[21] published tables of f_h/U:g relationships for the z values from 12 to 22 and accounted for the variations in the j value of the cooling curve. These relationships were arrived at by manually employing the general method of integration. Jen et al.[7] devised a computer program based on the finite difference method of Teixeira[24] for the general method and developed f_h/U:g tables. Purohit[9] refined these approaches and a series of f_h/U:g tables were developed by a universally acceptable computer program based on log-log interpolation and extrapolation.

Since the general method of integration was used to determine the value of U in the f_h/U:g relationships, it is important to note that for any given value of g, the corresponding value of U in the f_h/U:g ratio accounts for all the lethal heat available during heating and cooling parts of the process. The g value used in Equation 4 would also take into account all the lethal heat of both heating and cooling. These concepts are best understood by a step by step analysis of process calculations.

Process Evaluation for Conduction-Heating Products

If a low-acid food heats by conduction during processing there will be a lack of product movement and consequently there will be a temperature gradient from the geometrical center to the wall of the container. For this reason, the geometrical center is often considered as the slowest heating and the slowest cooling point in the container. The mathematical method of Ball[1,2] is based on the concept of integrating the lethal effects produced during the process at a single point in the container of food, generally the point of greatest temperature lag. The other points in the container receive more severe heat treatments and this was not accounted in evaluating the overall lethality per container with respect to the organism of concern. Stumbo[19] presented a mathematical procedure for integrating the lethal effects of the time-temperature combinations existing throughout a container of conduction-heating food during the process. The variation in severity of heating for conduction-heating food in a container from the wall to the geometrical center can be understood by picturing a series of imaginary concentric containers nested inside the real container. Different points on the surface of an imaginary container is supposed to receive the same amount of lethality and for this reason the container is considered to have an iso-F surface. The value of F depends on the value of g attained during the process. Since g can vary only if j varies, for any heating situation an iso-F surface is necessarily iso-j also.

The procedure adopted for conduction-heating low-acid foods is based on the basic hypothesis that an evaluation of the total lethality of a heat process, to reduce the number of bacteria in a container, should take into account the sum of all the lethal effects at all points throughout the container. There are several concepts involved in the development of suitable mathematical procedures for this purpose. For an understanding of these aspects the reader is advised to consult *Thermobacteriology in Food Processing*.[20] Proper application of these procedures generally yields accurate results; however, they are complex and tedious. A typical example of process evaluation for conduction-heating foods is presented here. The various mathematical steps involved are explained in detail for easy understanding.

The primary purpose is to determine the process time necessary to meet the minimum lethality requirements for safety with respect to spores of *C. botulinum* with a z value equal to 14, for a conduction-heating low-acid food. We will assume that the product is packed in a 300 × 407 can and is to be processed at a retort temperature of 240°F. The hypothetical variables involved in the processing are as follows:

Microbiological criteria	
The organism of concern	: *C. botulinum*
D_{250} Value	: 0.2 min
z Value	: 14 F°
Initial bacterial population (1/cm³)	: 432
Extent of reduction desired	: 12 log cycles
Heat penetration and processing parameters	
Heating rate function, f_h	: 52.82 min
Heating lag factor, j_{ch}	: 2.00
Cooling lag factor, j_{cc}	: 2.00
Initial food temperature, T_{ih}	: 140°F
Retort temperature, T_r	: 240°F

Step 1. To establish the process value (F_s) required.

The process value required can be established by Equation 2.

$$F_S = D_{250} (\log a - \log b)$$

Then

$$F_S = 0.20 (\log 432 - \log 10^{-12})$$

$$= 0.20 (2.636 + 12)$$

F_s required = $\underline{2.93}$

Now it is necessary to determine the process time to achieve F_s of 2.93 under the chosen processing conditions. For this purpose, F_c value corresponding to F_s required must be calculated and it is done by interpolation using the following equation:

$$F_c \text{ desired} = F_{c1} + \frac{F_{c2} - F_{c1}}{F_{s2} - F_{s1}} (F_s \text{ desired} - F_{s1}) \quad (5)$$

(F_{c1}, F_{s1}) and (F_{c2}, F_{s2}) correspond to two hypothetical situations chosen for the purpose of interpolation. Since the z value of *C. botulinum* in this case is 14F°, F_c and F_s, respectively, become F_c^{14} and F_s^{14}. Equation 5 is modified as

$$F_c^{14} \text{ desired} = F_{c1}^{14} + \frac{F_{c2}^{14} - F_{c1}^{14}}{F_{s2}^{14} - F_{s1}^{14}} (F_s^{14} \text{ desired} - F_{s1}^{14}) \quad (6)$$

Step 2. Selection of F_{c1} and F_{c2} values for interpolation.

The value of F_c is always less than F_s and the difference between F_s desired and F_c desired is generally more than one D_{250} value. Hence, F_c^{14} desired is likely to be lower than 2.73, viz., 2.93 − 0.2. The two hypothetical values F_{c1}^{14} and F_{c2}^{14} chosen should be close to F_c^{14} desired, however, one value should be higher and the other lower than F_c^{14} desired to facilitate interpolation. Hence, the following choice

$$F_{c1}^{14} = 2.00$$

$$F_{c2}^{14} = 3.00$$

The next step involves the calculation of F_{s1}^{14} from F_{c1}^{14} and F_{s2}^{14} from F_{c2}^{14}.

Step 3. Calculation of F_{s1}^{14} corresponding to F_{c1}^{14}.

$$U_c = F_c F_i$$

Since

$$U_{240}^{14} = F_c^{14} \cdot F_{i240}^{14}$$

$$F_i = \log^{-1} \frac{250 - T_r}{z}$$

Since $T_r = 240$ and $z = 14$,

$$F_{i240}^{14} = \log^{-1} \frac{250 - 240}{14} = \underline{5.179}$$

Also $F_{c1}^{14} = 2.00$

$$U_{c1} = F^{14}_{c1} \times F^{14}_{i240}$$

$$= 2.00 \times 5.179$$

$$U_{c1} = \underline{10.36}$$

Since $f_h = 52.82$

$$f_h / U_{c1} = \frac{52.82}{10.36} = \underline{5.099}$$

Now, from the f_h/U:g table for z of 14,[20] find the corresponding g value for

$$f_h / U_{c1} = 5.099 \text{ and } j_{cc} = 2.00$$

$$g_{c1} = \underline{5.424}$$

To calculate F_s desired from F_c the general equation[20] used is the following:

$$F_s = F_c + D_r \left(1.084 + \log \frac{F_\lambda - F_c}{D_r}\right) \tag{7}$$

F_λ represents the F value characterizing the heat treatment received by any iso-j region. It can be derived by using the following established relationships

$$g_\lambda = 0.5\, g_c \text{ and } j_\lambda = 0.5\, j_{cc}$$

To evaluate the F^{14}_{s1} value from F^{14}_{c1} Equation 7 may be written as

$$F^{14}_{s1} = F^{14}_{c1} + D_{250} \left(1.084 + \log \frac{F_{\lambda 1} - F^{14}_{c1}}{D_{250}}\right) \tag{8}$$

Also

$$g_{\lambda 1} = 0.5\, g_{c1}$$

And

$$j_{\lambda 1} = 0.5\, j_{cc}$$

Since $g_{c_1} = 5.424$ and $j_{cc} = 2.00$

$$g_{\lambda_1} = 0.5 \times 5.424 = \underline{2.712}$$

$$J_{\lambda_1} = 0.5 \times 2.00 = \underline{1.00}$$

Now from the f_h/U:g table for z of 14, find the corresponding f_h/U_{λ_1} for

$$g_{\lambda_1} = 2.712 \text{ and } j_{\lambda_1} = 1.00$$

$$f_h/U_{\lambda_1} = \underline{3.227}$$

Since $f_h = 52.82$

$$U_{\lambda_1} = \frac{52.82}{3.227} = \underline{16.37}$$

$$U_{\lambda_1} = F^{14}_{\lambda_1} \cdot F^{14}_{i240}$$

$$F_{\lambda_1} = \frac{U_{\lambda_1}}{F^{14}_{i240}}$$

Since $F^{14}_{i240} = 5.179$

$$F_{\lambda_1} = \frac{16.37}{5.179} = \underline{3.161}$$

Since

$$F^{14}_{c1} = 2.00$$

$$F_{\lambda_1} = 3.161 \quad \text{and}$$

$$D_{250} = 0.2$$

Equation 8 thus becomes

$$F^{14}_{s1} = 2.00 + 0.20\left(1.084 + \log \frac{3.161 - 2.00}{0.20}\right)$$

$$= \underline{2.369}$$

F^{14}_{s1} corresponding to F^{14}_{c1} is 2.369.

Step 4. Calculation of F^{14}_{s2} from F^{14}_{c2}.

The calculation of F^{14}_{s2} value from the chosen F^{14}_{c2} is similar to the steps involved in arriving at F^{14}_{s1} from F^{14}_{c1}.

$$F^{14}_{c2} = 3.00 \text{ and } F^{14}_{i240} = 5.179$$

$$U_{c2} = F^{14}_{c2} \times F^{14}_{i240}$$

$$= 3.00 \times 5.179$$

$$= \underline{15.54}$$

Since $f_h = 52.82$

$$f_h/U_{c2} = \frac{52.82}{15.54} = \underline{3.400}$$

Now from the f_h/U:g table for z of 14 find the corresponding g value for

$$f_h/U_{c2} = 3.400 \quad \text{and} \quad j_{cc} = 2.00$$

$$g_{c2} = \underline{3.682}$$

To evaluate the F_{S2}^{14} value from F_{C2}^{14} Equation 7 may be written as

$$F_{S2}^{14} = F_{C2}^{14} + D_{250}\left(1.084 + \log \frac{F_{\lambda 2} - F_{C2}^{14}}{D_{250}}\right) \qquad (9)$$

Also

$$g_{\lambda 2} = 0.5\, g_{c2}$$

$$j_{\lambda 2} = 0.5\, j_{cc}$$

Since $g_{c2} = 3.682$ and $j_{cc} = 2.00$

$$g_{\lambda 2} = 0.5 \times 3.682 = \underline{1.841}$$

$$j_{\lambda 2} = 0.5 \times 2.00 = \underline{1.00}$$

Now from the f_h/U:g table for z of 14, find the corresponding $f_h/U_{\lambda 2}$ for

$$g_{\lambda 2} = 1.841 \quad \text{and } j_{\lambda 2} = 1.00$$

$$f_h/U_{\lambda 2} = \underline{2.290}$$

Since $f_h = 52.82$

$$U_{\lambda 2} = \frac{52.82}{2.290} = \underline{23.07}$$

$$U_{\lambda 2} = F_{\lambda 2} \cdot F_{i240}^{14}$$

$$F_{\lambda 2} = \frac{U_{\lambda 2}}{F_{i240}^{14}}$$

Since $F_{i240}^{14} = 5.179$

$$F_{\lambda 2} = \frac{23.07}{5.179} = \underline{4.450}$$

The equation relating F_{c2}^{14} and F_{s2}^{14} is

$$F_{S2}^{14} = F_{C2}^{14} + D_{250}\left(1.084 + \log\frac{F_{\lambda 2} - F_{C2}^{14}}{D_{250}}\right) \qquad (9)$$

Since

$$F_{C2}^{14} = 3.00$$

$$F_{\lambda 2} = 4.45 \quad \text{and}$$

$$D_{250} = 0.20$$

Equation 9 thus becomes

$$F_{S2}^{14} = 3.00 + 0.2\left(1.084 + \log\frac{4.44 - 3.00}{0.20}\right)$$

$$= \underline{3.389}$$

F_{s2}^{14} corresponding to F_{c2}^{14} is 3.389.

Step 5. Determination of F_c desired from F_s desired, F_{s1} and F_{s2}.
The equation which relates F_c^{14}, F_s^{14}, F_{s1}^{14}, and F_{s2}^{14} is written as

$$F_C^{14}\text{ desired} = F_{C_1}^{14} + \frac{F_{C_2}^{14} - F_{C_1}^{14}}{F_{S_2}^{14} - F_{S_1}^{14}}\left(F_S^{14}\text{ desired} - F_{S_1}^{14}\right) \qquad (6)$$

$$\text{Established } F_S^{14}\text{ desired} = 2.93$$

$$\text{chosen } F_{C_1}^{14} = 2.00$$

$$F_{C_2}^{14} = 3.00$$

$$\text{calculated } F_{S_1}^{14} = 2.369$$

$$F_{S_2}^{14} = 3.389$$

Substituting above values in Equation 6

$$F_C^{14}\text{ desired} = 2.00 + \frac{3.00 - 2.00}{3.389 - 2.369}(2.93 - 2.369)$$

$$F_C^{14}\text{ desired} = \underline{2.549}$$

Step 6. Evaluation of process time (B) from F_c desired.
This step is similar to the procedure adopted for the convection heating products and the following equation is used.

$$B = f_h(\log j_{ch} I_h - \log g_c)$$

$$I_h = T_r - T_{ih}$$

Since $T_r = 240°F$ and $T_{ih} = 140°F$

$$I_h = 240 - 140 = \underline{100}$$

The value of g_c is identified through the use of $f_h/U{:}g$ tables. First the value of f_h/U is determined.

$$U_c = F_c F_i$$

$$U_{240}^{14} = F_c^{14} \times F_{i240}^{14}$$

Since $F_c^{14} = 2.549$ and $F_{i240}^{14} = 5.179$

$$U_{240}^{14} = 2.549 \times 5.179 = \underline{13.20}$$

Also $f_h = 52.82$

$$f_h/U_{240}^{14} = \frac{52.82}{13.20} = \underline{4.00}$$

Now from the $f_h/U{:}g$ table for z of 14, find corresponding g_c value for

$$f_h/U_c = 4.00 \quad \text{and} \quad j_{cc} = 2.00$$

$$g_c = \underline{4.361}$$

Substituting the values

$$f_h = 52.82$$

$$j_{ch} = 2.00$$

$$I_h = 100 \quad \text{and}$$

$$g_c = 4.361$$

in the equation

$$B = f_h(\log j_{ch} I_h - \log g_c)$$

$$= 52.82\,(\log(2.00 \times 100) - \log 4.361)$$

$$= 52.82\,(2.3010 - 0.6396)$$

$$= \underline{87.8 \text{ min}}$$

The B of 87.8 min represents the process time needed to achieve an acceptable probability of reduction of *C. botulinum* with z of 14F° for the processing of a low-acid food in 300 × 407 cans at a retort temperature of 240°F. The corresponding F_s desired, referred to F_{250}^{14} in this case, is 2.93. The process time necessary would have been different if the z value considered was any value other than 14F°.

Under similar processing conditions, the higher the z value, the lower will be the process time needed, and vice versa, to achieve the same level of lethality as long as the food temperature does not go above 255°F during processing. In the above process evaluation, the process time computed would be considerably less if the z value was assumed to be 18F°. Consequently, the process time of 87.8 min, under similar processing conditions, would reflect a higher processing value if the evaluations are based on z of 18 (F_{250}^{18}) instead of z of 14 (F_{250}^{14}). The influence of z values are expressed essentially through the f_h/U:g tables. Every z value has a different f_h/U:g table. The value of F_{250}^{18} can be determined using the g_c values.

Now, to evaluate F_{250}^{18}, find the f_h/U value for $g_c = 4.361$ from the table corresponding to z of 18.

$$f_h/U = \underline{3.035}$$

Since $f_h = 52.82$,

$$U = \frac{f_h}{3.035} = \frac{52.82}{3.035} = \underline{17.40}$$

$$U = F_o \cdot F_{i240}^{18}$$

$$F_o = \frac{U}{F_{i240}^{18}} = \frac{17.40}{3.594} = \underline{4.84}$$

The z value of an organism accounts for the relative resistance at different temperatures. The lower the z value the greater the resistance to a lower temperature as compared to a higher temperature, and consequently the process time will be longer. Similarly, a higher z value will result in a shorter process time. This relative influence of z on the process time would be true for any value of z whether it is above or below 18. This trend, however, would be reversed if the food temperature goes above 255°F during processing. The value of z employed in a process evaluation depends on the relative resistance of the strain of *C. botulinum* in the specified low-acid food.

For convenience, the unit of lethality is generally expressed at the reference temperature of 250°F. The most commonly used z value is 18. Thus, F_{250}^{18}, also written as F_o, is considered to be a standard reference. In the process lethality guide tables, the final process values for all the processes were expressed in terms of F_o. A process based on the z lower than 18, such as 12, 14, or 16, would have a higher F_o value than a similar process designed for z of 18. Also processes evaluated for z value higher than 18, such as 20, 22, or 24, would have lower F_o values. Expressing the process values on the basis of a standard reference should be very useful to food processors to compare the lethality of different thermal processes.

DEVELOPMENT OF COMPUTER PROGRAMS FOR THERMAL PROCESS EVALUATIONS AND THE ESTABLISHMENT OF PROCESS LETHALITY GUIDES

The preceding discussion on the thermal process evaluation procedures reveal the complexity involved in the process calculations particularly for conduction-heating products. An accurate evaluation of the process time to achieve safety or commercial sterility for a low-acid food packed in a particular container and to be processed under specified conditions involves several variables and numerous mathematical steps. First the target process value is established and the process time is evaluated using mathematical steps which necessitate repeated references to the f_h/U:g tables. The various mathematical steps involved have been logically treated by Stumbo.[20] In spite of the clarity of his presentation, the actual evaluation tends to be time consuming particularly due to the manual interpolation of appropriate values in the f_h/U:g tables. For these reasons, the conventional methods have not been as widely applied as their versatility merits to practical processing situations for evaluating the adequacy of existing processes or for the establishment of new processes.

It was thought that improving the quickness and accuracy of process calculations would benefit the food processors in the proper utilization of these methods. Process lethality guides, if they could be developed, would be very useful to understand the margin of safety, at least in approximate terms, involved in various processing schedules. Also, excessive processing situations could be identified. A better understanding of the status of the process schedules is essential to a proper management of time and fuel energy in the thermal processing area.

In order to make the process calculations reasonably simple, computer programs were developed to perform the various mathematical operations involved. The f_h/U:g tables corresponding to different z values were incorporated as a part of the overall program so that the necessary repeated references to the tables would be done automatically. There is sufficient flexibility to accommodate a wide range of values for the variables associated with the thermobacteriological considerations and processing conditions. These programs are geared to calculate the process time from the process value and also check the adequacy of processes. The versatility of these programs makes it possible to apply them successfully to almost any conceivable practical processing situation.

These computer programs were utilized to undertake a rather difficult task of making an extensive study in the thermal processing of low-acid foods. An accurate evaluation of the critical thermal resistance and process variables on the lethality requirements for safe thermal processes and commercial sterility was made. Foods of varying heat transfer properties, containers of different sizes and widely varying processing conditions were considered. Approximately 250,000 evaluations were made for both conduction and convection heating foods. The range of processing conditions for the establishment of the process lethality guide tables were chosen so that they would approximate the practical processing situations as closely as possible.

In developing the process lethality guides, the safety aspects were given the greatest importance. The safe thermal processes were based on minimum lethality requirements for heat processes designed to assure an acceptable remote possibility of survival of *C. botulinum* in low-acid foods. For commercial sterility, an assurance of a reasonable degree of freedom from economic spoilage was considered essential and it was based on the elimination of spore forming mesophilic bacteria, *C. sporogenes* group, with a D_{250} value as high as 1.5. The basic variables which were taken into consideration in the establishment of lethality guides are as follows:

41 can sizes
5 heating rates (f_h)
2 D_{250} values
6 z values
11 initial food temperatures (T_{ih})
4 retort temperatures (T_r)

The process lethality guides are intended to offer guidance to processors in assessing the status of the different process schedules. The variables characterizing the actual process schedule most likely will not exactly coincide with the corresponding variables in the tables. However, the tables would certainly be useful in an approximate assessment of most of the process schedules for the margin of safety or the degree of commercial sterility. The proper method of using the tables is described in detail in later parts of this book. If a particular process is to be evaluated precisely, the calculations should be done individually for the exact bacteriological criteria and processing conditions of every process schedule.

MICROBIOLOGICAL BASIS FOR THERMAL PROCESS LETHALITY GUIDES

In the establishment of processes for low-acid foods there are two basic aspects involved. The first one is to define the target F value based on the thermobacteriological criteria. The second one relates to achieving the target F value using appropriate processing conditions. In order to define the target F value, an understanding of the fundamentals of thermobacteriology of low-acid foods is very essential. The magnitude of F value needed would greatly depend upon the type of processing desired, whether to ensure a safe thermal process or commercial sterility. In any case, the safety aspects should be given the highest priority and it is based on the elimination of spores of *C. botulinum*. Commercial sterility could be designed to achieve different degrees of freedom from economic spoilage and the organism of importance in this respect is generally the spores of mesophilic and thermophilic anaerobes. The bacteria mentioned here are considered to be the major concern in the thermal processing of low-acid foods mainly because they grow well above pH 4.5 under the anaerobic conditions of the low-acid canned foods, and they also produce either a toxin or cause economic spoilage.

Before establishing the target F value, different kinds of information are needed on the microbiological aspects and they are as follows:

1. The organism of concern based on the type of processing desired.
2. The heat resistance characteristics of the organism of concern (D_{250} and z values).
3. The initial population of the organism.
4. The extent of reduction desired of the population of the organism.

Safe Thermal Processes

Because of its public health significance, the toxin-producing organism, *C. botulinum*, is considered to be of greatest importance in establishing safety in the thermal processing of low-acid foods. This organism is an obligate anaerobe and grows only in foods above pH 4.5. Low-acid canned foods can provide both these conditions. Type A, B, E, and F of *C. botulinum* are those known to affect humans. Spores of types A and B are more heat resistant than types E and F, therefore, types A and B are of greatest concern in the sterilization of foods. While establishing the process value for safety, it must always be assumed that *C. botulinum* spores of the highest resistance would be present. The public health significance of *C. botulinum* is due to the following unique properties.

1. The natural habitat of *C. botulinum* is the soil and, therefore, its contamination of foods cannot be avoided. Its presence in unprocessed foods must always be presumed.
2. It produces spores which are more resistant to heat than any other pathogenic or toxin producing microorganism.
3. Though not infectious, it produces one of the most deadly neuroparalytic toxins.

4. Most low-acid foods (pH above 4.5) are good media for its growth and toxin production. If its spores are not killed by the heat process applied, it must be presumed that they will germinate to give rise to vegetative growth and toxin production.

In order to evaluate the minimum target F value to achieve safety in any other thermal process, it is important to define the initial population, the heat resistant characteristics, and the extent of reduction desired for the organism, *C. botulinum*. For the establishment of process values for safe thermal processes in the process lethality guides, certain microbiological standards were adopted for spores of *C. botulinum*.

Initial population of *C. botulinum* — There is little information on the prevalence of *C. botulinum* in low-acid food products prior to processing. The available published information and our own experience indicates that population of the spores of *C. botulinum* would seldom be greater than one per gram of food.[5,6,10,14] Since most of the spores of *C. botulinum* encountered are not likely to have the maximum possible heat resistance, consideration of one spore per gram should provide a good basic assumption in the best interests of safety.

The D value — This reflects the heat resistant characteristics of an organism at a constant temperature. It is defined as the time required, at any designated temperature, to destroy 90% of the spores or vegetative cells of a given organism. Published and unpublished works for the last 55 years indicate that the most heat resistant spores are characterized by D_{250} values no greater than 0.20 min. This is for spores dispersed in low-acid foods, water, or neutral phosphate buffer solutions. Based on the established information it was considered safe to assume the D_{250} value of *C. botulinum* to be 0.20.[4,22,25,26]

The z value — This is defined as the number of Fahrenheit degrees required for the thermal destruction curve to traverse one log cycle. In thermal process evaluation, it accounts for the relative resistance of an organism to different lethal temperatures operative during the application of heat in a sterilization process. The literature published so far indicates that the z values for the types A and B of *C. botulinum* are generally in the range of 14 to 18F°.[4,22,25,26] When food temperatures attained during heat processing of low-acid canned foods normally do not exceed 255°F, the lower z values are usually employed in computation. Consequently the process time computed for an equivalent population reduction will be larger. If the food temperatures exceed 255°F, the reverse would be true and this would be applicable to processing done at a retort temperature of 260°F particularly for the convection-heating products. The relative resistance of bacteria at different temperatures would be greatly influenced by the strain of microorganism and the nature of the food in which they are suspended during heating. Different strains of *C. botulinum* spores isolated from various low-acid foods have been shown to have z values as low as 12 and as high as 24.[20] In order to cover a wide range of heat resistance of various strains of *C. botulinum*, z values from 12 to 24 were considered in the evaluation of safety aspects of foods.

Probability of survival — The order of death of bacteria subjected to moist heat, is essentially logarithmic. Based on this assumption, an acceptable probability of survival of *C. botulinum* spores in heat processed low-acid foods has been arbitrarily established to meet the minimum safety requirements, for public health considerations. It is now accepted that chance of survival should be no greater than one organism per 10^{12} containers. It can also be expressed that the probability of survival of a *C. botulinum* spore in any one heat processed container of low-acid food should be no more than 10^{-12}. This basic assumption is generally referred to as 12 D concept of sterilization and this forms the basis for the evaluations of safe thermal processes of low-acid foods presented in the process lethality guide tables.

Commercial Sterility

In industry, thermal processing of low-acid foods is directed to address the problems of both safety and economic spoilage. Commercial sterility is based on achieving an acceptable reduction in the probability of survival of spores of certain groups of spoilage organisms along with due consideration to the change in the economic value of the product because of processing. The organisms of importance in commercial sterility generally are more heat resistant than the types A and B of *C. botulinum*. Consequently, the processing is more severe and the reduction of *C. botulinum* spores achieved in commercial sterility is likely to be two to five times the minimum requirement for safety. If processed properly, low-acid canned foods subjected to commercial sterility should assure a high degree of safety.

The most important organisms of concern in the commercial sterility of low-acid foods are as follows:

***C. sporogenes* group (including P.A. 3679)** — They are obligate anaerobes with an optimum growth temperature in the mesophilic range (25 to 35°C).

C. thermosaccharolyticum — These organisms are also obligate anaerobes, thermophilic in nature, with an optimum growth temperature of about 131°F (55°C). They are saccharolytic and are important mainly in low-acid foods, such as corn, which provide a good source of carbohydrate.

***Bacillus stearothermophilus* and related species** — These flat sour producing organisms are facultative anaerobes and thermophilic with an optimum growth temperature ranging from 120 to 131°F (49 to 55°C). They are highly heat resistant and a number of strains and species are known to have D_{250} values in excess of 4.00 min.[20]

The thermophiles are relatively less important particularly if the products are cooled quickly and not exposed to high temperatures above 100°F (37.8°C) after processing. If the processed product is to be subjected to above average ambient temperatures or stored in a tropical climate, the processes should be designed to reduce the spores of thermophilic spoilage organisms to an acceptable level in the final product. Under normal conditions, the mesophilic organisms of *C. sporogenes* group are the most important in controlling economic spoilage of the low-acid canned foods. Accordingly, in the process lethality tables for commercial sterility the evaluations were based on the reduction of spores of the organisms of *C. sporogenes* group. In order to establish the target F value for commercial sterility, it is necessary to define the basic considerations of the thermobacteriological aspects of *C. sporogenes* group. These aspects are discussed in the following paragraphs.

Initial population — The population, prior to processing, of spores of mesophilic bacteria with a heat resistance more than *C. botulinum* should seldom be expected to be greater than one per gram of the low acid food.[5,6,10,14] Based on this information, the initial load of *C. sporogenes* was determined for every can size used in the establishment of process lethality guides.

The D value — The D_{250} value of *C. sporogenes* group including P.A. 3679 generally of the order of 0.50 to 1.5 min.[13,22] In all the process evaluations related to commercial sterility, a D_{250} value of 1.5 min was used to assure a high degree of freedom from economic spoilage.

The z value — Values of z, characterizing the relative resistance of the more resistant spores to temperatures of significant lethal value in heat processing of low-acid foods, generally range from 16 to 22F°.[13,22] It seemed appropriate to use z values in the range of 16 to 22F° in designing processes to achieve commercial sterility of low-acid canned foods.

Probability of survival — The D_{250} value of 1.5 considered for the *C. sporogenes* group represents a relatively higher heat resistance than most of the mesophilic organism of commercial importance one might encounter in low-acid foods. For the process lethality guide tables, reducing the probability of survival of any spore forming mesophilic bacteria more resistant than *C. botulinum* by four log cycles was recognized as adequate to achieve a reasonable commercial sterility of low-acid canned foods.

APPLICATION OF THE TABLES TO PRACTICAL PROCESSING SCHEDULES

The tables that follow are intended to serve only as a guide to the minimum process conditions for low-acid foods in the various sizes of metal containers specified. No attempt should be made to extrapolate the data in these tables to can sizes not appearing in the tables, nor to the processing of foods in glass containers.

It is not questioned that there may be occasions when it is necessary to employ process conditions more severe than those described by these tables. However, it is emphasized that the tables delineate minimum process times under specific conditions for the intended purpose. Therefore, it is cautioned that if these tables are used no process less severe than those represented within the tables should be employed by a food processor. Furthermore, the process times shown by the tables were computed for representative conduction-heating and convection-heating products with straight line semilogarithmic heating curves. Because of this, the process times shown by the tables should not be applied to food products that exhibit "broken" heating curves. For "broken-heating" products, it is suggested that appropriate processing schedules be determined by employing the established graphical procedures.[20]

Likewise, the data in these tables are not applicable where certain deviant variables such as steam failure, retort breakdown, etc. may be encountered during normal processing operations. In such instances, the proper process schedule must be separately determined by appropriate mathematical or graphical procedures,[20] or, if circumstances warrant, the product may either be reprocessed or discarded.

The tables that follow do not delineate process times for commercial sterility with respect to the thermal inactivation of thermophilic bacterial spores that may be of concern as a contributory cause of food spoilage. For such circumstances, processes more severe than those contained within the tables must be individually calculated, and no attempt should be made to extrapolate the process data from these tables.

There are several low-acid canned food items where a part of the product (brine, broth, or gravy) heats by convection or semiconvection and the solid portion of the product (vegetables, meatballs, etc.) heats by conduction. For those products, where internal contamination of the solid food particles is not likely, (e.g., diced carrots, peas, corn, potato cubes, etc.) the processing times contained in the tables may be applied with confidence.

For those products where internal contamination of the solid food masses is a definite possibility (pasta masses, meatballs, whole or sliced mushrooms, etc.), and wherein there is no reliable means to accurately measure heat penetration into the conduction heating food masses, the process conditions described in these tables are not applicable. With such products, the only reliable method for establishing process parameters is by properly designed spore population reduction studies.

There are certain heat transfer systems in which reliable heat penetration determinations are difficult or impossible to obtain. Included among these are such as flame sterilizers, hydrostatic cookers, and several different agitating cookers. These tables should not be applied to systems such as these, and it is recommended that such systems be evaluated by properly designed spore reduction studies.

The data in these tables are appropriately applicable for low-acid food items where the lowest food temperature during processing does not exceed 260°F. For those heating systems where the food temperature exceeds 260°F, processing times represented by those tables describing commercial sterility with either a moderate degree of assurance or a high degree of assurance should be employed as a minimum. This will ensure both safety with respect to inactivation of *C. botulinum* spores and adequate processing conditions to provide for the desired degree of commercial sterility within the food product.

Thermal Process Lethality Guides for Conduction-Heating Low-Acid Canned Foods

HEAT PENETRATION AND PROCESSING PARAMETERS

The primary purpose of establishing the thermal process lethality guides is to assist the food processors in assessing the status of their existing or new process schedules for the sterilization of low-acid canned foods. In the industry the parameters associated with heat penetration and processing differ widely from one situation to another. It is inconceivable that the thermal process lethality guides could cover all the different processing conditions. However, by proper usage of the guide tables an approximate evaluation of the process adequacy is possible in most cases. In designing these tables, the possible application to conduction-heating foods of varying heat transfer properties packed in different can sizes was considered. The parameters associated with the processing conditions per se included different combinations of retort and initial food temperatures. For every variable associated with the processing condition for a practical process schedule, in most cases a close approximation could be made to a corresponding variable in the guide tables. In deducing the process values from the guide tables, caution should be exercised as explained under method of using the tables. In any case, the guide tables are likely to be useful in an approximate evaluation of the margin of safety or the degree of commercial sterility.

For conduction-heating foods all the 41 can sizes, which are generally used in the food industry, were considered. For every can size, the combinations of other variables include 5 heating rates (f_h), 11 initial food temperatures (T_{ih}), 4 retort temperatures (T_r), and 1 standard value for the lag factors of heating (j_{ch}) and cooling (j_{cc}). The heat penetration and processing parameters used are the same for both safe thermal processes and commercial sterility. The rationale involved in the selection of these variables is discussed in the following paragraphs.

The heating rate function (f_h) — The heat transfer characteristics of a low-acid food packed in a container of a particular size is generally designated by the symbol, f_h. It is defined as the time, in minutes, required for the straight line portion of the conventionally plotted semi-log heating curve to traverse one log cycle. By definition, the f_h value takes into account the heat transfer properties of the food per se and the container size. The numerical value of f_h for a conduction-heating food depends on the following two factors.

1. Thermal diffusivity (k) of the food
2. Container dimensions

Thermal diffusivity refers to the flow of heat. For different conduction-heating foods in one container size, the value of f_h will vary directly as the reciprocal of k. The value of k itself is related to the nature of the food. For different conduction-heating foods in the same size container, the value of f_h will vary considerably even though all the products may be judged to have the same mechanism of heat transfer. Also, the same conduction-heating food in containers of varying sizes would have different f_h values.

To establish the process lethality tables, it was necessary to choose a range of f_h values appropriate to the container size and also relating, at least in approximate terms, to the practical processing situations. It was deemed advisable to choose a range of f_h values that might be observed for conduction-heating products packed in 603 × 700 cans. The range was covered by 5 different values and the f_h values selected were 170, 180, 190, 200, and 210 min. Five different equivalent f_h values for the other 40 can sizes were computed by the conversion equation[8,20] used for finite cylindrical food containers.

$$f' = \frac{(1/a^2) + (0.427/b^2)\, f}{(1/a'^2) + (0.427/b'^2)}$$

in which f′ = f of heating or cooling curve for a given product in can size other than 603 × 700, f = f of heating or cooling curve for the same product in 603 × 700 can, a = radius of 603 × 700 can (inside dimension), b = one half length of 603 × 700 can (inside dimension), a′ = radius of other can (inside dimension), and b′ = one half length of other can (inside dimension).

Theoretically, other things being equal, the numerical value of f_h should be equal to f_c, the cooling rate function. The value of f_c is not needed in the mathematical methods of evaluation, since the heat available during the early stages of cooling is accounted for conveniently through the f_h/U:g tables. However, f_c is generally considered to be equal f_h in most cases. Every can size will have a range of f_h covered by five different values which would increase gradually with the size of the can. In the lethality guide tables, the f_h values defined here were used only for conduction-heating low-acid foods. However, all the numerical values defining the heating rate functions are applicable to processes designed to achieve both safety and commercial sterility in conduction-heating low-acid canned foods.

The lag factors of heating (j_{ch}) and cooling (j_{cc}) — In theoretical terms, the value of j_{ch} for heating at the geometrical center of a conduction-heating food should be 2.04.[20] This is based on the assumption that the temperature distribution is uniform within the food at the beginning of heating. It is known that the experimentally determined values of j_{ch} is usually less than 2.04. In process calculations the larger the value of j_{ch} employed the longer will be the process time needed. It is generally considered appropriate to use a j_{ch} of 2.00 for most conduction-heating products. The actual j_{ch} is likely to be less and not more than 2.00. This assumption might result in slightly more processing than necessary. However, it is certainly advisable to be on the safe side. The cooling lag factor, j_{cc}, is an important value for deducing the correct values from the f_h/U:g tables. It is considered to be an appropriate procedure to assume that j_{cc} is equal to j_{ch} for most conduction-heating processes. In the process lethality guides, the evaluations for safety and commercial sterility for conduction-heating foods were done assuming the values of j_{ch} and j_{cc} to be 2.00 regardless of the can size.

Retort temperature and initial temperature of the food — In practice, the temperature of most of the conduction-heating low-acid canned foods at the beginning of the process range from 100 to 200°F. To achieve sterilization, under these conditions, the retort temperatures used range from 230 to 260°F. In the process lethality guides, the structure of the tables were designed to closely approximate the parameters of the practical processing situations. For this, 11 initial food temperatures were considered and they were 100, 110, 120, 130, 140, 150, 160, 170, 180, 190, and 200°F. Four widely used retort temperatures of 230, 240, 250, and 260°F were selected. These processing conditions were applicable to both safe thermal processes and commercial sterility.

USE OF THE TABLES FOR CONDUCTION-HEATING PRODUCTS

The tables that follow describe process times (B) that were computed for processing conduction-heating low-acid foods packaged in 41 different commercial can sizes. Process times for safe thermal processes employing z values from 12 to 18 are shown in the 164 tables of Section I; whereas, safe thermal processes based on z values from 18 to 24 are given in the 164 tables of Section II. In Section III, are found the 164 tables that describe process times for commercial sterility with a high degree of assurance when z values of 16 to 22 were utilized in the computations.

Proper use of the table dictates that the following process variables for the product be known: (1) the specific container size, (2) the retort temperature, (3) the initial food temperature at start of retorting, (4) the f_h for the product, and (5) the z for the organism of concern.

For example, assume the following data is known for processing a conduction-heating product.

1. Container size — 300 × 407
2. Retort temperature — 240°F
3. Initial food temperature — 180°F
4. Product f_h — 42.5 min
5. The z — 16F°

Now, assume that by using the tables it is desired to obtain the processing time required for a safe thermal process. Proceed by first locating the table in Section I that contains the data for the above process variables. In this case, the proper table is Table 74, and it is included as Figure 2. To use the table properly locate the following in stepwise procedure as shown by the example in Figure 2: (1) can size — 300 × 407; (2) retort temperature — 240°F; (3) initial food temperature — 180°F; (4) f_h — 42.76 (since the actual f_h of 42.5 is not in the table, proper use of the table dictates that, for reasons of safety, the next higher f_h of 42.76 be used); (5) z — 16F°, and then at (6) the proper processing time is determined to be 58.9 min for this product.

When using the guideline tables, it is very likely that a situation will be encountered, with an individual food product, wherein the value of a process variable, such as the f_h, initial food temperature, or retort temperature, does not coincide precisely, or nearly so as in the previous example, with values appearing in the tables, or a value may be intermediate between those that appear in a given table.

In such an event, to use the tables properly, it is suggested in the interest of safety that one proceed according to the following guidelines.

1. If the container size is not shown in these tables, do not proceed any further, or attempt to extrapolate data from the tables.
2. If the retort temperature is not exact, use the next lower retort temperature shown in the tables.
3. If the initial temperature lies between two given values, e.g., between 140 and 150°F, use the lower initial temperature (140°F).
4. If the product f_h does not exactly match with those appearing in the table, use the next higher value as was done in the preceding problem.
5. The z selected should always match precisely the values in the table.

By proceeding as outlined in the above guidelines, the necessary precautions have been taken to insure that the adequacy of the process will not be lessened.

As an example of the above, assume that from heat penetration data a conduction-heating food packaged in a 300 × 407 can was determined to have an f_h equal to 51.0 min, and it is desired to provide a safe thermal process for this product when the z is 16F° and the initial food temperature is 130°F. The retort temperature to be employed is 240°F. The processing times (B) for these conditions are shown in Figure 2. In viewing Figure 2 it is obvious that processing times for an f_h equal to 51.0 min are not given. However, f_h values of 50.3 and 52.82 appear in the table. In reviewing the process times that appear beneath the 130°F initial food temperature column on the horizontal line representing z of 16F° and f_h values of 50.3 and 52.82, it becomes obvious that the 82.2 min processing time specified for an f_h of 52.82 and z of 16 provides greater safety than does the process time of 79.2 min specified for an f_h of 50.3 and z of 16. Therefore, it seems only logical that the process time of 82.2 min would be more than adequate to provide the needed safety margin for the product with an f_h of 51.0 min.

TABLE 74 ②

Process Times (B) at Retort Temperature of 240°F for Conduction-Heating Foods in 300 x 407 Can ①

INITIAL FOOD TEMPERATURE (T_{ih})

f_h	z	100	110	120	130	140	150	160	170	180 ③	190	200	Equivalent F_c^{18}	Equivalent F_s^{18}
④	12	90.7	89.3	87.8	86.2	84.4	82.5	80.3	77.8	74.9	71.5	67.4	6.65	7.04
42.76	14	81.4	80.0	78.6	76.9	75.2	73.2	71.0	68.5	65.7	62.3	58.1	4.70	5.10
⑤	16	74.6	73.3	71.8	70.2	68.4	66.4	64.2	61.8	58.9 ⑥	55.5	51.4	3.40	3.79
	18	69.6	68.2	66.8	65.1	63.4	61.4	59.2	56.7	53.9	50.5	46.4	2.54	2.93
	12	94.6	93.2	91.6	89.9	88.0	85.9	83.6	81.0	77.9	74.4	70.0	6.78	7.17
45.27	14	85.0	83.6	82.0	80.3	78.4	76.3	74.0	71.4	68.4	64.8	60.4	4.74	5.15
	16	78.0	76.5	74.9	73.2	71.4	69.3	67.0	64.3	61.3	57.7	53.3	3.41	3.80
	18	72.7	71.3	69.7	68.0	66.1	64.0	61.7	59.1	56.1	52.5	48.1	2.54	2.93
	12	98.5	96.9	95.3	93.5	91.5	89.3	86.9	84.1	80.9	77.1	72.5	6.90	7.30
47.79	14	88.6	87.0	85.4	83.6	81.6	79.4	76.9	74.2	71.0	67.2	62.6	4.78	5.19
	16	81.3	79.7	78.1	76.3	74.3	72.1	69.7	66.9	63.7	59.9	55.3	3.42	3.82
	18	75.8	74.3	72.6	70.8	68.8	66.7	64.2	61.4	58.2	54.5	49.8	2.54	2.93
	12	102.3	100.7	98.9	97.0	94.9	92.6	90.0	87.1	83.8	79.8	74.9	7.02	7.42
50.30	14	92.0	90.4	88.7	86.8	84.7	82.4	79.8	76.9	73.5	69.5	64.7	4.82	5.23
	16	84.5	82.9	81.1	79.2	77.2	74.9	72.3	69.4	66.0	62.0	57.1	3.43	3.83
	18	78.9	77.3	75.5	73.6	71.6	69.3	66.7	63.8	60.4	56.4	51.5	2.53	2.93
	12	106.1	104.4	102.5	100.5	98.4	95.9	93.2	90.2	86.6	82.5	77.3	7.05	7.46
52.82	14	95.5	93.8	91.9	89.9	87.7	85.3	82.6	79.6	76.0	71.8	66.7	4.84	5.25
	16	87.7	86.0	84.2	82.2	80.0	77.6	74.9	71.8	68.3	64.1	59.0	3.42	3.83
	18	81.9	80.2	78.4	76.4	74.2	71.8	69.1	66.0	62.5	58.3	53.2	2.53	2.93

FIGURE 2. A typical page of data for conduction-heating foods to achieve a safe thermal process.

SECTION I: SAFE THERMAL PROCESSES WITH z VALUES FROM 12 TO 18; TABLES 1 TO 164

Hypothetical Processing Criteria To Achieve Safety in Conduction-Heating Products

Thermobacteriological considerations

Organism of concern	: *C. botulinum*
Initial population	: One per gram of food
Extent of reduction	: 12 log cycles
D_{250} Value	: 0.20 min
z Values	: 12, 14, 16, and 18F°

Processing conditions

Initial food temperatures (T_{ih})	: 100 to 200°F
Retort temperatures (T_r)	: 230 to 260°F
Heating rate function (f_h)	: Based on 5 values for No. 10 can
Heating lag factor (j_{ch})	: 2.00
Cooling lag factor (j_{cc})	: 2.00

TABLE 1

Process Times (B) at Retort Temperature of 230°F for Conduction-Heating Foods in 202 x 204 Can

f_h	z	INITIAL FOOD TEMPERATURE (T_{ih}) 100	110	120	130	140	150	160	170	180	190	200	Equivalent F_c^{18}	F_s^{18}
16.91	12	139.4	138.8	138.2	137.5	136.7	135.9	134.9	133.7	132.4	130.8	128.7	9.84	10.11
	14	100.7	100.2	99.5	98.8	98.0	97.2	96.2	95.1	93.7	92.1	90.0	5.62	5.85
	16	74.5	73.9	73.2	72.5	71.8	70.9	69.9	68.8	68.4	65.8	63.7	3.64	3.88
	18	60.1	59.5	58.9	58.2	57.4	56.5	55.5	54.4	53.1	51.4	49.3	2.57	2.79
17.90	12	143.5	142.9	142.2	141.4	140.6	139.7	138.7	137.5	136.1	134.3	132.1	9.84	10.12
	14	102.5	101.9	101.2	100.5	99.6	98.7	97.7	96.5	95.1	93.3	91.1	5.62	5.86
	16	75.8	75.1	74.5	73.7	72.9	72.0	71.0	69.8	68.3	66.6	64.4	3.63	3.87
	18	61.7	61.1	60.4	59.6	58.8	57.9	56.9	55.7	54.3	52.5	50.3	2.56	2.80
18.89	12	147.3	146.7	146.0	145.2	144.3	143.3	142.2	141.0	139.5	137.7	135.3	9.85	10.12
	14	104.0	103.4	102.7	101.9	101.0	100.0	98.9	97.7	96.2	94.4	92.0	5.62	5.86
	16	77.3	76.6	75.9	75.1	74.2	73.3	72.2	70.9	69.4	67.6	65.2	3.65	3.88
	18	63.1	62.5	61.8	61.0	60.1	59.2	58.1	56.8	55.3	53.5	51.1	2.56	2.80
19.89	12	151.0	150.3	149.5	148.7	147.8	146.8	145.6	144.3	142.7	140.8	138.3	9.85	10.13
	14	105.2	104.5	103.8	103.0	102.0	101.0	99.9	98.5	97.0	95.0	92.6	5.61	5.85
	16	78.9	78.2	77.5	76.6	75.7	74.7	73.6	72.2	70.6	68.7	66.2	3.64	3.89
	18	64.5	63.9	63.1	62.3	61.4	60.4	59.2	57.9	56.3	54.4	51.9	2.55	2.79
20.88	12	154.4	153.7	152.9	152.0	151.1	150.0	148.8	147.4	145.7	143.7	141.1	9.86	10.14
	14	106.2	105.5	104.7	103.8	102.9	101.8	100.6	99.2	97.5	95.5	92.9	5.60	5.84
	16	80.4	79.7	78.9	78.0	77.1	76.0	74.8	73.4	71.8	69.7	67.1	3.63	3.88
	18	66.1	65.4	64.6	63.8	62.8	61.7	60.5	59.1	57.5	55.4	52.8	2.55	2.80

TABLE 2

Process Time (B) at Retort Temperature of 240°F for Conduction-Heating Foods in 202 x 204 Can

f_h	z	INITIAL FOOD TEMPERATURE (T_{ih})											Equivalent	
		100	110	120	130	140	150	160	170	180	190	200	F_c^{18}	F_s^{18}
16.91	12	47.0	46.5	45.9	45.3	44.6	43.8	42.9	41.9	40.8	39.5	37.8	5.54	5.87
	14	42.2	41.7	41.1	40.4	39.7	39.0	38.1	37.1	36.0	34.6	33.0	4.18	4.52
	16	38.3	37.8	37.2	36.6	35.9	35.1	34.2	33.2	32.1	30.8	29.1	3.15	3.48
	18	35.1	34.6	34.0	33.3	32.6	31.9	31.0	30.0	28.9	27.5	25.9	2.49	2.80
17.90	12	48.9	48.3	47.7	47.0	46.3	45.5	44.5	43.5	42.3	40.9	39.1	5.63	5.96
	14	43.9	43.3	42.7	42.0	41.2	40.4	39.5	38.5	37.3	35.9	34.1	4.18	4.52
	16	39.8	39.2	38.6	37.9	37.1	36.3	35.4	34.4	33.2	31.8	30.0	3.15	3.48
	18	36.3	35.7	35.1	34.4	33.7	32.9	32.0	30.9	29.7	28.3	26.6	2.48	2.79
18.89	12	50.7	50.1	49.5	48.8	48.0	47.1	46.2	45.1	43.8	42.3	40.5	5.71	6.05
	14	45.5	44.9	44.2	43.5	42.7	41.8	40.9	39.8	38.5	37.0	35.2	4.18	4.53
	16	41.1	40.5	39.9	39.2	38.4	37.5	36.5	35.4	34.2	32.7	30.9	3.15	3.48
	18	37.8	37.2	36.5	35.8	35.0	34.1	33.2	32.1	30.8	29.3	27.5	2.48	2.80
19.89	12	52.6	51.9	51.2	50.5	49.7	48.7	47.7	46.6	45.2	43.7	41.7	5.79	6.13
	14	47.0	46.4	45.7	44.9	44.1	43.2	42.2	41.0	39.7	38.1	36.2	4.18	4.53
	16	42.5	41.8	41.1	40.4	39.6	38.7	37.6	36.5	35.1	33.6	31.6	3.15	3.48
	18	39.2	38.5	37.8	37.1	36.3	35.4	34.3	33.2	31.9	30.3	28.4	2.47	2.80
20.88	12	54.3	53.7	52.9	52.2	51.3	50.3	49.3	48.1	46.7	45.0	43.0	5.86	6.21
	14	48.6	47.9	47.2	46.4	45.5	44.5	43.5	42.3	40.9	39.2	37.2	4.18	4.53
	16	43.8	43.1	42.4	41.6	40.7	39.8	38.7	37.5	36.1	34.4	32.4	3.15	3.48
	18	40.6	39.9	39.2	38.4	37.5	36.5	35.5	34.3	32.9	31.2	29.2	2.47	2.80

TABLE 3

Process Times (B) at Retort Temperature of 250°F for Conduction-Heating Foods in 202 x 204 Can

f_h	z	INITIAL FOOD TEMPERATURE (T_{ih})											Equivalent	
		100	110	120	130	140	150	160	170	180	190	200	F_c^{18}	F_s^{18}
16.91	12	29.1	28.6	28.0	27.4	26.8	26.1	25.3	24.5	23.5	22.3	21.0	4.24	4.66
	14	27.6	27.1	26.6	26.0	25.3	24.6	23.9	23.0	22.0	20.9	19.6	3.39	3.80
	16	26.5	26.0	25.5	24.9	24.3	23.6	22.8	21.9	20.9	19.8	18.5	2.82	3.22
	18	25.7	25.2	24.6	24.0	23.4	22.7	21.9	21.0	20.1	18.9	17.6	2.39	2.80
17.90	12	30.5	29.9	29.3	28.7	28.0	27.3	26.5	25.6	24.5	23.3	21.9	4.29	4.71
	14	28.9	28.4	27.8	27.2	26.5	25.8	25.0	24.0	23.0	21.8	20.4	3.41	3.83
	16	27.8	27.3	26.7	26.1	25.4	24.6	23.8	22.9	21.9	20.7	19.3	2.82	3.23
	18	26.9	26.3	25.7	25.1	24.5	23.7	22.9	22.0	20.9	19.7	18.3	2.39	2.80
18.89	12	31.8	31.3	30.6	30.0	29.3	28.5	27.6	26.7	25.6	24.3	22.8	4.32	4.75
	14	30.2	29.7	29.1	28.4	27.7	26.9	26.0	25.1	24.0	22.7	21.1	3.43	3.85
	16	29.0	28.5	27.8	27.2	26.5	25.7	24.8	23.9	22.8	21.5	20.0	2.83	3.24
	18	28.0	27.5	26.9	26.2	25.5	24.7	23.8	22.9	21.8	20.5	19.0	2.39	2.80
19.89	12	33.2	32.6	32.0	31.3	30.5	29.7	28.8	27.8	26.6	25.3	23.7	4.37	4.80
	14	31.5	30.9	30.3	29.6	28.8	28.0	27.1	26.1	24.9	23.6	22.0	3.46	3.88
	16	30.3	29.7	29.0	28.3	27.6	26.8	25.8	24.8	23.7	22.3	20.8	2.85	3.26
	18	29.2	28.6	28.0	27.3	26.5	25.7	24.8	23.8	22.6	21.3	19.7	2.39	2.80
20.88	12	34.5	33.9	33.2	32.5	31.7	30.9	29.9	28.8	27.6	26.2	24.6	4.41	4.85
	14	32.8	32.2	31.5	30.8	30.0	29.1	28.2	27.1	25.9	24.5	22.8	3.49	3.91
	16	31.5	30.8	30.2	29.4	28.7	27.8	26.8	25.8	24.6	23.2	21.5	2.85	3.27
	18	30.4	29.7	29.1	28.3	27.6	26.7	25.7	24.7	23.5	22.1	20.4	2.38	2.80

TABLE 4

Process Times (B) at Retort Temperature of 260°F for Conduction-Heating Foods in 202 x 204 Can

f_h	z	INITIAL FOOD TEMPERATURE (T_{ih})											Equivalent	
		100	110	120	130	140	150	160	170	180	190	200	F_c^{18}	F_s^{18}
16.91	12	22.2	21.7	21.2	20.6	20.0	19.4	18.7	17.9	17.1	16.1	15.0	3.44	3.91
	14	21.8	21.4	20.9	20.3	19.7	19.1	18.4	17.6	16.7	15.8	14.6	3.15	3.62
	16	21.3	20.9	20.4	19.8	19.2	18.6	17.9	17.1	16.3	15.3	14.1	2.73	3.19
	18	20.8	20.4	19.9	19.3	18.7	18.1	17.4	16.6	15.8	14.8	13.6	2.35	2.80
17.90	12	23.3	22.8	22.3	21.7	21.1	20.4	19.7	18.9	17.9	16.9	15.7	3.51	3.99
	14	22.9	22.4	21.9	21.3	20.7	20.0	19.3	18.5	17.5	16.5	15.3	3.19	3.66
	16	22.4	21.9	21.4	20.8	20.2	19.5	18.8	18.0	17.0	16.0	14.8	2.75	3.21
	18	21.9	21.4	20.8	20.3	19.6	19.0	18.2	17.4	16.5	15.5	14.3	2.34	2.80
18.89	12	24.5	23.9	23.4	22.8	22.1	21.4	20.6	19.8	18.8	17.7	16.4	3.59	4.07
	14	24.0	23.5	23.0	22.3	21.7	21.0	20.2	19.3	18.4	17.3	16.0	3.21	3.69
	16	23.5	23.0	22.4	21.8	21.1	20.4	19.6	18.8	17.8	16.7	15.4	2.77	3.23
	18	22.9	22.4	21.8	21.2	20.5	19.8	19.1	18.2	17.2	16.1	14.9	2.34	2.80
19.89	12	25.6	25.1	24.5	23.8	23.1	22.4	21.6	20.7	19.6	18.5	17.1	3.66	4.14
	14	25.1	24.6	24.0	23.4	22.7	21.9	21.1	20.2	19.2	18.0	16.7	3.24	3.71
	16	24.5	24.0	23.4	22.8	22.1	21.3	20.5	19.6	18.6	17.4	16.1	2.78	3.25
	18	23.9	23.4	22.8	22.1	21.4	20.7	19.9	19.0	17.9	16.8	15.5	2.34	2.80
20.88	12	26.8	26.2	25.6	24.9	24.2	23.4	22.5	21.5	20.5	19.3	17.9	3.73	4.21
	14	26.2	25.7	25.0	24.4	23.6	22.8	22.0	21.0	20.0	18.7	17.3	3.27	3.75
	16	25.6	25.0	24.4	23.7	23.0	22.2	21.3	20.4	19.3	18.1	16.7	2.79	3.26
	18	24.9	24.4	23.7	23.1	22.3	21.5	20.7	19.7	18.7	17.4	16.1	2.34	2.80

TABLE 5

Process Times (B) at Retort Temperature of 230°F for Conduction-Heating Foods in 202 x 214 Can

f_h	z	Initial Food Temperature (T_{ih}) 100	110	120	130	140	150	160	170	180	190	200	Equivalent F_c^{18}	F_s^{18}
19.73	12	151.1	150.4	149.7	148.9	148.0	147.0	145.8	144.5	142.9	141.0	138.6	9.94	10.22
	14	105.8	105.1	104.4	103.6	102.7	101.7	100.5	99.2	97.6	95.7	93.3	5.66	5.91
	16	79.1	78.4	77.7	76.8	75.9	74.9	73.8	72.5	70.9	69.0	66.5	3.67	3.92
	18	64.6	64.0	63.2	62.4	61.5	60.5	59.3	58.0	56.5	54.6	52.1	2.58	2.82
20.89	12	155.2	154.5	153.7	152.8	151.8	150.8	149.6	148.2	146.5	144.5	141.9	9.95	10.23
	14	107.0	106.3	105.5	104.6	103.7	102.6	101.4	100.0	98.3	96.3	93.7	5.65	5.89
	16	80.9	80.1	79.4	78.5	77.5	76.5	75.3	73.9	72.2	70.2	67.6	3.66	3.92
	18	66.5	65.7	64.9	64.1	63.1	62.1	60.8	59.4	57.8	55.8	53.2	2.58	2.82
22.05	12	159.0	158.2	157.4	156.5	155.5	154.3	153.1	151.6	149.8	147.7	144.9	9.95	10.23
	14	108.9	108.2	107.3	106.4	105.4	104.3	103.0	101.5	99.8	97.6	94.9	5.71	5.95
	16	82.6	81.9	81.0	80.1	79.1	78.0	76.7	75.2	73.5	71.3	68.6	3.66	3.92
	18	68.2	67.5	66.6	65.7	64.7	63.6	62.3	60.8	59.1	56.9	54.2	2.57	2.82
23.21	12	162.5	161.7	160.9	159.9	158.8	157.6	156.3	154.7	152.9	150.7	147.8	9.96	10.24
	14	110.7	109.9	109.0	108.1	107.0	105.8	104.5	102.9	101.1	98.8	96.0	5.67	5.94
	16	84.3	83.5	82.6	81.6	80.6	79.4	78.1	76.5	74.7	72.4	69.5	3.66	3.91
	18	69.9	69.0	68.2	67.2	66.1	65.0	63.6	62.1	60.2	58.0	55.1	2.57	2.82
24.37	12	165.9	165.0	164.1	163.1	162.0	160.7	159.3	157.7	155.8	153.4	150.3	9.96	10.25
	14	112.8	111.9	111.0	110.0	108.9	107.6	106.2	104.6	102.7	100.3	97.3	5.67	5.94
	16	86.3	85.4	84.5	83.5	82.4	81.1	79.7	78.1	76.1	73.8	70.7	3.67	3.93
	18	71.7	70.8	69.9	68.9	67.8	66.5	65.1	63.5	61.5	59.2	56.1	2.57	2.82

TABLE 6

Process Times (B) at Retort Temperature of 240°F for Conduction-Heating Foods in 202 x 214 Can

f_h	z	INITIAL FOOD TEMPERATURE (T_{ih})											Equivalent	
		100	110	120	130	140	150	160	170	180	190	200	F_c^{18}	F_s^{18}
19.73	12	52.4	51.8	51.1	50.4	49.5	48.6	47.6	46.5	45.2	43.6	41.7	5.82	6.16
	14	46.9	46.3	45.6	44.9	44.1	43.1	42.1	41.0	39.7	38.1	36.2	4.22	4.57
	16	42.4	41.8	41.1	40.3	39.5	38.6	37.6	36.5	35.2	33.6	31.7	3.18	3.51
	18	39.1	38.4	37.7	37.0	36.2	35.3	34.3	33.1	31.8	30.2	28.3	2.50	2.82
20.89	12	54.5	53.8	53.1	52.3	51.5	50.5	49.4	48.2	46.8	45.2	43.2	5.90	6.25
	14	48.7	48.1	47.3	46.5	45.7	44.7	43.7	42.4	41.0	39.4	37.4	4.22	4.57
	16	43.9	43.2	42.5	41.7	40.9	39.9	38.8	37.6	36.2	34.6	32.6	3.18	3.51
	18	40.7	40.0	39.3	38.5	37.6	36.7	35.6	34.4	33.0	31.3	29.3	2.49	2.82
22.05	12	56.6	55.9	55.1	54.3	53.4	52.3	51.2	49.9	48.5	46.7	44.6	5.93	6.29
	14	50.5	49.8	49.0	48.2	47.2	46.2	45.1	43.8	42.4	40.6	38.5	4.22	4.57
	16	45.6	44.9	44.2	43.3	42.4	41.4	40.3	39.0	37.5	35.8	33.6	3.22	3.55
	18	42.3	41.6	40.8	40.0	39.0	38.0	36.9	35.6	34.2	32.4	30.3	2.48	2.82
23.21	12	58.6	57.9	57.0	56.2	55.2	54.1	53.0	51.6	50.1	48.2	46.0	5.94	6.30
	14	52.2	51.4	50.6	49.7	48.8	47.7	46.5	45.2	43.6	41.8	39.5	4.22	4.57
	16	47.4	46.6	45.8	44.9	44.0	42.9	41.7	40.4	38.8	37.0	34.7	3.27	3.60
	18	43.8	43.1	42.3	41.4	40.4	39.4	38.2	36.8	35.3	33.4	31.2	2.48	2.82
24.37	12	60.6	59.8	58.9	58.0	57.0	55.9	54.7	53.2	51.6	49.7	47.3	5.94	6.32
	14	53.8	53.0	52.2	51.3	50.2	49.1	47.9	46.5	44.8	42.9	40.6	4.22	4.57
	16	49.0	48.2	47.4	46.5	45.5	44.4	43.1	41.7	40.1	38.1	35.8	3.28	3.62
	18	45.3	44.6	43.7	42.8	41.8	40.7	39.4	38.0	36.4	34.5	32.1	2.47	2.82

TABLE 7

Process Times (B) at Retort Temperature of 250°F for Conduction-Heating Foods in 202 x 214 Can

f_h	z	INITIAL FOOD TEMPERATURE (T_{ih})											Equivalent	
		100	110	120	130	140	150	160	170	180	190	200	F_c^{18}	F_s^{18}
19.73	12	33.0	32.4	31.8	31.1	30.4	29.6	28.7	27.6	26.5	25.2	23.6	4.40	4.83
	14	31.4	30.8	30.1	29.5	28.7	27.9	27.0	26.0	24.8	23.5	22.0	3.48	3.90
	16	30.1	29.5	28.9	28.2	27.5	26.6	25.7	24.7	23.6	22.3	20.7	2.87	3.28
	18	29.1	28.5	27.9	27.2	26.4	25.6	24.7	23.7	22.5	21.2	19.7	2.41	2.82
20.89	12	34.6	34.0	33.3	32.6	31.8	30.9	30.0	28.9	27.7	26.3	24.6	4.45	4.88
	14	32.9	32.2	31.6	30.8	30.1	29.2	28.2	27.2	26.0	24.6	22.9	3.52	3.94
	16	31.5	30.9	30.2	29.5	28.7	27.9	26.9	25.8	24.6	23.2	21.6	2.88	3.30
	18	30.4	29.8	29.1	28.4	27.6	26.8	25.8	24.7	23.5	22.1	20.5	2.41	2.82
22.05	12	36.2	35.5	34.8	34.0	33.2	32.3	31.3	30.2	28.9	27.4	25.7	4.50	4.94
	14	34.4	33.7	33.0	32.2	31.4	30.5	29.5	28.3	27.1	25.6	23.8	3.54	3.97
	16	33.0	32.3	31.6	30.8	30.0	29.1	28.1	26.9	25.7	24.2	22.4	2.89	3.31
	18	31.8	31.1	30.4	29.6	28.8	27.9	26.9	25.8	24.5	23.0	21.3	2.41	2.82
23.21	12	37.7	37.0	36.3	35.5	34.6	33.7	32.6	31.4	30.1	28.5	26.7	4.55	4.99
	14	35.8	35.1	34.4	33.6	32.7	31.8	30.7	29.5	28.2	26.6	24.8	3.57	4.00
	16	34.4	33.7	32.9	32.1	31.2	30.3	29.2	28.0	26.7	25.1	23.3	2.90	3.33
	18	33.1	32.4	31.7	30.9	30.0	29.0	28.0	26.8	25.4	23.9	22.1	2.40	2.82
24.37	12	39.3	38.6	37.8	36.9	36.0	35.0	33.9	32.6	31.2	29.6	27.7	4.59	5.03
	14	37.3	36.6	35.8	35.0	34.0	33.0	31.9	30.7	29.3	27.6	25.7	3.60	4.04
	16	35.8	35.0	34.3	33.4	32.5	31.5	30.4	29.1	27.7	26.1	24.1	2.91	3.34
	18	34.5	33.7	33.0	32.1	31.2	30.2	29.1	27.8	26.4	24.8	22.8	2.40	2.82

TABLE 8

Process Times (B) at Retort Temperature of 260°F for Conduction-Heating Foods in 202 x 214 Can

f_h	z	INITIAL FOOD TEMPERATURE (T_{ih})											Equivalent	
		100	110	120	130	140	150	160	170	180	190	200	F_c^{18}	F_s^{18}
19.73	12	25.5	24.9	24.3	23.7	23.0	22.3	21.4	20.5	19.5	18.4	17.1	3.67	4.15
	14	25.0	24.4	23.9	23.2	22.5	21.8	21.0	20.1	19.1	17.9	16.6	3.26	3.74
	16	24.4	23.9	23.3	22.6	21.9	21.2	20.4	19.5	18.5	17.3	16.0	2.81	3.27
	18	23.8	23.2	22.6	22.0	21.3	20.6	19.8	18.9	17.9	16.7	15.4	2.36	2.82
20.89	12	26.8	26.2	25.6	24.9	24.2	23.4	22.5	21.6	20.5	19.3	17.9	3.75	4.24
	14	26.3	25.7	25.1	24.4	23.7	22.9	22.0	21.1	20.0	18.8	17.4	3.29	3.77
	16	25.6	25.1	24.4	23.8	23.0	22.2	21.4	20.4	19.4	18.1	16.7	2.81	3.28
	18	25.0	24.4	23.8	23.1	22.4	21.6	20.7	19.8	18.7	17.5	16.1	2.36	2.82
22.05	12	28.1	27.5	26.9	26.1	25.4	24.5	23.6	22.6	21.5	20.2	18.7	3.82	4.31
	14	27.5	26.9	26.3	25.6	24.8	24.0	23.0	22.0	20.9	19.6	18.2	3.33	3.81
	16	26.9	26.2	25.6	24.9	24.1	23.3	22.4	21.4	20.2	18.9	17.5	2.82	3.29
	18	26.2	25.5	24.9	24.2	23.4	22.6	21.7	20.7	19.5	18.3	16.8	2.36	2.82
23.21	12	29.5	28.8	28.1	27.4	26.6	25.7	24.7	23.7	22.5	21.1	19.6	3.88	4.37
	14	28.8	28.2	27.5	26.7	25.9	25.0	24.1	23.0	21.8	20.5	18.9	3.37	3.86
	16	28.1	27.4	26.7	26.0	25.2	24.3	23.3	22.3	21.1	19.8	18.2	2.84	3.31
	18	27.3	26.7	26.0	25.2	24.4	23.6	22.6	21.5	20.3	19.0	17.4	2.36	2.82
24.37	12	30.8	30.1	29.4	28.6	27.7	26.8	25.8	24.7	23.4	22.0	20.4	3.95	4.44
	14	30.1	29.4	28.7	27.9	27.0	26.1	25.1	24.0	22.7	21.3	19.7	3.40	3.88
	16	29.3	28.6	27.9	27.1	26.3	25.3	24.3	23.2	22.0	20.5	18.9	2.85	3.33
	18	28.5	27.8	27.1	26.3	25.5	24.5	23.5	22.4	21.2	19.8	18.1	2.36	2.82

TABLE 9

Process Times (B) at Retort Temperature of 230°F for Conduction-Heating Foods in 202 x 308 Can

f_h	z	INITIAL FOOD TEMPERATURE (T_{ih}) 100	110	120	130	140	150	160	170	180	190	200	Equivalent F_c^{18}	F_s^{18}
21.38	12	157.4	156.7	155.9	155.0	154.0	152.9	151.7	150.3	148.6	146.5	143.8	10.02	10.30
	14	108.1	107.3	106.5	105.7	104.7	103.6	102.3	100.9	99.2	97.1	94.5	5.69	5.94
	16	82.0	81.3	80.4	79.6	78.6	77.5	76.2	74.8	73.1	71.1	68.4	3.69	3.95
	18	67.5	66.7	65.9	65.0	64.1	63.0	61.7	60.3	58.6	56.5	53.9	2.59	2.84
22.64	12	161.5	160.7	159.8	158.9	157.9	156.7	155.4	153.9	152.1	149.9	147.1	10.02	10.31
	14	110.4	109.6	108.7	107.8	106.8	105.6	104.3	102.8	101.0	98.8	96.0	5.73	5.99
	16	83.8	83.0	82.2	81.3	80.2	79.1	77.7	76.2	74.4	72.2	69.4	3.68	3.94
	18	69.3	68.5	67.7	66.8	65.7	64.6	63.2	61.7	59.9	57.7	54.9	2.59	2.84
23.89	12	165.2	164.4	163.5	162.5	161.4	160.2	158.8	157.2	155.3	153.0	150.0	10.03	10.31
	14	112.4	111.6	110.7	109.7	108.6	107.4	106.0	104.4	102.5	100.2	97.2	5.71	5.99
	16	85.8	85.0	84.1	83.1	82.0	80.7	79.4	77.8	75.9	73.6	70.6	3.70	3.95
	18	71.2	70.3	69.4	68.4	67.4	66.1	64.7	63.1	61.3	58.9	56.0	2.59	2.84
25.15	12	168.7	167.8	166.9	165.8	164.7	163.4	161.9	160.3	158.3	155.8	152.7	10.04	10.32
	14	114.6	113.7	112.8	111.7	110.6	109.3	107.8	106.2	104.2	101.7	98.6	5.71	5.98
	16	87.9	87.0	86.0	85.0	83.8	82.5	81.1	79.4	77.4	75.0	71.8	3.69	3.96
	18	73.1	72.2	71.3	70.2	69.1	67.8	66.3	64.7	62.7	60.2	57.1	2.58	2.84
26.41	12	171.9	171.0	170.0	168.9	167.7	166.4	164.8	163.1	161.0	158.4	155.1	10.04	10.33
	14	116.6	115.6	114.6	113.5	112.3	111.0	109.5	107.7	105.6	103.0	99.7	5.70	5.98
	16	89.8	88.8	87.9	86.8	85.5	84.2	82.7	80.9	78.8	76.2	72.9	3.69	3.96
	18	74.9	74.0	73.0	71.9	70.7	69.3	67.8	66.0	64.0	61.4	58.1	2.58	2.84

TABLE 10

Process Times (B) at Retort Temperature of 240°F for Conduction-Heating Foods in 202 x 308 Can

f_h	z	INITIAL FOOD TEMPERATURE (T_{ih})											Equivalent	
		100	110	120	130	140	150	160	170	180	190	200	F_c^{18}	F_s^{18}
21.38	12	55.5	54.8	54.1	53.3	52.4	51.4	50.3	49.1	47.7	46.0	43.9	5.97	6.32
	14	49.6	48.9	48.2	47.4	46.5	45.5	44.4	43.2	41.7	40.0	38.0	4.25	4.60
	16	44.7	44.0	43.3	42.5	41.6	40.6	39.5	38.3	36.9	35.2	33.1	3.21	2.54
	18	41.4	40.8	40.0	39.2	38.3	37.3	36.2	35.0	33.6	31.9	29.8	2.51	2.84
22.64	12	57.7	57.0	56.2	55.4	54.4	53.4	52.2	50.9	49.4	47.6	45.4	5.98	6.34
	14	51.5	50.7	50.0	49.1	48.2	47.1	46.0	44.7	43.1	41.4	39.2	4.25	4.61
	16	46.6	45.9	45.1	44.2	43.3	42.3	41.1	39.8	38.3	36.5	34.3	3.26	3.60
	18	43.2	42.4	41.6	40.8	39.8	38.8	37.7	36.3	34.8	33.0	30.8	2.50	2.84
23.89	12	59.9	59.1	58.3	57.4	56.4	55.3	54.1	52.7	51.1	49.2	46.9	5.98	6.35
	14	53.3	52.5	51.7	50.8	49.8	48.7	47.5	46.1	44.5	42.6	40.3	4.25	4.61
	16	48.5	47.7	46.9	46.0	45.0	43.9	42.6	41.3	39.7	37.8	35.5	3.31	3.64
	18	44.8	44.1	43.2	42.3	41.3	40.2	39.0	37.6	36.0	34.1	31.8	2.49	2.84
25.15	12	62.0	61.2	60.4	59.4	58.4	57.2	55.9	54.5	52.8	50.8	48.4	5.99	6.37
	14	55.0	54.2	53.4	52.4	51.4	50.2	48.9	47.5	45.8	43.8	41.4	4.25	4.61
	16	50.3	49.4	48.6	47.6	46.6	45.4	44.1	42.7	41.0	39.0	36.6	3.30	3.64
	18	46.5	45.7	44.8	43.8	42.8	41.7	40.4	38.9	37.2	35.2	32.8	2.49	2.84
26.41	12	64.1	63.3	62.4	61.4	60.3	59.1	57.7	56.2	54.4	52.3	49.8	6.00	6.38
	14	56.8	56.0	55.1	54.1	53.0	51.8	50.4	48.9	47.1	45.0	42.5	4.27	4.63
	16	52.0	51.2	50.3	49.3	48.2	47.0	45.6	44.1	42.3	40.2	37.7	3.29	3.63
	18	48.1	47.2	46.3	45.3	44.2	43.0	41.7	40.1	38.4	36.3	33.7	2.49	2.84

TABLE 11

Process Times (B) at Retort Temperature of 250°F for Conduction-Heating Foods in 202 x 308 Can

f_h	z	INITIAL FOOD TEMPERATURE (T_{ih})											Equivalent	
		100	110	120	130	140	150	160	170	180	190	200	F_c^{18}	F_s^{18}
21.38	12	35.3	34.7	34.0	33.3	32.4	31.6	30.6	29.5	28.2	26.8	25.1	4.50	4.93
	14	33.5	32.9	32.2	31.5	30.7	29.8	28.8	27.7	26.5	25.0	23.3	3.55	3.98
	16	32.2	31.5	30.9	30.1	29.3	28.4	27.4	26.3	25.1	23.7	22.0	2.90	3.32
	18	31.1	30.4	29.7	29.0	28.2	27.3	26.3	25.2	24.0	22.6	20.9	2.43	2.84
22.64	12	37.0	36.3	35.6	34.8	34.0	33.0	32.0	30.8	29.5	28.0	26.2	4.56	5.00
	14	35.2	34.5	33.8	33.0	32.1	31.2	30.1	29.0	27.7	26.2	24.4	3.58	4.01
	16	33.7	33.0	32.3	31.5	30.7	29.7	28.7	27.5	26.2	24.7	22.9	2.92	3.34
	18	32.5	31.8	31.1	30.3	29.5	28.5	27.5	26.3	25.0	23.5	21.7	2.42	2.84
23.89	12	38.7	38.0	37.2	36.4	35.5	34.5	33.4	32.2	30.8	29.2	27.3	4.60	5.04
	14	36.8	36.0	35.3	34.4	33.5	32.6	31.5	30.2	28.9	27.3	25.4	3.61	4.04
	16	35.2	34.5	33.8	32.9	32.0	31.0	29.9	28.7	27.3	25.7	23.8	2.93	3.35
	18	34.0	33.2	32.5	31.6	30.7	29.8	28.7	27.4	26.1	24.5	22.6	2.42	2.84
25.15	12	40.4	39.7	38.8	38.0	37.0	36.0	34.8	33.5	32.1	30.4	28.4	4.66	5.10
	14	38.4	37.6	36.8	35.9	35.0	34.0	32.8	31.5	30.1	28.4	26.4	3.65	4.09
	16	36.8	36.0	35.2	34.3	33.4	32.3	31.2	29.9	28.5	26.8	24.8	2.95	3.38
	18	35.4	34.7	33.9	33.0	32.0	31.0	29.9	28.6	27.1	25.4	23.4	2.42	2.84
26.41	12	42.1	41.3	40.5	39.5	38.5	37.5	36.2	34.9	33.4	31.6	29.5	4.72	5.17
	14	40.0	39.2	38.4	37.4	36.4	35.4	34.1	32.8	31.3	29.5	27.4	3.70	4.14
	16	38.3	37.5	36.7	35.8	34.8	33.7	32.5	31.1	29.6	27.8	25.7	2.98	3.41
	18	36.9	36.1	35.3	34.3	33.3	32.2	31.0	29.7	28.2	26.4	24.3	2.42	2.84

TABLE 12

Process Times (B) at Retort Temperature of 260°F for Conduction-Heating Foods in 202 x 308 Can

f_h	z	INITIAL FOOD TEMPERATURE (T_{ih})											Equivalent	
		100	110	120	130	140	150	160	170	180	190	200	F_c^{18}	F_s^{18}
21.38	12	27.4	26.8	26.1	25.5	24.7	23.9	23.0	22.0	21.0	19.7	18.3	3.80	4.29
	14	26.8	26.2	25.6	24.9	24.2	23.4	22.5	21.5	20.4	19.2	17.7	3.33	3.81
	16	26.2	25.6	25.0	24.3	23.5	22.7	21.8	20.8	19.8	18.5	17.1	2.84	3.31
	18	25.5	24.9	24.3	23.6	22.8	22.0	21.2	20.2	19.1	17.8	16.4	2.38	2.84
22.64	12	28.8	28.2	27.5	26.8	26.0	25.2	24.2	23.2	22.0	20.7	19.2	3.87	4.36
	14	28.2	27.6	26.9	26.2	25.4	24.5	23.6	22.6	21.4	20.1	18.6	3.37	3.85
	16	27.5	26.9	26.2	25.5	24.7	23.8	22.9	21.9	20.7	19.4	17.9	2.85	3.32
	18	26.8	26.2	25.5	24.7	24.0	23.1	22.2	21.1	20.0	18.7	17.1	2.38	2.84
23.89	12	30.3	29.6	28.9	28.1	27.3	26.4	25.4	24.3	23.1	21.7	20.1	3.94	4.43
	14	29.6	28.9	28.2	27.4	26.6	25.7	24.7	23.6	22.4	21.0	19.4	3.42	3.90
	16	28.8	28.2	27.4	26.7	25.8	24.9	24.0	22.9	21.6	20.3	18.7	2.87	3.35
	18	28.1	27.4	26.7	25.9	25.1	24.2	23.2	22.1	20.9	19.5	17.9	2.38	2.84
25.15	12	31.7	31.0	30.2	29.4	28.6	27.6	26.6	25.4	24.1	22.7	21.0	4.01	4.51
	14	30.9	30.2	29.5	28.7	27.8	26.9	25.8	24.7	23.4	21.9	20.2	3.44	3.92
	16	30.1	29.4	28.7	27.9	27.0	26.0	25.0	23.9	22.6	21.1	19.4	2.88	3.35
	18	29.3	28.6	27.9	27.1	26.2	25.2	24.2	23.0	21.7	20.3	18.6	2.37	2.84
26.41	12	33.1	32.4	31.6	30.7	29.8	28.8	27.7	26.5	25.2	23.6	21.9	4.09	4.59
	14	32.3	31.5	30.8	29.9	29.0	28.0	26.9	25.7	24.3	22.8	21.0	3.46	3.94
	16	31.4	30.7	29.9	29.1	28.1	27.1	26.1	24.8	23.5	22.0	20.2	2.89	3.37
	18	30.6	29.8	29.0	28.2	27.3	26.3	25.2	24.0	22.6	21.1	19.3	2.37	2.84

TABLE 13

Process Times (B) at Retort Temperature of 230°F for Conduction-Heating Foods in 202 x 314 Can

f_h	z	INITIAL FOOD TEMPERATURE (T_{ih})											Equivalent	
		100	110	120	130	140	150	160	170	180	190	200	F_c^{18}	F_s^{18}
22.04	12	159.9	159.2	158.3	157.4	156.4	155.3	154.0	152.5	150.8	148.6	145.9	10.06	10.34
	14	109.7	108.9	108.1	107.1	106.1	105.0	103.7	102.3	100.5	98.4	95.6	5.75	6.00
	16	83.2	82.4	81.6	80.7	79.7	78.5	77.3	75.8	74.0	71.9	69.1	3.70	3.96
	18	68.6	67.8	67.0	66.1	65.1	64.0	62.7	61.2	59.5	57.3	54.6	2.60	2.85
23.34	12	163.9	163.1	162.2	161.3	160.2	159.0	157.7	156.1	154.3	152.0	149.1	10.06	10.35
	14	111.7	110.9	110.0	109.1	108.0	106.8	105.5	103.9	102.1	99.8	96.9	5.74	6.01
	16	85.0	84.2	83.3	82.3	81.3	80.1	78.7	77.2	75.3	73.1	70.1	3.70	3.95
	18	70.5	69.6	68.8	67.8	66.7	65.5	64.2	62.6	60.8	58.5	55.6	2.60	2.85
24.64	12	167.7	166.8	165.9	164.9	163.7	162.5	161.0	159.4	157.4	155.1	152.0	10.07	10.35
	14	114.0	113.1	112.2	111.2	110.1	108.8	107.4	105.7	103.8	101.4	98.3	5.73	6.01
	16	87.2	86.3	85.4	84.4	83.3	82.0	80.6	78.9	77.0	74.6	71.5	3.71	3.97
	18	72.4	71.6	70.7	69.6	68.5	67.3	65.8	64.2	62.2	59.2	56.8	2.59	2.85
25.93	12	171.1	170.2	169.2	168.2	167.0	165.6	164.1	162.4	160.3	157.8	154.6	10.07	10.36
	14	116.1	115.2	114.2	113.2	112.0	110.7	109.2	107.4	105.4	102.8	99.6	5.73	6.00
	16	89.2	88.3	87.4	86.3	85.1	83.8	82.3	80.5	78.5	76.0	72.7	3.70	3.97
	18	74.4	73.5	72.5	71.4	70.2	68.9	67.4	65.7	63.6	61.1	57.9	2.59	2.85
27.23	12	174.3	173.4	172.3	171.2	170.0	168.6	167.0	165.2	163.0	160.4	157.0	10.08	10.37
	14	117.9	117.0	116.0	114.8	113.6	112.2	110.6	108.8	106.6	104.0	100.6	5.72	5.99
	16	91.1	90.2	89.2	88.0	86.8	85.4	83.8	82.0	79.8	77.2	73.8	3.70	3.97
	18	76.3	75.3	74.3	73.2	71.9	70.5	69.0	67.1	65.0	62.3	58.9	2.59	2.85

TABLE 14

Process Times (B) at Retort Temperature of 240°F for Conduction-Heating Foods in 202 x 314 Can

f_h	z	INITIAL FOOD TEMPERATURE (T_{ih})											Equivalent	
		100	110	120	130	140	150	160	170	180	190	200	F_c^{18}	F_s^{18}
	12	56.8	56.1	55.3	54.5	53.5	52.5	51.4	50.1	48.7	46.9	44.8	6.00	6.36
22.04	14	50.7	50.0	49.2	48.4	47.4	46.4	45.3	44.0	42.6	40.8	38.7	4.27	4.62
	16	45.8	45.1	44.3	43.5	42.6	41.5	40.4	39.1	37.7	35.9	33.8	3.25	3.58
	18	42.4	41.7	40.9	40.1	39.2	38.2	37.0	35.8	34.3	32.5	30.4	2.51	2.85
	12	59.0	58.3	57.5	56.6	55.6	54.6	53.4	52.0	50.5	48.6	46.3	6.00	6.37
23.34	14	52.6	51.8	51.0	50.1	49.2	48.1	46.9	45.5	44.0	42.1	39.9	4.27	4.62
	16	47.7	46.9	46.1	45.3	44.3	43.2	42.0	40.7	39.1	37.3	35.0	3.30	3.63
	18	44.1	43.4	42.6	41.7	40.7	39.7	38.5	37.1	35.6	33.7	31.4	2.51	2.85
	12	61.3	60.5	59.6	58.7	57.7	56.5	55.3	53.8	52.2	50.2	47.9	6.01	6.38
24.64	14	54.4	53.6	52.8	51.8	50.8	49.7	48.4	47.0	45.3	43.4	41.0	4.27	4.62
	16	49.6	48.8	47.9	47.0	46.0	44.9	43.6	42.2	40.5	38.6	36.2	3.32	3.65
	18	45.9	45.1	44.2	43.3	42.3	41.1	39.9	38.4	36.8	34.8	32.5	2.50	2.85
	12	63.4	62.6	61.7	60.7	59.6	58.4	57.1	55.6	53.9	51.8	49.3	6.02	6.40
25.93	14	56.2	55.3	54.4	53.5	52.4	51.2	49.9	48.4	46.6	44.6	42.1	4.27	4.62
	16	51.4	50.6	49.7	48.7	47.6	46.4	45.1	43.6	41.9	39.8	37.3	3.30	3.65
	18	47.5	46.7	45.8	44.8	43.8	42.6	41.2	39.7	38.0	35.9	33.4	2.50	2.85
	12	65.5	64.7	63.7	62.7	61.6	60.3	58.9	57.3	55.5	53.4	50.7	6.03	6.41
27.23	14	58.2	57.3	56.4	55.3	54.2	53.0	51.6	50.0	48.2	46.0	43.4	4.32	4.68
	16	53.2	52.3	51.4	50.4	49.2	48.0	46.6	45.0	43.2	41.0	38.4	3.29	3.64
	18	49.2	48.3	47.4	46.4	45.2	44.0	42.6	41.0	39.2	37.0	34.4	2.50	2.85

TABLE 15

Process Times (B) at Retort Temperature of 250°F for Conduction-Heating Foods in 202 x 314 Can

f_h	z	INITIAL FOOD TEMPERATURE (T_{ih})											Equivalent	
		100	110	120	130	140	150	160	170	180	190	200	F_c^{18}	F_s^{18}
22.04	12	36.2	35.6	34.9	34.1	33.3	32.4	31.4	30.2	29.0	27.5	25.7	4.54	4.98
	14	34.4	33.8	33.1	32.3	31.5	30.5	29.5	28.4	27.1	25.6	23.9	3.58	4.00
	16	33.0	32.4	31.6	30.9	30.0	29.1	28.1	27.0	25.7	24.2	22.5	2.92	3.34
	18	31.9	31.2	30.5	29.7	28.9	28.0	27.0	25.8	24.6	23.1	21.3	2.44	2.85
23.34	12	38.0	37.3	36.5	35.7	34.9	33.9	32.8	31.6	30.3	28.7	26.9	4.60	5.04
	14	36.1	35.4	34.6	33.8	32.9	32.0	30.9	29.7	28.4	26.8	24.9	3.61	4.04
	16	34.6	33.9	33.1	32.3	31.5	30.5	29.4	28.2	26.9	25.3	23.5	2.94	3.36
	18	33.4	32.7	31.9	31.1	30.2	29.2	28.2	27.0	25.6	24.1	22.2	2.43	2.85
24.64	12	39.7	39.0	38.2	37.3	36.4	35.4	34.3	33.0	31.6	29.9	28.0	4.64	5.09
	14	37.7	37.0	36.2	35.3	34.4	33.4	32.3	31.0	29.6	27.9	26.0	3.64	4.08
	16	36.2	35.4	34.6	33.8	32.8	31.8	30.7	29.4	28.0	26.4	24.4	2.95	3.38
	18	34.9	34.1	33.3	32.5	31.5	30.5	29.4	28.1	26.7	25.0	23.1	2.43	2.85
25.93	12	41.5	40.7	39.9	39.0	38.0	36.9	35.7	34.4	32.9	31.2	29.1	4.71	5.16
	14	39.4	38.6	37.8	36.9	35.9	34.9	33.7	32.3	30.8	29.1	27.0	3.70	4.14
	16	37.8	37.0	36.2	35.3	34.3	33.2	32.0	30.7	29.2	27.4	25.4	2.98	3.41
	18	36.4	35.6	34.8	33.9	32.9	31.8	30.6	29.3	27.8	26.0	24.0	2.43	2.85
27.23	12	43.2	42.4	41.5	40.6	39.6	38.4	37.2	35.8	34.2	32.4	30.2	4.77	5.22
	14	41.1	40.3	39.4	38.4	37.4	36.3	35.0	33.6	32.1	30.2	28.1	3.74	4.18
	16	39.3	38.5	37.6	36.7	35.7	34.5	33.3	31.9	30.3	28.5	26.3	3.01	3.44
	18	37.9	37.1	36.2	35.2	34.2	33.1	31.8	30.4	28.9	27.0	24.9	2.42	2.85

TABLE 16

Process Times (B) at Retort Temperature of 260°F for Conduction-Heating Foods in 202 x 314 Can

f_h	z	INITIAL FOOD TEMPERATURE (T_{ih})											Equivalent	
		100	110	120	130	140	150	160	170	180	190	200	F_c^{18}	F_s^{18}
22.04	12	28.2	27.5	26.9	26.2	25.4	24.6	23.7	22.7	21.5	20.3	18.8	3.85	4.34
	14	27.6	27.0	26.3	25.6	24.8	24.0	23.1	22.1	21.0	19.7	18.2	3.36	3.85
	16	26.9	26.3	25.6	24.9	24.2	23.3	22.4	21.4	20.3	19.0	17.5	2.85	3.33
	18	26.2	25.6	24.9	24.2	23.5	22.6	21.7	20.7	19.6	18.3	16.8	2.39	2.85
23.34	12	29.6	29.0	28.3	27.5	26.7	25.9	24.9	23.8	22.6	21.3	19.7	3.92	4.41
	14	29.0	28.3	27.6	26.9	26.1	25.2	24.2	23.2	22.0	20.6	19.1	3.41	3.89
	16	28.3	27.6	26.9	26.2	25.2	24.5	23.5	22.4	21.2	19.9	18.3	2.87	3.35
	18	27.5	26.9	26.2	25.4	24.6	23.7	22.7	21.7	20.5	19.1	17.6	2.39	2.85
24.64	12	31.1	30.4	29.7	28.9	28.0	27.1	26.1	25.0	23.7	22.3	20.6	3.99	4.49
	14	30.4	29.7	29.0	28.2	27.3	26.4	25.4	24.3	23.0	21.6	19.9	3.44	3.93
	16	29.6	28.9	28.2	27.4	26.5	25.6	24.6	23.5	22.2	20.8	19.1	2.89	3.36
	18	28.8	28.1	27.4	26.6	25.7	24.8	23.8	22.7	21.4	20.0	18.3	2.38	2.85
25.93	12	32.6	31.9	31.1	30.3	29.4	28.4	27.3	26.1	24.8	23.3	21.6	4.07	4.57
	14	31.8	31.1	30.3	29.5	28.6	27.6	26.5	25.3	24.0	22.5	20.8	3.46	3.95
	16	31.0	30.2	29.5	28.6	27.7	26.7	25.7	24.5	23.2	21.7	19.9	2.90	3.37
	18	30.1	29.4	28.6	27.8	26.9	25.9	24.8	23.6	22.3	20.8	19.1	2.38	2.85
27.23	12	34.1	33.3	32.5	31.6	30.7	29.6	28.5	27.3	25.9	24.3	22.5	4.15	4.65
	14	33.2	32.4	31.6	30.7	29.8	28.7	27.6	26.4	25.0	23.4	21.6	3.48	3.97
	16	32.3	31.5	30.7	29.9	28.9	27.9	26.8	25.5	24.1	22.5	20.7	2.91	3.39
	18	31.4	30.6	29.8	28.9	28.0	27.0	25.8	24.6	23.2	21.6	19.8	2.38	2.85

TABLE 17

Process Times (B) at Retort Temperature of 230°F for Conduction-Heating Foods in 211 x 200 Can

f_h	z	INITIAL FOOD TEMPERATUE (T_{ih})											Equivalent	
		100	110	120	130	140	150	160	170	180	190	200	F_c^{18}	F_s^{18}
20.00	12	152.3	151.6	150.8	150.0	149.1	148.0	146.9	145.6	144.0	142.0	139.5	9.96	10.24
	14	106.3	105.6	104.8	104.0	103.1	102.1	100.9	99.6	98.0	96.1	93.6	5.67	5.92
	16	79.6	78.9	78.2	77.3	76.4	75.4	74.2	72.9	71.3	69.4	66.9	3.68	3.93
	18	65.1	64.4	63.7	62.8	61.9	60.9	59.7	58.4	56.8	54.9	52.4	2.58	2.82
21.18	12	156.3	155.6	154.8	153.9	152.9	151.9	150.6	149.2	147.5	145.5	142.8	9.97	10.25
	14	107.5	106.7	105.9	105.0	104.1	103.0	101.8	100.3	98.7	96.6	94.0	5.66	5.91
	16	81.4	80.7	79.9	79.0	78.0	77.0	75.7	74.3	72.6	70.6	67.9	3.67	3.93
	18	67.0	66.2	65.4	64.6	63.6	62.5	61.3	59.9	58.2	56.1	53.5	2.58	2.83
22.35	12	160.1	159.4	158.5	157.6	156.6	155.4	154.1	152.6	150.9	148.7	145.9	9.97	10.26
	14	109.5	108.8	107.9	107.0	106.0	104.8	103.5	102.0	100.3	98.1	95.3	5.71	5.96
	16	83.2	82.4	81.6	80.6	79.6	78.5	77.2	75.7	73.9	71.7	68.9	3.67	3.92
	18	68.7	68.0	67.1	66.2	65.2	64.0	62.7	61.2	59.5	57.3	54.5	2.58	2.83
23.53	12	163.7	162.9	162.0	161.0	159.9	158.7	157.4	155.8	153.9	151.6	148.7	9.98	10.26
	14	111.4	110.6	109.7	108.8	107.7	106.5	105.1	103.5	101.7	99.4	96.5	5.68	5.96
	16	84.9	84.1	83.2	82.3	81.2	80.0	78.6	77.0	75.2	72.9	70.0	3.67	3.93
	18	70.4	69.6	68.7	67.7	66.7	65.5	64.1	62.5	60.7	58.4	55.4	2.57	2.83
24.71	12	167.0	166.1	165.2	164.2	163.0	161.8	160.4	158.7	156.7	154.3	151.3	9.98	10.27
	14	113.5	112.6	111.7	110.7	109.6	108.3	106.9	105.2	103.2	100.9	97.8	5.68	5.96
	16	86.9	86.0	85.1	84.1	83.0	81.7	80.3	78.6	76.7	74.3	71.2	3.68	3.94
	18	72.2	71.4	70.5	69.4	68.3	67.0	65.6	64.0	62.0	59.6	56.5	2.57	2.83

TABLE 18

Process Times (B) at Retort Temperature of 240°F for Conduction-Heating Foods in 211 x 200 Can

f_h	z	INITIAL FOOD TEMPERATURE (T_{ih})											Equivalent	
		100	110	120	130	140	150	160	170	180	190	200	F_c^{18}	F_s^{18}
	12	53.0	52.3	51.6	50.9	50.0	49.1	48.1	46.9	45.6	44.0	42.1	5.85	6.19
20.00	14	47.4	46.8	46.1	45.3	43.6	43.6	42.5	41.4	40.0	38.5	36.5	4.23	4.58
	16	42.8	42.2	41.5	40.7	39.9	39.0	37.9	36.8	35.4	33.9	31.9	3.19	3.52
	18	39.5	38.8	38.1	37.4	36.5	35.6	34.6	33.4	32.1	30.5	28.6	2.50	2.83
	12	55.1	54.4	53.7	52.9	52.0	51.0	49.9	48.7	47.3	45.6	43.6	5.93	6.28
21.18	14	49.2	48.5	47.8	47.0	46.1	45.1	44.1	42.8	41.4	39.7	37.7	4.23	4.58
	16	44.4	43.7	42.9	42.1	41.3	40.3	39.2	38.0	36.6	34.9	32.8	3.19	3.52
	18	41.1	40.4	39.7	38.9	38.0	37.0	36.0	34.7	33.3	31.6	29.6	2.50	2.83
	12	57.2	56.4	55.7	54.8	53.9	52.9	51.7	50.4	48.9	47.2	45.0	5.95	6.31
22.35	14	51.0	50.2	49.5	48.6	47.7	46.7	45.5	44.2	42.7	41.0	38.8	4.23	4.58
	16	46.1	45.4	44.6	43.8	42.9	41.8	40.7	39.4	37.9	36.1	34.0	3.24	3.57
	18	42.7	42.0	41.2	40.4	39.4	38.4	37.3	36.0	34.5	32.7	30.5	2.49	2.83
	12	59.2	58.4	57.6	56.7	55.8	54.7	53.5	52.1	50.5	48.7	46.4	5.95	6.32
23.53	14	52.7	51.9	51.1	50.2	49.2	48.2	46.9	45.6	44.0	42.1	39.9	4.23	4.58
	16	47.9	47.1	46.3	45.4	44.4	43.3	42.1	40.8	39.2	37.3	35.1	3.29	3.62
	18	44.3	43.5	42.7	41.8	40.8	39.8	38.6	37.2	35.6	33.8	31.5	2.48	2.83
	12	61.2	60.4	59.5	58.6	57.6	56.5	55.2	53.8	52.1	50.1	47.8	5.96	6.33
24.71	14	54.3	53.5	52.7	51.7	50.7	49.6	48.3	46.9	45.2	43.3	40.9	4.23	4.58
	16	49.5	48.8	47.9	47.0	45.9	44.8	43.5	42.1	40.5	38.5	36.1	3.28	3.62
	18	45.8	45.0	44.2	43.2	42.2	41.1	39.8	38.4	36.7	34.8	32.4	2.48	2.83

TABLE 19

Process Times (B) at Retort Temperature of 250°F for Conduction-Heating Foods in 211 x 200 Can

f_h	z	INITIAL FOOD TEMPERATURE (T_{ih}) 100	110	120	130	140	150	160	170	180	190	200	Equivalent F_c^{18}	F_s^{18}
20.00	12	33.4	32.8	32.2	31.5	30.7	29.9	29.0	28.0	26.8	25.5	23.9	4.42	4.85
	14	31.7	31.1	30.5	29.8	29.0	28.2	27.3	26.3	25.1	23.8	22.2	3.50	3.92
	16	30.5	29.9	29.2	28.5	27.8	26.9	26.0	25.0	23.8	22.5	20.9	2.88	3.30
	18	29.4	28.8	28.2	27.5	26.7	25.9	25.0	24.0	22.8	21.5	19.9	2.42	2.83
21.18	12	35.0	34.4	33.7	33.0	32.2	31.3	30.3	29.2	28.0	26.6	24.9	4.47	4.90
	14	33.3	32.6	31.9	31.2	30.4	29.5	28.6	27.5	26.2	24.8	23.1	3.53	3.96
	16	31.9	31.3	30.6	29.9	29.1	28.2	27.2	26.1	24.9	23.5	21.8	2.89	3.31
	18	30.8	30.2	29.5	28.7	27.9	27.1	26.1	25.0	23.8	22.4	20.7	2.41	2.83
22.35	12	36.6	35.9	35.2	34.4	33.6	32.7	31.6	30.5	29.2	27.7	25.9	4.53	4.96
	14	34.8	34.1	33.4	32.6	31.8	30.8	29.8	28.7	27.4	25.9	24.1	3.55	3.98
	16	33.3	32.7	31.9	31.2	30.3	29.4	28.4	27.2	25.9	24.4	22.7	2.90	3.32
	18	32.2	31.5	30.8	30.0	29.1	28.2	27.2	26.1	24.8	23.3	21.5	2.41	2.83
23.53	12	38.2	37.5	36.7	35.9	35.0	34.0	33.0	31.8	30.4	28.8	27.0	4.57	5.01
	14	36.3	35.6	34.8	34.0	33.1	32.1	31.0	29.8	28.5	26.9	25.0	3.58	4.02
	16	34.8	34.1	33.3	32.5	31.6	30.6	29.5	28.3	27.0	25.4	23.5	2.91	3.34
	18	33.5	32.8	32.0	31.2	30.3	29.4	28.3	27.1	25.7	24.1	22.3	2.41	2.83
24.71	12	39.8	39.0	38.2	37.4	36.4	35.4	34.3	33.0	31.6	29.9	28.0	4.62	5.06
	14	37.8	37.0	36.2	35.4	34.4	33.4	32.3	31.0	29.6	27.9	26.0	3.62	4.06
	16	36.2	35.5	34.7	33.8	32.9	31.8	30.7	29.5	28.0	26.4	24.4	2.93	3.36
	18	34.9	34.1	33.3	32.5	31.5	30.5	29.4	28.1	26.7	25.0	23.1	2.41	2.83

TABLE 20

Process Times (B) at Retort Temperature of 260°F for Conduction-Heating Foods in 211 x 200 Can

f_h	z	INITIAL FOOD TEMPERATURE (T_{ih})											Equivalent	
		100	110	120	130	140	150	160	170	180	190	200	F_c^{18}	F_s^{18}
20.00	12	25.8	25.2	24.6	24.0	23.3	22.5	21.7	20.8	19.8	18.6	17.3	3.69	4.18
	14	25.3	24.7	24.1	23.5	22.8	22.1	21.2	20.3	19.3	18.1	16.8	3.28	3.75
	16	24.7	24.1	23.5	22.9	22.2	21.5	20.6	19.7	18.7	17.5	16.2	2.81	3.28
	18	24.1	23.5	22.9	22.3	21.6	20.8	20.0	19.1	18.1	16.9	15.6	2.37	2.83
21.18	12	27.1	26.5	25.9	25.2	24.5	23.7	22.8	21.8	20.8	19.5	18.1	3.78	4.26
	14	26.6	26.0	25.4	24.7	24.0	23.2	22.3	21.3	20.2	19.0	17.6	3.31	3.79
	16	26.0	25.4	24.7	24.0	23.3	22.5	21.6	20.7	29.6	18.4	16.9	2.82	3.29
	18	25.3	24.7	24.1	23.4	22.6	21.8	21.0	20.0	18.9	17.7	16.3	2.37	2.83
22.35	12	28.5	27.9	27.2	26.5	25.7	24.9	23.9	22.9	21.8	20.5	19.0	3.84	4.33
	14	27.9	27.3	26.6	25.9	25.1	24.3	23.3	22.3	21.2	19.9	18.4	3.35	3.83
	16	27.2	26.6	25.9	25.2	24.4	23.6	22.6	21.6	20.5	19.2	17.7	2.83	3.30
	18	26.5	25.9	25.2	24.5	23.7	22.8	21.9	20.9	19.8	18.5	17.0	2.37	2.83
23.53	12	29.8	29.2	28.5	27.7	26.9	26.0	25.0	24.0	22.8	21.4	19.8	3.90	4.40
	14	29.2	28.5	27.8	27.0	26.2	25.3	24.4	23.3	22.1	20.7	19.1	3.39	3.87
	16	28.4	27.8	27.1	26.3	25.5	24.6	23.6	22.6	21.3	20.0	18.4	2.85	3.33
	18	27.7	27.0	26.3	25.5	24.7	23.8	22.9	21.8	20.6	19.2	17.6	2.36	2.83
24.71	12	31.2	30.5	29.7	28.9	28.1	27.2	26.1	25.0	23.7	22.3	20.7	3.97	4.47
	14	30.4	29.8	29.0	28.2	27.4	26.4	25.4	24.3	23.0	21.6	19.9	3.41	3.90
	16	29.7	29.0	28.2	27.4	26.6	25.6	24.6	23.5	22.2	20.8	19.1	2.86	3.34
	18	28.9	28.2	27.4	26.6	25.8	24.8	23.8	22.7	21.4	20.0	18.3	2.36	2.83

TABLE 21

Process Times (B) at Retort Temperature of 230°F for Conduction-Heating Foods in 211 x 210 Can

f_h	z	INITIAL FOOD TEMPERATURE (T_{ih})											Equivalent	
		100	110	120	130	140	150	160	170	180	190	200	F_c^{18}	F_s^{18}
	12	172.8	171.9	170.9	169.8	168.6	167.2	165.7	163.9	161.8	159.2	155.9	10.09	10.38
26.54	14	117.2	116.2	115.2	114.1	112.9	111.6	110.0	108.2	106.1	103.6	110.3	5.73	6.01
	16	90.2	89.3	88.3	87.2	86.0	84.6	83.1	81.3	79.2	76.6	73.3	3.71	3.98
	18	75.3	74.4	73.4	72.3	71.1	69.7	68.2	66.4	64.3	61.7	58.4	2.59	2.86
	12	176.5	175.5	174.4	173.3	172.0	170.6	168.9	167.0	164.8	162.1	158.6	10.10	10.39
28.10	14	119.2	118.2	117.1	116.0	114.7	113.3	111.6	109.8	107.5	104.8	101.3	5.72	6.00
	16	92.6	91.6	90.5	89.4	88.1	86.6	85.0	83.1	80.9	78.2	74.7	3.71	3.98
	18	77.6	76.7	75.6	74.4	73.2	71.7	70.1	68.2	66.0	63.3	59.8	2.59	2.86
	12	179.8	178.8	177.7	176.4	175.1	173.6	171.8	169.9	167.5	164.6	160.9	10.10	10.39
29.66	14	121.9	120.9	119.8	118.5	117.2	115.7	113.9	112.0	109.6	106.7	103.0	5.77	6.05
	16	95.1	94.1	93.0	91.7	90.4	88.9	87.1	85.2	82.8	79.9	76.2	3.72	3.99
	18	79.9	78.9	77.8	76.5	75.2	73.7	72.0	70.0	67.6	64.7	61.0	2.59	2.86
	12	182.8	181.7	180.5	179.2	177.8	176.2	174.4	172.3	169.9	166.8	162.9	10.11	10.40
31.22	14	124.5	123.4	122.2	120.9	119.5	117.9	116.1	114.0	111.5	108.5	104.6	5.76	6.05
	16	97.5	96.4	95.3	94.0	92.5	91.0	89.1	87.1	84.6	81.6	77.7	3.71	3.99
	18	82.3	81.2	80.0	78.7	77.3	75.7	73.9	71.8	69.3	66.3	62.4	2.58	2.86
	12	185.5	184.3	183.1	181.8	180.3	178.6	176.7	174.5	171.9	168.7	164.6	10.11	10.41
32.78	14	127.0	125.8	124.6	123.2	121.7	120.0	118.1	115.9	113.4	110.2	106.1	5.75	6.05
	16	99.9	98.8	97.5	96.2	94.7	93.0	91.1	88.9	86.3	83.1	79.0	3.72	4.00
	18	84.5	83.4	82.1	80.8	79.3	77.6	75.7	73.5	70.9	67.7	63.6	2.58	2.85

TABLE 22

Process Times (B) at Retort Temperature of 240°F for Conduction-Heating Foods in 211 x 210 Can

f_h	z	INITIAL FOOD TEMPERATURE (T_{ih})											Equivalent	
		100	110	120	130	140	150	160	170	180	190	200	F_c^{18}	F_s^{18}
26.54	12	64.5	63.6	62.7	61.7	60.6	59.4	58.0	56.5	54.7	52.6	50.0	6.03	6.42
	14	57.1	56.3	55.4	54.4	53.3	52.0	50.7	49.1	47.4	45.3	42.7	4.29	4.65
	16	52.3	51.4	50.5	49.5	48.4	47.2	45.8	44.3	42.5	40.4	37.9	3.30	3.65
	18	48.3	47.5	46.6	45.6	44.5	43.3	41.9	40.4	38.6	36.5	33.9	2.50	2.86
28.10	12	67.0	66.1	65.1	64.0	62.9	61.6	60.1	58.5	56.6	54.4	51.7	6.04	6.42
	14	59.6	58.7	57.7	56.6	55.5	54.2	52.7	51.1	49.2	47.0	44.3	4.37	4.72
	16	54.4	53.5	52.6	51.5	50.3	49.1	47.6	46.0	44.1	41.9	39.2	3.29	3.65
	18	50.4	49.5	48.5	47.5	46.3	45.0	43.6	42.0	40.1	37.9	35.1	2.50	2.86
29.66	12	69.4	68.5	67.4	66.3	65.1	63.7	62.2	60.5	58.5	56.2	53.3	6.05	6.43
	14	62.0	61.0	60.0	58.9	57.6	56.3	54.8	53.0	51.0	48.7	45.8	4.44	4.80
	16	56.5	55.6	54.6	53.4	52.2	50.9	49.3	47.6	45.6	43.3	40.4	3.28	3.64
	18	52.5	51.6	50.5	49.4	48.2	46.8	45.3	43.6	41.6	39.3	36.4	2.50	2.86
31.22	12	71.8	70.8	69.7	68.5	67.2	65.8	64.2	62.4	60.3	57.8	54.8	6.06	6.44
	14	64.3	63.3	62.2	61.0	59.7	58.3	56.7	54.9	52.8	50.3	47.3	4.50	4.86
	16	58.6	57.6	56.5	55.4	54.1	52.6	51.0	49.2	47.1	44.7	41.6	3.27	3.64
	18	54.6	53.6	52.5	51.3	50.0	48.6	47.0	45.2	43.1	40.6	37.6	2.49	2.86
32.78	12	74.1	73.1	71.9	70.7	69.3	67.8	66.2	64.3	62.1	59.5	56.3	6.06	6.45
	14	66.6	65.5	64.4	63.2	61.8	60.3	58.6	56.7	54.5	51.9	48.8	4.57	4.93
	16	60.8	59.7	58.6	57.4	56.0	54.5	52.8	50.9	48.7	46.1	43.0	3.29	3.66
	18	56.6	55.5	54.4	53.1	51.8	50.3	48.6	46.7	44.5	41.9	38.7	2.49	2.86

TABLE 23

Process Times (B) at Retort Temperature of 250°F for Conduction-Heating Foods in 211 x 210 Can

f_h	z	INITIAL FOOD TEMPERATURE (T_{ih})											Equivalent	
		100	110	120	130	140	150	160	170	180	190	200	F_c^{18}	F_s^{18}
26.54	12	42.3	41.5	40.7	39.7	38.7	37.6	36.4	35.1	33.5	31.8	29.7	4.75	5.19
	14	40.2	39.4	38.6	37.6	36.6	35.5	34.3	33.0	31.4	29.6	27.5	3.72	4.16
	16	38.5	37.7	36.9	35.9	34.9	33.8	32.6	31.3	29.7	28.0	25.9	3.00	3.43
	18	37.1	36.3	35.4	34.5	33.5	32.4	31.2	29.8	28.3	26.5	24.4	2.43	2.86
28.10	12	44.4	43.6	42.6	41.7	40.6	39.4	38.2	36.7	35.1	33.2	31.0	4.82	5.27
	14	42.2	41.4	40.4	39.5	38.4	37.2	36.0	34.5	32.9	31.0	28.8	3.77	4.21
	16	40.4	39.6	38.7	37.7	36.6	35.5	34.2	32.7	31.1	29.2	27.0	3.02	3.46
	18	38.9	38.0	37.1	36.1	35.1	33.9	32.6	31.2	29.6	27.7	25.5	2.43	2.86
29.66	12	46.4	45.6	44.6	43.6	42.4	41.2	39.9	38.3	36.6	34.6	32.3	4.88	5.33
	14	44.2	43.3	42.3	41.3	40.2	38.9	37.6	36.1	34.3	32.4	30.0	3.81	4.26
	16	42.3	41.4	40.4	39.4	38.3	37.0	35.7	34.2	32.4	30.5	28.1	3.04	3.48
	18	40.6	39.7	38.8	37.8	36.6	35.4	34.0	32.5	30.8	28.8	26.5	2.42	2.86
31.22	12	48.5	47.5	46.5	45.4	44.3	43.0	41.5	39.9	38.1	36.0	33.6	4.92	5.38
	14	46.1	45.1	44.1	43.1	41.9	40.6	39.2	37.6	35.8	33.7	31.2	3.85	4.30
	16	44.1	43.2	42.1	41.1	39.9	38.6	37.2	35.6	33.8	31.7	29.2	3.05	3.49
	18	42.4	41.4	40.4	39.3	38.2	36.9	35.4	33.8	32.0	29.9	27.5	2.42	2.86
32.78	12	50.4	49.5	48.4	47.3	46.0	44.7	43.2	41.5	39.6	37.4	34.8	4.96	5.42
	14	48.0	47.0	46.0	44.8	43.6	42.2	40.7	39.0	37.1	34.9	32.3	3.87	4.32
	16	45.9	44.9	43.9	42.7	41.5	40.1	38.6	36.9	35.0	32.8	30.2	3.03	3.48
	18	44.1	43.1	42.0	40.9	39.6	38.3	36.8	35.1	33.2	31.0	28.4	2.42	2.86

TABLE 24

Process Times (B) at Retort Temperature of 260°F for Conduction-Heating Foods in 211 x 210 Can

f_h	z	INITIAL FOOD TEMPERATURE (T_{ih})											Equivalent	
		100	110	120	130	140	150	160	170	180	190	200	F_c^{18}	F_s^{18}
	12	33.3	32.5	31.8	30.9	30.0	29.0	27.9	26.7	25.3	23.8	22.0	4.11	4.61
26.54	14	32.4	31.7	30.9	30.1	29.1	28.1	27.0	25.8	24.5	22.9	21.1	3.48	3.96
	16	31.6	30.9	30.1	29.2	28.3	27.3	26.2	25.0	23.6	22.1	20.3	2.91	3.39
	18	30.7	30.0	29.2	28.3	27.4	26.4	25.3	24.1	22.7	21.2	19.4	2.39	2.86
	12	35.1	34.3	33.4	32.5	31.5	30.5	29.3	28.0	26.6	25.0	23.1	4.20	4.71
28.10	14	34.1	33.3	32.5	31.6	30.6	29.5	28.4	27.1	25.7	24.0	22.1	3.51	4.00
	16	33.2	32.4	31.6	30.7	29.7	28.6	27.5	26.2	24.7	23.1	21.2	2.92	3.40
	18	32.3	31.5	30.6	29.7	28.8	27.7	26.5	25.3	23.8	22.2	20.3	2.39	2.86
	12	36.8	36.0	35.1	34.1	33.1	32.0	30.8	29.4	27.9	26.2	24.2	4.30	4.81
29.66	14	35.8	34.9	34.1	33.1	32.1	30.9	29.7	28.4	26.8	25.1	23.1	3.56	4.05
	16	34.8	34.0	33.1	32.1	31.1	30.0	28.8	27.4	25.9	24.2	22.2	2.94	3.42
	18	33.8	33.0	32.1	31.1	30.1	29.0	27.8	26.4	24.9	23.2	21.2	2.38	2.86
	12	38.6	37.7	36.7	35.7	34.7	33.5	32.2	30.7	29.2	27.3	25.3	4.38	4.88
31.22	14	37.4	36.5	35.6	34.6	33.5	32.3	31.0	29.6	28.0	26.2	24.1	3.57	4.07
	16	36.4	35.5	34.6	33.6	32.5	31.3	30.0	28.6	27.0	25.2	23.1	2.95	3.44
	18	35.3	34.5	33.5	32.5	31.4	30.3	29.0	27.5	25.9	24.1	22.0	2.38	2.86
	12	40.3	39.4	38.4	37.3	36.2	35.0	33.6	32.1	30.4	28.5	26.3	4.45	4.96
32.78	14	39.1	38.1	37.2	36.1	35.0	33.7	32.4	30.9	29.2	27.3	25.1	3.60	4.10
	16	38.0	37.1	36.1	35.0	33.9	32.6	31.3	29.8	28.1	26.2	24.0	2.96	3.45
	18	36.9	35.9	35.0	33.9	32.8	31.5	30.2	28.7	27.0	25.1	22.9	2.38	2.86

TABLE 25

Process Times (B) at Retort Temperature of 230°F for Conduction-Heating Foods in 211 x 212 Can

f_h	z	INITIAL FOOD TEMPERATURE (T_{ih}) 100	110	120	130	140	150	160	170	180	190	200	Equivalent F_c^{18}	F_s^{18}
	12	175.4	174.4	173.4	172.3	171.0	169.6	168.0	166.2	164.0	161.3	157.9	10.11	10.40
27.54	14	118.6	117.7	116.6	115.5	114.2	112.8	111.2	109.4	107.2	104.5	101.1	5.74	6.01
	16	91.8	90.8	89.8	88.6	87.4	86.0	84.4	82.5	80.3	77.7	74.2	3.71	3.98
	18	76.9	75.9	74.9	73.7	72.5	71.1	69.5	67.6	65.4	62.8	59.3	2.60	2.86
	12	179.0	178.0	176.9	175.7	174.3	172.8	171.2	169.2	166.9	164.1	160.4	10.12	10.41
29.16	14	121.1	120.1	119.0	117.8	116.5	115.0	113.3	111.3	109.0	106.2	102.5	5.76	6.03
	16	94.4	93.4	92.3	91.1	89.7	88.3	86.6	84.6	82.3	79.5	75.8	3.73	4.00
	18	79.3	78.3	77.2	76.0	74.6	73.1	71.4	69.5	67.2	64.4	60.7	2.59	2.86
	12	182.2	181.1	180.0	178.7	177.3	175.7	173.9	171.9	169.4	166.5	162.6	10.13	10.41
30.78	14	123.9	122.8	121.7	120.4	119.0	117.4	115.6	113.6	111.1	108.1	104.3	5.77	6.06
	16	97.0	95.9	94.7	93.5	92.0	90.5	88.7	86.6	84.2	81.2	77.4	3.72	4.00
	18	81.7	80.6	79.4	78.2	76.7	75.2	73.4	71.3	68.9	65.9	62.1	2.59	2.86
	12	185.1	184.0	182.7	181.4	179.9	178.3	176.4	174.2	171.6	168.5	164.5	10.13	10.42
32.40	14	126.5	125.3	124.1	122.8	121.3	119.6	117.8	115.6	113.0	109.9	105.8	5.76	6.06
	16	99.4	98.3	97.0	95.7	94.2	92.5	90.7	88.5	85.9	82.8	78.7	3.72	4.00
	18	84.0	82.9	81.7	80.3	78.9	77.2	75.3	73.2	70.6	67.4	63.4	2.58	2.86
	12	187.6	186.5	185.2	183.8	182.2	180.5	178.5	176.2	173.5	170.2	166.0	10.14	10.43
34.02	14	129.0	127.8	126.5	125.1	123.5	121.8	119.8	117.5	114.8	111.5	107.3	5.75	6.05
	16	102.0	100.8	99.5	98.1	96.6	94.8	92.9	90.6	87.9	84.6	80.3	3.73	4.02
	18	86.5	85.3	84.0	82.6	81.1	79.3	77.4	75.1	72.4	69.1	64.8	2.58	2.86

TABLE 26

Process Times (B) at Retort Temperature of 240°F for Conduction-Heating Foods in 211 x 212 Can

f_h	z	INITIAL FOOD TEMPERATURE (T_{ih})											Equivalent	
		100	110	120	130	140	150	160	170	180	190	200	F_c^{18}	F_s^{18}
	12	66.1	65.2	64.3	63.2	62.1	60.8	59.4	57.8	56.0	53.8	51.1	6.05	6.43
27.54	14	58.7	57.9	56.9	55.9	54.7	53.5	52.0	50.4	48.6	46.4	43.8	4.35	4.70
	16	53.7	52.8	51.9	50.8	49.7	48.4	47.0	45.4	43.6	41.4	38.7	3.30	3.66
	18	49.7	48.8	47.8	46.8	45.7	44.4	43.0	41.4	39.6	37.4	34.7	2.51	2.86
	12	68.7	67.8	66.7	65.6	64.4	63.1	61.6	59.9	58.0	55.7	52.8	6.06	6.44
29.16	14	61.2	60.3	59.3	58.2	57.0	55.6	54.2	52.5	50.5	48.2	45.4	4.42	4.78
	16	55.9	55.0	54.0	52.9	51.7	50.3	48.8	47.1	45.2	42.9	40.0	3.29	3.65
	18	51.9	50.9	49.9	48.8	47.6	46.3	44.8	43.1	41.1	38.8	36.0	2.50	2.86
	12	71.2	70.2	69.1	68.0	66.7	65.3	63.7	61.9	59.9	57.4	54.4	6.06	6.45
30.78	14	63.7	62.7	61.6	60.5	59.2	57.8	56.2	54.4	52.4	49.9	46.9	4.49	4.85
	16	58.1	57.1	56.0	54.9	53.6	52.2	50.6	48.8	46.8	44.3	41.3	3.28	3.65
	18	54.0	53.0	52.0	50.8	49.5	48.1	46.5	44.8	42.7	40.3	37.3	2.50	2.86
	12	73.6	72.6	71.5	70.2	68.9	67.4	65.7	63.9	61.7	59.1	56.0	6.07	6.46
32.40	14	66.1	65.0	63.9	62.7	61.3	59.9	58.2	56.3	54.2	51.6	48.4	4.56	4.92
	16	60.3	59.2	58.1	56.9	55.6	54.1	52.4	50.5	48.4	45.8	42.7	3.39	3.66
	18	56.1	55.1	54.0	52.7	51.4	49.9	48.2	46.4	44.2	41.6	38.5	2.50	2.86
	12	76.0	74.9	73.7	72.4	71.0	69.4	67.7	65.7	63.5	60.8	57.5	6.08	6.46
34.02	14	68.4	67.3	66.2	64.9	63.5	61.9	60.2	58.2	55.9	53.2	49.9	4.57	4.94
	16	62.5	61.4	60.3	59.0	57.6	56.0	54.3	52.3	50.0	47.3	44.0	3.31	3.69
	18	58.2	57.1	55.9	54.6	53.2	51.7	49.9	47.9	45.7	43.0	39.7	2.49	2.86

TABLE 27

Process Times (B) at Retort Temperature of 250°F for Conduction-Heating Foods in 211 x 212 Can

f_h	z	INITIAL FOOD TEMPERATURE (T_{ih})											Equivalent	
		100	110	120	130	140	150	160	170	180	190	200	F_c^{18}	F_s^{18}
	12	43.7	42.8	42.0	41.0	40.0	38.8	37.6	36.2	34.6	32.7	30.5	4.80	5.25
27.54	14	41.5	40.7	39.8	38.8	37.8	36.7	35.4	34.0	32.4	30.5	28.4	3.76	4.20
	16	39.7	38.9	38.0	37.1	36.0	34.9	33.6	32.2	30.6	28.8	26.6	3.02	3.46
	18	38.2	37.4	36.5	35.6	34.5	33.4	32.1	30.7	29.1	27.3	25.1	2.43	2.86
	12	45.8	44.9	44.0	43.0	41.9	40.7	39.3	37.8	36.2	34.2	31.9	4.87	5.33
29.16	14	43.5	42.7	41.7	40.7	39.6	38.4	37.1	35.6	33.9	31.9	29.6	3.80	4.25
	16	41.7	40.8	39.9	38.9	37.8	36.5	35.2	33.7	32.0	30.1	27.8	3.04	3.48
	18	40.1	39.2	38.3	37.3	36.2	35.0	33.6	32.1	30.4	28.5	26.2	2.43	2.86
	12	47.9	47.0	46.0	44.9	43.8	42.5	41.1	39.5	37.7	35.7	33.2	4.92	5.37
30.78	14	45.6	44.6	43.6	42.6	41.4	40.1	38.7	37.2	35.4	33.3	30.9	3.85	4.29
	16	43.6	42.7	41.7	40.6	39.4	38.2	36.8	35.2	33.4	31.3	28.9	3.06	3.50
	18	41.9	41.0	40.0	38.9	37.7	36.5	35.1	33.5	31.7	29.6	27.2	2.43	2.86
	12	50.0	49.0	48.0	46.8	45.6	44.3	42.8	41.1	39.3	37.1	34.5	4.95	5.42
32.40	14	47.5	46.6	45.5	44.4	43.2	41.8	40.4	38.7	36.8	34.7	32.1	3.87	4.32
	16	45.5	44.5	43.5	42.3	41.1	39.8	38.3	36.6	34.7	32.6	30.0	3.04	3.49
	18	43.7	42.7	41.7	40.5	39.3	38.0	36.5	34.8	32.9	30.8	28.2	2.43	2.86
	12	52.0	51.0	49.9	48.7	47.4	46.0	44.5	42.7	40.8	38.5	35.8	4.99	5.46
34.02	14	49.5	48.5	47.4	46.2	44.9	43.5	42.0	40.2	38.2	36.0	33.3	3.89	4.35
	16	47.3	46.3	45.2	44.0	42.7	41.3	39.8	38.0	36.1	33.8	31.1	3.03	3.48
	18	45.4	44.4	43.3	42.1	40.8	39.4	37.9	36.1	34.2	31.9	29.2	2.42	2.86

TABLE 28

Process Times (B) at Retort Temperature of 260°F for Conduction-Heating Foods in 211 x 212 Can

f_h	z	INITIAL FOOD TEMPERATURE (T_{ih})											Equivalent	
		100	110	120	130	140	150	160	170	180	190	200	F_c^{18}	F_s^{18}
	12	34.4	33.7	32.8	31.9	31.0	29.9	28.8	27.5	26.1	24.5	22.7	4.17	4.67
27.54	14	33.5	32.7	31.9	31.0	30.1	29.0	27.9	26.6	25.2	23.6	21.8	3.50	3.99
	16	32.6	31.9	31.0	30.2	29.2	28.2	27.0	25.8	24.4	22.8	20.9	2.92	3.40
	18	31.7	31.0	30.1	29.2	28.3	27.3	26.1	24.9	23.4	21.8	20.0	2.39	2.86
	12	36.3	35.4	34.6	33.6	32.6	31.5	30.3	29.0	27.5	25.8	23.8	4.28	4.78
29.16	14	35.3	34.4	33.6	32.6	31.6	30.5	29.3	28.0	26.5	24.8	22.8	3.55	4.04
	16	34.3	33.5	32.6	31.7	30.7	29.6	28.4	27.0	25.5	23.8	21.9	2.94	3.43
	18	33.3	32.5	31.6	30.7	29.7	28.6	27.4	26.0	24.6	22.9	20.9	2.39	2.86
	12	38.1	37.2	36.3	35.3	34.2	33.1	31.8	30.4	28.8	27.0	25.0	4.36	4.87
30.78	14	37.0	36.1	35.2	34.2	33.1	32.0	30.7	29.3	27.7	25.9	23.9	3.58	4.07
	16	36.0	35.1	34.2	33.2	32.1	31.0	29.7	28.3	26.7	24.9	22.9	2.95	3.44
	18	34.9	34.1	33.1	32.1	31.1	29.9	28.6	27.2	25.7	23.9	21.8	2.39	2.86
	12	39.9	39.0	38.0	37.0	35.8	34.6	33.3	31.8	30.1	28.3	26.1	4.44	4.95
32.40	14	38.7	37.8	36.8	35.7	34.6	33.4	32.0	30.6	28.9	27.0	24.9	3.60	4.10
	16	37.6	36.7	35.7	34.7	33.6	32.3	31.0	29.5	27.8	26.0	23.8	2.96	3.45
	18	36.5	35.6	34.6	33.6	32.4	31.2	29.9	28.4	26.7	24.9	22.7	2.39	2.86
	12	41.7	40.7	39.7	38.6	37.4	36.1	34.7	33.2	31.4	29.5	27.2	4.52	5.03
34.02	14	40.4	39.4	38.4	37.3	36.1	34.8	33.4	31.9	30.1	28.1	25.9	3.63	4.13
	16	39.2	38.3	37.3	36.2	35.0	33.7	32.3	30.7	29.0	27.0	24.7	2.97	3.45
	18	38.1	37.1	36.1	35.0	33.8	32.5	31.1	29.6	27.8	25.9	23.6	2.38	2.86

TABLE 29

Process Times (B) at Retort Temperature of 230°F for Conduction-Heating Foods in 211 x 214 Can

f_h	z	INITIAL FOOD TEMPERATURE (T_{ih}) 100	110	120	130	140	150	160	170	180	190	200	Equivalent F_c^{18}	F_s^{18}
28.46	12	117.7	176.7	175.6	174.4	173.1	171.7	170.0	168.1	165.9	163.1	159.5	10.13	10.42
	14	119.9	118.9	117.8	116.7	115.4	113.9	112.3	110.4	108.1	105.3	101.8	5.74	6.01
	16	93.3	92.3	91.3	90.1	88.8	87.3	85.7	83.8	81.5	78.8	75.2	3.72	4.00
	18	78.3	77.3	76.3	75.1	73.8	72.3	70.7	68.8	66.5	63.7	60.2	2.60	2.86
30.14	12	181.2	180.1	179.0	177.7	176.4	174.8	173.1	171.0	168.7	165.7	162.0	10.14	10.43
	14	123.0	121.9	120.8	119.5	118.1	116.6	114.9	112.8	110.5	107.5	103.8	5.79	6.07
	16	96.0	95.0	93.9	92.6	91.2	89.7	87.9	85.9	83.5	80.6	76.8	3.73	4.01
	18	80.7	79.7	78.6	77.3	75.9	74.4	72.6	70.6	68.2	65.3	61.5	2.59	2.86
31.81	12	184.3	183.2	182.0	180.7	179.2	177.6	175.7	173.6	171.1	168.0	164.0	10.14	10.44
	14	125.7	124.5	123.3	122.0	120.6	118.9	117.1	115.0	112.5	109.4	105.4	5.77	6.07
	16	98.6	97.5	96.3	95.0	93.5	91.9	90.0	87.9	85.4	82.3	78.3	3.72	4.01
	18	83.3	82.2	81.0	79.6	78.2	76.6	74.7	72.6	70.1	67.0	63.0	2.59	2.87
33.49	12	187.0	185.9	184.6	183.2	181.7	180.0	178.0	175.8	173.2	169.9	165.7	10.15	10.44
	14	128.3	127.1	125.9	124.5	123.0	121.2	119.3	117.1	114.4	111.2	107.0	5.77	6.06
	16	101.2	100.1	98.8	97.4	95.9	94.2	92.2	90.0	87.3	84.1	79.9	3.74	4.02
	18	85.6	84.5	83.2	81.8	80.3	78.6	76.6	74.4	71.8	68.5	64.3	2.58	2.86
35.16	12	189.3	188.1	186.7	185.3	183.7	181.9	179.8	177.5	174.7	171.3	166.9	10.14	10.44
	14	130.7	129.5	128.2	126.7	125.1	123.3	121.3	118.9	116.1	112.7	108.3	5.76	6.05
	16	103.9	102.6	101.3	99.9	98.3	96.5	94.4	92.1	89.3	85.9	81.5	3.74	4.03
	18	88.5	87.3	85.9	84.5	82.9	81.1	79.0	76.7	73.9	70.5	66.1	2.58	2.87

TABLE 30

Process Times (B) at Retort Temperature of 240°F for Conduction-Heating Foods in 211 x 214 Can

f_h	z	INITIAL FOOD TEMPERATURE (T_{ih}) 100	110	120	130	140	150	160	170	180	190	200	Equivalent F_c^{18}	F_s^{18}
	12	67.6	66.7	65.7	64.7	63.5	62.2	60.7	59.1	57.2	54.9	52.1	6.06	6.45
28.46	14	60.2	59.3	58.3	57.2	56.0	54.7	53.3	51.6	49.7	47.5	44.7	4.40	4.75
	16	55.0	54.1	53.1	52.0	50.8	49.5	48.1	46.4	44.5	42.3	39.5	3.30	3.66
	18	51.0	50.1	49.1	48.0	46.8	45.5	44.0	42.4	40.5	38.2	35.5	2.51	2.86
	12	70.2	69.3	68.2	67.1	65.8	64.5	62.9	61.2	59.2	56.8	53.9	6.07	6.46
30.14	14	62.7	61.8	60.7	59.6	58.3	57.0	55.4	53.7	51.7	49.3	46.3	4.47	4.83
	16	57.2	56.3	55.2	54.1	52.8	51.5	49.9	48.2	46.2	43.8	40.8	3.29	3.65
	18	53.2	52.2	51.2	50.0	48.8	47.4	45.9	44.1	42.1	39.7	36.8	2.51	2.87
	12	72.8	71.8	70.7	69.5	68.1	66.7	65.1	63.2	61.1	58.6	55.5	6.08	6.46
31.81	14	65.2	64.2	63.1	61.9	60.6	59.1	57.5	55.7	53.5	51.0	47.9	4.54	4.90
	16	59.5	58.5	57.4	56.2	54.8	53.4	51.8	49.9	47.8	45.3	42.2	3.28	3.66
	18	55.4	54.4	53.3	52.1	50.7	49.3	47.7	45.8	43.7	41.2	38.1	2.50	2.87
	12	75.3	74.2	73.0	71.8	70.4	68.8	67.1	65.2	62.9	60.3	57.0	6.09	6.47
33.49	14	67.7	66.6	65.4	64.2	62.8	61.3	59.6	57.6	55.4	52.7	49.5	4.58	4.95
	16	61.8	60.7	59.6	58.3	56.9	55.4	53.7	51.7	49.5	46.9	43.6	3.31	3.68
	18	57.5	56.5	55.3	54.0	52.6	51.1	49.4	47.5	45.2	42.6	39.3	2.50	2.87
	12	77.8	76.7	75.5	74.1	72.7	71.1	69.3	67.2	64.9	62.1	58.7	6.13	6.51
35.16	14	70.1	69.0	67.7	66.4	65.0	63.3	61.5	59.5	57.2	54.4	51.0	4.57	4.94
	16	64.1	63.0	61.8	60.5	59.0	57.4	55.6	53.6	51.2	48.4	45.0	3.33	3.71
	18	59.6	58.5	57.3	56.0	54.5	52.9	51.1	49.1	46.7	43.9	40.5	2.50	2.87

TABLE 31

Process Times (B) at Retort Temperature of 250°F for Conduction-Heating Foods in 211 x 214 Can

f_h	z	INITIAL FOOD TEMPERATURE (T_{ih})											Equivalent	
		100	110	120	130	140	150	160	170	180	190	200	F_c^{18}	F_s^{18}
	12	44.9	44.1	43.1	42.1	41.1	39.9	38.6	37.1	35.5	33.6	31.3	4.85	5.30
28.46	14	42.7	41.8	40.9	39.9	38.8	37.7	36.4	34.9	33.3	31.4	29.1	3.79	4.23
	16	40.9	40.0	39.1	38.1	37.0	35.8	34.5	33.1	31.4	29.5	27.3	3.04	3.47
	18	39.3	38.5	37.5	36.6	35.5	34.3	33.0	31.5	29.9	28.0	25.7	2.44	2.86
	12	47.1	46.2	45.2	44.2	43.0	41.8	40.4	38.9	37.1	35.1	32.7	4.91	5.36
30.14	14	44.8	43.9	42.9	41.9	40.7	39.5	38.1	36.5	34.8	32.8	30.4	3.83	4.28
	16	42.8	41.9	41.0	39.9	38.8	37.5	36.2	34.6	32.9	30.9	28.5	3.06	3.50
	18	41.2	40.3	39.3	38.3	37.1	35.9	34.5	33.0	31.2	29.2	26.8	2.43	2.86
	12	49.2	48.3	47.3	46.2	45.0	43.6	42.2	40.6	38.7	36.6	34.1	4.95	5.41
31.81	14	46.8	45.9	44.9	43.8	42.6	41.2	39.8	38.2	36.3	34.2	31.7	3.87	4.32
	16	44.8	43.9	42.8	41.7	40.5	39.2	37.7	36.1	34.3	32.1	29.6	3.05	3.50
	18	43.0	42.1	41.1	40.0	38.8	37.4	36.0	34.4	32.5	30.4	27.9	2.43	2.86
	12	51.4	50.4	49.3	48.1	46.9	45.5	43.9	42.2	40.3	38.0	35.4	4.99	5.45
33.49	14	48.9	47.9	46.8	45.6	44.4	43.0	41.4	39.7	37.8	35.5	32.9	3.89	4.34
	16	46.7	45.7	44.6	43.5	42.2	40.8	39.3	37.6	35.6	33.4	30.7	3.04	3.49
	18	44.9	43.9	42.8	41.6	40.3	39.0	37.4	35.7	33.8	31.5	28.9	2.43	2.86
	12	53.5	52.4	51.3	50.1	48.7	47.3	45.7	43.9	41.8	39.5	36.7	5.02	5.49
35.16	14	50.9	49.8	48.7	47.5	46.1	44.7	43.1	41.3	39.2	36.9	34.1	3.91	4.37
	16	48.6	47.6	46.4	45.2	43.9	42.4	40.8	39.0	37.0	34.6	31.8	3.03	3.48
	18	46.6	45.6	44.5	43.2	41.9	40.5	38.8	37.0	35.0	32.7	29.9	2.43	2.86

TABLE 32

Process Times (B) at Retort Temperature of 260°F for Conduction-Heating Foods in 211 x 214 Can

f_h	z	INITIAL FOOD TEMPERATURE (T_{ih})											Equivalent	
		100	110	120	130	140	150	160	170	180	190	200	F_c^{18}	F_s^{18}
	12	35.5	34.7	33.8	32.9	31.9	30.8	29.7	28.4	26.9	25.3	23.4	4.24	4.74
28.46	14	34.5	33.7	32.9	31.9	31.0	29.9	28.7	27.4	25.9	24.3	22.4	3.53	4.02
	16	33.6	32.8	31.9	31.0	30.0	29.0	27.8	26.5	25.0	23.4	21.5	2.94	3.42
	18	32.7	31.9	31.0	30.1	29.1	28.0	26.8	25.5	24.1	22.4	20.5	2.39	2.86
	12	37.4	36.5	35.6	34.6	33.6	32.5	31.2	29.8	28.3	26.5	24.5	4.34	4.84
30.14	14	36.3	35.5	34.5	33.6	32.5	31.4	30.1	28.8	27.2	25.5	23.5	3.57	4.07
	16	35.3	34.5	33.6	32.6	31.6	30.4	29.2	27.8	26.2	24.5	22.5	2.95	3.44
	18	34.3	33.5	32.5	31.6	30.5	29.4	28.1	26.8	25.2	23.5	21.5	2.39	2.86
	12	39.2	38.3	37.4	36.4	35.3	34.1	32.7	31.3	29.7	27.8	25.7	4.42	4.92
31.81	14	38.1	37.2	36.2	35.2	34.1	32.9	31.6	30.1	28.5	26.6	24.5	3.59	4.09
	16	37.0	36.1	35.2	34.1	33.0	31.8	30.5	29.1	27.4	25.6	23.5	2.96	3.45
	18	35.9	35.0	34.1	33.1	32.0	30.8	29.4	28.0	26.4	24.5	22.4	2.39	2.87
	12	41.1	40.2	39.2	38.1	36.9	35.6	34.3	32.7	31.0	29.1	26.8	4.50	5.01
33.49	14	39.8	38.9	37.9	36.8	35.6	34.4	33.0	31.4	29.7	27.8	25.5	3.63	4.12
	16	38.7	37.8	36.8	35.7	34.5	33.2	31.9	30.3	28.6	26.7	24.4	2.97	3.46
	18	37.6	36.6	35.6	34.5	33.4	32.1	30.7	29.2	27.5	25.5	23.3	2.39	2.87
	12	43.0	42.0	40.9	39.8	38.6	37.2	35.8	34.2	32.4	30.3	28.0	4.58	5.10
35.16	14	41.6	40.6	39.5	38.4	37.2	35.8	34.4	32.8	31.0	28.9	26.6	3.66	4.16
	16	40.4	39.4	38.3	37.2	36.0	34.7	33.2	31.6	29.8	27.8	25.4	2.98	3.47
	18	39.2	38.2	37.1	36.0	34.8	33.5	32.0	30.4	28.6	26.6	24.2	2.39	2.87

TABLE 33

Process Times (B) at Retort Temperature of 230°F for Conduction-Heating Foods in 211 x 300 Can

f_h	z	INITIAL FOOD TEMPERATURE (T_{ih}) 100	110	120	130	140	150	160	170	180	190	200	Equivalent F_c^{18}	Equivalent F_s^{18}
	12	179.7	178.6	177.5	176.3	175.0	173.5	171.8	169.8	167.5	164.7	161.0	10.15	10.44
29.31	14	121.6	120.6	119.5	118.3	116.9	115.4	113.7	111.8	109.4	106.6	102.9	5.78	6.05
	16	94.8	93.8	92.7	91.5	90.1	88.6	86.9	85.0	82.6	79.8	76.1	3.74	4.01
	18	79.6	78.6	77.5	76.3	74.9	73.4	71.7	69.8	67.4	64.6	60.9	2.60	2.87
	12	183.1	182.0	180.8	179.5	178.1	176.5	174.7	172.6	170.2	167.2	163.3	10.16	10.45
31.03	14	124.5	123.5	122.3	121.0	119.6	118.0	116.2	114.1	111.7	108.6	104.8	5.79	6.08
	16	97.5	96.4	95.3	94.0	92.5	91.0	89.2	87.1	84.6	81.6	77.7	3.73	4.01
	18	82.2	81.1	79.9	78.6	77.2	75.6	73.8	71.7	69.3	66.3	62.4	2.60	2.87
	12	186.1	184.9	183.7	182.4	180.9	179.2	177.3	175.1	172.5	169.3	165.2	10.16	10.45
32.76	14	127.3	126.1	124.9	123.5	122.1	120.4	118.5	116.3	113.7	110.5	106.4	5.78	6.07
	16	100.1	99.0	97.7	96.4	94.9	93.2	91.3	89.1	86.5	83.3	79.3	3.73	4.02
	18	84.7	83.5	82.3	80.9	79,4	77.7	75.8	73.7	71.1	67.9	63.8	2.59	2.87
	12	188.7	187.5	186.2	184.8	183.2	181.4	179.4	177.1	174.4	171.1	166.8	10.17	10.46
34.48	14	129.9	128.7	127.4	126.0	124.4	122.6	120.6	118.3	115.6	112.2	107.9	5.77	6.07
	16	102.9	101.7	100.4	99.0	97.4	95.6	93.6	91.3	88.6	85.2	80.9	3.75	4.03
	18	87.4	86.2	84.9	83.4	81.9	80.1	78.1	75.8	73.1	69.7	65.4	2.58	2.87
	12	190.7	189.4	188.0	186.5	184.9	183.0	180.9	178.5	175.6	172.1	167.6	10.15	10.44
36.20	14	132.6	131.4	130.0	128.5	126.9	125.0	122.9	120.5	117.6	114.1	109.6	5.79	6.08
	16	105.5	104.3	102.9	101.4	99.7	97.9	95.8	93.4	90.5	87.0	82.5	3.74	4.03
	18	90.2	89.0	87.6	86.1	84.5	82.6	80.5	78.1	75.2	71.7	67.2	2.58	2.87

TABLE 34

Process Times (B) at Retort Temperature of 240°F for Conduction-Heating Foods in 211 x 300 Can

f_h	z	INITIAL FOOD TEMPERATURE (T_{ih})											Equivalent	
		100	110	120	130	140	150	160	170	180	190	200	F_c^{18}	F_s^{18}
	12	69.0	68.1	67.0	65.9	64.7	63.4	61.9	60.2	58.2	55.9	53.1	6.08	6.46
29.31	14	61.5	60.6	59.6	58.4	57.2	55.9	54.4	52.7	50.7	48.4	45.6	4.44	4.80
	16	56.2	55.2	54.2	53.1	51.9	50.5	49.0	47.3	45.4	43.1	40.2	3.30	3.66
	18	52.1	51.2	50.2	49.0	47.8	46.5	45.0	43.4	41.3	39.0	36.2	2.51	2.87
	12	71.7	70.7	69.6	68.4	67.1	65.7	64.1	62.3	60.2	57.8	54.8	6.09	6.47
31.03	14	64.1	63.1	62.0	60.9	59.6	58.2	56.6	54.8	52.7	50.2	47.2	4.51	4.87
	16	58.5	57.5	56.4	55.2	53.9	52.5	50.9	49.1	47.0	44.6	41.6	3.29	3.66
	18	54.4	53.4	52.3	51.1	49.9	48.4	46.8	45.0	43.0	40.5	37.5	2.51	2.87
	12	74.2	73.2	72.0	70.8	69.4	67.9	66.3	64.4	62.2	59.6	56.4	6.09	6.48
32.76	14	66.7	65.6	64.5	63.2	61.9	60.4	58.7	56.8	54.6	52.0	48.8	4.58	4.95
	16	60.8	59.8	58.6	57.4	56.0	54.5	52.9	51.0	48.8	46.2	43.0	3.30	3.68
	18	56.6	55.6	54.4	53.2	51.8	50.3	48.7	46.8	44.6	42.0	38.8	2.50	2.87
	12	76.7	75.6	74.4	73.1	71.7	70.1	68.3	66.3	64.0	61.3	58.0	6.10	6.48
34.48	14	69.2	68.0	66.8	65.5	64.1	62.5	60.8	58.8	56.5	53.7	50.4	4.58	4.95
	16	63.2	62.1	60.9	59.6	58.2	56.6	54.8	52.8	50.5	47.8	44.5	3.33	3.70
	18	58.8	57.7	56.5	55.2	53.8	52.2	50.4	48.4	46.1	43.4	40.1	2.50	2.87
	12	79.6	78.4	77.2	75.8	74.3	72.6	70.8	68.7	66.3	63.4	59.9	6.20	6.58
36.20	14	71.6	70.4	69.2	67.8	66.3	64.6	62.8	60.7	58.3	55.4	51.9	4.57	4.94
	16	65.6	64.4	63.2	61.8	60.3	58.6	56.8	54.7	52.3	49.4	45.9	3.35	3.73
	18	61.0	59.8	58.6	57.2	55.7	54.0	52.2	50.1	47.7	44.8	41.3	2.50	2.87

TABLE 35

Process Times (B) at Retort Temperature of 250°F for Conduction-Heating Foods in 211 x 300 Can

f_h	z	INITIAL FOOD TEMPERATURE (T_{ih}) 100	110	120	130	140	150	160	170	180	190	200	Equivalent F_c^{18}	F_s^{18}
29.31	12	46.0	45.1	44.2	43.2	42.1	40.9	39.5	38.0	36.3	34.4	32.0	4.89	5.34
	14	43.8	42.9	41.9	40.9	39.8	38.6	37.3	35.8	34.1	32.1	29.8	3.82	4.26
	16	41.9	41.0	40.1	39.0	37.9	36.7	35.4	33.9	32.2	30.2	27.9	3.05	3.49
	18	40.3	39.4	38.5	37.4	36.3	35.1	33.8	32.3	30.6	28.6	26.3	2.44	2.87
31.03	12	48.3	47.3	46.3	45.3	44.1	42.8	41.4	39.8	38.0	35.9	33.5	4.94	5.39
	14	45.9	45.0	44.0	42.9	41.7	40.4	39.0	37.4	35.6	33.5	31.1	3.86	4.31
	16	43.9	43.0	42.0	40.9	39.7	38.4	37.0	35.4	33.6	31.6	29.1	3.07	3.51
	18	42.2	41.3	40.3	39.2	38.0	36.7	35.3	33.7	31.9	29.8	27.4	2.44	2.87
32.76	12	50.5	49.5	48.4	47.3	46.1	44.7	43.2	41.5	39.6	37.4	34.8	4.98	5.44
	14	48.0	47.0	46.0	44.8	43.6	42.2	40.7	39.1	37.2	35.0	32.4	3.89	4.34
	16	45.9	44.9	43.9	42.7	41.5	40.1	38.6	37.0	35.1	32.9	30.3	3.05	3.50
	18	44.1	43.1	42.0	40.9	39.7	38.3	36.8	35.1	33.2	31.0	28.5	2.43	2.87
34.48	12	52.6	51.6	50.5	49.3	48.0	46.6	45.0	43.2	41.2	38.9	36.2	5.02	5.48
	14	50.1	49.0	47.9	46.7	45.4	44.0	42.4	40.7	38.7	36.4	33.6	3.91	4.36
	16	47.9	46.8	45.7	44.5	43.2	41.8	40.2	38.5	36.5	34.1	31.4	3.04	3.49
	18	45.9	44.9	43.8	42.6	41.3	39.9	38.3	36.5	34.5	32.2	29.5	2.43	2.87
36.20	12	54.8	53.7	52.5	51.3	49.9	48.4	46.7	44.9	42.8	40.4	37.5	5.04	5.51
	14	52.1	51.0	49.9	48.6	47.2	45.7	44.1	42.2	40.1	37.7	34.9	3.92	4.38
	16	49.8	48.7	47.6	46.3	44.9	43.4	41.8	39.9	37.8	35.4	32.5	3.03	3.48
	18	47.8	46.7	45.5	44.2	42.9	41.4	39.7	37.9	35.8	33.4	30.5	2.43	2.87

TABLE 36

Process Times (B) at Retort Temperature of 260°F for Conduction-Heating Foods in 211 x 300 Can

f_h	z	INITIAL FOOD TEMPERATURE (T_{ih})											Equivalent	
		100	110	120	130	140	150	160	170	180	190	200	F_c^{18}	F_s^{18}
	12	36.4	35.6	34.7	33.8	32.8	31.7	30.5	29.1	27.6	25.9	23.9	4.29	4.80
29.31	14	35.4	34.6	33.7	32.8	31.8	30.7	29.4	28.1	26.6	24.9	22.9	3.56	4.05
	16	34.5	33.7	32.8	31.8	30.8	29.7	28.5	27.2	25.7	24.0	22.0	2.95	3.44
	18	33.5	32.7	31.8	30.8	29.8	28.7	27.5	26.2	24.7	23.0	21.0	2.40	2.87
	12	38.4	37.5	36.6	35.6	34.5	33.3	32.0	30.6	29.0	27.2	25.1	4.38	4.89
31.03	14	37.2	36.4	35.4	34.4	33.4	32.2	30.9	29.5	27.9	26.1	24.0	3.59	4.09
	16	36.2	35.4	34.4	33.4	32.4	31.2	29.9	28.5	26.9	25.1	23.0	2.96	3.45
	18	35.2	34.3	33.4	32.4	31.3	30.1	28.8	27.4	25.8	24.0	22.0	2.40	2.87
	12	40.3	39.4	38.4	37.3	36.2	35.0	33.6	32.1	30.4	28.5	26.3	4.47	4.98
32.76	14	39.1	38.1	37.2	36.1	35.0	33.7	32.4	30.9	29.2	27.3	25.1	3.62	4.11
	16	38.0	37.1	36.1	35.0	33.9	32.6	31.3	29.8	28.1	26.2	24.0	2.97	3.46
	18	36.9	35.9	35.0	33.9	32.8	31.5	30.2	28.7	27.0	25.1	22.9	2.39	2.87
	12	42.2	41.2	40.2	39.1	37.9	36.6	35.2	33.6	31.8	29.8	27.5	4.55	5.06
34.48	14	40.9	39.9	38.9	37.7	36.5	35.2	33.8	32.2	30.5	28.5	26.2	3.65	4.15
	16	39.7	38.7	37.7	36.6	35.4	34.1	32.7	31.1	29.3	27.3	25.0	2.98	3.47
	18	38.5	37.6	36.5	35.4	34.2	32.9	31.5	29.9	28.2	26.2	23.8	2.39	2.87
	12	44.1	43.1	42.0	40.9	39.6	38.2	36.7	35.1	33.2	31.1	28.7	4.65	5.16
36.20	14	42.6	41.6	40.5	39.4	38.1	36.7	35.2	33.6	31.7	29.6	27.2	3.68	4.18
	16	41.4	40.4	39.3	38.2	36.9	35.5	34.0	32.4	30.5	28.4	26.0	3.00	3.49
	18	40.2	39.2	38.1	36.9	35.7	34.3	32.8	31.2	29.3	27.2	24.8	2.39	2.87

TABLE 37

Process Times (B) at Retort Temperature of 230°F for Conduction-Heating Foods in 211 x 304 Can

f_h	z	INITIAL FOOD TEMPERATURE (T_{ih}) 100	110	120	130	140	150	160	170	180	190	200	Equivalent F_c^{18}	F_s^{18}
30.79	12	183.0	181.9	180.7	179.5	178.0	176.5	174.7	172.6	170.2	167.2	163.4	10.19	10.48
	14	124.4	123.3	122.1	120.8	119.4	117.9	116.1	114.0	111.6	108.6	104.7	5.81	6.09
	16	97.3	96.2	95.0	93.8	92.4	90.8	89.0	86.9	84.5	81.5	77.7	3.74	4.02
	18	81.9	80.8	79.7	78.4	77.0	75.4	73.6	71.6	69.1	66.1	62.3	2.60	2.88
32.60	12	186.2	185.1	183.8	182.5	181.0	179.3	177.4	175.3	172.7	169.5	165.4	10.19	10.48
	14	127.2	126.1	124.9	123.5	122.0	120.4	118.5	116.3	113.7	110.6	106.5	5.79	6.09
	16	100.0	98.9	97.6	96.3	94.8	93.1	91.2	89.0	86.5	83.3	79.2	3.74	4.03
	18	84.5	83.4	82.2	80.8	79.3	77.7	75.8	73.6	71.0	67.9	63.8	2.60	2.88
34.41	12	189.0	187.8	186.5	185.1	183.5	181.8	179.8	177.5	174.8	171.4	167.1	10.20	10.49
	14	130.0	128.8	127.5	126.1	124.5	122.8	120.8	118.5	115.7	112.4	108.1	5.79	6.08
	16	102.9	101.7	100.4	99.0	97.4	95.7	93.7	91.4	88.6	85.3	81.0	3.76	4.04
	18	87.3	86.2	84.9	83.4	81.9	80.1	78.1	75.8	73.1	69.7	65.4	2.59	2.88
36.22	12	191.1	189.9	188.5	187.0	185.3	183.5	181.4	179.0	176.1	172.6	168.1	10.18	10.47
	14	132.9	131.6	130.2	128.7	127.1	125.2	123.1	120.7	117.8	114.3	109.8	5.80	6.10
	16	105.7	104.4	103.1	101.6	99.9	98.1	96.0	93.5	90.7	87.2	82.6	3.75	4.04
	18	90.4	89.1	87.7	86.2	84.6	82.7	80.6	78.2	75.3	71.8	67.3	2.58	2.88
38.03	12	193.7	192.4	190.9	189.3	187.6	185.7	183.5	180.9	177.9	174.2	169.5	10.22	10.51
	14	136.0	134.7	133.2	131.6	129.9	128.0	125.7	123.2	120.2	116.5	111.8	5.84	6.13
	16	108.5	107.2	105.8	104.2	102.5	100.5	98.3	95.8	92.8	89.1	84.3	3.76	4.06
	18	93.3	92.0	90.5	88.9	87.2	85.3	83.1	80.5	77.5	73.8	69.1	2.58	2.88

TABLE 38

Process Times (B) at Retort Temperature of 240°F for Conduction-Heating Foods in 211 x 304 Can

f_h	z	INITIAL FOOD TEMPERATURE (T_{ih})											Equivalent	
		100	110	120	130	140	150	160	170	180	190	200	F_c^{18}	F_s^{18}
30.79	12	71.4	70.4	69.3	68.1	66.9	65.4	63.9	62.1	60.0	57.6	54.6	6.10	6.49
	14	63.8	62.8	61.7	60.6	59.3	57.9	56.3	54.5	52.5	50.0	47.1	4.51	4.87
	16	58.2	57.2	56.1	55.0	53.7	52.3	50.7	48.9	46.9	44.4	41.4	3.30	3.67
	18	54.1	53.1	52.1	50.9	49.6	48.2	46.6	44.8	42.8	40.3	37.4	2.52	2.88
32.60	12	74.1	73.0	71.9	70.7	69.3	67.8	66.2	64.3	62.1	59.5	56.3	6.11	6.50
	14	66.5	65.4	64.3	63.1	61.7	60.2	58.6	56.7	54.5	51.9	48.8	4.59	4.95
	16	60.7	59.6	58.5	57.2	55.9	54.4	52.7	50.8	48.7	46.1	42.9	3.31	3.68
	18	56.5	55.4	54.3	53.1	51.7	50.2	48.5	46.7	44.5	41.9	38.7	2.51	2.88
34.41	12	76.7	75.6	74.4	73.1	71.7	70.1	68.3	66.3	64.0	61.3	58.0	6.11	6.50
	14	69.1	68.0	66.8	65.5	64.1	62.5	60.7	58.8	56.5	53.7	50.4	4.60	4.97
	16	63.2	62.1	60.9	59.6	58.2	56.6	54.8	52.8	50.5	47.8	44.5	3.33	3.71
	18	58.8	57.7	56.5	55.2	53.7	52.2	50.4	48.4	46.1	43.4	40.1	2.51	2.88
36.22	12	79.7	78.5	77.3	75.9	74.4	72.7	70.9	68.8	66.4	63.5	60.0	6.21	6.60
	14	71.7	70.5	69.3	67.9	66.4	64.7	62.9	60.8	58.4	55.5	52.0	4.58	4.96
	16	65.7	64.5	63.2	61.9	60.4	58.7	56.9	54.8	52.3	49.5	45.9	3.36	3.74
	18	61.1	59.9	58.6	57.3	55.8	54.1	52.3	50.2	47.7	44.9	41.3	2.51	2.88
38.03	12	82.7	81.4	80.1	78.7	77.1	75.4	73.4	71.2	68.7	65.7	62.0	6.31	6.70
	14	74.2	73.0	71.7	70.2	68.7	66.9	65.0	62.8	60.2	57.2	53.5	4.57	4.95
	16	68.1	66.9	65.6	64.1	62.5	60.8	58.8	56.6	54.1	51.1	47.4	3.35	3.73
	18	63.4	62.2	60.8	59.4	57.8	56.1	54.1	51.9	49.4	46.4	42.7	2.50	2.88

TABLE 39

Process Times (B) at Retort Temperature of 250°F for Conduction-Heating Foods in 211 x 304 Can

f_h	z	INITIAL FOOD TEMPERATURE (T_{ih})											Equivalent	
		100	110	120	130	140	150	160	170	180	190	200	F_c^{18}	F_s^{18}
	12	48.0	47.1	46.1	45.0	43.8	42.6	41.1	39.6	37.8	35.7	33.3	4.94	5.40
30.79	14	45.6	44.7	43.7	42.6	41.5	40.2	38.8	37.2	35.4	33.4	30.9	3.87	4.31
	16	43.6	42.7	41.7	40.7	39.5	38.2	36.8	35.2	33.5	31.4	29.0	3.08	3.52
	18	42.0	41.0	40.0	39.0	37.8	36.5	35.1	33.5	31.8	29.7	27.3	2.44	2.88
	12	50.3	49.3	48.3	47.1	45.9	44.6	43.1	41.4	39.5	37.3	34.7	4.99	5.45
32.60	14	47.8	46.9	45.8	44.7	43.4	42.1	40.6	38.9	37.0	34.9	32.3	3.89	4.35
	16	45.8	44.8	43.7	42.6	41.4	40.0	38.5	36.9	35.0	32.8	30.2	3.06	3.51
	18	43.9	43.0	41.9	40.8	39.5	38.2	36.7	35.0	33.1	31.0	28.4	2.44	2.88
	12	52.6	51.5	50.4	49.2	47.9	46.5	44.9	43.2	41.2	38.9	36.2	5.03	5.49
34.41	14	50.0	49.0	47.9	46.7	45.4	44.0	42.4	40.6	38.6	36.3	33.6	3.92	4.37
	16	47.8	46.8	45.7	44.5	43.2	41.8	40.2	38.4	36.4	34.1	31.4	3.05	3.50
	18	45.9	44.9	43.8	42.6	41.3	39.8	38.3	36.5	34.5	32.2	29.5	2.44	2.88
	12	54.8	53.7	52.6	51.3	49.9	48.4	46.8	44.9	42.8	40.4	37.5	5.05	5.52
36.22	14	52.2	51.5	49.9	48.7	47.3	45.8	44.1	42.3	40.2	37.8	34.9	3.93	4.39
	16	49.9	48.8	47.6	46.3	45.0	43.5	41.8	40.0	37.9	35.4	32.6	3.04	3.49
	18	47.8	46.7	45.6	44.3	42.9	41.4	39.8	37.9	35.8	33.4	30.5	2.44	2.88
	12	57.1	56.0	54.8	53.4	52.0	50.4	48.7	46.7	44.5	42.0	39.0	5.11	5.58
38.03	14	54.4	53.2	52.0	50.7	49.3	47.7	45.9	44.0	41.8	39.2	36.2	3.98	4.44
	16	51.9	50.8	49.6	48.3	46.8	45.2	43.5	41.6	39.4	36.8	33.8	3.06	3.51
	18	49.8	48.7	47.4	46.1	44.7	43.1	41.4	39.4	37.2	34.7	31.6	2.44	2.88

TABLE 40

Process Times (B) at Retort Temperature of 260°F for Conduction-Heating Foods in 211 x 304 Can

f_h	z	INITIAL FOOD TEMPERATURE (T_{ih}) 100	110	120	130	140	150	160	170	180	190	200	Equivalent F_c^{18}	F_s^{18}
	12	38.1	37.2	36.3	35.3	34.3	33.1	31.8	30.4	28.8	27.0	25.0	4.38	4.89
30.79	14	37.0	36.1	35.2	34.2	33.2	32.0	30.7	29.3	27.7	25.9	23.9	3.60	4.09
	16	36.0	35.1	34.2	33.2	32.2	31.0	29.7	28.3	26.7	25.0	22.9	2.97	3.46
	18	35.0	34.1	33.2	32.2	31.1	29.9	28.7	27.3	25.7	23.9	21.8	2.40	2.88
	12	40.1	39.2	38.2	37.2	36.1	34.8	33.5	32.0	30.3	28.4	26.2	4.47	4.98
32.60	14	38.9	38.0	37.0	36.0	34.8	33.6	32.2	30.8	29.1	27.2	25.0	3.62	4.12
	16	37.8	36.9	35.9	34.9	33.8	32.5	31.2	29.7	28.0	26.1	23.9	2.98	3.47
	18	36.7	35.8	34.8	33.8	32.7	31.4	30.1	28.6	26.9	25.0	22.8	2.40	2.88
	12	42.1	41.2	40.1	39.0	37.8	36.5	35.1	33.5	31.8	29.8	27.5	4.56	5.07
34.41	14	40.8	39.8	38.8	37.7	36.5	35.2	33.8	32.2	30.4	28.4	26.1	3.66	4.16
	16	39.6	38.7	37.7	36.5	35.3	34.0	32.6	31.0	29.3	27.3	25.0	2.99	3.48
	18	38.5	37.5	36.5	35.4	34.2	32.9	31.5	29.9	28.1	26.1	23.8	2.40	2.88
	12	44.2	43.2	42.1	40.9	39.6	38.3	36.8	35.1	33.3	31.2	28.7	4.66	5.17
36.22	14	42.7	41.7	40.6	39.4	38.1	36.8	35.3	33.6	31.8	29.7	27.2	3.69	4.19
	16	41.5	40.5	39.4	38.2	36.9	35.6	34.1	32.4	30.6	28.5	26.0	3.00	3.50
	18	40.2	39.2	38.1	37.0	35.7	34.3	32.8	31.2	29.3	27.2	24.8	2.40	2.88
	12	46.2	45.1	44.0	42.8	41.4	40.0	38.4	36.7	34.7	32.5	30.0	4.76	5.28
38.03	14	44.5	43.5	42.3	41.1	39.8	38.4	36.8	35.0	33.1	30.9	28.3	3.71	4.22
	16	43.3	42.2	41.1	39.8	38.5	37.1	35.5	33.8	31.8	29.6	27.1	3.02	3.51
	18	42.0	40.9	39.8	38.5	37.2	35.8	34.2	32.5	30.5	28.3	25.8	2.40	2.88

TABLE 41

Process Times (B) at Retort Temperature of 230°F for Conduction-Heating Foods in 211 x 306 Can

f_h	z	INITIAL FOOD TEMPERATURE (T_{ih})											Equivalent	
		100	100	120	130	140	150	160	170	180	190	200	F_c^{18}	F_s^{18}
	12	184.3	183.3	182.1	180.8	179.3	177.7	175.9	173.8	171.3	168.3	164.3	10.20	10.49
31.44	14	125.5	124.4	123.2	121.9	120.5	118.9	117.0	114.9	112.5	109.4	105.5	5.81	6.10
	16	98.3	97.2	96.1	94.8	93.3	91.7	89.9	87.8	85.3	82.2	78.3	3.75	4.03
	18	82.9	81.8	80.6	79.3	77.9	76.3	74.5	72.4	69.9	66.8	62.9	2.61	2.88
	12	187.5	186.3	185.1	183.7	182.2	180.5	178.6	176.3	173.7	170.5	166.3	10.21	10.50
33.29	14	128.5	127.3	126.0	124.7	123.1	121.4	119.5	117.3	114.6	111.4	107.3	5.80	6.10
	16	101.2	100.0	98.8	97.4	95.9	94.2	92.2	90.0	87.4	84.1	80.0	3.75	4.04
	18	85.6	84.4	83.1	81.8	80.2	78.5	76.6	74.4	71.8	68.5	64.4	2.60	2.88
	12	190.1	188.9	187.6	186.1	184.5	182.7	180.7	178.3	175.5	172.1	167.7	10.20	10.50
35.14	14	131.2	129.9	128.6	127.2	125.5	123.8	121.7	119.4	116.6	113.2	108.8	5.79	6.09
	16	104.1	102.9	101.6	100.1	98.5	96.7	94.7	92.3	89.5	86.1	81.8	3.76	4.05
	18	88.6	87.4	86.1	84.6	83.0	81.2	79.2	76.8	74.0	70.6	66.2	2.59	2.88
	12	192.2	190.9	189.5	187.9	186.2	184.4	182.2	179.7	176.8	173.2	168.6	10.19	10.48
36.99	14	134.3	133.0	131.6	130.1	128.4	126.5	124.4	121.9	118.9	115.4	110.7	5.83	6.12
	16	106.9	105.6	104.2	102.7	101.0	99.1	97.0	94.5	91.6	88.0	83.4	3.76	4.05
	18	91.6	90.4	89.0	87.4	85.7	83.8	81.7	79.2	76.3	72.7	68.1	2.59	2.88
	12	195.5	194.2	192.7	191.1	189.3	187.3	185.1	182.5	179.4	175.6	170.8	10.28	10.58
38.84	14	137.4	136.0	134.6	133.0	131.2	129.2	126.9	124.3	121.3	117.5	112.7	5.84	6.14
	16	109.9	108.5	107.1	105.5	103.7	101.7	99.4	96.8	93.8	90.0	85.2	3.77	4.07
	18	94.6	93.2	91.8	90.2	88.4	86.4	84.2	81.6	78.5	74.7	69.9	2.58	2.88

TABLE 42

Process Times (B) at Retort Temperature of 240°F for Conduction-Heating Foods in 211 x 306 Can

f_h	z	INITIAL FOOD TEMPERATURE (T_{ih})											Equivalent	
		100	110	120	130	140	150	160	170	180	190	200	F_c^{18}	F_s^{18}
	12	72.4	71.4	70.3	69.1	67.8	66.3	64.7	62.9	60.8	58.3	55.3	6.11	6.50
31.44	14	64.8	63.8	62.7	61.5	60.2	58.8	57.2	55.3	53.2	50.7	47.7	4.54	4.90
	16	59.1	58.1	57.0	55.8	54.5	53.1	51.4	49.6	47.5	45.0	42.0	3.30	3.67
	18	55.0	54.0	52.9	51.7	50.4	49.0	47.3	45.5	43.4	40.9	37.9	2.52	2.88
	12	75.1	74.1	72.9	71.6	70.3	68.7	67.0	65.1	62.9	60.2	57.0	6.12	6.51
33.29	14	67.5	66.4	65.3	64.0	62.7	61.1	59.4	57.5	55.3	52.6	49.4	4.62	4.98
	16	61.6	60.6	59.4	58.2	56.8	55.3	53.6	51.6	49.4	46.8	43.5	3.32	3.70
	18	57.4	56.3	55.1	53.9	52.5	51.0	49.3	47.4	45.1	42.5	39.3	2.51	2.88
	12	77.9	76.8	75.5	74.2	72.8	71.2	69.4	67.3	65.0	62.2	58.8	6.15	6.54
35.14	14	70.2	69.0	67.8	66.5	65.0	63.4	61.6	59.6	57.2	54.5	51.1	4.60	4.97
	16	64.2	63.1	61.8	60.5	59.1	57.5	55.7	53.6	51.3	48.5	45.1	3.35	3.73
	18	59.7	58.6	57.4	56.0	54.6	53.0	51.2	49.1	46.8	44.0	40.6	2.51	2.88
	12	81.0	79.8	78.5	77.1	75.6	73.9	72.0	69.8	67.4	64.4	60.9	6.26	6.65
36.99	14	72.8	71.6	70.3	68.9	67.4	65.7	63.8	61.7	59.2	56.2	52.7	4.58	4.96
	16	66.7	65.5	64.2	62.8	61.3	59.6	57.7	55.6	53.1	50.2	46.6	3.36	3.74
	18	62.1	60.9	59.6	58.2	56.7	55.0	53.1	50.9	48.5	45.5	41.9	2.51	2.88
	12	84.0	82.8	81.4	79.9	78.3	76.5	74.6	72.3	69.7	66.6	62.9	6.36	6.75
38.84	14	75.4	74.1	72.8	71.3	69.7	67.9	65.9	63.7	61.1	58.0	54.2	4.57	4.96
	16	69.2	67.9	66.6	65.1	64.5	61.7	59.7	57.5	54.9	51.8	48.1	3.35	3.74
	18	64.4	63.2	61.8	60.4	58.7	57.0	55.0	52.7	50.1	47.1	43.3	2.50	2.88

TABLE 43

Process Times (B) at Retort Temperature of 250°F for Conduction-Heating Foods in 211 x 306 Can

f_h	z	INITIAL FOOD TEMPERATURE ($_{ih}$)											Equivalent	
		100	110	120	130	140	150	160	170	180	190	200	F_c^{18}	F_s^{18}
	12	48.8	47.9	46.9	45.8	44.6	43.3	41.8	40.2	38.4	36.3	33.8	4.97	5.42
31.44	14	46.4	45.5	44.5	43.4	42.2	40.9	39.5	37.8	36.0	33.9	31.4	3.88	4.33
	16	44.4	43.5	42.5	41.4	40.2	38.9	37.4	35.8	34.0	31.9	29.4	3.08	3.52
	18	42.7	41.7	40.7	39.6	38.4	37.1	35.7	34.1	32.3	30.2	27.7	2.45	2.88
	12	51.2	50.2	49.1	48.0	46.7	45.3	43.8	42.1	40.2	37.9	35.3	5.01	5.47
33.29	14	48.7	47.7	46.6	45.5	44.2	42.8	41.3	39.6	37.7	35.4	32.8	3.91	4.36
	16	46.6	45.6	44.5	43.3	42.1	40.7	39.2	37.5	35.5	33.3	30.7	3.06	3.51
	18	44.7	43.7	42.6	41.5	40.2	38.8	37.3	35.6	33.7	31.5	28.8	2.45	2.88
	12	53.5	52.4	51.3	50.1	48.8	47.3	45.7	43.9	41.9	39.5	36.7	5.05	5.52
35.14	14	50.9	49.9	48.7	47.5	46.2	44.7	43.1	41.3	39.3	36.9	34.1	3.93	4.39
	16	48.7	47.6	46.5	45.2	43.9	42.5	40.9	39.1	37.0	34.7	31.9	3.05	3.50
	18	46.7	45.6	44.5	43.3	41.9	40.5	38.9	37.1	35.0	32.7	29.9	2.44	2.88
	12	55.8	54.7	53.5	52.2	50.8	49.3	47.6	45.7	43.6	41.1	38.2	5.08	5.54
36.99	14	53.1	52.0	50.8	49.5	48.1	46.6	44.9	43.0	40.9	38.4	35.5	3.95	4.41
	16	50.7	49.6	48.4	47.1	45.8	44.2	42.5	40.6	38.5	36.0	33.1	3.05	3.50
	18	48.6	47.5	46.3	45.1	43.7	42.1	40.4	38.5	36.4	33.9	31.0	2.44	2.88
	12	58.2	57.0	55.8	54.4	52.9	51.3	49.6	47.6	45.3	42.7	39.6	5.14	5.61
38.84	14	55.4	54.2	53.0	51.6	50.1	48.5	46.8	44.8	42.5	39.9	36.8	4.00	4.46
	16	52.9	51.7	50.5	49.1	47.7	46.0	44.3	42.3	40.0	37.4	34.4	3.07	3.53
	18	50.7	49.5	48.3	46.9	45.5	43.8	42.1	40.1	37.8	35.2	32.2	2.44	2.88

TABLE 44

Process Times (B) at Retort Temperature of 260°F for Conduction-Heating Foods in 211 x 306 Can

f_h	z	INITIAL FOOD TEMPERATURE (T_{ih})											Equivalent	
		100	110	120	130	140	150	160	170	180	190	200	F_c^{18}	F_s^{18}
31.44	12	38.8	38.0	37.0	36.0	34.9	33.7	32.4	31.0	29.4	27.5	25.4	4.42	4.92
	14	37.7	36.8	35.9	34.9	33.8	32.6	31.3	29.8	28.2	26.4	24.3	3.61	4.11
	16	36.7	35.8	34.8	33.8	32.7	31.6	30.3	28.8	27.2	25.4	23.3	2.98	3.47
	18	35.6	34.7	33.8	32.8	31.7	30.5	29.2	27.7	26.1	24.3	22.2	2.41	2.88
33.29	12	40.9	40.0	39.0	37.9	36.7	35.5	34.1	32.6	30.9	29.0	26.7	4.51	5.02
	14	39.6	38.7	37.7	36.6	35.5	34.2	32.8	31.3	29.6	27.7	25.5	3.64	4.14
	16	38.5	37.6	36.6	35.5	34.4	33.1	31.7	30.2	28.5	26.6	24.4	2.99	3.48
	18	37.4	36.5	35.5	34.4	33.2	32.0	30.6	29.1	27.4	25.4	23.2	2.40	2.88
35.14	12	43.0	42.0	40.9	39.8	38.6	37.2	35.8	34.2	32.4	30.3	28.0	4.60	5.11
	14	41.6	40.6	39.5	38.4	37.2	35.8	34.4	32.8	31.0	28.9	26.6	3.68	4.18
	16	40.4	39.4	38.4	37.2	36.0	34.7	33.2	31.6	29.8	27.8	25.4	3.00	3.49
	18	39.2	38.2	37.2	36.0	34.8	33.5	32.0	30.4	28.6	26.6	24.2	2.40	2.88
36.99	12	45.0	44.0	42.9	41.7	40.4	39.0	37.5	35.8	33.9	31.7	29.3	4.71	5.22
	14	43.5	42.4	41.3	40.1	38.8	37.5	35.9	34.2	32.3	30.2	27.7	3.70	4.20
	16	42.2	41.2	40.1	38.9	37.6	36.2	34.7	33.0	31.1	29.0	26.5	3.02	3.51
	18	41.0	39.9	38.8	37.6	36.4	35.0	33.4	31.7	29.8	27.7	25.2	2.40	2.88
38.84	12	47.1	46.0	44.8	43.6	42.2	40.8	39.2	37.4	35.4	33.1	30.5	4.81	5.33
	14	45.4	44.3	43.1	41.9	40.5	39.1	37.5	35.7	33.7	31.4	28.8	3.73	4.24
	16	44.1	43.0	41.8	40.6	39.2	37.8	36.1	34.4	32.4	30.1	27.5	3.02	3.52
	18	42.7	41.7	40.5	39.2	37.9	36.4	34.8	33.0	31.0	28.8	26.2	2.40	2.88

TABLE 45

Process Times (B) at Retort Temperature of 230°F for Conduction-Heating Foods in 211 x 400 Can

f_h	z	INITIAL FOOD TEMPERATURE (T_{ih})											Equivalent	
		100	110	120	130	140	150	160	170	180	190	200	F_c^{18}	F_s^{18}
	12	189.4	188.2	186.9	185.5	184.0	182.2	180.2	178.0	175.3	172.0	167.7	10.27	10.56
33.98	14	130.0	128.8	127.5	126.1	124.5	122.8	120.8	118.6	115.9	112.6	108.3	5.83	6.13
	16	102.6	101.4	100.1	98.7	97.2	95.4	93.5	91.2	88.5	85.2	80.9	3.78	4.07
	18	86.8	85.7	84.4	83.0	81.4	79.7	77.7	75.4	72.7	69.4	65.2	2.61	2.89
	12	192.0	190.7	189.4	187.9	186.2	184.4	182.3	179.9	177.0	173.6	169.1	10.26	10.55
35.98	14	132.9	131.7	130.3	128.8	127.2	125.4	123.3	120.9	118.0	114.5	110.0	5.83	6.13
	16	105.7	104.5	103.1	101.6	100.0	98.1	96.0	93.6	90.8	87.3	82.8	3.78	4.07
	18	90.2	88.9	87.6	86.1	84.5	82.6	80.5	78.1	75.3	71.8	67.3	2.61	2.90
	12	194.4	193.0	191.6	190.0	188.3	186.3	184.1	181.6	178.6	174.9	170.2	10.26	10.56
37.98	14	136.4	135.1	133.7	132.1	130.4	128.4	126.2	123.7	120.7	117.0	112.2	5.88	6.18
	16	108.8	107.5	106.1	104.5	102.7	100.8	98.6	96.1	93.1	89.4	84.6	3.79	4.08
	18	93.4	92.1	90.7	89.1	87.4	85.4	83.2	80.7	77.7	74.0	69.3	2.60	2.90
	12	198.2	196.8	195.3	193.6	191.8	189.8	187.4	184.8	181.6	177.7	172.7	10.39	10.69
39.98	14	139.7	138.3	136.8	135.1	133.3	131.2	128.9	126.2	123.1	119.2	114.2	5.87	6.18
	16	112.0	110.6	109.1	107.4	105.6	103.5	101.2	98.5	95.4	91.5	86.5	3.80	4.09
	18	96.6	95.2	93.7	92.1	90.2	88.2	85.9	83.2	80.0	76.1	71.2	2.59	2.90
	12	201.6	200.2	198.6	196.8	194.9	192.8	190.3	187.5	184.2	180.1	174.9	10.37	10.69
41.98	14	142.7	141.2	139.6	137.9	136.0	133.8	131.4	128.6	125.3	121.2	116.0	5.86	6.17
	16	115.0	113.5	112.0	110.2	108.3	106.1	103.7	100.9	97.6	93.5	88.3	3.79	4.09
	18	99.8	98.3	96.7	95.0	93.0	90.9	88.5	85.7	82.3	78.3	73.0	2.59	2.90

TABLE 46

Process Times (B) at Retort Temperature of 240°F for Conduction-Heating Foods in 211 x 400 Can

f_h	z	INITIAL FOOD TEMPERATURE (T_{ih})											Equivalent	
		100	110	120	130	140	150	160	170	180	190	200	F_c^{18}	F_s^{18}
33.98	12	76.3	75.2	74.0	72.7	71.3	69.8	68.0	66.1	63.8	61.1	57.8	6.16	6.55
	14	68.6	67.6	66.4	65.1	63.7	62.1	60.4	58.4	56.1	53.5	50.2	4.64	5.01
	16	62.7	61.6	60.4	59.1	57.7	56.2	54.4	52.5	50.2	47.5	44.2	3.35	3.73
	18	58.4	57.3	56.1	54.8	53.4	51.8	50.1	48.1	45.8	43.2	39.9	2.53	2.90
35.98	12	79.4	78.3	77.0	75.7	74.2	72.5	70.7	68.6	66.2	63.3	59.9	6.23	6.61
	14	71.5	70.3	69.1	67.7	66.2	64.6	62.8	60.7	58.3	55.4	51.9	4.62	5.00
	16	65.5	64.3	63.0	61.7	60.2	58.6	56.7	54.6	52.2	49.4	45.9	3.38	3.76
	18	60.9	59.7	58.5	57.1	55.6	54.0	52.1	50.0	47.6	44.8	41.3	2.53	2.90
37.98	12	82.7	81.5	80.2	78.8	77.2	75.4	73.5	71.3	68.8	65.8	62.1	6.34	6.73
	14	74.3	73.1	71.8	70.3	68.8	67.0	65.1	62.9	60.3	57.3	53.6	4.61	4.99
	16	68.2	66.9	65.6	64.2	62.6	60.9	58.9	56.7	54.2	51.2	47.5	3.38	3.76
	18	63.4	62.2	60.9	59.4	57.9	56.1	54.2	52.0	49.5	46.4	42.8	2.52	2.90
39.98	12	86.0	84.7	83.3	81.8	80.1	78.3	76.3	73.9	71.3	68.1	64.2	6.45	6.84
	14	77.1	75.9	74.5	73.0	71.3	69.5	67.4	65.1	62.4	59.3	55.4	4.61	5.00
	16	70.8	69.5	68.1	66.6	65.0	63.1	61.1	58.8	56.1	52.9	49.1	3.37	3.75
	18	66.0	64.7	63.3	61.8	60.1	58.3	56.2	53.9	51.2	48.1	44.2	2.52	2.90
41.98	12	89.2	87.8	86.4	84.8	83.0	81.1	79.0	76.5	73.7	70.4	66.3	6.56	6.95
	14	80.1	78.7	77.3	75.7	73.9	72.0	69.9	67.4	64.6	61.3	57.2	4.65	5.04
	16	73.4	72.1	70.6	69.0	67.3	65.4	63.2	60.8	58.0	54.6	50.6	3.36	3.75
	18	68.5	67.1	65.6	64.1	62.3	60.4	58.3	55.8	53.0	49.7	45.6	2.51	2.90

TABLE 47

Process Times (B) at Retort Temperature of 250°F for Conduction-Heating Foods in 211 x 400 Can

f_h	z	INITIAL FOOD TEMPERATURE (T_{ih}) 100	110	120	130	140	150	160	170	180	190	200	Equivalent F_c^{18}	F_s^{18}
33.98	12	52.1	51.1	50.0	48.8	47.5	46.1	44.6	42.8	40.9	38.6	35.9	5.05	5.52
	14	49.6	48.6	47.5	46.3	45.0	43.6	42.0	40.3	38.3	36.1	33.4	3.94	4.40
	16	47.4	46.4	45.3	44.1	42.8	41.4	39.9	38.1	36.2	33.9	31.2	3.08	3.53
	18	45.5	44.5	43.4	42.2	40.9	39.5	38.0	36.2	34.3	32.0	29.3	2.46	2.90
35.98	12	54.6	53.5	52.4	51.1	49.8	48.3	46.6	44.8	42.7	40.3	37.4	5.09	5.56
	14	52.0	50.9	49.7	48.5	47.1	45.6	44.0	42.1	40.1	37.6	34.8	3.96	4.42
	16	49.7	48.6	47.4	46.2	44.8	43.3	41.7	39.8	37.7	35.3	32.5	3.07	3.52
	18	47.6	46.6	45.4	44.1	42.8	41.3	39.6	37.8	35.7	33.3	30.5	2.46	2.90
37.98	12	57.1	56.0	54.8	53.4	52.0	50.4	48.7	46.8	44.6	42.0	39.0	5.14	5.61
	14	54.4	53.2	52.0	50.7	49.3	47.7	46.0	44.0	41.8	39.3	36.3	4.00	4.46
	16	51.9	50.8	49.6	48.3	46.8	45.3	43.5	41.6	39.4	36.8	33.8	3.08	3.53
	18	49.8	48.7	47.4	46.1	44.7	43.1	41.4	39.4	37.2	34.7	31.7	2.46	2.90
39.98	12	59.7	58.5	57.2	55.8	54.3	52.6	50.8	48.8	46.4	43.8	40.6	5.20	5.68
	14	56.8	55.6	54.3	52.9	51.4	49.8	48.0	45.9	43.6	40.9	37.7	4.05	4.52
	16	54.3	53.1	51.8	50.4	48.9	47.2	45.4	43.3	41.0	38.3	35.2	3.11	3.56
	18	52.0	50.8	49.5	48.1	46.6	44.9	43.1	41.1	38.8	36.1	32.9	2.46	2.90
41.98	12	62.2	60.9	59.6	58.1	56.5	54.8	52.9	50.7	48.3	45.5	42.2	5.27	5.74
	14	59.2	58.0	56.6	55.2	53.6	51.8	49.9	47.8	45.3	42.5	39.2	4.08	4.55
	16	56.5	55.3	53.9	52.5	50.9	49.2	47.2	45.1	42.6	39.8	36.5	3.13	3.59
	18	54.1	52.9	51.5	50.1	48.5	46.7	44.8	42.7	40.2	37.4	34.1	2.45	2.90

TABLE 48

Process Times (B) at Retort Temperature of 260°F for Conduction-Heating Foods in 211 x 400 Can

f_h	z	INITIAL FOOD TEMPERATURE (T_{ih})											Equivalent	
		100	110	120	130	140	150	160	170	180	190	200	F_c^{18}	F_s^{18}
33.98	12	41.7	40.7	39.7	38.6	37.5	36.2	34.8	33.2	31.5	29.5	27.2	4.56	5.07
	14	40.4	39.4	38.4	37.3	36.1	34.9	33.5	31.9	30.2	28.2	25.9	3.68	4.17
	16	39.3	38.3	37.3	36.2	35.0	33.7	32.3	30.8	29.0	27.1	24.8	3.01	3.50
	18	38.1	37.2	36.1	35.0	33.9	32.6	31.2	29.6	27.9	25.9	23.6	2.42	2.90
35.98	12	43.9	42.9	41.8	40.7	39.4	38.1	36.6	34.9	33.1	31.0	28.6	4.67	5.18
	14	42.5	41.5	40.4	39.2	38.0	36.6	35.1	33.5	31.6	29.6	27.1	3.71	4.22
	16	41.3	40.3	39.2	38.0	36.8	35.4	33.9	32.3	30.4	28.4	25.9	3.02	3.52
	18	40.0	39.0	38.0	36.8	35.6	34.2	32.7	31.1	29.2	27.1	24.7	2.42	2.90
37.98	12	46.2	45.1	44.0	42.7	41.4	40.0	38.4	36.7	34.7	32.5	30.0	4.78	5.30
	14	44.5	43.5	42.3	41.1	39.8	38.4	36.8	35.0	33.1	30.9	28.4	3.74	4.24
	16	43.3	42.2	41.1	39.8	38.5	37.1	35.5	33.8	31.8	29.6	27.1	3.04	3.53
	18	42.0	40.9	39.8	38.5	37.2	35.8	34.2	32.5	30.5	28.3	25.8	2.42	2.90
39.98	12	48.4	47.2	46.1	44.8	43.4	41.9	40.2	38.4	36.3	34.0	31.3	4.89	5.41
	14	46.6	45.5	44.3	43.0	41.6	40.1	38.4	36.6	34.6	32.2	29.6	3.77	4.28
	16	45.2	44.1	42.9	41.6	40.2	38.7	37.1	35.2	33.2	30.9	28.2	3.04	3.54
	18	43.9	42.7	41.5	40.3	38.9	37.4	35.7	33.9	31.8	29.5	26.8	2.41	2.90
41.98	12	50.6	49.4	48.1	46.8	45.3	43.7	42.0	40.1	37.9	35.5	32.7	4.98	5.51
	14	48.6	47.5	46.2	44.9	43.4	41.8	40.1	38.2	36.0	33.6	30.8	3.80	4.31
	16	47.2	46.0	44.8	43.4	42.0	40.4	38.7	36.7	34.6	32.1	29.3	3.06	3.56
	18	45.8	44.6	43.3	42.0	40.5	38.9	37.2	35.3	33.1	30.7	27.9	2.41	2.90

TABLE 49

Process Times (B) at Retort Temperature of 230°F for Conduction-Heating Foods in 211 x 413 Can

f_h	z	INITIAL FOOD TEMPERATURE (T_{ih})											Equivalent	
		100	110	120	130	140	150	160	170	180	190	200	F_c^{18}	F_s^{18}
36.09	12	193.1	191.8	190.4	188.9	187.3	185.4	183.3	180.9	178.1	174.6	170.1	10.32	10.62
	14	133.6	132.3	131.0	129.5	127.8	126.0	123.9	121.5	118.6	115.1	110.6	5.87	6.16
	16	106.2	105.0	103.6	102.1	100.5	98.6	96.5	94.1	91.2	87.8	83.2	3.81	4.10
	18	90.6	89.3	88.0	86.5	84.8	83.0	80.9	78.5	75.6	72.1	67.6	2.62	2.92
38.22	12	195.6	194.2	192.8	191.2	189.5	187.5	185.3	182.7	179.7	176.0	171.2	10.33	10.62
	14	137.3	136.0	134.5	132.9	131.2	129.2	127.0	124.5	121.4	117.7	112.9	5.92	6.22
	16	109.5	108.2	106.7	105.1	103.4	101.4	99.2	96.7	93.6	89.9	85.2	3.81	4.11
	18	94.0	92.7	91.3	89.7	87.9	86.0	83.8	81.2	78.2	74.5	69.7	2.61	2.92
40.34	12	199.6	198.2	196.7	195.0	193.2	191.1	188.8	186.1	182.9	179.0	173.9	10.46	10.76
	14	140.7	139.3	137.8	136.1	134.3	132.2	129.9	127.2	124.0	120.1	115.0	5.91	6.22
	16	112.8	111.4	109.9	108.2	106.4	104.3	102.0	99.3	96.1	92.2	87.2	3.82	4.12
	18	97.4	96.0	94.5	92.8	91.0	88.9	86.6	83.9	80.7	76.8	71.7	2.61	2.92
42.46	12	203.3	201.8	200.2	198.5	196.5	194.4	191.9	189.1	185.7	181.6	176.3	10.44	10.76
	14	143.9	142.5	140.8	139.1	137.1	135.0	132.5	129.7	126.3	122.2	116.9	5.90	6.21
	16	116.1	114.6	113.0	111.2	109.3	107.1	104.7	101.8	98.5	94.3	89.0	3.82	4.12
	18	100.7	99.3	97.6	95.9	93.9	91.8	89.3	86.5	83.1	79.0	73.7	2.61	2.92
44.59	12	207.1	205.6	203.9	202.0	200.0	197.7	195.1	192.1	188.6	184.3	178.7	10.43	10.76
	14	147.5	146.0	144.3	142.4	140.4	138.1	135.5	132.6	129.0	124.7	119.1	5.93	6.24
	16	119.4	117.9	116.2	114.3	112.3	110.0	107.4	104.5	100.9	96.6	91.0	3.84	4.14
	18	104.0	102.4	100.7	98.9	96.9	94.6	92.0	89.0	85.5	81.2	75.6	2.60	2.91

TABLE 50

Process Times (B) at Retort Temperature of 240°F for Conduction-Heating Foods in 211 x 413 Can

f_h	z	INITIAL FOOD TEMPERATURE (T_{ih}) 100	110	120	130	140	150	160	170	180	190	200	Equivalent F_c^{18}	F_s^{18}
	12	79.7	78.6	77.3	76.0	74.5	72.8	71.0	68.9	66.5	63.6	60.1	6.26	6.65
36.09	14	71.8	70.6	69.4	68.0	66.5	64.9	63.0	60.9	58.5	55.7	52.2	4.65	5.03
	16	65.7	64.6	63.3	61.9	60.4	58.8	56.9	54.9	52.4	49.6	46.1	3.40	3.78
	18	61.1	60.0	58.7	57.3	55.8	54.2	52.3	50.3	47.8	45.0	41.5	2.54	2.91
	12	83.3	82.0	80.7	79.3	77.7	75.9	74.0	71.8	69.2	66.2	62.5	6.38	6.77
38.22	14	74.8	73.5	72.2	70.8	69.2	67.4	65.5	63.3	60.7	57.7	54.0	4.64	5.02
	16	68.6	67.4	66.0	64.6	63.0	61.3	59.3	57.1	54.5	51.5	47.8	3.40	3.78
	18	63.8	62.6	61.3	59.8	58.2	56.5	54.5	52.3	49.8	46.7	43.0	2.54	2.91
	12	86.7	85.4	84.0	82.5	80.8	79.0	76.9	74.6	71.9	68.7	64.8	6.50	6.89
40.34	14	77.8	76.5	75.1	73.6	71.9	70.1	68.0	65.7	63.0	59.8	55.9	4.65	5.03
	16	71.4	70.1	68.7	67.2	65.5	63.7	61.6	59.3	36.6	53.4	49.5	3.39	3.78
	18	66.5	65.2	63.8	62.3	60.6	58.8	56.7	54.4	51.7	48.5	44.6	2.53	2.91
	12	90.1	88.7	87.3	85.6	83.9	81.9	79.8	77.3	74.5	71.1	67.0	6.61	7.01
42.46	14	80.9	79.5	78.1	76.4	74.7	72.7	70.6	68.1	65.3	61.9	57.8	4.68	5.08
	16	74.2	72.8	71.3	69.7	68.0	66.0	63.8	61.4	58.5	55.2	51.1	3.38	3.77
	18	69.2	67.8	66.3	64.7	63.0	61.0	58.9	56.4	53.5	50.2	46.1	2.53	2.92
	12	93.4	92.0	90.4	88.8	86.9	84.9	82.6	80.0	77.0	73.5	69.2	6.72	7.12
44.59	14	83.9	82.5	81.0	79.3	77.4	75.4	73.1	70.5	67.5	64.0	59.7	4.71	5.11
	16	77.0	75.5	74.0	72.3	70.5	68.4	66.1	63.6	60.6	57.0	52.7	3.39	3.78
	18	71.8	70.4	68.8	67.1	65.3	63.2	61.0	58.4	55.4	51.9	47.5	2.53	2.91

TABLE 51

Process Times (B) at Retort Temperature of 250°F for Conduction-Heating Foods in 211 x 413 Can

f_h	z	INITIAL FOOD TEMPERATURE (T_{ih})											Equivalent	
		100	110	120	130	140	150	160	170	180	190	200	F_c^{18}	F_s^{18}
	12	54.8	53.7	52.6	51.3	50.0	48.5	46.8	45.0	42.9	40.5	37.6	5.12	5.59
36.09	14	52.2	51.1	49.9	48.7	47.3	45.8	44.2	42.3	40.2	37.8	34.9	3.99	4.45
	16	49.8	48.8	47.6	46.4	45.0	43.5	41.8	40.0	37.9	35.5	32.6	3.09	3.54
	18	47.8	46.7	45.6	44.3	43.0	41.5	39.8	38.0	35.9	33.5	30.6	2.48	2.91
	12	57.5	56.3	55.1	53.8	52.3	50.8	49.0	47.1	44.8	42.3	39.3	5.17	5.64
38.22	14	54.7	53.6	52.3	51.0	49.6	48.0	46.2	44.3	42.1	39.5	36.5	4.02	4.49
	16	52.3	51.1	49.9	48.6	47.1	45.5	43.8	41.8	39.6	37.1	34.0	3.10	3.55
	18	50.1	49.0	47.7	46.4	45.0	43.4	41.6	39.7	37.5	34.9	31.9	2.47	2.92
	12	60.2	59.0	57.7	56.3	54.8	53.1	51.2	49.2	46.8	44.1	40.9	5.24	5.72
40.34	14	57.3	56.1	54.8	53.4	51.9	50.2	48.4	46.3	44.0	41.3	38.1	4.08	4.55
	16	54.7	53.5	52.2	50.8	49.3	47.6	45.8	43.7	41.4	38.7	35.5	3.13	3.58
	18	52.4	51.2	49.9	48.5	47.0	45.3	43.5	41.4	39.1	36.4	33.2	2.47	2.92
	12	62.9	61.6	60.2	58.7	57.1	55.4	53.4	51.3	48.8	46.0	42.6	5.31	5.79
42.46	14	59.9	58.6	57.2	55.8	54.2	52.4	50.5	48.3	45.8	43.0	39.6	4.11	4.58
	16	57.2	55.9	54.5	53.0	51.4	49.7	47.7	45.6	43.1	40.3	36.9	3.16	3.62
	18	54.7	53.4	52.1	50.6	49.0	47.2	45.3	43.1	40.7	37.8	34.5	2.47	2.91
	12	65.5	64.2	62.7	61.2	59.5	57.6	55.6	53.3	50.7	47.8	44.2	5.36	5.84
44.59	14	62.4	61.1	59.6	58.1	56.3	54.6	52.5	50.2	47.7	44.7	41.1	4.13	4.60
	16	59.5	58.2	56.8	55.2	53.5	51.7	49.7	47.4	44.8	41.8	38.3	3.19	3.65
	18	57.0	55.6	54.2	52.7	51.0	49.1	47.1	44.8	42.2	39.2	35.7	2.47	2.91

TABLE 52

Process Times (B) at Retort Temperature of 260°F for Conduction-Heating Foods in 211 x 413 Can

f_h	z	INITIAL FOOD TEMPERATURE (T_{ih})											Equivalent	
		100	110	120	130	140	150	160	170	180	190	200	F_c^{18}	F_s^{18}
	12	44.1	43.1	42.0	40.8	39.6	38.2	36.7	35.1	33.2	31.1	28.7	4.69	5.21
36.09	14	42.6	41.6	40.5	39.4	38.1	36.7	35.3	33.6	31.8	29.7	27.2	3.74	4.24
	16	41.4	40.4	39.3	38.2	36.9	35.5	34.1	32.4	30.6	28.5	26.0	3.04	3.54
	18	40.2	39.2	38.1	36.9	35.7	34.3	32.8	31.2	29.3	27.2	24.8	2.43	2.91
	12	46.4	45.4	44.2	43.0	41.7	40.2	38.6	36.9	34.9	32.7	30.2	4.81	5.33
38.22	14	44.8	43.7	42.6	41.4	40.0	38.6	37.0	35.3	33.3	31.1	28.5	3.76	4.27
	16	43.5	42.5	41.3	40.1	38.8	37.3	35.7	34.0	32.0	29.8	27.3	3.06	3.56
	18	42.2	41.2	40.0	38.8	37.5	36.0	34.4	32.7	30.7	28.5	26.0	2.43	2.91
	12	48.8	47.7	46.5	45.2	43.8	42.2	40.6	38.7	36.7	34.3	31.6	4.93	5.45
40.34	14	47.0	45.9	44.7	43.4	42.0	40.4	38.8	36.9	34.9	32.5	29.8	3.80	4.30
	16	45.6	44.5	43.3	42.0	40.6	39.1	37.4	35.6	33.5	31.2	28.5	3.07	3.56
	18	44.2	43.1	41.9	40.6	39.2	37.7	36.0	34.2	32.1	29.8	27.1	2.43	2.91
	12	51.1	49.9	48.7	47.3	45.8	44.2	42.5	40.5	38.3	35.9	33.0	5.03	5.55
42.46	14	49.2	48.0	46.7	45.4	43.9	42.3	40.5	38.6	36.4	33.9	31.1	3.83	4.34
	16	47.7	46.5	45.3	43.9	42.4	40.8	39.1	37.1	35.0	32.5	29.7	3.08	3.58
	18	46.3	45.1	43.8	42.4	41.0	39.4	37.6	35.7	33.5	31.0	28.2	2.43	2.92
	12	53.4	52.2	50.8	49.4	47.9	46.2	44.3	42.3	40.0	37.4	34.4	5.11	5.63
44.59	14	51.4	50.1	48.8	47.3	45.8	44.1	42.3	40.2	37.9	35.3	32.4	3.86	4.37
	16	49.8	48.6	47.2	45.8	44.2	42.6	40.7	38.7	36.4	33.8	30.8	3.09	3.59
	18	48.3	47.0	45.7	44.2	42.7	41.0	39.2	37.1	34.8	32.3	29.3	2.43	2.91

TABLE 53

Process Times (B) at Retort Temperature of 230°F for Conduction-Heating Foods in 211 x 414 Can

f_h	z	INITIAL FOOD TEMPERATURE (T_{ih})											Equivalent	
		100	110	120	130	140	150	160	170	180	190	200	F_c^{18}	F_s^{18}
36.22	12	193.3	192.0	190.6	189.1	187.5	185.6	183.5	181.1	178.2	174.7	170.2	10.33	10.62
	14	133.8	132.6	131.2	129.7	128.1	126.2	124.1	121.7	118.8	115.3	110.8	5.87	6.17
	16	106.4	105.2	103.8	102.3	100.7	98.8	96.7	94.3	91.4	87.9	83.4	3.81	4.10
	18	90.8	89.5	88.2	86.7	85.0	83.2	81.1	78.6	75.8	72.3	67.7	2.62	2.92
38.35	12	195.9	194.6	193.1	191.5	189.8	187.8	185.6	183.0	180.0	176.3	171.5	10.34	10.64
	14	137.5	136.2	134.8	133.2	131.4	129.5	127.2	124.7	121.6	117.9	113.1	5.92	6.22
	16	109.7	108.4	107.0	105.4	103.6	101.7	99.4	96.9	93.8	90.1	85.3	3.81	4.11
	18	94.3	92.9	91.5	89.9	88.1	86.2	83.9	81.4	78.3	74.6	69.8	2.62	2.92
40.48	12	199.9	198.5	197.0	195.3	193.4	191.4	189.0	186.3	183.1	179.2	174.1	10.47	10.77
	14	141.0	139.6	138.0	136.4	134.5	132.4	130.1	127.4	124.2	120.3	115.2	5.91	6.22
	16	113.1	111.7	110.1	108.5	106.6	104.5	102.2	99.5	96.3	92.4	87.3	3.82	4.12
	18	97.6	96.2	94.7	93.0	91.2	89.1	86.8	84.0	80.8	76.9	71.9	2.61	2.92
42.61	12	203.6	202.2	200.5	198.8	196.8	194.7	192.2	189.3	186.0	181.8	176.5	10.44	10.76
	14	144.2	142.7	141.1	139.3	137.4	135.2	132.7	129.9	126.5	122.4	117.0	5.90	6.21
	16	116.3	114.9	113.2	111.5	109.5	107.4	104.9	102.0	98.7	94.5	89.2	3.82	4.12
	18	101.0	99.5	97.9	96.1	94.2	92.0	89.5	86.7	83.3	79.2	73.8	2.61	2.92
44.74	12	207.4	205.9	204.2	202.3	200.3	198.0	195.4	192.4	188.9	184.5	178.9	10.44	10.76
	14	147.8	146.3	144.6	142.7	140.7	138.4	135.8	132.8	129.3	124.9	119.3	5.93	6.25
	16	119.7	118.1	116.4	114.6	112.5	110.3	107.7	104.7	101.1	96.8	91.2	3.84	4.14
	18	104.2	102.7	101.0	99.1	97.1	94.8	92.2	89.2	85.7	81.3	75.7	2.61	2.92

TABLE 54

Process Times (B) at Retort Temperature of 240°F for Conduction-Heating Foods in 211 x 414 Can

f_h	z	INITIAL FOOD TEMPERATURE (T_{ih}) 100	110	120	130	140	150	160	170	180	190	200	Equivalent F_c^{18}	F_s^{18}
36.22	12	80.0	78.8	77.5	76.2	74.7	73.0	71.2	69.1	66.6	63.8	60.3	6.27	6.66
	14	72.0	70.8	69.6	68.2	66.7	65.0	63.2	61.1	58.7	55.8	52.3	4.66	5.03
	16	65.9	64.7	63.5	62.1	60.6	58.9	57.1	55.0	52.6	49.7	46.2	3.40	3.78
	18	61.3	60.1	58.9	57.7	56.0	54.3	52.5	50.4	48.0	45.1	41.6	2.54	2.92
38.35	12	83.5	82.3	80.9	79.5	77.9	76.1	74.2	71.9	69.4	66.3	62.6	6.39	6.78
	14	75.0	73.7	72.4	71.0	69.4	67.6	65.7	63.4	60.9	57.8	54.1	4.64	5.02
	16	68.8	67.5	66.2	64.8	63.2	61.4	59.4	57.2	54.7	51.6	47.9	3.40	3.78
	18	64.0	62.8	61.4	60.0	58.4	56.6	54.7	52.5	49.9	46.9	43.1	2.54	2.92
40.48	12	86.9	85.6	84.2	82.7	81.0	79.2	77.1	74.8	72.0	68.8	64.9	6.51	6.90
	14	78.0	76.7	75.3	73.8	72.1	70.2	68.2	65.8	63.1	59.9	56.0	4.65	5.04
	16	71.6	70.3	68.9	67.3	65.7	63.8	61.8	59.4	56.7	53.5	49.6	3.39	3.78
	18	66.7	65.4	64.0	62.5	60.8	58.9	56.9	54.5	51.8	48.6	44.7	2.54	2.92
42.61	12	90.3	89.0	87.5	85.9	84.1	82.2	80.0	77.5	74.7	71.3	67.2	6.62	7.02
	14	81.1	79.7	78.3	76.7	74.9	72.9	70.8	68.3	65.4	62.1	57.9	4.68	5.08
	16	74.4	73.0	71.5	69.9	68.1	66.2	64.0	61.5	58.7	55.3	51.2	3.38	3.77
	18	69.4	68.0	66.5	64.9	63.1	61.2	59.0	56.5	53.7	50.3	46.2	2.53	2.92
44.74	12	93.7	92.2	90.7	89.0	87.1	85.1	82.8	80.2	77.2	73.7	69.3	6.73	7.13
	14	84.2	82.7	81.2	79.5	77.6	75.6	73.3	70.7	67.7	64.2	59.8	4.72	5.12
	16	77.2	75.7	74.2	72.5	70.6	68.6	66.3	63.7	60.7	57.2	52.8	3.39	3.79
	18	72.0	70.5	69.0	67.3	65.4	63.4	61.1	58.5	55.5	52.0	47.6	2.53	2.92

TABLE 55

Process Times (B) at Retort Temperature of 250°F for Conduction-Heating Foods in 211 x 414 Can

f_h	z	INITIAL FOOD TEMPERATURE (T_{ih})											Equivalent	
		100	110	120	130	140	150	160	170	180	190	200	F_c^{18}	F_s^{18}
36.22	12	55.0	53.9	52.7	51.5	50.1	48.6	46.9	45.1	43.0	40.6	37.7	5.13	5.60
	14	52.3	51.2	50.1	48.8	47.4	45.9	44.3	42.4	40.3	37.9	35.0	3.99	4.45
	16	50.0	48.9	47.7	46.5	45.1	43.6	42.0	40.1	38.0	35.6	32.7	3.09	3.54
	18	48.0	46.9	45.7	44.4	43.1	41.6	39.9	38.1	36.0	33.5	30.7	2.48	2.92
38.35	12	57.7	56.5	55.3	53.9	52.5	50.9	49.2	47.2	45.0	42.4	39.4	5.18	5.65
	14	54.9	53.7	52.5	51.2	49.7	48.1	46.4	44.4	42.2	39.6	36.6	4.03	4.49
	16	52.4	51.3	50.0	48.7	47.3	45.7	43.9	42.0	39.7	37.2	34.1	3.10	3.55
	18	50.3	49.1	47.9	46.5	45.1	43.5	41.8	39.8	37.6	35.0	32.0	2.48	2.92
40.48	12	60.4	59.2	57.9	56.5	54.9	53.2	51.4	49.3	47.0	44.3	41.1	5.25	5.72
	14	57.5	56.3	55.0	53.6	52.0	50.4	48.5	46.4	44.1	41.4	38.2	4.09	4.55
	16	54.9	53.7	52.4	51.0	49.4	47.8	45.9	43.8	41.5	38.8	35.6	3.13	3.59
	18	52.6	51.4	50.1	48.7	47.1	45.5	43.6	41.5	39.2	36.5	33.3	2.47	2.92
42.61	12	63.1	61.8	60.4	58.9	57.3	55.5	53.6	51.4	48.9	46.1	42.7	5.32	5.79
	14	60.1	58.8	57.4	55.9	54.3	52.6	50.6	48.4	46.0	43.1	39.7	4.11	4.58
	16	57.3	56.0	54.7	53.2	51.6	49.8	47.9	45.7	43.2	40.4	37.0	3.16	3.62
	18	54.9	53.6	52.2	50.8	49.1	47.4	45.4	43.3	40.8	37.9	34.6	2.47	2.92
44.74	12	65.7	64.4	62.9	61.4	59.7	57.8	55.8	53.5	50.9	47.9	44.3	5.36	5.84
	14	62.6	61.3	59.8	58.3	56.6	54.7	52.7	50.4	47.8	44.8	41.2	4.13	4.60
	16	59.7	58.4	56.9	55.4	53.7	51.8	49.8	47.5	44.9	41.9	38.4	3.19	3.65
	18	57.1	55.8	54.4	52.8	51.1	49.3	47.2	44.9	42.3	39.3	35.8	2.47	2.92

TABLE 56

Process Times (B) at Retort Temperature of 260°F for Conduction-Heating Foods in 211 x 414 Can

f_h	z	INITIAL FOOD TEMPERATURE (T_{ih})											Equivalent	
		100	110	120	130	140	150	160	170	180	190	200	F_c^{18}	F_s^{18}
36.22	12	44.2	43.2	42.1	41.0	39.7	38.3	36.8	35.2	33.3	31.2	28.8	4.70	5.21
	14	42.8	41.7	40.7	39.5	38.2	36.9	35.4	33.7	31.9	29.8	27.3	3.74	4.24
	16	41.5	40.5	39.4	38.3	37.0	35.7	34.2	32.5	30.6	28.5	26.1	3.05	3.54
	18	40.3	39.3	38.2	37.0	35.8	34.4	32.9	31.3	29.4	27.3	24.9	2.44	2.92
38.35	12	46.6	45.5	44.4	43.1	41.8	40.4	38.8	37.0	35.1	32.8	30.3	4.82	5.34
	14	45.0	43.9	42.7	41.5	40.2	38.7	37.1	35.4	33.4	31.2	28.6	3.77	4.27
	16	43.7	42.6	41.5	40.2	38.9	37.4	35.8	34.1	32.1	29.9	27.3	3.06	3.56
	18	42.4	41.3	40.1	38.9	37.6	36.1	34.5	32.8	30.8	28.6	26.0	2.43	2.92
40.48	12	49.0	47.8	46.6	45.3	43.9	42.4	40.7	38.8	36.8	34.4	31.7	4.94	5.46
	14	47.2	46.0	44.8	43.5	42.1	40.6	38.9	37.0	35.0	32.6	29.9	3.80	4.31
	16	45.8	44.6	43.4	42.1	40.7	39.2	37.5	35.7	33.6	31.2	28.5	3.07	3.56
	18	44.4	43.2	42.0	40.7	39.3	37.8	36.1	34.3	32.2	29.8	27.1	2.43	2.92
42.61	12	51.3	50.1	48.8	47.4	46.0	44.4	42.6	40.6	38.5	36.0	33.1	5.03	5.56
	14	49.3	48.1	46.9	45.5	44.0	42.4	40.6	38.7	36.5	34.0	31.2	3.84	4.35
	16	47.9	46.7	45.4	44.0	42.6	41.0	39.2	37.2	35.1	32.6	29.7	3.09	3.58
	18	46.4	45.2	43.9	42.6	41.1	39.5	37.7	35.8	33.6	31.1	28.3	2.43	2.92
44.74	12	53.6	52.3	51.0	49.6	48.0	46.3	44.5	42.4	40.1	37.5	34.5	5.11	5.64
	14	51.5	50.3	48.9	47.5	45.9	44.2	42.4	40.3	38.0	35.4	32.5	3.86	4.38
	16	50.0	48.7	47.4	45.9	44.4	42.7	40.8	38.8	36.5	33.9	30.9	3.09	3.59
	18	48.4	47.2	45.8	44.4	42.8	41.1	39.3	37.2	34.9	32.4	29.4	2.43	2.92

TABLE 57

Process Times (B) at Retort Temperature of 230°F for Conduction-Heating Foods in 211 x 600 Can

f_h	z	INITIAL FOOD TEMPERATURE (T_{ih})											Equivalent	
		100	110	120	130	140	150	160	170	180	190	200	F_c^{18}	F_s^{18}
37.88	12	196.1	194.8	193.4	191.8	190.1	188.1	185.9	183.4	180.4	176.7	172.0	10.39	10.68
	14	137.2	135.9	134.5	132.9	131.2	129.3	127.1	124.5	121.5	117.9	113.1	5.95	6.25
	16	109.3	108.0	106.6	105.0	103.3	101.3	99.1	96.6	93.6	89.9	85.2	3.83	4.13
	18	93.7	92.4	91.0	89.4	87.7	85.7	83.6	81.0	78.0	74.3	69.6	2.64	2.94
40.10	12	200.2	198.8	197.3	195.6	193.8	191.7	189.4	186.7	183.5	179.7	174.6	10.51	10.81
	14	140.9	139.5	138.0	136.4	134.5	132.5	130.1	127.5	124.3	120.4	115.4	5.96	6.26
	16	112.9	111.5	110.0	108.3	106.5	104.4	102.1	99.4	96.2	92.3	87.3	3.85	4.15
	18	97.3	95.9	94.4	92.7	90.9	88.8	86.5	83.8	80.6	76.8	71.7	2.63	2.94
42.33	12	204.0	202.5	200.9	199.2	197.2	195.1	192.6	189.8	186.4	182.3	177.0	10.51	10.83
	14	144.3	142.9	141.3	139.5	137.6	135.4	133.0	130.1	126.8	122.7	117.4	5.94	6.26
	16	116.2	114.8	113.2	111.4	109.5	107.3	104.9	102.0	98.7	94.6	89.3	3.85	4.15
	18	100.8	99.3	97.7	96.0	94.0	91.9	89.4	86.6	83.2	79.1	73.8	2.63	2.94
44.56	12	208.0	206.5	204.8	202.9	200.9	198.6	196.0	193.1	189.5	185.2	179.6	10.51	10.84
	14	148.0	146.5	144.8	142.9	140.9	138.6	136.0	133.1	129.5	125.2	119.6	5.97	6.28
	16	119.8	118.2	116.5	114.7	112.6	110.4	107.8	104.8	101.3	97.0	91.4	3.86	4.17
	18	104.2	102.7	101.0	99.1	97.1	94.8	92.2	89.3	85.7	81.4	75.8	2.62	2.94
46.79	12	211.7	210.1	208.3	206.4	204.3	201.9	199.2	196.0	192.3	187.8	181.9	10.50	10.83
	14	151.7	150.1	148.3	146.4	144.2	141.9	139.1	136.0	132.3	127.8	121.9	6.00	6.31
	16	123.1	121.5	119.7	117.8	115.6	113.2	110.5	107.4	103.7	99.2	93.3	3.86	4.17
	18	107.6	105.9	104.2	102.2	100.1	97.7	95.0	91.9	88.1	83.6	77.8	2.62	2.94

TABLE 58

Process Times (B) at Retort Temperature of 240°F for Conduction-Heating Foods in 211 x 600 Can

f_h	z	INITIAL FOOD TEMPERATURE (T_{ih})											Equivalent	
		100	110	120	130	140	150	160	170	180	190	200	F_c^{18}	F_s^{18}
	12	82.9	81.6	80.3	78.9	77.3	75.6	73.7	71.5	68.9	65.9	62.3	6.40	6.79
37.88	14	74.5	73.3	71.9	70.5	68.9	67.2	65.3	63.1	60.5	57.5	53.9	4.68	5.06
	16	68.3	67.0	65.7	64.3	62.7	61.0	59.1	56.9	54.3	51.3	47.7	3.43	3.81
	18	63.5	62.3	61.0	59.5	58.0	56.2	54.3	52.1	49.6	46.6	42.9	2.56	2.94
	12	86.5	85.2	83.8	82.3	80.6	78.8	76.7	74.4	71.7	68.6	64.7	6.52	6.91
40.10	14	77.6	76.3	74.9	73.4	71.7	69.9	67.8	65.5	62.8	59.7	55.8	4.67	5.06
	16	71.2	69.9	68.5	67.0	65.4	63.5	61.5	59.2	56.5	53.3	49.4	3.42	3.81
	18	66.3	65.1	63.7	62.1	60.5	58.7	56.6	54.3	51.6	48.4	44.5	2.56	2.94
	12	90.1	88.7	87.2	85.6	83.9	81.9	79.8	77.3	74.5	71.1	67.0	6.64	7.03
42.33	14	80.9	79.5	78.0	76.4	74.7	72.7	70.6	68.1	65.3	61.9	57.8	4.71	5.10
	16	74.1	72.8	71.3	69.7	68.0	66.0	63.9	61.4	58.6	55.2	51.1	3.41	3.80
	18	69.1	67.8	66.3	64.7	63.0	61.0	58.8	56.4	53.6	50.2	46.1	2.55	2.94
	12	93.6	92.1	90.6	88.9	87.1	85.0	82.7	80.2	77.2	73.6	69.3	6.76	7.15
44.56	14	84.1	82.6	81.1	79.4	77.6	75.5	73.2	70.7	67.7	64.1	59.8	4.74	5.15
	16	77.1	75.6	74.1	72.4	70.6	68.5	66.2	63.7	60.7	57.2	52.8	3.42	3.81
	18	71.9	70.5	68.9	67.2	65.4	63.3	61.1	58.5	55.5	52.0	47.7	2.55	2.94
	12	97.0	95.5	93.9	92.1	90.2	88.0	85.7	82.9	79.8	76.1	71.6	6.87	7.26
46.79	14	87.2	85.7	84.1	82.3	80.4	78.2	75.9	73.1	70.0	66.3	61.8	4.78	5.18
	16	80.0	78.5	76.9	75.1	73.2	71.0	68.6	65.9	62.8	59.1	54.6	3.43	3.82
	18	74.6	73.1	71.5	69.7	67.8	65.7	63.3	60.6	57.4	53.7	49.2	2.55	2.94

TABLE 59

Process Times (B) at Retort Temperature of 250°F for Conduction-Heating Foods in 211 x 600 Can

f_h	z	INITIAL FOOD TEMPERATURE (T_{ih}) 100	110	120	130	140	150	160	170	180	190	200	Equivalent F_c^{18}	F_s^{18}
37.88	12	57.1	56.0	54.8	53.4	52.0	50.5	48.7	46.8	44.6	42.0	39.0	5.19	5.66
	14	54.4	53.2	52.0	50.7	49.3	47.7	46.0	44.0	41.8	39.3	36.3	4.04	4.50
	16	51.9	50.8	49.6	48.3	46.8	45.3	43.5	41.6	39.4	36.9	33.9	3.11	3.57
	18	49.8	48.7	47.4	46.1	44.7	43.1	41.4	39.5	37.3	34.7	31.7	2.50	2.94
40.10	12	60.0	58.8	57.5	56.1	54.6	52.9	51.1	49.0	46.7	44.0	40.8	5.27	5.74
	14	57.1	55.9	54.6	53.2	51.7	50.0	48.2	46.1	43.8	41.1	38.0	4.10	4.56
	16	54.5	53.3	52.0	50.6	49.1	47.5	45.6	43.6	41.3	38.6	35.4	3.15	3.60
	18	52.2	51.0	49.8	48.4	46.8	45.2	43.4	41.3	39.0	36.3	33.1	2.49	2.94
42.33	12	62.8	61.5	60.1	58.7	57.1	55.3	53.4	51.2	48.8	45.9	42.6	5.34	5.82
	14	59.8	58.5	57.2	55.7	54.1	52.3	50.4	48.2	45.8	42.9	39.6	4.14	4.61
	16	57.1	55.8	54.4	53.0	51.4	49.6	47.7	45.5	43.1	40.2	36.9	3.18	3.64
	18	54.7	53.4	52.0	50.6	49.0	47.2	45.3	43.1	40.6	37.8	34.5	2.49	2.94
44.56	12	65.6	64.2	62.8	61.2	59.5	57.7	55.7	53.4	50.8	47.8	44.3	5.39	5.87
	14	62.5	61.1	59.7	58.1	56.5	54.6	52.6	50.3	47.7	44.7	41.2	4.16	4.63
	16	59.6	58.3	56.8	55.3	53.6	51.7	49.7	47.4	44.8	41.9	38.3	3.21	3.67
	18	57.0	55.7	54.3	52.7	51.0	49.2	47.1	44.9	42.3	39.3	35.8	2.49	2.94
46.79	12	68.3	66.9	65.4	63.7	62.0	60.0	57.9	55.5	52.8	49.7	46.0	5.44	5.92
	14	65.1	63.7	62.2	60.5	58.8	56.8	54.7	52.3	49.6	46.5	42.8	4.17	4.65
	16	62.1	60.7	59.2	57.5	55.8	53.8	51.7	49.3	46.6	43.5	39.8	3.23	3.69
	18	59.4	58.0	56.5	54.8	53.1	51.1	49.0	46.6	43.9	40.7	37.0	2.49	2.94

TABLE 60

Process Times (B) at Retort Temperature of 260°F for Conduction-Heating Foods in 211 x 600 Can

f_h	z	INITIAL FOOD TEMPERATURE (T_{ih})											Equivalent	
		100	110	120	130	140	150	160	170	180	190	200	F_c^{18}	F_s^{18}
	12	46.1	45.0	43.9	42.7	41.4	39.9	38.4	36.6	34.7	32.5	30.0	4.82	5.33
37.88	14	44.5	43.4	42.3	41.1	39.8	38.3	36.8	35.0	33.1	30.9	28.4	3.78	4.29
	16	43.2	42.2	41.1	39.8	38.5	37.1	35.5	33.8	31.8	29.7	27.1	3.08	3.58
	18	42.0	40.9	39.8	38.5	37.2	35.8	34.2	32.5	30.5	28.4	25.8	2.45	2.93
	12	48.6	47.4	46.2	45.0	43.6	42.0	40.4	38.6	36.5	34.2	31.5	4.94	5.46
40.10	14	46.8	45.7	44.5	43.2	41.8	40.3	38.6	36.8	34.7	32.4	29.7	3.82	4.33
	16	45.5	44.3	43.1	41.8	40.4	38.9	37.3	35.4	33.4	31.1	28.4	3.09	3.58
	18	44.1	42.9	41.7	40.5	39.1	37.5	35.9	34.0	32.0	29.7	27.0	2.45	2.93
	12	51.0	49.8	48.6	47.2	45.7	44.1	42.4	40.4	38.3	35.8	33.0	5.05	5.57
42.33	14	49.1	47.9	46.6	45.3	43.8	42.2	40.5	38.5	36.3	33.9	31.1	3.85	4.36
	16	47.7	46.5	45.2	43.8	42.4	40.8	39.0	37.1	34.9	32.5	29.6	3.11	3.60
	18	46.2	45.0	43.7	42.4	40.9	39.3	37.5	35.6	33.4	31.0	28.2	2.45	2.94
	12	53.4	52.2	50.9	49.4	47.9	46.2	44.4	42.3	40.0	37.4	34.5	5.13	5.66
44.56	14	51.4	50.1	48.8	47.4	45.8	44.1	42.3	40.2	38.0	35.4	32.4	3.89	4.40
	16	49.8	48.6	47.3	45.8	44.3	42.6	40.7	38.7	36.4	33.8	30.9	3.11	3.61
	18	48.3	47.0	45.7	44.3	42.7	41.0	39.2	37.2	34.9	32.3	29.3	2.45	2.94
	12	55.9	54.5	53.1	51.6	50.0	48.2	46.3	44.2	41.8	39.1	35.9	5.21	5.74
46.79	14	53.6	52.3	50.9	49.4	47.8	46.0	44.1	41.9	39.5	36.8	33.7	3.91	4.43
	16	52.0	50.7	49.3	47.8	46.2	44.4	42.5	40.3	37.9	35.2	32.1	3.12	3.62
	18	50.4	49.1	47.7	46.2	44.5	42.8	40.8	38.7	36.3	33.6	30.4	2.45	2.94

TABLE 61

Process Times (B) at Retort Temperature of 230°F for Conduction-Heating Foods in 300 x 206 Can

f_h	z	INITIAL FOOD TMEPERATURE (T_{ih}) 100	110	120	130	140	150	160	170	180	190	200	Equivalent F_c^{18}	F_s^{18}
27.58	12	175.7	174.7	173.7	172.5	171.3	169.9	168.3	166.4	164.2	161.6	158.1	10.13	10.42
	14	118.8	117.9	116.8	115.7	114.4	113.0	111.4	109.6	107.4	104.7	101.3	5.75	6.02
	16	91.9	91.0	89.9	88.8	87.5	86.1	84.5	82.7	80.5	77.8	74.4	3.72	3.99
	18	77.0	76.0	75.0	73.8	72.6	71.2	69.6	67.7	65.5	62.9	59.4	2.60	2.87
29.20	12	179.3	178.3	177.2	176.0	174.6	173.1	171.4	169.5	167.2	164.3	160.7	10.14	10.43
	14	121.3	120.3	119.2	118.0	116.6	115.1	113.5	111.5	109.2	106.4	102.7	5.77	6.04
	16	94.6	93.5	92.4	91.2	89.9	88.4	86.7	84.7	82.4	79.6	76.0	3.73	4.01
	18	79.4	78.4	77.3	76.1	74.7	73.2	71.5	69.6	67.3	64.5	60.8	2.60	2.87
30.82	12	182.5	181.4	180.3	179.0	177.6	176.0	174.2	172.2	169.7	166.7	162.9	10.14	10.43
	14	124.1	123.0	121.9	120.6	119.2	117.6	115.8	113.7	111.3	108.3	104.5	5.78	6.07
	16	97.1	96.0	94.9	93.6	92.2	90.6	88.8	86.8	84.3	81.3	77.5	3.73	4.01
	18	81.8	80.7	79.5	78.3	76.9	75.3	73.5	71.4	69.0	66.0	62.2	2.59	2.87
32.44	12	185.4	184.3	183.0	181.7	180.2	178.6	176.7	174.5	171.9	168.8	164.7	10.15	10.44
	14	126.7	125.5	124.3	123.0	121.5	119.8	117.9	115.8	113.2	110.1	106.0	5.77	6.07
	16	99.5	98.4	97.2	95.8	94.4	92.7	90.8	88.6	86.1	82.9	78.9	3.72	4.01
	18	84.2	83.0	81.8	80.5	79.0	77.3	75.4	73.3	70.7	67.6	63.5	2.59	2.86
34.06	12	188.0	186.8	185.5	184.1	182.5	180.8	178.8	176.5	173.8	170.5	166.3	10.15	10.45
	14	129.2	128.0	126.7	125.3	123.7	122.0	120.0	117.7	115.0	111.7	107.5	5.76	6.06
	16	102.2	101.0	99.7	98.3	96.7	95.0	93.0	90.7	88.0	84.7	80.5	3.74	4.03
	18	86.6	85.4	84.2	82.8	81.2	79.5	77.5	75.2	72.5	69.2	64.9	2.58	2.86

TABLE 62

Process Times (B) at Retort Temperature of 250°F for Conduction-Heating Foods in 300 x 206 Can

f_h	z	INITIAL FOOD TEMPERATURE (T_{ih})											Equivalent	
		100	110	120	130	140	150	160	170	180	190	200	F^{18}_c	F^{18}_s
	12	66.2	65.3	64.4	63.3	62.2	60.9	59.5	57.9	56.1	53.9	51.2	6.06	6.44
27.58	14	58.8	57.9	57.0	55.9	54.8	53.5	52.1	50.5	48.7	46.5	43.8	4.35	4.71
	16	53.8	52.9	51.9	50.9	49.8	48.5	47.1	45.5	43.6	41.5	38.8	3.31	3.66
	18	49.8	48.9	47.9	46.9	45.7	44.5	43.1	41.5	39.6	37.4	34.8	2.51	2.86
	12	68.8	67.9	66.8	65.7	64.5	63.2	61.7	60.0	58.0	55.7	52.9	6.07	6.45
29.20	14	61.3	60.4	59.4	58.3	57.1	55.7	54.2	52.5	50.6	48.3	45.4	4.43	4.79
	16	56.0	55.1	54.0	52.9	51.7	50.4	48.9	47.2	45.2	42.9	40.1	3.29	3.66
	18	51.9	51.0	50.0	48.9	47.7	46.3	44.9	43.2	41.2	38.9	36.1	2.51	2.87
	12	71.3	70.3	69.2	68.1	66.8	65.4	63.8	62.0	60.0	57.5	54.5	6.03	6.46
30.82	14	63.8	62.8	61.7	60.5	59.3	57.9	56.3	54.5	52.4	50.0	47.0	4.50	4.86
	16	58.2	57.2	56.1	54.9	53.7	52.2	50.7	48.9	46.8	44.4	41.4	3.29	3.65
	18	54.1	53.1	52.0	50.9	49.6	48.2	46.6	44.8	42.8	40.3	37.3	2.50	2.87
	12	73.7	72.7	71.6	70.3	69.0	67.5	65.8	64.0	61.8	59.2	56.1	6.08	6.47
32.44	14	66.2	65.1	64.0	62.8	61.4	59.9	58.3	56.4	54.2	51.7	48.5	4.57	4.93
	16	60.4	59.3	58.2	57.0	55.6	54.1	52.5	50.6	48.4	45.9	42.7	3.29	3.67
	18	56.2	55.2	54.0	52.8	51.5	50.0	48.3	46.4	44.3	41.7	38.5	2.50	2.87
	12	76.1	75.0	73.8	72.5	71.1	69.5	67.8	65.8	63.5	60.9	57.6	6.09	6.47
34.06	14	68.5	67.4	66.2	65.0	63.5	62.0	60.2	58.3	56.0	53.3	50.0	4.58	4.95
	16	62.6	61.5	60.3	59.1	57.7	56.1	54.4	52.4	50.1	47.4	44.1	3.32	3.69
	18	58.3	57.2	56.0	54.7	53.3	51.7	50.0	48.0	45.7	43.0	39.7	2.50	2.87

TABLE 63

Process Times (B) at Retort Temperature of 250°F for Conduction-Heating foods in 300 x 206 Can

f_h	z	INITIAL FOOD TEMPERATURE (T_{ih})											Equivalent	
		100	110	120	130	140	150	160	170	180	190	200	F_c^{18}	F_s^{18}
	12	43.7	42.9	42.0	41.1	40.0	38.9	37.6	36.2	34.6	32.8	30.6	4.81	5.26
27.58	14	41.6	40.7	39.8	38.9	37.8	36.7	35.4	34.0	32.4	30.6	28.4	3.76	4.21
	16	39.8	39.0	38.1	37.1	36.1	34.9	33.7	32.3	30.7	28.8	26.6	3.03	3.46
	18	38.3	37.5	36.6	35.6	34.6	33.4	32.2	30.8	29.2	27.3	25.1	2.44	2.87
	12	45.9	45.0	44.1	43.0	41.9	40.7	39.4	37.9	36.2	34.3	31.9	4.88	5.33
29.20	14	43.6	42.7	41.8	40.8	39.7	38.5	37.1	35.6	33.9	32.0	29.7	3.81	4.26
	16	41.7	40.9	39.9	38.9	37.8	36.6	35.3	33.8	32.1	30.1	27.8	3.05	3.49
	18	40.1	39.3	38.3	37.3	36.2	35.0	33.7	32.2	30.5	28.5	26.2	2.43	2.87
	12	48.0	47.1	46.1	45.0	43.8	42.5	41.1	39.6	37.8	35.7	33.3	4.92	5.38
30.82	14	45.6	44.7	43.7	42.6	41.5	40.2	38.8	37.2	35.4	33.4	30.9	3.85	4.30
	16	43.6	42.7	41.7	40.7	39.5	38.2	36.8	35.2	33.4	31.4	28.9	3.06	3.50
	18	4.19	41.0	40.0	39.0	37.8	36.5	35.1	33.5	31.7	29.7	27.2	2.43	2.87
	12	50.1	49.1	48.0	46.9	45.7	44.3	42.9	41.2	39.3	37.1	34.6	4.96	5.43
32.44	14	47.6	46.6	45.6	44.5	43.2	41.9	40.4	38.8	36.9	34.7	32.1	3.88	4.33
	16	45.5	44.6	43.5	42.4	41.2	39.8	38.3	36.7	34.8	32.6	30.1	3.05	3.49
	18	43.7	42.8	41.7	40.6	39.4	38.0	36.5	34.9	33.0	30.8	28.2	2.43	2.87
	12	52.1	51.1	50.0	48.8	47.5	46.1	44.5	42.8	40.8	38.5	35.8	5.00	5.46
34.06	14	49.6	48.5	47.4	46.3	45.0	43.6	42.0	40.3	38.3	36.0	33.3	3.90	4.35
	16	47.4	46.4	45.3	44.1	42.8	41.4	39.8	38.1	36.1	33.8	31.1	3.04	3.48
	18	45.5	44.5	43.4	42.2	40.9	39.5	37.9	36.2	34.2	31.9	29.2	2.43	2.87

TABLE 64

Process Times (B) at Retort Temperature of 260°F for Conduction-Heating Foods in 300 x 206 Can

f_h	z	INITIAL FOOD TEMPERATURE (T_{ih})											Equivalent	
		100	110	120	130	140	150	160	170	180	190	200	F_c^{18}	F_s^{18}
27.58	12	34.5	33.7	32.9	32.0	31.0	30.0	28.8	27.6	26.2	24.6	22.7	4.18	4.68
	14	33.6	32.8	32.0	31.1	30.1	29.1	27.9	26.7	25.3	23.7	21.8	3.50	3.99
	16	32.7	31.9	31.1	30.2	29.2	28.2	27.1	25.8	24.4	22.8	20.9	2.93	3.41
	18	31.8	31.0	30.2	29.3	28.3	27.3	26.1	24.9	23.5	21.9	20.0	2.40	2.87
29.20	12	36.3	35.5	34.6	33.7	32.7	31.6	30.3	29.0	27.5	25.8	23.9	4.28	4.79
	14	35.3	34.5	33.6	32.7	31.7	30.5	29.3	28.0	25.5	24.8	22.9	3.55	4.05
	16	34.4	33.5	32.7	31.7	30.7	29.6	28.4	27.1	25.6	23.9	21.9	2.95	3.43
	18	33.4	32.6	31.7	30.7	29.7	28.6	27.4	26.1	24.6	22.9	20.9	2.39	2.87
30.82	12	38.1	37.3	36.3	35.3	34.3	33.1	31.8	30.4	28.8	27.1	25.0	4.37	4.88
	14	37.0	36.1	35.2	34.2	33.2	32.0	30.7	29.3	27.7	25.9	23.9	3.58	4.08
	16	36.0	35.2	34.2	33.2	32.2	31.0	29.7	28.3	26.7	25.0	22.9	2.96	3.45
	18	35.0	34.1	33.2	32.2	31.1	30.0	28.7	27.3	25.7	23.9	21.8	2.39	2.87
32.44	12	39.9	39.0	38.1	37.0	35.9	34.7	33.3	31.8	30.2	28.3	26.1	4.45	4.96
	14	38.7	37.8	36.8	35.8	34.7	33.4	32.1	30.6	28.9	27.1	24.9	3.61	4.10
	16	37.7	36.7	35.8	34.7	33.6	32.4	31.0	29.5	27.9	26.0	23.8	2.97	3.46
	18	36.5	35.6	34.7	33.6	32.5	31.3	29.9	28.4	26.8	24.9	22.7	2.39	2.87
34.06	12	41.7	40.8	39.8	38.7	37.5	36.2	34.8	33.2	31.5	29.5	27.2	4.53	5.04
	14	40.4	39.5	38.4	37.3	36.2	34.9	33.5	31.9	30.2	28.2	25.9	3.64	4.14
	16	39.3	38.3	37.3	36.2	35.0	33.7	32.3	30.8	29.0	27.0	24.8	2.97	3.46
	18	38.1	37.2	36.1	35.0	33.9	32.6	31.2	29.6	27.9	25.9	23.6	2.39	2.87

TABLE 65

Process Times (B) at Retort Temperature of 230°F for Conduction-Heating Foods in 300 x 308 Can

f_h	z	INITIAL FOOD TEMPERATURE (T_{ih})											Equivalent	
		100	110	120	130	140	150	160	170	180	190	200	F_c^{18}	F_s^{18}
	12	195.0	193.6	192.2	190.6	188.9	186.9	184.7	182.1	179.1	175.4	170.7	10.29	10.59
38.12	14	136.9	135.5	134.1	132.5	130.8	128.8	126.6	124.1	121.0	117.3	112.6	5.90	6.19
	16	109.2	107.8	106.4	104.8	103.1	101.1	98.9	96.4	93.4	89.7	84.9	3.80	4.09
	18	93.8	92.4	91.0	89.4	87.7	85.7	83.5	81.0	77.9	74.2	69.5	2.60	2.90
	12	199.2	197.8	196.2	194.6	192.7	190.7	188.3	185.6	182.4	178.5	173.5	10.43	10.73
40.37	14	140.5	139.1	137.6	135.9	134.0	132.0	129.6	126.9	123.7	119.8	114.8	5.89	6.19
	16	112.7	111.3	109.8	108.1	106.2	104.2	101.8	99.1	95.9	92.0	87.0	3.81	4.10
	18	97.3	95.9	94.4	92.7	90.9	88.8	86.5	83.8	80.6	76.7	71.6	2.60	2.91
	12	203.1	201.6	200.0	198.3	196.3	194.1	191.7	188.8	185.4	181.3	176.0	10.40	10.72
42.61	14	143.8	142.4	140.7	139.0	137.0	134.9	132.4	129.5	126.2	122.0	116.7	5.87	6.19
	16	116.1	114.6	113.0	111.3	109.3	107.1	104.7	101.8	98.4	94.3	89.0	3.81	4.11
	18	100.8	99.3	97.7	96.0	94.0	91.8	89.4	86.5	83.1	79.0	73.7	2.60	2.91
	12	207.1	205.5	203.8	202.0	199.9	197.6	195.0	192.0	188.5	184.1	178.5	10.39	10.72
44.85	14	147.7	146.1	144.4	142.6	140.5	138.2	135.6	132.6	129.1	124.7	119.1	5.91	6.23
	16	119.6	118.1	116.4	114.5	112.5	110.2	107.6	104.6	101.0	96.7	91.1	3.82	4.13
	18	104.2	102.7	101.0	99.1	97.1	94.8	92.2	98.2	85.6	81.3	75.7	2.59	2.90
	12	210.6	209.9	207.2	205.3	203.1	200.7	198.0	194.8	191.1	186.5	180.6	10.38	10.71
47.10	14	151.4	149.7	147.9	146.0	143.8	141.4	138.7	135.5	131.8	127.3	121.4	5.93	6.24
	16	123.2	121.5	119.8	117.8	115.7	113.2	110.5	107.4	103.6	99.1	93.2	3.83	4.14
	18	107.6	105.9	104.2	102.2	100.1	97.6	94.9	91.8	88.0	83.5	77.6	2.59	2.90

TABLE 66

Process Times (B) at Retort Temperature of 240° F for Conduction-Heating Foods in 300 x 308 Can

f_h	z	INITIAL FOOD TEMPERATURE (T_{ih})											Equivalent	
		100	110	120	130	140	150	160	170	180	190	200	F_c^{18}	F_s^{18}
38.12	12	83.0	81.8	80.5	79.0	77.5	75.7	73.8	71.6	69.0	66.0	62.3	6.36	6.75
	14	74.6	73.3	72.0	70.6	69.0	67.2	65.3	63.1	60.5	57.5	53.8	4.62	5.00
	16	68.4	67.2	65.8	64.4	62.8	61.1	59.1	56.9	54.4	51.3	47.7	3.39	3.37
	18	63.7	62.4	61.1	59.7	58.1	56.3	54.4	52.2	49.6	46.6	42.9	2.53	2.90
40.37	12	86.7	85.4	84.0	82.4	80.8	78.9	76.9	74.5	71.8	68.6	64.7	6.48	6.88
	14	77.8	76.5	75.1	73.5	71.9	70.0	68.0	65.6	62.9	59.7	55.8	4.63	5.02
	16	71.4	70.1	68.7	67.1	65.5	63.6	61.6	59.2	56.5	53.5	49.4	3.38	3.76
	18	66.5	65.2	63.8	62.3	60.6	58.7	56.7	54.3	51.6	48.4	44.5	2.52	2.90
42.61	12	90.2	88.9	87.4	85.8	84.0	82.1	79.9	77,4	74.6	71.2	67.1	6.60	7.00
	14	81.0	79.7	78.2	76.6	74.8	72.9	70.7	68.2	65.3	62.0	57.8	4.67	5.06
	16	74.3	72.9	71.4	69.8	68.0	66.1	63.9	61.4	58.6	55.2	51.1	3.37	3.76
	18	69.3	67.9	66.4	64.8	63.1	61.1	58.9	56.5	53.6	50.2	46.1	2.52	2.90
44.85	12	93.7	92.3	90.7	89.0	87.2	85.1	82.8	80.2	77.2	73.7	69.3	6.72	7.11
	14	84.2	82.8	81.2	79.5	77.7	75.6	73.3	70.7	67.7	64.2	59.8	4.70	5.10
	16	77.3	75.8	74.3	72.6	70.7	68.6	66.4	63.8	60.8	57.2	52.9	3.38	3.77
	18	72.0	70.6	69.0	67.3	65.5	63.4	61.1	58.5	55.5	52.0	47.6	2.52	2.90
47.10	12	97.2	95.7	94.0	92.3	90.3	88.2	85.7	83.0	79.9	76.1	71.6	6.83	7.23
	14	87.4	85.9	84.2	82.5	80.5	78.4	76.0	73.2	70.1	66.3	61.8	4.74	5.14
	16	80.2	78.7	77.0	75.3	73.3	71.2	68.8	66.0	62.9	59.1	54.6	3.39	3.79
	18	74.8	73.3	71.7	69.9	67.9	65.8	63.4	60.6	57.5	53.8	49.2	2.52	2.90

TABLE 67

Process Times (B) at Retort Temperature of 250°F for Conduction-Heating Foods in 300 x 308 Can

f_h	z	INITIAL FOOD TEMPERATURE (T_{ih})											Equivalent	
		100	110	120	130	140	150	160	170	180	190	200	F^{18}_c	F^{18}_z
38.12	12	57.3	56.2	55.0	53.6	52.2	50.6	48.9	46.9	44.7	42.2	39.1	5.15	5.62
	14	54.6	53.4	52.2	50.9	49.4	47.9	46.1	44.2	42.0	39.4	36.4	4.01	4.47
	16	52.1	51.0	49.8	48.4	47.0	45.4	43.7	41.7	39.5	37.0	33.9	3.09	3.54
	18	50.0	48.8	47.6	46.3	44.8	43.3	41.5	39.6	37.4	34.8	31.8	2.46	2.90
40.37	12	60.2	59.0	57.7	56.3	54.8	53.1	51.2	49.2	46.8	44.1	40.9	5.23	5.70
	14	57.3	56.1	54.8	53.4	51.8	50.2	48.4	46.3	44.4	41.3	38.1	4.07	4.53
	16	54.7	53.5	52.2	50.8	49.3	47.6	45.8	43.7	41.4	38.7	35.5	3.12	3.57
	18	52.4	51.2	49.9	48.5	47.0	45.3	43.5	41.4	39.1	36.4	33.2	2.46	2.90
42.61	12	63.0	61.7	60.4	58.9	57.3	55.5	53.6	51.4	48.9	46.1	42.7	5.30	5.77
	14	60.0	58.7	57.4	55.9	54.3	52.5	50.6	48.4	45.9	43.1	39.7	4.10	4.56
	16	57.3	56.0	54.6	53.2	51.5	49.8	47.8	45.7	43.2	40.3	37.0	3.15	3.61
	18	54.8	53.6	52.2	50.7	49.1	47.3	45.4	43.2	40.7	37.9	34.5	2.46	2.90
44.85	12	65.8	64.4	63.0	61.4	59.7	57.9	55.8	53.5	50.9	47.9	44.4	5.34	5.82
	14	62.7	61.3	59.9	58.3	56.6	54.8	52.7	50.4	47.8	44.8	41.3	4.11	4.58
	16	59.8	58.5	57.0	55.5	53.8	51.9	49.9	47.6	45.0	42.0	38.4	3.18	3.64
	18	57.2	55.9	54.4	52.9	51.2	49.3	47.3	45.0	42.4	39.4	35.8	2.46	2.90
47.10	12	68.5	67.1	65.6	64.0	62.2	60.2	58.1	55.7	52.9	49.8	46.1	5.39	5.87
	14	65.3	63.9	62.4	60.7	59.0	57.0	54.9	52.5	49.7	46.6	42.8	4.13	4.60
	16	62.3	60.9	59.4	57.7	55.9	54.0	51.8	49.4	46.7	43.5	39.8	3.20	3.67
	18	59.6	58.1	56.6	55.0	53.2	51.3	49.1	46.7	44.0	40.8	37.1	2.46	2.90

TABLE 68

Process Times (B) at Retort Temperature of 260°F for Conduction-Heating Foods in 300 x 308 Can

f_h	z	INITIAL FOOD TEMPERATURE (T_{ih})											Equivalent	
		100	110	120	130	140	150	160	170	180	190	200	F_c^{18}	F_s^{18}
	12	46.3	45.3	44.1	42.9	41.6	40.1	38.5	36.8	34.9	32.6	30.1	4.80	5.31
38.12	14	44.7	43.6	42.5	41.3	39.9	38.5	36.9	35.2	33.2	31.0	28.5	3.75	4.25
	16	43.4	42.4	41.2	40.0	38.7	37.2	35.6	33.9	32.0	29.7	27.2	3.05	3.54
	18	42.1	41.0	39.9	38.7	37.4	35.9	34.3	32.6	30.6	28.4	25.9	2.42	2.90
	12	48.8	47.7	46.5	45.2	43.8	42.2	40.6	38.7	36.7	34.3	31.6	4.92	5.44
40.37	14	47.0	45.9	44.7	43.4	42.0	40.4	38.8	36.9	34.9	32.5	29.8	3.78	4.29
	16	45.6	44.5	43.3	42.0	40.6	39.1	37.4	35.6	33.5	31.1	28.4	3.05	3.55
	18	44.2	43.1	41.9	40.6	39.2	37.7	36.0	34.2	32.1	29.7	27.0	2.42	2.90
	12	51.3	50.1	48.8	47.4	45.9	44.3	42.6	40.6	38.4	36.0	33.1	5.02	5.54
42.61	14	49.3	48.1	46.8	45.5	44.0	42.4	40.6	38.7	36.5	34.0	31.2	3.82	4.33
	16	47.9	46.7	45.4	44.0	42.5	40.9	39.2	37.2	35.0	32.6	29.7	3.07	3.57
	18	46.4	45.2	43.9	42.5	41.1	39.4	37.7	35.7	33.6	31.1	28.2	2.42	2.90
	12	53.7	52.4	51.1	49.7	48.1	46.4	44.5	42.5	40.2	37.6	34.6	5.10	5.63
44.85	14	51.6	50.3	49.0	47.6	46.0	44.3	42.4	40.4	38.1	35.5	32.5	3.85	4.36
	16	50.0	48.8	47.4	46.0	44.4	42.7	40.9	38.8	36.5	33.9	30.9	3.07	3.57
	18	48.5	47.2	45.9	44.4	42.9	41.2	39.3	37.3	35.0	32.4	29.4	2.42	2.90
	12	56.1	54.8	53.4	51.9	50.2	48.4	46.5	44.3	41.9	39.2	36.0	5.18	5.70
47.10	14	53.9	52.6	51.2	49.6	48.0	46.2	44.3	42.1	39.7	37.0	33.8	3.89	4.40
	16	52.2	50.9	49.5	48.0	46.4	44.6	42.6	40.5	38.1	35.3	32.2	3.08	3.58
	18	50.6	49.3	47.8	46.3	44.7	42.9	41.0	38.8	36.4	33.7	30.5	2.42	2.90

TABLE 69

Process Times (B) at Retort Temperature of 230°F for Conduction-Heating Foods in 300 x 400 Can

f_h	z	INITIAL FOOD TEMPERATURE (T_{ih})											Equivalent	
		100	110	120	130	140	150	160	170	180	190	200	F_c^{18}	F_s^{18}
	12	200.7	199.3	197.7	196.0	194.1	192.1	189.7	186.9	183.7	179.7	174.6	10.47	10.77
40.91	14	141.7	140.3	138.7	137.0	135.1	133.1	130.7	127.9	124.7	120.7	115.6	5.91	6.22
	16	113.8	112.3	110.8	109.1	107.2	105.1	102.8	100.0	96.8	92.8	87.7	3.82	4.12
	18	98.3	96.9	95.4	93.7	91.8	89.7	87.3	84.6	81.4	77.4	72.3	2.61	2.92
	12	205.0	203.5	201.8	200.1	198.1	195.9	193.3	190.4	187.0	182.8	177.4	10.44	10.77
43.32	14	145.4	143.9	142.3	140.5	138.5	136.3	133.8	130.9	127.4	123.2	117.8	5.91	6.22
	16	117.5	116.0	114.3	112.6	110.6	108.4	105.8	102.9	99.5	95.3	89.9	3.83	4.13
	18	102.1	100.6	98.9	97.1	95.2	92.9	90.4	87.5	84.1	79.9	74.5	2.61	2.92
	12	209.1	207.5	205.8	203.9	201.8	199.5	196.8	193.8	190.2	185.7	180.0	10.44	10.77
45.73	14	149.5	147.9	146.2	144.3	142.2	139.9	137.2	134.1	130.5	126.1	120.4	5.95	6.26
	16	121.2	119.6	117.9	116.0	113.9	111.5	108.9	105.8	102.2	97.8	92.1	3.83	4.14
	18	105.7	104.1	102.4	100.5	98.4	96.1	93.4	90.4	86.8	82.3	76.6	2.61	2.92
	12	212.7	211.1	209.3	207.3	205.1	202.6	199.8	196.6	192.8	188.1	182.1	10.42	10.75
48.13	14	153.4	151.7	149.9	147.9	145.7	143.2	140.4	137.2	133.4	128.7	122.7	5.95	6.27
	16	125.2	123.5	121.7	119.7	117.5	115.0	112.2	109.0	105.2	100.5	94.5	3.86	4.17
	18	109.3	107.6	105.8	103.8	101.6	99.1	96.3	93.1	89.3	84.6	78.6	2.61	2.92
	12	216.1	214.3	212.4	210.3	208.0	205.4	202.5	199.1	195.1	190.2	183.9	10.41	10.74
50.54	14	157.2	155.4	153.5	151.4	149.1	146.5	143.6	140.2	136.2	131.3	125.0	5.96	6.28
	16	129.3	127.6	125.7	123.6	121.3	118.7	115.7	112.4	108.4	103.5	97.1	3.90	4.22
	18	112.7	111.0	109.1	107.0	104.7	102.1	99.2	95.8	91.8	86.9	80.6	2.61	2.92

TABLE 70

Process Times (B) at Retort Temperature of 240°F for Conduction-Heating Foods in 300 x 400 Can

f_h	z	INITIAL FOOD TEMPERATURE (T_{ih})											Equivalent	
		100	110	120	130	140	150	160	170	180	190	200	F_c^{18}	F_s^{18}
	12	87.6	86.3	84.9	83.4	81.7	79.8	77.7	75.3	72.6	69.4	65.4	6.53	6.93
40.91	14	78.7	77.3	75.9	74.4	72.7	70.8	68.7	66.3	63.6	60.4	56.4	4.66	5.05
	16	72.2	70.9	69.4	67.9	66.2	64.3	62.2	59.9	57.1	53.9	49.9	3.39	3.78
	18	67.3	65.9	64.5	63.0	61.3	59.4	57.3	54.9	52.2	49.0	45.0	2.54	2.92
	12	91.5	90.1	88.6	86.9	85.1	83.2	80.9	78.4	75.5	72.1	67.9	6.66	7.05
43.32	14	82.1	80.8	79.2	77.6	75.8	73.8	71.6	69.1	66.2	62.8	58.6	4.70	5.09
	16	75.3	73.9	72.4	70.8	69.0	67.0	64.8	62.3	59.4	55.9	51.7	3.39	3.78
	18	70.3	68.9	67.3	65.7	63.9	61.9	59.7	57.2	54.3	50.9	46.7	2.53	2.92
	12	95.2	93.7	92.2	90.4	88.5	86.4	84.1	81.5	78.4	74.8	70.3	6.78	7.18
45.73	14	85.6	84.1	82.5	80.8	78.9	76.8	74.5	71.8	68.8	65.1	60.7	4.73	5.14
	16	78.5	77.0	75.4	73.7	71.8	69.7	67.4	64.7	61.7	58.1	53.6	3.40	3.79
	18	73.2	71.7	70.1	68.4	66.5	64.4	62.1	59.4	56.4	52.8	48.3	2.53	2.92
	12	98.9	97.4	95.7	93.9	91.9	89.7	87.2	84.4	81.2	77.4	72.7	6.90	7.30
48.13	14	89.0	87.4	85.7	83.9	81.9	79.7	77.3	74.5	71.2	67.4	62.8	4.77	5.18
	16	81.6	80.1	78.4	76.6	74.6	72.4	69.9	67.2	63.9	60.1	55.5	3.41	3.81
	18	76.2	74.6	73.0	71.1	69.2	67.0	64.5	61.7	58.5	54.7	50.0	2.53	2.92
	12	102.5	100.9	99.1	97.2	95.1	92.8	90.2	87.3	83.9	79.9	75.0	7.01	7.41
50.54	14	92.3	90.6	88.9	87.1	84.9	82.6	80.0	77.1	73.7	69.7	64.8	4.80	5.21
	16	84.7	83.1	81.4	79.4	77.4	75.0	72.5	69.5	66.1	62.1	57.2	3.42	3.82
	18	79.1	77.5	75.7	73.8	71.7	69.4	66.8	63.9	60.5	56.5	51.6	2.52	2.92

TABLE 71

Process Times (B) at Retort Temperature of 250°F for Conduction-Heating Foods in 300 x 400 Can

f_h	z	INITIAL FOOD TEMPERATURE (T_{ih})											Equivalent	
		100	110	120	130	140	150	160	170	180	190	200	F_c^{18}	F_s^{18}
40.91	12	60.9	59.7	58.4	57.0	55.4	53.7	51.9	49.8	47.4	44.6	41.4	5.27	5.74
	14	58.0	56.8	55.5	54.1	52.5	50.8	48.9	46.9	44.5	41.7	38.5	4.10	4.56
	16	55.4	54.2	52.9	51.4	49.9	48.2	46.3	44.2	41.9	39.1	35.9	3.14	3.60
	18	53.1	51.8	50.5	49.1	47.6	45.9	44.0	41.9	39.5	36.8	33.5	2.47	2.92
43.32	12	63.9	62.6	61.3	59.7	58.1	56.3	54.3	52.1	49.6	46.7	43.3	5.33	5.81
	14	60.9	59.6	58.2	56.7	55.1	53.3	51.3	49.1	46.6	43.7	40.2	4.12	4.59
	16	58.1	56.8	55.4	53.9	52.3	50.5	48.5	46.3	43.8	40.9	37.5	3.17	3.63
	18	55.6	54.3	53.0	51.4	49.8	48.0	46.0	43.8	41.3	38.4	35.0	2.47	2.92
45.73	12	66.9	65.5	64.1	62.5	60.8	58.9	56.8	54.4	51.8	48.7	45.1	5.38	5.86
	14	63.8	62.4	60.9	59.3	57.6	55.7	53.6	51.3	48.6	45.6	41.9	4.14	4.61
	16	60.8	59.5	58.0	56.4	54.7	52.8	50.7	48.3	45.7	42.6	39.0	3.20	3.66
	18	58.2	56.8	55.3	53.8	52.0	50.1	48.0	45.7	43.1	40.0	36.4	2.47	2.92
48.13	12	69.8	68.4	66.8	65.2	63.4	61.4	59.2	56.7	53.9	50.7	46.9	5.43	5.91
	14	66.6	65.1	63.6	61.9	60.1	58.1	55.9	53.4	50.6	47.4	43.6	4.15	4.63
	16	63.5	62.0	60.5	58.8	57.0	55.0	52.8	50.3	47.5	44.3	40.5	3.23	3.69
	18	60.7	59.2	57.7	56.0	54.2	52.2	50.0	47.5	44.8	41.5	37.7	2.47	2.92
50.54	12	72.8	71.3	69.6	67.9	66.0	63.9	61.6	59.0	56.0	52.7	48.7	5.48	5.97
	14	69.4	67.9	66.3	64.5	62.6	60.5	58.2	55.6	52.7	49.3	45.3	4.19	4.66
	16	66.1	64.6	63.0	61.2	59.4	57.2	54.9	52.3	49.4	46.0	42.0	3.23	3.70
	18	63.2	61.7	60.1	58.3	56.4	54.3	52.0	49.4	46.5	43.1	39.1	2.47	2.92

TABLE 72

Process Times (B) at Retort Temperature of 260°F for Conduction-Heating Foods in 300 x 400 Can

f_h	z	INITIAL FOOD TEMPERATURE (T_{ih})											Equivalent	
		100	110	120	130	140	150	160	170	180	190	200	F_c^{18}	F_s^{18}
	12	49.4	48.3	47.1	45.7	44.3	42.8	41.1	39.2	37.1	34.7	32.0	4.96	5.48
40.91	14	47.6	46.5	45.2	43.9	42.5	40.9	39.2	37.4	35.3	32.9	30.2	3.81	4.32
	16	46.2	45.1	43.8	42.5	41.1	39.6	37.9	36.0	33.9	31.5	28.8	3.07	3.57
	18	44.8	43.6	42.4	41.1	39.7	38.1	36.4	34.6	32.5	30.1	27.4	2.43	2.92
	12	52.1	50.9	49.6	48.2	46.7	45.0	43.2	41.2	39.0	36.5	33.6	5.06	5.59
43.32	14	50.1	48.9	47.6	46.2	44.7	43.0	41.2	39.2	37.0	34.5	31.6	3.85	4.36
	16	48.6	47.4	46.1	44.7	43.2	41.5	39.7	37.8	35.5	33.0	30.1	3.09	3.59
	18	47.1	45.9	44.6	43.2	41.7	40.0	38.2	36.3	34.0	31.5	28.6	2.43	2.92
	12	54.7	53.4	52.0	50.5	49.0	47.2	45.3	43.2	40.9	38.3	35.2	5.15	5.68
45.73	14	52.5	51.2	49.9	48.4	46.8	45.1	43.2	41.1	38.8	36.1	33.0	3.88	4.39
	16	50.9	49.6	48.3	46.8	45.2	43.5	41.6	39.5	37.2	34.5	31.5	3.09	3.59
	18	49.3	48.1	46.7	45.2	43.6	41.9	40.0	37.9	35.6	32.9	29.9	2.43	2.92
	12	57.2	55.9	54.5	52.9	51.2	49.4	47.4	45.2	42.8	40.0	36.7	5.23	5.76
48.13	14	55.0	53.6	52.2	50.7	49.0	47.2	45.2	43.0	40.5	37.7	34.5	3.93	4.45
	16	53.3	51.9	50.5	48.9	47.3	45.4	43.5	41.3	38.8	36.0	32.8	3.10	3.61
	18	51.6	50.2	48.8	47.2	45.6	43.8	41.8	39.6	37.1	34.3	31.1	2.43	2.92
	12	59.8	58.4	56.9	55.2	53.5	51.6	49.5	47.2	44.6	41.7	38.3	5.30	5.84
50.54	14	57.5	56.1	54.5	52.9	51.2	49.2	47.2	44.8	42.3	39.3	35.9	3.99	4.51
	16	55.6	54.2	52.7	51.1	49.3	47.4	45.3	43.0	40.4	37.5	34.1	3.12	3.62
	18	53.8	52.4	50.9	49.3	47.5	45.6	43.5	41.2	38.6	35.7	32.3	2.43	2.92

TABLE 73

Process Times (B) at Retort Temperature of 230°F for Conduction-Heating Foods in 300 x 407 Can

f_h	z	INITIAL FOOD TEMPERATURE (T_{ih})											Equivalent	
		100	110	120	130	140	150	160	170	180	190	200	F_c^{18}	F_s^{18}
	12	204.4	202.9	20.13	199.5	197.6	195.4	192.9	190.1	186.7	182.5	177.2	10.48	10.81
42.76	14	144.7	143.2	141.6	139.9	137.9	135.7	133.2	130.4	127.0	122.8	117.5	5.92	6.24
	16	116.8	115.3	113.7	111.9	109.9	107.8	105.3	102.4	99.0	94.9	89.5	3.84	4.14
	18	101.3	99.9	98.2	96.5	94.5	92.3	89.9	87.0	83.6	79.5	74.1	2.62	2.93
	12	208.9	207.3	205.6	203.7	201.6	199.3	196.7	193.6	190.1	185.7	180.0	10.48	10.81
45.27	14	149.0	147.4	145.7	143.9	141.8	139.5	136.8	133.8	130.2	125.8	120.2	5.96	6.28
	16	120.7	119.1	117.4	115.5	113.5	111.2	108.5	105.5	101.9	97.5	91.9	3.85	4.16
	18	105.2	103.6	101.9	100.0	98.0	95.6	93.0	90.0	86.4	82.0	76.4	2.62	2.93
	12	212.8	211.1	209.3	207.3	205.2	202.7	199.9	196.7	193.0	188.3	182.4	10.46	10.79
47.79	14	153.1	151.4	149.6	147.7	145.5	143.0	140.3	137.1	133.3	128.6	122.7	5.98	6.29
	16	124.7	123.1	121.3	119.3	117.1	114.7	111.9	108.7	104.9	100.3	94.3	3.87	4.18
	18	108.9	107.3	105.5	103.5	101.3	98.8	96.1	92.9	89.1	84.5	78.5	2.62	2.93
	12	216.1	214.4	212.5	210.4	208.1	205.5	202.6	199.3	195.3	190.4	184.1	10.44	10.76
50.30	14	157.0	155.3	153.4	151.3	149.0	146.4	143.5	140.1	136.2	131.3	125.0	5.97	6.30
	16	129.1	127.3	125.4	123.4	121.1	118.5	115.6	112.2	108.2	103.3	97.1	3.91	4.23
	18	112.6	110.8	108.9	106.8	104.5	102.0	99.0	95.7	91.7	86.8	80.5	2.62	2.93
	12	220.9	219.0	217.0	214.8	212.4	209.7	206.7	203.1	198.9	193.8	187.2	10.53	10.86
52.82	14	161.2	159.4	157.4	155.2	152.8	150.1	147.0	143.5	139.3	134.2	127.6	6.01	6.33
	16	133.3	131.5	129.5	127.3	124.9	122.2	119.1	115.6	111.4	106.3	99.7	3.91	4.23
	18	116.1	114.3	112.3	110.1	107.7	105.0	101.9	98.4	94.2	89.1	82.5	2.62	2.93

TABLE 74

Process Times (B) at Retort Temperature of 240°F for Conduction-Heating Foods in 300 x 407 Can

f_h	z	INITIAL FOOD TEMPERATURE (T_{ih})											Equivalent	
		100	110	120	130	140	150	160	170	180	190	200	F_c^{18}	F_s^{18}
	12	90.7	89.3	87.8	86.2	84.4	82.5	80.3	77.8	74.9	71.5	67.4	6.65	7.04
42.76	14	81.4	80.0	78.6	76.9	75.2	73.2	71.0	68.5	65.7	62.3	58.1	4.70	5.10
	16	74.6	73.3	71.8	70.2	68.4	66.4	64.2	61.8	58.9	55.5	51.4	3.40	3.79
	18	69.6	68.2	66.8	65.1	63.4	61.4	59.2	56.7	53.9	50.5	46.4	2.54	2.93
	12	94.6	93.2	91.6	89.9	88.0	85.9	83.6	81.0	77.9	74.4	70.0	6.78	7.17
45.27	14	85.0	83.6	82.0	80.3	78.4	76.3	74.0	71.4	68.4	64.8	60.4	4.74	5.15
	16	78.0	76.5	74.9	73.2	71.4	69.3	67.0	64.3	61.3	57.7	53.3	3.41	3.80
	18	72.7	71.3	69.7	68.0	66.1	64.0	61.7	59.1	56.1	52.5	48.1	2.54	2.93
	12	98.5	96.9	95.3	93.5	91.5	89.3	86.9	84.1	80.9	77.1	72.5	6.90	7.30
47.79	14	88.6	87.0	85.4	83.6	81.6	79.4	76.9	74.2	71.0	67.2	62.6	4.78	5.19
	16	81.3	79.7	78.1	76.3	74.3	72.1	69.7	66.9	63.7	59.9	55.3	3.42	3.82
	18	75.8	74.3	72.6	70.8	68.8	66.7	64.2	61.4	58.2	54.5	49.8	2.54	2.93
	12	102.3	100.7	98.9	97.0	94.9	92.6	90.0	87.1	83.8	79.8	74.9	7.02	7.42
50.30	14	92.0	90.4	88.7	86.8	84.7	82.4	79.8	76.9	73.5	69.5	64.7	4.82	5.23
	16	84.5	82.9	81.1	79.2	77.2	74.9	72.3	69.4	66.0	62.0	57.1	3.43	3.83
	18	78.9	77.3	75.5	73.6	71.6	69.3	66.7	63.8	60.4	56.4	51.5	2.53	2.93
	12	106.1	104.4	102.5	100.5	98.4	95.9	93.2	90.2	86.6	82.5	77.3	7.05	7.46
52.82	14	95.5	93.8	91.9	89.9	87.7	85.3	82.6	79.6	76.0	71.8	66.7	4.84	5.25
	16	87.7	86.0	84.2	82.2	80.0	77.6	74.9	71.8	68.3	64.1	59.0	3.42	3.83
	18	81.9	80.2	78.4	76.4	74.2	71.8	69.1	66.0	62.5	58.3	53.2	2.53	2.93

TABLE 75

Process Times (B) at Retort Temperature of 250°F for Conduction-Heating Foods in 300 x 407 Can

f_h	z	INITIAL FOOD TEMPERATURE (T_{ih}) 100	110	120	130	140	150	160	170	180	190	200	Equivalent F_c^{18}	F_s^{18}
42.76	12	63.3	62.0	60.6	59.1	57.5	55.8	53.8	51.6	49.1	46.3	42.9	5.34	5.82
	14	60.3	59.0	57.6	56.1	54.5	52.7	50.8	48.6	46.1	43.3	39.9	4.13	4.60
	16	57.5	56.3	54.9	53.4	51.8	50.0	48.0	45.9	43.4	40.5	37.1	3.18	3.63
	18	55.1	53.8	52.4	50.9	49.3	47.6	45.6	43.4	40.9	38.1	34.7	2.48	2.93
45.27	12	66.4	65.0	63.6	62.0	60.3	58.4	56.4	54.0	51.4	48.4	44.8	5.39	5.87
	14	63.3	61.9	60.5	58.9	57.2	55.3	53.2	50.9	48.3	45.3	41.7	4.15	4.62
	16	60.4	59.0	57.5	56.0	54.3	52.4	50.3	48.0	45.4	42.3	38.8	3.21	3.67
	18	57.7	56.4	54.9	53.4	51.7	49.8	47.7	45.4	42.8	39.7	36.1	2.48	2.93
47.79	12	69.5	68.0	66.5	64.8	63.0	61.0	58.9	56.4	53.6	50.4	46.7	5.44	5.92
	14	66.2	64.8	63.2	61.6	59.8	57.8	55.6	53.2	50.4	47.2	43.4	4.17	4.64
	16	63.1	61.7	60.2	58.5	56.7	54.7	52.5	50.1	47.3	44.1	40.3	3.24	3.70
	18	60.4	58.9	57.4	55.7	53.9	52.0	49.8	47.3	44.6	41.4	37.6	2.48	2.93
50.30	12	72.5	71.0	69.4	67.6	65.7	63.7	61.4	58.8	55.9	52.5	48.5	5.49	5.98
	14	69.1	67.6	66.0	64.3	62.4	60.3	58.0	55.4	52.5	49.1	45.1	4.19	4.67
	16	65.9	64.4	62.8	61.0	59.1	57.1	54.8	52.2	49.3	45.9	41.9	3.24	3.71
	18	63.0	61.5	59.9	58.1	56.2	54.1	51.8	49.3	46.3	43.0	39.0	2.48	2.93
52.82	12	75.6	74.0	72.3	70.5	68.5	66.3	63.9	61.2	58.1	54.6	50.4	5.56	6.05
	14	72.1	70.5	68.8	67.0	65.0	62.8	60.4	57.7	54.6	51.1	46.9	4.24	4.72
	16	68.7	67.1	65.4	63.6	61.6	59.4	57.0	54.3	51.2	47.7	43.5	3.26	3.72
	18	65.6	64.1	62.4	60.5	58.5	56.3	53.9	51.2	48.2	44.6	40.4	2.47	2.93

TABLE 76

Process Times (B) at Retort Temperature of 260°F for Conduction-Heating Foods in 300 x 407 Can

f_h	z	INITIAL FOOD TEMPERATURE (T_{ih})											Equivalent	
		100	110	120	130	140	150	160	170	180	190	200	F_c^{18}	F_s^{18}
42.76	12	51.5	50.3	49.0	47.6	46.1	44.5	42.7	40.8	38.6	36.1	33.3	5.06	5.58
	14	49.5	48.3	47.0	45.7	44.2	42.6	40.8	38.8	36.6	34.2	31.3	3.85	4.36
	16	48.1	46.9	45.6	44.2	42.7	41.1	39.3	37.4	35.2	32.7	29.8	3.10	3.60
	18	46.6	45.4	44.1	42.7	41.2	39.6	37.8	35.9	33.7	31.2	28.4	2.44	2.93
45.27	12	54.2	52.9	51.6	50.1	48.5	46.8	45.0	42.9	40.6	37.9	34.9	5.15	5.67
	14	52.1	50.8	49.5	48.0	46.4	44.7	42.8	40.8	38.5	35.8	32.8	3.89	4.40
	16	50.5	49.2	47.9	46.4	44.9	43.1	41.3	39.2	36.9	34.3	31.2	3.10	3.60
	18	48.9	47.7	46.3	44.9	43.3	41.6	39.7	37.6	35.3	32.7	29.7	2.44	2.93
47.79	12	56.9	55.6	54.1	52.6	50.9	49.1	47.2	45.0	42.5	39.7	36.5	5.23	5.76
	14	54.7	53.3	51.9	50.3	48.7	46.9	44.9	42.7	40.3	37.5	34.3	3.93	4.45
	16	53.0	51.6	50.2	48.7	47.0	45.2	43.2	41.0	38.6	35.8	32.6	3.11	3.61
	18	51.3	49.9	48.5	47.0	45.3	43.5	41.5	39.3	36.9	34.1	30.9	2.44	2.93
50.30	12	59.6	58.2	56.7	55.0	53.3	51.4	49.3	47.0	44.4	41.5	38.2	5.31	5.84
	14	57.2	55.8	54.3	52.7	51.0	49.1	47.0	44.7	42.1	39.2	35.8	4.00	4.51
	16	55.4	54.0	52.5	50.9	49.1	47.2	45.1	42.8	40.3	37.3	34.0	3.13	3.63
	18	53.6	52.2	50.7	49.1	47.4	45.5	43.4	41.1	38.5	35.6	32.2	2.44	2.93
52.82	12	62.2	60.7	59.2	57.5	55.6	53.6	51.4	49.0	46.3	43.3	39.7	5.38	5.92
	14	59.8	58.3	56.8	55.1	53.2	51.2	49.0	46.6	43.9	40.9	37.3	4.04	4.56
	16	57.8	56.4	54.8	53.1	51.2	49.2	47.0	44.6	41.9	38.9	35.3	3.14	3.65
	18	56.0	54.5	52.9	51.2	49.4	47.4	45.2	42.8	40.1	37.0	33.5	2.44	2.93

TABLE 77

Process Times (B) at Retort Temperature of 230°F for Conduction-Heating Foods in 301 x 411 Can

f_h	z	INITIAL FOOD TEMPERATURE (T_{ih})											Equivalent	
		100	110	120	130	140	150	160	170	180	190	200	F_c^{18}	F_s^{18}
45.22	12	209.2	207.6	205.9	204.0	202.0	199.7	197.0	194.0	190.4	186.0	180.4	10.51	10.84
	14	149.2	147.6	145.9	144.0	141.9	139.6	137.0	134.0	130.4	126.0	120.4	5.98	6.29
	16	120.8	119.2	117.5	115.6	113.6	111.3	108.6	105.6	102.0	97.7	92.0	3.86	4.17
	18	105.2	103.7	101.9	100.1	98.0	95.7	93.1	90.0	86.5	82.1	76.4	2.62	2.94
47.88	12	213.4	211.7	209.9	207.9	205.7	203.3	200.5	197.3	193.5	188.9	182.9	10.50	10.83
	14	153.5	151.8	150.0	148.0	145.9	143.4	140.6	137.4	133.6	129.0	123.0	6.00	6.31
	16	125.0	123.4	121.6	119.6	117.4	114.9	112.2	109.0	105.2	100.5	94.5	3.88	4.19
	18	109.2	107.5	105.7	103.7	101.5	99.1	96.3	93.1	89.3	84.7	78.7	2.62	2.94
50.54	12	216.9	215.2	213.3	211.2	208.9	206.3	203.3	200.0	196.0	191.1	184.7	10.47	10.80
	14	157.7	155.9	154.0	151.9	149.6	147.0	144.1	140.7	136.7	131.8	125.5	5.99	6.32
	16	129.5	127.9	126.0	123.9	121.6	119.0	116.1	112.7	108.7	103.8	97.5	3.93	4.24
	18	113.0	111.3	109.4	107.3	105.0	102.4	99.4	96.1	92.1	87.2	80.8	2.62	2.94
53.20	12	221.9	220.1	218.1	215.9	213.4	210.7	207.6	204.1	199.9	194.7	188.1	10.57	10.90
	14	162.1	160.3	158.3	156.1	153.6	150.9	147.8	144.3	140.0	134.9	128.2	6.03	6.35
	16	134.1	132.3	130.3	128.1	125.6	122.9	119.8	116.3	112.0	106.9	100.2	3.92	4.25
	18	116.8	114.9	112.9	110.7	108.3	105.5	102.5	98.9	94.7	89.5	82.9	2.62	2.94
55.86	12	226.4	224.4	222.3	220.0	217.5	214.6	211.4	207.6	203.2	197.8	190.8	10.61	10.94
	14	166.4	164.4	162.3	160.0	157.4	154.6	151.3	147.6	143.2	137.8	130.8	6.04	6.37
	16	138.5	136.6	134.4	132.1	129.6	126.7	123.5	119.7	115.3	109.9	102.9	3.91	4.24
	18	120.4	118.4	116.3	114.0	111.5	108.6	105.4	101.6	97.2	91.8	84.8	2.62	2.94

TABLE 78

Process Times (B) at Retort Temperature of 240°F for Conduction-Heating Foods in 301 x 411 Can

f_h	z	INITIAL FOOD TEMPERATURE (T_{ih})											Equivalent	
		100	110	120	130	140	150	160	170	180	190	200	F_c^{18}	F_s^{18}
45.22	12	94.6	93.2	91.6	89.9	88.0	85.9	83.6	81.0	78.0	74.4	70.0	6.79	7.19
	14	85.0	83.6	82.0	80.3	78.4	76.3	74.0	71.4	68.4	64.8	60.4	4.76	5.16
	16	78.0	76.5	74.9	73.2	71.4	69.3	67.0	64.4	61.3	57.7	53.4	3.42	3.81
	18	72.7	71.3	69.7	68.0	66.1	64.0	61.7	59.1	56.1	52.5	48.1	2.55	2.94
47.88	12	98.7	97.2	95.5	93.7	91.7	89.5	87.1	84.3	81.1	77.3	72.7	6.92	7.32
	14	88.8	87.2	85.6	83.7	81.8	79.6	77.1	74.3	71.1	67.4	62.7	4.80	5.20
	16	81.5	79.9	78.2	76.4	74.5	72.3	69.8	67.0	63.8	60.0	55.4	3.44	3.83
	18	76.0	74.5	72.8	71.0	69.0	66.8	64.4	61.6	58.4	54.6	50.0	2.55	2.94
50.54	12	102.7	101.1	99.3	97.4	95.4	93.0	90.4	87.5	84.1	80.1	75.2	7.05	7.45
	14	92.4	90.8	89.1	87.1	85.1	82.7	80.2	77.2	73.8	69.8	64.9	4.83	5.24
	16	84.9	83.3	81.5	79.6	77.5	75.2	72.6	69.7	66.3	62.3	57.4	3.44	3.84
	18	79.3	77.6	75.9	74.0	71.9	69.6	67.0	64.0	60.7	56.7	51.8	2.54	2.94
53.20	12	106.8	105.0	103.2	101.2	99.0	96.5	93.8	90.7	87.2	83.0	77.8	7.08	7.49
	14	96.1	94.4	92.5	90.5	88.3	85.9	83.1	80.1	76.5	72.3	67.1	4.86	5.27
	16	88.3	86.6	84.7	82.7	80.5	78.1	75.3	72.3	68.7	64.5	59.3	3.43	3.84
	18	82.5	80.8	78.9	76.9	74.7	72.3	69.5	66.5	62.9	58.7	53.5	2.54	2.94
55.86	12	110.9	109.1	107.2	105.1	102.8	100.2	97.3	94.1	90.4	85.9	80.5	7.15	7.56
	14	99.8	98.0	96.0	93.9	91.6	89.1	86.2	83.0	79.2	74.8	69.4	4.88	5.29
	16	91.7	89.9	88.0	85.8	83.5	81.0	78.1	74.9	71.1	66.7	61.3	3.44	3.85
	18	85.7	83.9	81.9	79.8	77.5	74.9	72.1	68.8	65.1	60.7	55.3	2.54	2.94

TABLE 79

Process Times (B) at Retort Temperature of 250°F for Conduction-Heating Foods in 301 x 411 Can

f_h	z	INITIAL FOOD TEMPERATURE (T_{ih})											Equivalent	
		100	110	120	130	140	150	160	170	180	190	200	F_c^{18}	F_s^{18}
	12	66.4	65.0	63.6	62.0	60.3	58.4	56.3	54.0	51.4	48.4	44.8	5.41	5.89
45.22	14	63.2	61.9	60.4	58.9	57.2	55.3	53.2	50.9	48.3	45.2	41.7	4.16	4.63
	16	60.3	59.0	57.5	56.0	54.2	52.4	50.3	48.0	45.4	42.3	38.8	3.22	3.68
	18	57.7	56.4	54.9	53.4	51.6	49.8	47.7	45.4	42.8	39.7	36.2	2.49	2.94
	12	69.6	68.2	66.6	65.0	63.2	61.2	59.0	56.5	53.8	50.6	46.8	5.46	5.94
47.88	14	66.4	64.9	63.4	61.7	59.9	57.9	55.7	53.3	50.5	47.3	43.5	4.18	4.66
	16	63.3	61.9	60.3	58.6	56.8	54.9	52.7	50.2	47.4	44.2	40.4	3.25	3.71
	18	60.5	59.1	57.5	55.9	54.1	52.1	49.9	47.4	44.7	41.5	37.7	2.49	2.94
	12	72.9	71.3	69.7	68.0	66.0	63.9	61.6	59.1	56.1	52.7	48.7	5.51	6.00
50.54	14	69.5	68.0	66.3	64.6	62.7	60.6	58.3	55.7	52.7	49.4	45.4	4.21	4.69
	16	66.2	64.7	63.1	61.3	59.4	57.3	55.0	52.4	49.5	46.1	42.1	3.25	3.72
	18	63.3	61.8	60.1	58.4	56.5	54.4	52.1	49.5	46.5	43.2	39.2	2.49	2.94
	12	76.1	74.5	72.8	71.0	69.0	66.8	64.3	61.6	58.5	55.0	50.7	5.58	6.07
53.20	14	72.6	71.0	60.3	67.5	65.4	63.2	60.8	58.1	55.0	51.4	47.2	4.26	4.74
	16	69.2	67.6	65.9	64.0	62.0	59.8	57.4	54.7	51.6	48.0	43.8	3.27	3.74
	18	66.1	64.5	62.8	60.9	58.9	56.7	54.3	51.6	48.5	44.9	40.7	2.48	2.94
	12	79.4	77.7	75.9	74.0	71.8	69.5	67.0	64.1	60.9	57.1	52.7	5.65	6.14
55.86	14	75.7	74.0	72.2	70.3	68.2	65.9	63.3	60.5	57.2	53.5	49.1	4.31	4.79
	16	72.1	70.4	68.7	66.7	64.6	62.3	59.7	56.9	53.6	49.9	45.5	3.28	3.75
	18	68.8	67.2	65.4	63.4	61.3	59.0	56.5	53.6	50.4	46.6	42.2	2.48	2.94

TABLE 80

Process Times (B) at Retort Temperature of 260°F for Conduction-Heating Foods in 301 x 411 Can

f_h	z	INITIAL FOOD TEMPERATURE (T_{ih})											Equivalent	
		100	110	120	130	140	150	160	170	180	190	200	F_c^{18}	F_s^{18}
	12	54.2	52.9	51.5	50.1	48.5	46.8	44.9	42.9	40.6	37.9	34.9	5.16	5.69
45.22	14	52.1	50.8	49.4	48.0	46.4	44.7	42.8	40.8	38.4	35.8	32.8	3.90	4.41
	16	50.5	49.2	47.9	46.4	44.8	43.1	41.3	39.2	36.9	34.3	31.2	3.11	3.61
	18	48.9	47.7	46.3	44.8	43.3	41.6	39.7	37.6	35.3	32.7	29.7	2.45	2.94
	12	57.0	55.7	54.3	52.7	51.0	49.2	47.3	45.1	42.6	39.8	36.6	5.25	5.78
47.88	14	54.8	53.4	52.0	50.5	48.8	47.0	45.0	42.8	40.4	37.6	34.4	3.95	4.46
	16	53.1	51.7	50.3	48.8	47.1	45.3	43.3	41.1	38.7	35.9	32.7	3.12	3.63
	18	51.4	50.1	48.6	47.1	45.4	43.6	41.6	39.4	37.0	34.2	31.0	2.45	2.94
	12	59.9	58.4	56.9	55.3	53.5	51.6	49.5	47.2	44.6	41.7	38.3	5.33	5.87
50.54	14	57.5	56.1	54.6	53.0	51.2	49.3	47.2	44.9	42.3	39.4	36.0	4.01	4.53
	16	55.7	54.2	52.7	51.1	49.3	47.4	45.3	43.0	40.4	37.5	34.1	3.14	3.64
	18	53.9	52.5	51.0	49.3	47.6	45.7	43.6	41.3	38.7	35.7	32.4	2.45	2.94
	12	62.7	61.2	59.6	57.9	56.0	54.0	51.8	49.4	46.6	43.6	40.0	5.41	5.94
53.20	14	60.2	58.7	57.1	55.4	53.6	51.6	49.4	46.9	44.2	41.1	37.6	4.06	4.58
	16	58.2	56.7	55.1	53.4	51.6	49.6	47.4	44.9	42.2	39.1	35.6	3.16	3.66
	18	56.3	54.9	53.3	51.5	49.7	47.7	45.5	43.0	40.3	37.2	33.7	2.44	2.94
	12	65.5	63.9	62.3	60.5	58.5	56.4	54.1	51.6	48.7	45.5	41.7	5.50	6.04
55.86	14	62.9	61.4	59.7	57.9	55.9	53.8	51.5	49.0	46.1	42.9	39.1	4.11	4.63
	16	60.8	59.2	57.2	55.7	53.8	51.7	49.4	46.8	44.0	40.7	37.0	3.16	3.67
	18	58.8	57.2	55.6	53.8	51.8	49.7	47.4	44.8	42.0	38.7	35.0	2.44	2.94

TABLE 81

Process Times (B) at Retort Temperature of 230°F for Conduction-Heating Foods in 303 x 406 Can

f_h	z	INITIAL FOOD TEMPERATURE (T_{ih})											Equivalent	
		100	110	120	130	140	150	160	170	180	190	200	F_c^{18}	F_s^{18}
	12	212.3	210.7	208.9	206.9	204.8	202.4	199.6	196.5	192.7	188.2	182.3	10.51	10.84
47.10	14	152.3	150.6	148.9	146.9	144.7	142.3	139.6	136.5	132.7	128.2	122.3	6.00	6.31
	16	123.7	122.0	120.3	118.3	116.2	113.7	111.0	107.9	104.1	99.6	93.7	3.86	4.17
	18	108.1	106.4	104.6	102.7	100.5	98.1	95.4	92.2	88.5	83.9	78.1	2.63	2.94
	12	216.1	214.4	212.5	210.4	208.2	205.6	202.7	199.4	195.4	190.6	184.4	10.48	10.81
49.87	14	156.6	154.9	153.0	150.9	148.6	146.1	143.2	139.8	135.9	131.1	124.8	5.99	6.31
	16	128.5	126.8	124.9	122.8	120.5	118.0	115.1	111.8	107.8	103.0	96.7	3.92	4.23
	18	112.1	110.4	108.5	106.4	104.1	101.6	98.7	95.3	91.4	86.0	80.3	2.61	2.94
	12	221.0	219.2	217.2	215.0	212.6	209.9	206.8	203.3	199.2	194.1	187.5	10.56	10.88
52.64	14	161.2	159.4	157.4	155.2	152.8	150.1	147.1	143.5	139.4	134.3	127.7	6.02	6.35
	16	133.2	131.4	129.4	127.2	124.8	122.1	119.0	115.5	111.4	106.3	99.7	3.92	4.25
	18	116.0	114.2	112.2	110.0	107.6	104.9	101.8	98.3	94.2	89.1	82.5	2.62	2.94
	12	225.7	223.8	221.7	219.4	216.8	214.0	210.8	207.1	202.7	197.3	190.4	10.62	10.95
55.42	14	165.7	163.7	161.7	159.4	156.8	154.0	150.8	147.1	142.7	137.3	130.4	6.04	6.37
	16	137.8	135.9	133.8	131.5	128.9	126.1	122.9	119.2	114.8	109.4	102.5	3.91	4.24
	18	119.8	117.9	115.8	113.5	110.9	108.1	104.9	101.2	96.8	91.4	84.5	2.62	2.94
	12	230.2	228.2	226.0	223.6	221.0	218.0	214.6	210.7	206.1	200.5	193.2	10.59	10.94
58.19	14	170.1	168.1	165.9	163.5	160.9	157.9	154.5	150.6	146.0	140.4	133.1	6.05	6.38
	16	142.3	140.2	138.0	135.6	133.0	130.0	126.6	122.7	118.1	112.5	105.2	3.90	4.24
	18	123.5	121.5	119.3	116.8	114.2	111.2	107.8	103.9	99.3	93.7	86.4	2.62	2.94

TABLE 82

Process Times (B) at Retort Temperature of 240°F for Conduction-Heating Foods in 303 x 406 Can

f_h	z	INITIAL FOOD TEMPERATURE (T_{ih})											Equivalent	
		100	110	120	130	140	150	160	170	180	190	200	F_c^{18}	F_s^{18}
	12	97.5	96.0	94.4	92.6	90.6	88.5	86.1	83.3	80.2	76.5	71.9	6.89	7.28
47.10	14	87.7	86.2	84.5	82.7	80.8	78.6	76.2	73.5	70.3	66.6	62.0	4.79	5.19
	16	80.4	78.9	77.3	75.5	73.6	71.4	69.0	66.3	63.1	59.4	54.8	3.43	3.83
	18	75.0	73.5	71.9	70.1	68.2	66.0	63.6	60.9	57.7	54.0	49.4	2.55	2.94
	12	101.7	100.1	98.4	96.5	94.4	92.2	89.6	86.7	83.4	79.4	74.6	7.02	7.42
49.87	14	91.5	89.9	88.2	86.3	84.2	82.0	79.4	76.5	73.2	69.2	64.4	4.83	5.23
	16	84.0	82.4	80.7	78.8	76.7	74.5	71.9	69.0	65.7	61.7	56.9	3.44	3.84
	18	78.4	76.8	75.1	73.2	71.2	68.9	66.3	63.4	60.1	56.1	51.3	2.54	2.94
	12	105.9	104.2	102.4	100.4	98.2	95.8	93.1	90.0	86.5	82.3	77.2	7.07	7.48
52.64	14	95.3	93.6	91.8	89.8	87.6	85.2	82.5	79.5	75.9	71.8	66.7	4.86	5.27
	16	87.6	85.9	84.1	82.1	79.9	77.5	74.8	71.7	68.2	64.0	58.9	3.44	3.84
	18	81.8	80.1	78.3	76.3	74.1	71.7	69.0	66.0	62.4	58.3	53.2	2.54	2.94
	12	110.2	108.4	106.5	104.4	102.1	99.6	96.8	93.5	89.8	85.4	80.1	7.14	7.55
55.42	14	99.2	97.4	95.5	93.4	91.1	88.5	85.7	82.5	78.8	74.4	69.0	4.87	5.29
	16	91.1	89.3	87.4	85.3	83.0	80.5	77.7	74.4	70.7	66.3	61.0	3.44	3.85
	18	85.1	83.3	81.4	79.3	77.0	74.5	71.7	68.4	64.7	60.3	55.0	2.54	2.94
	12	114.5	112.6	110.6	108.4	106.0	103.3	100.4	97.0	93.1	88.5	82.8	7.21	7.63
58.19	14	103.0	101.1	99.1	96.9	94.5	91.8	88.8	85.5	81.6	77.0	71.3	4.89	5.31
	16	94.7	92.8	90.8	88.6	86.2	83.5	80.5	77.2	73.3	68.7	63.0	3.45	3.86
	18	88.4	86.6	84.6	82.4	79.9	77.3	74.3	70.9	67.0	62.4	56.8	2.54	2.94

TABLE 83

Process Times (B) at Retort Temperature of 250°F for Conduction-Heating Foods in 303 x 406 Can

f_h	z	INITIAL FOOD TEMPERATURE (T_{ih}) 100	110	120	130	140	150	160	170	180	190	200	Equivalent F_c^{18}	F_s^{18}
47.10	12	68.7	67.3	65.7	64.1	62.3	60.4	58.2	55.8	53.1	49.9	46.2	5.44	5.93
	14	65.5	64.0	62.5	60.9	59.1	57.2	55.0	52.6	49.9	46.7	43.0	4.18	4.65
	16	62.4	61.0	59.5	57.9	56.1	54.1	52.0	49.6	46.8	43.7	40.0	3.24	3.70
	18	59.7	58.3	56.8	55.1	53.4	51.4	49.3	46.8	44.1	41.0	37.2	2.49	2.94
49.87	12	72.0	70.5	68.9	67.2	65.3	63.2	61.0	58.4	55.5	52.2	48.2	5.49	5.98
	14	68.7	67.2	65.6	63.8	62.0	59.9	57.6	55.1	52.2	48.8	44.9	4.19	4.67
	16	65.5	64.0	62.4	60.6	58.7	56.7	54.4	51.8	49.0	45.6	41.7	3.25	3.71
	18	62.6	61.1	59.5	57.7	55.8	53.8	51.5	48.9	46.1	42.7	38.8	2.49	2.94
52.64	12	75.4	73.9	72.2	70.3	68.4	66.2	63.8	61.1	58.0	54.5	50.3	5.57	6.06
	14	72.0	70.4	68.7	66.9	64.9	62.7	60.3	57.6	54.5	51.0	46.8	4.25	4.73
	16	68.6	67.0	65.3	63.5	61.5	59.3	56.3	54.2	51.1	47.6	43.5	3.27	3.73
	18	65.5	63.9	62.2	60.4	58.4	56.2	53.8	51.1	48.1	44.5	40.4	2.48	2.94
55.42	12	78.8	77.2	75.4	73.5	71.4	69.1	66.5	63.7	60.5	56.8	52.4	5.64	6.13
	14	75.2	73.5	71.8	69.8	67.7	65.4	62.9	60.1	56.9	53.1	48.8	4.30	3.75
	16	71.6	70.0	68.2	66.3	64.2	61.9	59.3	56.5	53.3	49.6	45.2	3.28	3.75
	18	68.4	66.7	64.9	63.0	60.9	58.6	56.1	53.3	50.0	46.3	41.9	2.48	2.94
58.19	12	82.2	80.4	78.6	76.5	74.3	71.9	69.3	66.3	62.9	59.0	54.4	5.68	6.18
	14	78.4	76.7	74.8	72.8	70.6	68.2	65.5	62.5	59.1	55.2	50.6	4.35	4.84
	16	74.7	72.9	71.0	69.0	66.8	64.4	61.7	58.8	55.4	51.5	46.9	3.30	3.77
	18	71.2	69.5	67.6	65.6	63.4	61.0	58.3	55.3	52.0	48.1	43.5	2.48	2.94

TABLE 84

Process Times (B) at Retort Temperature of 260°F for Conduction-Heating Foods in 303 x 406 Can

f_h	z	INITIAL FOOD TEMPERATURE (T_{ih})											Equivalent	
		100	110	120	130	140	150	160	170	180	190	200	F_c^{18}	F_s^{18}
	12	56.2	54.9	53.5	51.9	50.3	48.5	46.6	44.4	42.0	39.3	36.1	5.22	5.75
47.10	14	54.0	52.6	51.2	49.7	48.1	46.3	44.3	42.2	39.8	37.1	33.9	3.92	4.44
	16	52.3	51.0	49.6	48.1	46.4	44.7	42.7	40.6	38.1	35.4	32.3	3.12	3.62
	18	50.7	49.4	47.9	46.4	44.8	43.0	41.1	38.9	36.5	33.8	30.6	2.45	2.94
	12	59.1	57.8	56.3	54.7	52.9	51.0	49.0	46.7	44.1	41.2	37.9	5.31	5.85
49.87	14	56.8	55.4	53.9	52.3	50.6	48.7	46.6	44.4	41.8	38.9	35.6	4.00	4.52
	16	55.0	53.6	52.1	50.5	48.8	46.9	44.8	42.6	40.0	37.1	33.8	3.14	3.64
	18	53.3	51.9	50.4	48.8	47.0	45.2	43.1	40.8	38.3	35.4	32.0	2.45	2.94
	12	62.1	60.6	59.0	57.3	55.5	53.5	51.3	48.9	46.2	43.2	39.5	5.39	5.93
52.64	14	59.7	58.2	56.6	54.9	53.1	51.1	48.9	46.5	43.8	40.8	37.2	4.05	4.57
	16	57.7	56.2	54.6	52.9	51.1	49.1	46.9	44.5	41.8	38.8	35.3	3.16	3.66
	18	55.8	54.4	52.8	51.1	49.3	47.3	45.1	42.7	40.0	36.9	33.4	2.45	2.94
	12	65.0	63.5	61.8	60.0	58.1	56.0	53.7	51.2	48.4	45.1	41.4	5.49	6.03
55.42	14	62.5	60.9	59.3	57.5	55.5	53.4	51.2	48.6	45.6	42.6	38.9	4.10	4.62
	16	60.4	58.8	57.1	55.4	53.4	51.3	49.0	46.5	43.7	40.5	36.7	3.16	3.67
	18	58.4	56.8	55.2	53.4	51.5	49.4	47.1	44.5	41.7	38.5	34.8	2.44	2.94
	12	68.0	66.4	64.6	62.7	60.7	58.5	56.1	53.4	50.5	47.1	43.2	5.58	6.12
58.19	14	65.2	63.6	61.9	60.0	58.0	55.8	53.4	50.7	47.7	44.4	40.5	4.14	4.67
	16	63.0	61.4	59.6	57.8	55.7	53.5	51.1	48.5	45.5	42.1	38.2	3.17	3.68
	18	60.9	59.3	57.5	55.7	53.7	51.5	49.0	46.4	43.4	40.0	36.1	2.44	2.94

TABLE 85

Process Times (B) at Retort Temperature of 230°F for Conduction-Heating Foods in 303 x 509 Can

f_h	z	INITIAL FOOD TEMPERATURE (T_{ih})											Equivalent	
		100	110	120	130	140	150	160	170	180	190	200	F_c^{18}	F_s^{18}
	12	219.3	217.5	215.6	213.4	211.1	208.5	205.5	202.1	198.0	193.0	186.6	10.56	10.89
51.26	14	159.5	157.7	155.8	153.7	151.3	148.7	145.7	142.3	138.2	133.3	126.9	6.05	6.37
	16	131.2	129.5	127.5	125.4	123.1	120.4	117.5	114.0	110.0	105.0	98.6	3.97	4.28
	18	114.4	112.6	110.7	108.6	106.2	103.6	100.6	97.2	93.1	88.2	81.8	2.65	2.96
	12	224.9	223.0	220.9	218.7	216.2	213.4	210.3	206.6	202.3	197.1	190.3	10.68	11.01
54.28	14	164.5	162.6	160.6	158.3	115.8	153.1	149.9	146.3	142.0	136.7	129.9	6.09	6.41
	16	136.3	134.4	132.4	130.1	127.6	124.9	121.7	118.1	113.8	108.5	101.7	3.95	4.28
	18	118.6	116.7	114.7	112.4	109.9	107.2	104.0	100.4	96.1	90.8	84.1	2.65	2.96
	12	229.8	227.8	225.7	223.3	220.7	217.7	214.4	210.6	206.1	200.5	193.3	10.68	11.02
57.29	14	169.3	167.3	165.1	162.7	160.1	157.2	153.9	150.0	145.5	139.9	132.8	6.09	6.42
	16	141.2	139.2	137.1	134.7	132.1	129.2	125.8	122.0	117.5	111.9	104.7	3.94	4.28
	18	122.7	120.7	118.5	116.2	113.5	110.6	107.3	103.4	98.9	93.4	86.2	2.65	2.96
	12	234.7	232.6	230.4	227.9	225.1	222.0	218.5	214.5	209.7	203.9	196.3	10.67	11.02
60.31	14	174.3	172.2	169.9	167.4	164.6	161.5	158.1	154.0	149.2	143.4	135.9	6.12	6.45
	16	146.1	144.0	141.7	139.2	136.4	133.4	129.9	125.8	121.0	115.2	107.7	3.94	4.28
	18	126.6	124.5	122.3	119.8	117.0	113.9	110.4	106.4	101.6	95.8	88.2	2.65	2.96
	12	239.2	237.0	234.6	232.0	229.1	225.8	222.2	217.9	212.9	206.8	198.9	10.64	10.99
63.33	14	179.1	176.9	174.5	171.9	169.0	165.7	162.0	157.8	152.8	146.7	138.7	6.15	6.48
	16	150.8	148.6	146.2	143.6	140.7	137.5	133.8	129.6	124.6	118.4	110.5	3.93	4.28
	18	130.4	128.2	125.9	123.2	120.3	117.1	113.4	109.2	104.2	98.0	90.1	2.65	2.96

TABLE 86

Process Times (B) at Retort Temperature of 240°F for Conduction-Heating Foods in 303 x 509 Can

f_h	z	INITIAL FOOD TEMPERATURE (T_{ih})											Equivalent	
		100	110	120	130	140	150	160	170	180	190	200	F_c^{18}	F_s^{18}
	12	104.0	102.4	100.6	98.7	96.5	94.2	91.6	88.6	85.2	81.1	76.1	7.12	7.52
51.26	14	93.6	92.0	90.2	88.3	86.1	83.8	81.2	78.2	74.8	70.7	65.7	4.88	5.29
	16	86.0	84.3	82.6	80.6	78.5	76.2	73.5	70.6	67.1	63.1	58.1	3.47	3.87
	18	80.3	78.6	76.9	74.9	72.8	70.5	67.8	64.9	61.4	57.4	52.4	2.57	2.96
	12	108.6	106.9	105.0	103.0	100.7	98.2	95.5	92.3	88.7	84.4	79.1	7.16	7.57
54.28	14	97.8	96.0	94.1	92.1	89.8	87.4	84.6	81.4	77.8	73.5	68.2	4.91	5.32
	16	89.8	88.1	86.2	84.1	81.9	79.4	76.6	73.5	69.9	65.6	60.3	3.46	3.87
	18	83.9	82.2	80.3	78.2	76.0	73.5	70.7	67.6	63.9	59.7	54.4	2.56	2.96
	12	113.3	111.5	109.5	107.3	105.0	102.3	99.4	96.1	92.3	87.7	82.2	7.24	7.65
57.29	14	102.0	100.1	98.1	96.0	93.6	91.0	88.0	84.7	80.9	76.3	70.8	4.92	5.34
	16	93.7	91.9	89.9	87.7	85.3	82.7	79.8	76.5	72.6	68.1	62.5	3.47	3.89
	18	87.5	85.7	83.7	81.5	79.2	76.5	73.6	70.3	66.5	61.9	56.4	2.56	2.96
	12	118.0	116.0	113.9	111.7	109.2	106.4	103.3	99.8	95.8	91.0	85.2	7.31	7.73
60.31	14	106.1	104.1	102.0	99.8	97.3	94.5	91.4	87.9	83.9	79.1	73.3	4.94	5.36
	16	97.5	95.6	93.5	91.2	88.7	86.0	82.9	79.4	75.3	70.6	64.7	3.49	3.90
	18	91.1	89.2	87.1	84.8	82.3	79.6	76.5	73.0	68.9	64.2	58.3	2.56	2.96
	12	122.5	120.5	118.3	115.9	113.3	110.4	107.1	103.5	99.2	94.2	88.1	7.38	7.81
63.33	14	110.1	108.1	105.9	103.5	100.9	98.0	94.8	91.1	86.8	81.8	75.7	4.96	5.38
	16	101.3	99.3	97.1	94.7	92.1	89.2	85.9	82.3	78.0	73.0	66.9	3.49	3.91
	18	94.7	92.6	90.4	88.0	85.4	82.5	79.3	75.6	71.4	66.4	60.2	2.55	2.96

TABLE 87

Process Times (B) at Retort Temperature of 250°F for Conduction-Heating Foods in 303 x 509 Can

f_h	z	INITIAL FOOD TEMPERATURE (T_{ih})											Equivalent	
		100	110	120	130	140	150	160	170	180	190	200	F_c^{18}	F_s^{18}
	12	73.8	72.3	70.6	68.9	66.9	64.8	62.5	59.8	56.9	53.4	49.4	5.57	6.05
51.26	14	70.4	68.9	67.2	65.4	63.5	61.4	59.0	56.4	53.4	50.0	45.9	4.25	4.73
	16	67.1	65.6	63.9	62.1	60.2	58.1	55.7	53.1	50.1	46.7	42.7	3.29	3.75
	18	64.1	62.6	60.9	59.2	57.2	55.1	52.8	50.1	47.2	43.7	39.7	2.51	2.96
	12	77.5	75.9	74.2	72.3	70.2	68.0	65.6	62.7	59.6	55.9	51.6	5.65	6.14
54.28	14	74.0	72.3	70.6	68.7	66.7	64.4	61.9	59.1	56.0	52.4	48.1	4.31	4.79
	16	70.5	68.8	67.1	65.2	63.2	60.9	58.4	55.7	52.5	48.9	44.6	3.30	3.77
	18	67.3	65.7	63.9	62.0	60.0	57.7	55.3	52.5	49.3	45.7	41.4	2.51	2.96
	12	81.2	79.5	77.6	75.7	73.5	71.1	68.5	65.6	62.2	58.4	53.9	5.72	6.22
57.29	14	77.5	75.8	73.9	71.9	69.8	67.4	64.8	61.8	58.5	54.7	50.1	4.37	4.85
	16	73.8	72.1	70.2	68.2	66.1	63.7	61.1	58.1	54.8	51.0	46.5	3.32	3.79
	18	70.4	68.7	66.9	64.9	62.7	60.3	57.7	54.8	51.5	47.6	43.1	2.50	2.96
	12	84.8	83.0	81.1	79.0	76.7	74.2	71.4	68.4	64.9	60.8	56.0	5.74	6.24
60.31	14	80.9	79.1	77.2	75.1	72.8	70.3	67.6	64.6	61.0	56.9	52.2	4.42	4.90
	16	77.1	75.2	73.3	71.2	68.9	66.4	63.7	60.6	57.1	53.1	48.3	3.33	3.81
	18	73.5	71.7	69.8	67.7	65.4	62.9	60.1	57.0	53.5	49.5	44.7	2.50	2.96
	12	88.4	86.5	84.5	82.3	79.9	77.3	74.4	71.1	67.4	63.2	58.2	5.77	6.27
63.33	14	84.4	82.5	80.4	78.2	75.8	73.2	70.3	67.1	63.4	59.2	54.2	4.47	4.96
	16	80.3	78.4	76.4	74.2	71.8	69.2	66.3	63.0	59.3	55.1	50.1	3.35	3.83
	18	76.6	74.7	72.6	70.4	68.0	65.4	62.5	59.3	55.6	51.4	46.4	2.50	2.96

TABLE 88

Process Times (B) at Retort Temperature of 260°F for Conduction-Heating Foods in 303 x 509 Can

f_h	z	INITIAL FOOD TEMPERATURE (T_{ih})											Equivalent	
		100	110	120	130	140	150	160	170	180	190	200	F_c^{18}	F_s^{18}
51.26	12	60.7	59.2	57.7	56.1	54.3	52.3	50.2	47.9	45.2	42.3	38.8	5.39	5.92
	14	58.3	56.9	55.3	53.7	51.9	50.0	47.8	45.5	42.9	39.9	36.5	4.06	4.57
	16	56.4	55.0	53.4	51.8	50.0	48.1	46.0	43.6	41.0	38.0	34.6	3.17	3.67
	18	54.6	53.2	51.6	50.0	48.2	46.3	44.2	41.8	39.2	36.2	32.8	2.47	2.96
54.28	12	63.9	62.3	60.7	59.0	57.1	55.0	52.8	50.3	47.5	44.4	40.7	5.48	6.02
	14	61.4	59.9	58.2	56.5	54.6	52.5	50.3	47.8	45.0	41.9	38.3	4.11	3.69
	16	59.3	57.8	56.2	54.4	52.5	50.5	48.2	45.8	43.0	39.8	36.2	3.19	3.69
	18	57.4	55.9	54.2	52.5	50.6	48.6	46.3	43.8	41.1	37.9	34.3	2.47	2.96
57.29	12	67.1	65.5	63.8	61.9	59.9	57.8	55.4	52.8	49.8	46.5	42.7	5.58	6.12
	14	64.4	62.8	61.1	59.2	57.3	55.1	52.7	50.1	47.2	43.8	40.0	4.16	4.69
	16	62.2	60.6	58.9	57.0	55.1	52.9	50.5	47.9	45.0	41.6	37.8	3.19	3.70
	18	60.2	58.6	56.9	55.0	53.0	50.9	48.5	45.9	42.9	39.6	35.8	2.47	2.96
60.31	12	70.3	68.6	66.8	64.8	62.7	60.5	58.0	55.2	52.1	48.6	44.6	5.68	6.22
	14	67.4	65.7	63.9	62.0	59.9	57.6	55.1	52.4	49.3	45.8	41.7	4.19	4.72
	16	65.1	63.4	61.6	59.7	57.6	55.3	52.8	50.1	47.0	43.5	39.4	3.22	3.73
	18	62.9	61.2	59.4	57.5	55.4	53.1	50.6	47.9	44.8	41.3	37.2	2.46	2.96
63.33	12	73.4	71.7	69.8	67.7	65.5	63.1	60.5	57.6	54.4	50.7	46.5	5.77	6.31
	14	70.4	68.6	66.7	64.7	62.5	60.1	57.5	54.6	51.3	47.7	43.4	4.22	4.74
	16	68.0	66.3	64.4	62.3	60.1	57.7	55.1	52.2	49.0	45.3	41.1	3.26	3.77
	18	65.7	63.9	62.0	60.0	57.8	55.4	52.7	49.8	46.6	42.9	38.7	2.46	2.96

TABLE 89

Process Times (B) at Retort Temperature of 230°F for Conduction-Heating Foods in 307 x 113 Can

f_h	z	INITIAL FOOD TEMPERATURE (T_{ih})											Equivalent	
		100	110	120	130	140	150	160	170	180	190	200	F_c^{18}	F_s^{18}
	12	157.1	156.4	155.6	154.7	153.7	152.7	151.4	150.0	148.3	146.3	143.7	10.09	10.37
21.09	14	108.4	107.7	106.9	106.0	105.1	104.0	102.8	101.4	99.7	97.6	95.0	5.73	5.98
	16	81.9	81.2	80.4	79.5	78.5	77.5	76.2	74.8	73.2	71.1	68.5	3.72	3.98
	18	67.3	66.5	65.7	64.9	63.9	62.8	61.6	60.2	58.5	56.5	53.8	2.61	2.86
	12	161.2	160.4	159.6	158.6	157.6	156.5	155.2	153.7	151.9	149.7	147.0	10.10	10.38
22.33	14	110.4	109.7	108.8	107.9	106.9	105.7	104.4	102.9	101.2	99.0	96.2	5.79	6.03
	16	83.8	83.0	82.2	81.3	80.2	79.1	77.8	76.3	74.5	72.4	69.6	3.71	3.97
	18	69.2	68.4	67.6	66.6	65.6	64.5	63.2	61.7	59.9	57.7	55.0	2.61	2.86
	12	165.0	164.2	163.3	162.3	161.2	160.0	158.6	157.1	155.2	152.9	150.0	10.10	10.39
23.57	14	112.4	111.6	110.7	109.7	108.6	107.4	106.0	104.5	102.6	100.3	97.4	5.75	6.03
	16	85.6	84.8	83.9	82.9	81.8	80.6	79.2	77.7	75.8	73.5	70.6	3.71	3.97
	18	70.9	70.1	69.2	68.2	67.2	66.0	64.6	63.0	61.1	58.9	55.9	2.61	2.86
	12	168.5	167.7	166.7	165.7	164.6	163.3	161.9	160.2	158.2	155.8	152.7	10.11	10.39
24.81	14	114.6	113.7	112.8	111.8	110.6	109.3	107.9	106.2	104.3	101.9	98.8	5.75	6.03
	16	87.7	86.8	85.9	84.8	83.7	82.4	81.0	79.3	77.4	75.0	71.9	3.72	3.99
	18	72.9	72.0	71.1	70.0	68.9	67.6	66.2	64.5	62.6	60.2	57.1	2.60	2.86
	12	171.8	170.9	169.9	168.8	167.7	166.3	164.8	163.1	161.0	158.5	155.2	10.11	10.40
26.05	14	116.6	115.7	114.7	113.6	112.4	111.1	109.6	107.8	105.8	103.3	100.0	5.75	6.03
	16	89.6	88.7	87.7	86.7	85.5	84.1	82.6	80.9	78.8	76.3	73.0	3.72	3.99
	18	74.7	73.8	72.8	71.7	70.5	69.2	67.7	65.9	63.9	61.4	58.1	2.60	2.86

TABLE 90

Process Times (B) at Retort Temperature of 240°F for Conduction-Heating Foods in 307 x 113 Can

f_h	z	INITIAL FOOD TEMPERATURE (T_{ih})											Equivalent	
		100	110	120	130	140	150	160	170	180	190	200	F_c^{18}	F_s^{18}
21.09	12	55.1	54.5	53-7	52.9	52.1	51.1	50.0	48.8	47.4	45.7	43.7	5.98	6.33
	14	49.3	48.6	47.9	47.1	46.2	45.3	44.2	42.9	41.5	39.9	37.8	4.28	4.64
	16	44.4	43.8	43.0	42.2	41.4	40.4	39.3	38.1	36.7	35.0	33.0	3.23	3.56
	18	41.1	40.5	39.7	38.9	38.1	37.1	36.0	34.8	33.4	31.7	29.7	2.53	2.86
22.33	12	57.3	56.6	55.9	55.0	54.1	53.1	51.9	50.6	49.1	47.4	45.2	6.02	6.38
	14	51.2	50.4	49.7	48.8	47.9	46.9	45.7	44.4	42.9	41.2	39.0	4.28	4.64
	16	46.3	45.4	44.8	43.9	43.0	42.0	40.8	39.5	38.0	36.3	34.1	3.27	3.60
	18	42.8	42.1	41.3	40.5	39.6	38.6	37.4	36.1	34.6	32.9	30.7	2.52	2.86
23.57	12	59.5	58.8	57.9	57.0	56.1	55.0	53.8	52.4	50.8	49.0	46.7	6.03	6.40
	14	53.0	52.2	51.4	50.5	49.5	48.5	47.2	45.9	44.3	42.4	40.2	4.29	4.64
	16	48.1	47.3	46.5	45.6	44.6	43.6	42.4	41.0	39.4	37.6	35.3	3.32	3.65
	18	44.5	43.7	42.9	42.0	41.1	40.0	38.8	37.4	35.8	34.0	31.7	2.52	2.86
24.81	12	61.6	60.8	60.0	59.0	58.0	56.9	55.6	54.2	52.5	50.5	48.1	6.03	6.41
	14	54.7	53.9	53.1	52.1	51.1	50.0	48.7	47.3	45.6	43.6	41.2	4.29	4.64
	16	49.9	49.1	48.2	47.3	46.3	45.1	43.9	42.4	40.8	38.8	36.4	3.33	3.67
	18	46.1	45.3	44.5	43.5	42.5	41.4	40.1	38.7	37.0	35.0	32.6	2.51	2.86
26.05	12	63.7	62.9	62.0	61.0	59.9	58.7	57.4	55.9	54.1	52.1	49.5	6.04	6.42
	14	56.4	55.6	54.7	53.7	52.6	51.4	50.1	48.6	46.8	44.8	42.3	4.28	4.64
	16	51.6	50.8	49.9	48.9	47.8	46.6	45.3	43.8	42.1	40.0	37.5	3.32	3.66
	18	47.8	46.9	46.0	45.0	43.9	42.8	41.4	39.9	38.2	36.1	33.6	2.51	2.86

TABLE 91

Process Times (B) at Retort Temperature of 250°F for Conduction-Heating Foods in 307 x 113 Can

f_h	z	INITIAL FOOD TEMPERATURE (T_{ih})											Equivalent	
		100	110	120	130	140	150	160	170	180	190	200	F_c^{18}	F_s^{18}
21.09	12	35.0	34.4	33.7	32.9	32.1	31.3	30.3	29.2	28.0	26.6	24.9	4.51	4.95
	14	33.2	32.6	31.9	31.2	30.4	29.5	28.5	27.5	26.2	24.8	23.2	3.57	4.00
	16	31.9	31.2	30.6	29.8	29.0	28.2	27.2	26.1	24.9	23.5	21.8	2.92	3.34
	18	30.8	30.1	29.5	28.7	27.9	27.1	26.1	25.0	23.8	22.4	20.7	2.45	2.86
22.33	12	36.7	36.0	35.3	34.5	33.7	32.7	31.7	30.6	29.3	27.8	26.0	4.57	5.01
	14	34.8	34.1	33.4	32.7	31.8	30.9	29.9	28.7	27.4	25.9	24.2	3.60	4.03
	16	33.4	32.7	32.0	31.2	30.4	29.5	28.4	27.3	26.0	24.5	22.7	2.93	3.36
	18	32.2	31.5	30.8	30.0	29.2	28.3	27.3	26.1	24.8	23.3	21.6	2.44	2.86
23.57	12	38.3	37.6	36.9	36.0	35.2	34.2	33.1	31.9	30.5	29.0	27.1	4.62	5.06
	14	36.4	35.7	34.9	34.1	33.2	32.3	31.2	30.0	28.6	27.0	25.2	3.62	4.06
	16	34.9	34.2	33.4	32.6	31.7	30.8	29.7	28.5	27.1	25.5	23.7	2.95	3.38
	18	33.6	32.9	32.2	31.4	30.5	29.5	28.4	27.2	25.8	24.3	22.4	2.44	2.86
24.81	12	40.0	39.3	38.5	37.6	36.7	35.6	34.5	33.2	31.8	30.1	28.2	4.67	5.11
	14	38.0	37.2	36.4	35.6	34.6	33.6	32.5	31.2	29.8	28.1	26.1	3.66	4.10
	16	36.4	35.7	34.9	34.0	33.1	32.0	30.9	29.6	28.2	26.5	24.6	2.96	3.39
	18	35.1	34.3	33.5	32.7	31.7	30.7	29.6	28.3	26.9	25.2	23.2	2.44	2.86
26.05	12	41.7	40.9	40.1	39.2	38.2	37.1	35.9	34.6	33.1	31.3	29.3	4.73	5.18
	14	39.6	38.8	38.0	37.1	36.1	35.0	33.8	32.5	31.0	29.2	27.2	3.71	4.15
	16	37.9	37.2	36.3	35.4	34.4	33.3	32.2	30.8	29.3	27.6	25.5	2.99	3.42
	18	36.5	35.8	34.9	34.0	33.0	31.9	30.8	29.4	27.9	26.2	24.1	2.44	2.86

TABLE 92

Process Times (B) at Retort Temperature of 260°F for Conduction-Heating Foods in 307 x 113 Can

f_h	z	INITIAL FOOD TEMPERATURE (T_{ih})											Equivalent	
		100	110	120	130	140	150	160	170	180	190	200	F_c^{18}	F_s^{18}
21.09	12	27.1	26.5	25.9	25.2	24.4	23.6	22.8	21.8	20.7	19.5	18.1	3.80	4.29
	14	26.6	26.0	25.3	24.7	23.9	23.1	22.2	21.3	20.2	19.0	17.6	3.34	3.82
	16	25.9	25.3	24.7	24.0	23.3	22.5	21.6	20.6	19.6	18.3	16.9	2.86	3.33
	18	25.3	24.7	24.0	23.4	22.6	21.8	21.0	20.0	18.9	17.7	16.3	2.40	2.86
22.33	12	28.5	27.9	27.2	26.5	25.7	24.9	24.0	22.9	21.8	20.5	19.0	3.88	4.37
	14	27.9	27.3	26.6	25.9	25.1	24.3	23.4	22.3	21.2	19.9	18.4	3.38	3.87
	16	27.2	26.6	25.9	25.2	24.4	23.6	22.7	21.6	20.5	19.2	17.7	2.87	3.34
	18	26.5	25.9	25.2	24.5	23.7	22.9	22.0	20.9	19.8	18.5	17.0	2.40	2.86
23.57	12	29.9	29.3	28.6	27.8	27.0	26.1	25.1	24.0	22.8	21.5	19.9	3.94	4.44
	14	29.3	28.6	27.9	27.1	26.3	25.4	24.5	23.4	22.2	20.8	19.2	3.43	3.91
	16	28.5	27.9	27.2	26.4	25.6	24.7	23.7	22.6	21.4	20.1	18.5	2.89	3.36
	18	27.8	27.1	26.4	25.6	24.8	23.9	23.0	21.9	20.7	19.3	17.7	2.40	2.86
24.81	12	31.3	30.6	29.9	29.1	28.2	27.3	26.3	25.1	23.9	22.4	20.8	4.01	4.51
	14	30.6	29.9	29.2	28.4	27.5	26.6	25.5	24.4	23.1	21.7	20.0	3.46	3.94
	16	29.8	29.1	28.4	27.6	26.7	25.8	24.8	23.6	22.4	20.9	19.3	2.90	3.38
	18	29.0	28.3	27.6	26.8	25.9	25.0	24.0	22.8	21.5	20.1	18.4	2.39	2.86
26.05	12	32.8	32.0	31.2	30.4	29.5	28.5	27.4	26.2	24.9	23.4	21.7	4.09	4.59
	14	31.9	31.2	30.4	29.6	28.7	27.7	26.6	25.4	24.1	22.6	20.8	3.48	3.96
	16	31.1	30.4	29.6	28.8	27.9	26.9	25.8	24.6	23.3	21.8	20.0	2.91	3.39
	18	30.3	29.5	28.7	27.9	27.0	26.0	24.9	23.7	22.4	20.9	19.2	2.39	2.86

TABLE 93

Process Times (B) at Retort Temperature of 230°F for Conduction-Heating Foods in 307 x 203 Can

f_h	z	INITIAL FOOD TEMPERATURE (T_{ih})											Equivalent	
		100	110	120	130	140	150	160	170	180	190	200	F_c^{18}	F_s^{18}
	12	178.2	177.2	176.2	175.0	173.7	172.2	170.6	168.7	166.4	163.7	160.1	10.19	10.48
28.40	14	120.4	119.4	118.3	117.1	115.8	114.4	112.7	110.8	108.6	105.8	102.3	5.77	6.05
	16	93.5	92.5	91.4	90.3	89.0	87.5	85.9	84.0	81.7	79.0	75.4	3.74	4.02
	18	78.4	77.5	76.4	75.2	73.9	72.5	70.8	68.9	66.7	63.9	60.4	2.61	2.88
	12	181.8	180.7	179.6	178.3	177.0	175.4	173.7	171.7	169.3	166.4	162.6	10.20	10.49
30.07	14	123.3	122.2	121.1	119.9	118.5	116.9	115.2	113.2	110.8	107.9	104.1	5.83	6.11
	16	96.2	95.2	94.1	92.8	91.4	89.9	88.1	86.1	83.8	80.8	77.1	3.75	4.03
	18	80.9	79.8	78.7	77.5	76.1	74.5	72.8	70.8	68.4	65.5	61.7	2.61	2.88
	12	184.9	183.8	182.6	181.3	179.9	178.2	176.4	174.3	171.8	168.7	164.7	10.20	10.50
31.74	14	126.0	124.9	123.7	122.4	120.9	119.3	117.5	115.3	112.8	109.8	105.8	5.81	6.10
	16	98.8	97.7	96.5	95.2	93.7	92.1	90.3	88.1	85.6	82.6	78.6	3.75	4.03
	18	83.4	82.3	81.1	79.8	78.3	76.7	74.8	72.7	70.2	67.1	63.2	2.61	2.88
	12	187.7	186.6	185.3	183.9	182.4	180.7	178.8	176.5	173.9	170.6	166.5	10.21	10.50
33.41	14	128.7	127.5	126.2	124.9	123.3	121.6	119.7	117.4	114.8	111.6	107.4	5.80	6.10
	16	101.4	100.2	99.0	97.6	96.1	94.4	92.4	90.2	87.5	84.3	80.1	3.76	4.04
	18	85.8	84.6	83.3	81.9	80.4	78.7	76.8	74.5	71.9	68.6	64.5	2.60	2.88
	12	190.1	188.9	187.6	186.1	184.5	182.7	180.7	178.3	175.5	172.1	167.8	10.21	10.50
35.08	14	131.1	129.9	128.6	127.1	125.5	123.7	121.7	119.3	116.6	113.2	108.8	5.79	6.09
	16	104.1	102.8	101.5	100.1	98.5	96.7	94.6	92.3	89.5	86.1	81.7	3.76	4.05
	18	88.5	87.3	86.0	84.5	82.9	81.1	79.1	76.7	74.0	70.6	66.2	2.59	2.88

TABLE 94

Process Times (B) at Retort Temperature of 250°F for Conduction-Heating Foods in 307 x 203 Can

f_h	z	INITIAL FOOD TEMPERATURE (T_{ih})											Equivalent	
		100	110	120	130	140	150	160	170	180	190	200	F_c^{18}	F_s^{18}
	12	67.7	66.8	65.8	64.7	63.5	62.2	60.8	59.1	57.2	55.0	52.2	6.10	6.49
28.40	14	60.2	59.3	58.3	57.2	56.1	54.8	53.3	51.7	49.8	47.5	44.8	4.41	4.77
	16	55.0	54.1	53.1	52.0	50.9	49.6	48.1	46.5	44.6	42.3	39.6	3.32	3.68
	18	51.0	50.0	49.1	48.0	46.8	45.5	44.1	42.4	40.5	38.3	35.5	2.53	2.88
	12	70.3	69.3	68.3	67.1	65.9	64.5	63.0	61.2	59.2	56.8	53.9	6.11	6.49
30.07	14	62.8	61.8	60.7	59.6	58.4	57.0	55.4	53.7	51.7	49.3	46.4	4.49	4.85
	16	57.3	56.3	55.3	54.1	52.9	51.5	50.0	48.2	46.2	43.8	40.9	3.31	3.67
	18	53.2	52.2	51.2	50.0	48.8	47.4	45.9	44.1	42.1	39.7	36.8	2.52	2.88
	12	72.8	71.8	70.7	69.5	68.2	66.8	65.1	63.3	61.2	58.6	55.6	6.12	6.50
31.74	14	65.3	64.2	63.1	61.9	60.6	59.2	57.5	55.7	53.6	51.1	48.0	4.56	4.92
	16	59.5	58.5	57.4	56.2	54.9	53.4	51.8	49.9	47.8	45.3	42.2	3.30	3.67
	18	55.4	54.4	53.3	52.1	50.7	49.3	47.7	45.8	43.7	41.2	38.1	2.52	2.88
	12	75.3	74.2	73.1	71.8	70.4	68.9	67.2	65.3	63.0	60.4	57.1	6.12	6.51
33.41	14	67.7	66.6	65.5	64.2	62.8	61.3	59.6	57.6	55.4	52.8	49.5	4.62	4.98
	16	61.8	60.7	59.6	58.3	56.9	55.4	53.7	51.8	49.5	46.9	43.6	3.33	3.70
	18	57.5	56.5	55.3	54.0	52.7	51.1	49.4	47.5	45.2	42.6	39.4	2.52	2.88
	12	77.8	76.7	75.5	74.1	72.7	71.1	69.3	67.3	64.9	62.1	58.7	6.15	6.54
35.08	14	70.1	69.0	67.8	66.4	65.0	63.4	61.6	59.5	57.2	54.4	51.0	4.60	4.97
	16	64.1	63.0	61.8	60.5	59.0	57.4	55.6	53.6	51.2	48.4	45.0	3.35	3.73
	18	59.7	58.5	57.3	56.0	54.5	52.9	51.1	49.1	46.7	44.0	40.6	2.51	2.88

TABLE 95

Process Times (B) at Retort Temperature of 250°F for Conduction-Heating Foods in 307 x 203 Can

f_h	z	INITIAL FOOD TEMPERATURE (T_{ih})											Equivalent	
		100	110	120	130	140	150	160	170	180	190	200	F_c^{18}	F_s^{18}
	12	44.9	44.0	43.1	42.1	41.0	39.9	38.6	37.1	35.5	33.6	31.3	4.87	5.32
28.40	14	42.6	41.8	40.9	39.9	38.8	37.6	36.3	34.9	33.2	31.3	29.1	3.81	4.25
	16	40.8	40.0	39.1	38.1	37.0	35.8	34.5	33.1	31.4	29.5	27.3	3.05	3.49
	18	39.3	38.4	37.5	36.5	35.5	34.3	33.0	31.5	29.9	28.0	25.7	2.45	2.88
	12	47.1	46.2	45.2	44.1	43.0	41.8	40.4	38.9	37.1	35.1	32.7	4.93	5.39
30.07	14	44.7	43.8	42.9	41.8	40.7	39.4	38.1	36.5	34.8	32.8	30.4	3.85	4.30
	16	42.8	41.9	41.0	39.9	38.8	37.5	36.1	34.6	32.9	30.9	28.5	3.08	3.52
	18	41.2	40.3	39.3	38.3	37.1	35.9	34.5	33.0	31.2	29.2	26.8	2.45	2.88
	12	49.2	48.3	47.2	46.1	44.9	43.6	42.2	40.6	38.7	36.6	34.1	4.97	5.43
31.74	14	46.8	45.9	44.8	43.7	42.5	41.2	39.8	38.1	36.3	34.2	31.7	3.89	4.34
	16	44.8	43.8	42.8	41.7	40.5	39.2	37.7	36.1	34.3	32.1	29.6	3.08	3.52
	18	43.0	42.1	41.0	39.9	38.7	37.4	36.0	34.4	32.5	30.4	27.9	2.45	2.88
	12	51.3	50.3	49.3	48.1	46.8	45.5	43.9	42.2	40.3	38.0	35.4	5.01	5.48
33.41	14	48.8	47.8	46.8	45.6	44.3	43.0	41.4	39.7	37.8	35.5	32.9	3.91	4.37
	16	46.7	45.7	44.6	43.5	42.2	40.8	39.3	37.6	35.6	33.4	30.8	3.06	3.51
	18	44.8	43.8	42.8	41.6	40.3	39.0	37.4	35.7	33.8	31.5	28.9	2.45	2.88
	12	53.4	52.4	51.3	50.0	48.7	47.3	45.7	43.9	41.8	39.5	36.7	5.05	5.52
35.08	14	50.8	49.8	48.7	47.4	46.1	44.7	43.1	41.3	39.2	36.9	34.1	3.93	4.39
	16	48.6	47.5	46.4	45.2	43.9	42.4	40.8	39.0	37.0	34.6	31.9	3.05	3.50
	18	46.6	45.6	44.4	43.2	41.9	40.4	38.8	37.0	35.0	32.7	29.9	2.44	2.88

TABLE 96

Process Times (B) at Retort Temperature of 260°F for Conduction-Heating Foods in 307 x 203 Can

f_h	z	INITIAL FOOD TEMPERATURE (T_{ih}) 100	110	120	130	140	150	160	170	180	190	200	Equivalent F_c^{18}	F_s^{18}
28.40	12	35.4	34.6	33.8	32.9	31.9	30.8	29.6	28.3	26.9	25.2	23.3	4.25	4.75
	14	34.5	33.7	32.8	31.9	30.9	29.9	28.7	27.4	25.9	24.3	22.4	3.55	4.04
	16	33.6	32.8	31.9	31.0	30.0	28.9	27.8	26.5	25.0	23.4	21.5	2.95	3.44
	18	32.6	31.8	31.0	30.1	29.1	28.0	26.8	25.5	24.1	22.4	20.5	2.41	2.88
30.07	12	37.3	36.5	35.6	34.6	33.6	32.4	31.2	29.8	28.3	26.5	24.5	4.35	4.86
	14	36.3	35.4	34.5	33.5	32.5	31.4	30.1	28.7	27.2	25.5	23.4	3.60	4.09
	16	35.3	34.4	33.5	32.6	31.5	30.4	29.1	27.8	26.2	24.5	22.5	2.97	3.46
	18	34.3	33.4	32.5	31.5	30.5	29.4	28.1	26.7	25.2	23.5	21.5	2.41	2.88
31.74	12	39.2	38.3	37.3	36.3	35.2	34.0	32.7	31.2	29.6	27.8	25.7	4.43	4.94
	14	38.0	37.1	36.2	35.1	34.0	32.8	31.5	30.1	28.5	26.6	24.5	3.61	4.11
	16	37.0	36.1	35.1	34.1	33.0	31.8	30.5	29.0	27.4	25.6	23.5	2.98	3.47
	18	35.9	35.0	34.1	33.0	31.9	30.7	29.4	28.0	26.3	24.5	22.4	2.41	2.88
33.41	12	41.0	40.1	39.1	38.0	36.9	35.6	34.2	32.7	31.0	29.0	26.8	4.52	5.03
	14	39.8	38.8	37.8	36.8	35.6	34.3	32.9	31.4	29.7	27.8	25.5	3.64	4.14
	16	38.7	37.7	36.7	35.6	34.5	33.2	31.8	30.3	28.6	26.7	24.4	2.99	3.48
	18	37.5	36.6	35.6	34.5	33.3	32.1	30.7	29.2	27.5	25.5	23.3	2.41	2.88
35.08	12	42.9	41.9	40.9	39.7	38.5	37.2	35.7	34.1	32.3	0.3	28.0	4.60	5.11
	14	41.5	40.5	39.5	38.3	37.1	35.8	34.3	32.7	30.9	28.9	26.6	3.68	4.18
	16	40.3	39.4	38.3	37.2	36.0	34.6	33.2	31.6	29.8	27.7	25.4	3.00	3.49
	18	39.1	38.2	37.1	36.0	34.8	33.4	32.0	30.4	28.6	26.6	24.2	2.40	2.88

TABLE 97

Process Times (B) at Retort Temperature of 230°F for Conduction-Heating Foods in 307 x 214 Can

f_h	z	INITIAL FOOD TEMPERATURE (T_{ih})											Equivalent	
		100	110	120	130	140	150	160	170	180	190	200	F_c^{18}	F_s^{18}
	12	197.8	196.4	194.9	193.3	191.5	189.5	187.2	184.5	181.4	177.6	172.7	10.40	10.69
39.38	14	139.1	137.7	136.2	134.6	132.8	130.8	128.5	125.8	122.7	118.9	114.0	5.90	6.20
	16	111.3	109.9	108.4	106.8	105.0	103.0	100.7	98.0	94.9	91.1	86.2	3.81	4.11
	18	95.8	94.5	93.0	91.3	89.5	87.5	85.2	82.6	79.5	75.7	70.7	2.61	2.91
	12	201.6	200.2	198.6	196.9	195.0	192.9	190.4	187.6	184.3	180.3	175.1	10.42	10.73
41.70	14	142.6	141.2	139.6	137.9	136.0	133.8	131.4	128.6	125.3	121.3	116.1	5.89	6.20
	16	114.8	113.3	111.8	110.0	108.1	106.0	103.6	110.8	97.5	93.4	88.2	3.81	4.11
	18	99.5	98.0	96.5	94.7	92.8	90.7	88.3	85.5	82.2	78.1	72.9	2.60	2.91
	12	205.9	204.3	202.7	200.9	198.8	196.6	194.0	191.1	187.6	183.3	117.8	10.41	10.74
44.01	14	146.4	144.9	143.2	141.4	139.4	137.1	134.6	131.6	128.1	123.9	118.4	5.91	6.22
	16	118.4	116.9	115.2	113.4	111.4	109.2	106.6	103.7	100.2	95.9	90.4	3.82	4.13
	18	103.0	101.5	99.8	98.0	96.0	93.8	91.2	88.3	84.8	80.5	75.0	2.60	2.91
	12	209.7	208.1	206.4	204.5	202.3	200.0	197.3	194.2	190.5	186.0	180.2	10.41	10.74
46.33	14	150.3	148.7	146.9	145.0	142.9	140.5	137.8	134.7	131.0	126.6	120.8	5.94	6.25
	16	121.9	120.3	118.6	116.6	114.5	112.2	109.5	106.4	102.7	98.2	92.4	3.83	4.13
	18	106.5	104.9	103.2	101.2	99.1	96.8	94.1	91.0	87.3	82.8	77.0	2.60	2.91
	12	213.0	211.4	209.5	207.5	205.3	202.8	200.0	196.7	192.9	188.1	182.1	10.38	10.71
48.65	14	153.9	152.2	150.4	148.4	146.2	143.7	140.8	137.6	133.7	129.0	122.9	5.93	6.25
	16	126.0	124.3	122.4	120.4	118.2	115.7	112.9	109.6	105.8	101.1	95.0	3.86	4.17
	18	109.9	108.2	106.4	104.4	102.1	99.7	96.8	93.6	89.7	85.0	78.9	2.60	2.91

TABLE 98

Process Times (B) at Retort Temperature of 240°F for Conduction-Heating Foods in 307 x 214 Can

f_h	z	INITIAL FOOD TEMPERATURE (T_{ih})											Equivalent	
		100	110	120	130	140	150	160	170	180	190	200	F_c^{18}	F_s^{18}
	12	85.1	83.8	82.5	81.0	79.4	77.6	75.5	73.3	70.6	67.5	63.7	6.44	6.83
39.38	14	76.4	75.1	73.7	72.2	70.6	68.8	66.8	64.5	61.9	58.7	54.9	4.62	5.01
	16	70.1	68.8	67.5	66.0	64.3	62.5	60.5	58.2	55.6	52.5	48.7	3.39	3.77
	18	65.3	64.0	62.6	61.2	59.5	57.7	55.7	53.4	50.8	47.7	43.9	2.53	2.91
	12	88.8	87.5	86.0	84.5	82.7	80.8	78.7	76.3	73.5	70.2	66.1	6.56	6.96
41.70	14	79.7	78.4	77.0	75.4	73.7	71.7	69.6	67.2	64.4	61.1	57.1	4.66	5.05
	16	73.1	71.8	70.3	68.8	67.0	65.1	63.0	60.6	57.8	54.5	50.4	3.38	3.77
	18	68.2	66.8	65.4	63.8	62.1	60.2	58.1	55.6	52.8	49.5	45.5	2.53	2.91
	12	92.5	91.1	89.5	87.9	86.1	84.0	81.8	79.2	76.3	72.8	68.5	6.68	7.08
44.01	14	83.1	81.7	80.1	78.5	76.7	74.6	72.4	69.8	66.9	63.4	59.1	4.70	5.10
	16	76.2	74.8	73.2	71.6	69.7	67.7	65.5	62.9	60.0	56.5	52.2	3.38	3.77
	18	71.1	69.6	68.1	66.4	64.6	62.6	60.4	57.8	54.9	51.4	47.1	2.52	2.91
	12	96.1	94.6	93.0	91.2	89.3	87.2	84.8	82.1	79.0	75.4	70.9	6.80	7.20
46.33	14	86.4	84.9	83.3	81.5	79.6	77.5	75.1	72.4	60.3	65.7	61.2	4.73	5.14
	16	79.2	77.7	76.1	74.4	72.5	70.3	68.0	65.3	62.2	58.5	54.0	3.39	3.79
	18	73.9	72.4	70.8	69.1	67.1	65.0	62.7	60.0	56.9	53.2	48.7	2.52	2.91
	12	99.6	98.0	96.3	94.5	92.5	90.3	87.8	85.0	81.7	77.9	73.1	6.91	7.31
48.65	14	89.6	88.0	86.3	84.5	82.5	80.3	77.8	75.0	71.7	67.8	63.1	4.77	5.17
	16	82.2	80.7	79.0	77.2	75.1	72.9	70.4	67.6	64.3	60.5	55.8	3.41	3.80
	18	76.8	75.2	73.5	71.7	69.7	67.4	64.9	62.1	58.9	55.0	50.3	2.52	2.91

TABLE 99

Process Times (B) at Retort Temperature of 250°F for Conduction-Heating Foods in 307 x 214 Can

f_h	z	INITIAL FOOD TEMPERATURE (T_{ih})											Equivalent	
		100	110	120	130	140	150	160	170	180	190	200	F_c^{18}	F_s^{18}
39.38	12	59.0	57.8	56.5	55.1	53.7	52.0	50.2	48.2	45.9	43.3	40.2	5.20	5.68
	14	56.1	55.0	53.7	53.7	50.8	49.2	47.4	45.4	43.1	40.5	37.3	4.05	4.51
	16	53.6	52.4	51.2	49.8	48.3	46.7	44.9	42.9	40.6	37.9	34.8	3.11	3.56
	18	51.4	50.2	48.9	47.6	46.1	44.4	42.6	40.6	38.3	35.7	32.6	2.47	2.91
41.70	12	61.9	60.6	59.3	57.8	56.3	54.5	52.6	50.5	48.1	45.3	42.0	5.28	5.75
	14	58.9	57.7	56.4	54.9	53.3	51.6	49.7	47.6	45.1	42.4	39.0	4.10	4.56
	16	56.3	55.0	53.7	52.2	50.7	48.9	47.0	44.9	42.5	39.7	36.4	3.14	3.60
	18	53.9	52.6	51.3	49.8	48.3	46.5	44.6	42.5	40.1	37.3	34.0	2.47	2.91
44.01	12	64.8	63.5	62.0	60.5	58.8	57.0	55.0	52.8	50.2	47.3	43.8	5.34	5.81
	14	61.7	60.4	59.0	57.4	55.8	54.0	51.9	49.7	47.1	44.2	40.7	4.11	4.58
	16	58.9	57.6	56.2	54.6	53.0	51.1	49.1	46.9	44.3	41.4	37.9	3.17	3.63
	18	56.4	55.0	53.6	52.1	50.4	48.6	46.6	44.3	41.8	38.8	35.4	2.46	2.91
46.33	12	67.6	66.2	64.7	63.1	61.4	59.5	57.3	55.0	52.3	49.2	45.4	5.38	5.86
	14	64.4	63.1	61.6	60.0	58.2	56.3	54.2	51.8	49.1	46.0	42.3	4.13	4.60
	16	61.5	60.1	58.6	57.0	55.2	53.3	51.2	48.8	46.1	43.0	39.4	3.20	3.66
	18	58.8	57.4	55.9	54.3	52.5	50.6	48.5	46.1	43.5	40.3	36.7	2.46	2.91
48.65	12	70.4	69.0	67.4	65.7	63.9	61.9	59.6	57.1	54.3	51.1	47.2	5.42	5.91
	14	67.1	65.7	64.1	62.4	60.6	58.6	56.3	53.9	51.0	47.8	43.9	4.15	4.62
	16	64.0	62.6	61.0	59.3	57.5	55.4	53.2	50.7	47.9	44.7	40.8	3.22	3.68
	18	61.2	59.7	58.2	56.5	54.6	52.6	50.4	47.9	45.1	41.8	38.0	2.46	2.91

TABLE 100

Process Times (B) at Retort Temperature of 260°F for Conduction-Heating Foods in 307 x 214 Can

f_h	z	INITIAL FOOD TEMPERATURE (T_{ih})											Equivalent	
		100	110	120	130	140	150	160	170	180	190	200	F_c^{18}	F_s^{18}
39.38	12	47.7	46.6	45.4	44.2	42.8	41.3	39.7	37.9	35.9	33.6	31.0	4.87	5.39
	14	46.0	44.9	43.7	42.5	41.1	39.6	38.0	36.2	34.2	31.9	29.2	3.78	4.28
	16	44.7	43.6	42.4	41.1	39.8	38.3	36.6	34.8	32.8	30.5	27.9	3.06	3.55
	18	43.3	42.2	41.0	39.8	38.4	36.9	35.3	33.5	31.5	29.2	26.5	2.43	2.91
41.70	12	50.3	49.1	47.9	46.5	45.1	43.5	41.8	39.9	37.7	35.3	32.5	4.99	5.51
	14	48.4	47.2	46.0	44.6	43.2	41.6	39.9	38.0	35.8	33.4	30.6	3.81	4.32
	16	47.0	45.8	44.6	43.2	41.8	40.2	38.5	36.6	34.4	32.0	29.2	3.07	3.57
	18	45.5	44.4	43.1	41.8	40.3	38.7	37.0	35.1	33.0	30.6	27.8	2.43	2.91
44.01	12	52.8	51.6	50.3	48.8	47.3	45.6	43.8	41.8	39.6	37.0	34.1	5.08	5.60
	14	50.8	49.5	48.2	46.8	45.3	43.6	41.8	39.8	37.5	35.0	32.0	3.85	3.58
	16	49.2	48.0	46.7	45.3	43.7	42.1	40.3	38.2	36.0	33.4	30.5	3.08	3.58
	18	47.7	46.5	45.2	43.8	42.2	40.6	38.7	36.7	34.5	31.9	29.0	2.42	2.91
46.33	12	55.3	54.0	52.6	51.1	49.5	47.8	45.8	43.7	41.4	38.7	35.6	5.16	5.69
	14	53.1	51.8	50.4	48.9	47.3	45.6	43.7	41.5	39.2	36.5	33.4	3.87	4.39
	16	51.5	50.2	48.8	47.3	45.7	44.0	42.0	39.9	37.6	34.9	31.8	3.08	3.59
	18	49.9	48.6	47.2	45.7	44.1	42.3	40.4	38.3	35.9	33.3	30.1	2.42	2.91
48.65	12	57.8	56.4	55.0	53.4	51.7	49.9	47.8	45.6	43.1	40.3	37.1	5.23	5.76
	14	55.5	54.1	52.7	51.1	49.4	47.6	45.6	43.4	40.9	38.0	34.8	3.94	4.45
	16	53.8	52.4	50.9	49.4	47.7	45.8	43.8	41.6	39.1	36.3	33.0	3.10	3.60
	18	52.0	50.7	49.2	47.7	46.0	44.1	42.1	39.9	37.4	34.6	31.3	2.42	2.91

TABLE 101

Process Times (B) at Retort Temperature of 230°F for Conduction-Heating Foods in 307 x 306 Can

f_h	z	INITIAL FOOD TEMPERATURE (T_{ih}) 100	110	120	130	140	150	160	170	180	190	200	Equivalent F_c^{18}	F_s^{18}
45.31	12	208.8	207.3	205.5	203.7	201.6	199.3	196.7	193.6	190.0	185.6	180.0	10.47	10.80
	14	149.0	147.5	145.7	143.9	141.8	139.5	136.8	133.8	130.2	125.8	120.2	5.96	6.27
	16	120.7	119.2	117.4	115.6	113.5	111.2	108.5	105.5	101.9	97.5	91.9	3.85	4.16
	18	105.2	103.6	101.9	100.1	98.0	95.7	93.0	90.0	86.4	82.0	76.4	2.61	2.93
47.98	12	213.0	211.3	209.5	207.5	205.3	202.8	200.1	196.9	193.1	188.4	182.4	10.45	10.78
	14	153.3	151.7	149.9	147.9	145.7	143.2	140.4	137.2	133.4	128.8	112.8	5.97	6.29
	16	125.0	123.4	121.6	119.6	117.4	114.9	112.1	108.9	105.1	100.5	94.5	3.87	4.18
	18	109.2	107.5	105.7	103.7	101.5	99.1	96.3	93.1	89.3	84.6	78.6	2.61	2.93
50.64	12	216.6	214.9	213.0	210.9	208.6	206.0	203.0	199.6	195.6	190.7	184.4	10.44	10.77
	14	157.6	155.8	153.9	151.8	149.5	146.9	144.0	140.6	136.6	131.6	125.3	5.97	6.30
	16	129.6	127.9	126.0	123.9	121.6	119.0	116.0	112.6	108.6	103.7	97.4	3.92	4.23
	18	113.0	111.3	109.3	107.2	104.9	102.3	99.4	96.0	92.0	87.1	80.8	2.61	2.93
53.31	12	221.6	219.8	217.8	215.5	213.1	210.4	207.3	203.7	199.5	194.3	187.7	10.54	10.87
	14	162.0	160.2	158.1	155.9	153.5	150.8	147.7	114.1	139.9	134.7	128.1	6.01	6.33
	16	134.1	132.3	130.3	128.0	125.6	122.9	119.8	116.2	112.0	106.8	100.2	3.90	4.23
	18	116.7	114.9	112.9	110.7	108.2	105.5	102.4	98.8	94.6	89.5	82.8	2.61	2.93
55.97	12	226.0	224.1	222.0	219.7	217.1	214.2	211.0	207.3	202.8	197.4	190.4	10.56	10.90
	14	166.2	164.3	162.2	159.8	157.3	154.4	151.2	147.4	143.0	137.6	130.6	6.02	6.35
	16	138.5	136.5	134.4	132.1	129.6	126.7	123.4	119.7	115.3	109.8	102.8	3.89	4.23
	18	120.4	118.4	116.3	114.0	111.4	108.6	105.3	101.6	97.1	91.7	84.7	2.61	2.93

TABLE 102

Process Times (B) at Retort Temperature of 240°F for Conduction-Heating Foods in 307 x 306 Can

f_h	z	INITIAL FOOD TEMPERATURE (T_{ih})											Equivalent	
		100	110	120	130	140	150	160	170	180	190	200	F_c^{18}	F_s^{18}
45.31	12	94.7	93.2	91.6	89.9	88.0	86.0	83.6	81.0	78.0	74.4	70.0	6.78	7.17
	14	85.1	83.6	82.0	80.3	78.4	76.4	74.0	71.4	68.4	64.8	60.4	4.74	5.14
	16	78.0	76.6	75.0	73.3	71.4	69.3	67.0	64.4	61.3	57.7	53.4	3.41	3.80
	18	72.7	71.3	69.7	68.0	66.1	64.1	61.7	59.1	56.1	52.5	48.1	2.54	2.93
47.98	12	98.7	97.2	95.5	93.7	91.7	89.5	87.1	84.3	81.1	77.3	72.6	6.91	7.31
	14	88.8	87.3	85.6	83.8	81.8	79.6	77.1	74.4	71.2	67.4	62.7	4.78	5.19
	16	81.5	80.0	78.3	76.5	74.5	72.3	69.8	67.1	63.8	60.0	55.4	3.42	3.82
	18	76.1	74.5	72.8	71.0	69.0	66.8	64.4	61.6	58.4	54.6	49.9	2.54	2.93
50.64	12	102.8	101.1	99.4	97.5	95.4	93.0	90.5	87.5	84.1	80.1	75.2	7.03	7.43
	14	92.5	90.9	89.1	87.2	85.1	82.8	80.2	77.2	73.9	69.8	64.9	4.82	5.23
	16	84.9	83.3	81.5	79.6	77.5	75.2	72.6	69.7	66.3	62.3	57.4	3.43	3.83
	18	79.3	77.7	75.9	74.0	71.9	69.6	67.0	64.1	60.7	56.7	51.8	2.53	2.93
53.31	12	106.8	105.1	103.3	101.2	99.0	96.6	93.9	90.8	87.2	83.0	77.8	7.06	7.47
	14	96.1	94.4	92.6	90.5	88.3	85.9	83.2	80.1	76.5	72.3	67.1	4.84	5.25
	16	88.3	86.6	84.8	82.7	80.5	78.1	75.4	72.3	68.7	64.5	59.3	3.42	3.82
	18	82.5	80.8	79.0	76.9	74.7	72.3	69.6	66.5	62.9	58.7	53.5	2.53	2.93
55.97	12	111.0	109.2	107.2	105.1	102.8	100.2	97.4	94.1	90.4	86.0	80.5	7.13	7.54
	14	99.8	98.0	96.1	94.0	91.7	89.1	86.2	83.0	79.2	74.8	69.4	4.86	5.27
	16	91.8	90.0	88.0	85.9	83.6	81.0	78.2	74.9	71.2	68.7	61.3	3.43	3.84
	18	85.7	83.9	82.0	79.9	77.5	75.0	72.1	68.9	65.1	60.7	55.3	2.53	2.93

TABLE 103

Process Times (B) at Retort Temperature of 250°F for Conduction-Heating Foods in 307 x 306 Can

f_h	z	INITIAL FOOD TEMPERATURE (T_{ih})											Equivalent	
		100	110	120	130	140	150	160	170	180	190	200	F_c^{18}	F_s^{18}
45.31	12	66.4	65.1	63.6	62.0	60.3	58.5	56.4	54.1	51.4	48.4	44.8	5.39	5.87
	14	63.3	62.0	60.5	58.9	57.2	55.3	53.3	50.9	48.3	45.3	41.7	4.15	4.62
	16	60.4	59.0	57.6	56.0	54.3	52.4	50.3	48.0	45.4	42.4	38.8	3.21	3.67
	18	57.8	56.4	55.0	53.4	51.7	49.8	47.7	45.4	42.8	39.8	36.2	2.48	2.93
47.98	12	69.7	68.2	66.7	65.0	63.2	61.2	59.0	56.6	53.8	50.6	46.8	5.44	5.92
	14	66.4	65.0	63.4	61.8	60.0	58.0	55.8	53.3	50.5	47.3	43.5	4.16	4.64
	16	63.3	61.9	60.4	58.7	56.9	54.9	52.7	50.2	47.5	44.3	40.5	3.24	3.70
	18	60.6	59.1	57.6	55.9	54.1	52.1	49.9	47.5	44.7	41.5	37.7	2.48	2.93
50.64	12	72.9	71.4	69.8	68.0	66.1	64.0	61.7	59.1	56.2	52.8	48.8	5.50	5.98
	14	69.5	68.0	66.4	64.6	62.7	60.6	58.3	55.7	52.8	49.4	45.4	4.20	4.68
	16	66.3	64.8	63.1	61.4	59.5	57.4	55.1	52.5	49.5	46.1	42.1	3.24	3.71
	18	63.3	61.8	60.2	58.4	56.5	54.4	52.1	49.5	46.6	43.2	39.2	2.47	2.93
53.31	12	76.2	74.6	72.9	71.0	69.0	66.8	64.4	61.7	58.6	55.0	50.8	5.57	6.06
	14	72.7	71.1	69.4	67.5	65.5	63.3	60.9	58.1	55.0	51.5	47.3	4.25	4.73
	16	69.3	67.7	66.0	64.1	62.1	59.9	57.4	54.7	51.6	48.1	43.8	3.26	3.73
	18	66.1	64.5	62.8	61.0	59.0	56.8	54.3	51.6	48.5	44.9	40.7	2.47	2.93
55.97	12	79.5	77.8	76.0	74.0	71.9	69.6	67.0	64.2	60.9	57.2	52.7	5.64	6.13
	14	75.8	74.1	72.3	70.4	68.3	65.9	63.4	60.5	57.3	53.5	49.1	4.30	4.78
	16	72.2	70.5	68.7	66.8	64.7	62.3	59.8	56.9	53.7	49.9	45.5	3.27	3.74
	18	68.9	67.2	65.4	63.5	61.4	59.1	56.5	53.6	50.4	46.6	42.2	2.47	2.93

TABLE 104

Process Times (B) at Retort Temperature of 260°F for Conduction-Heating Foods in 307 x 306 Can

f_h	z	INITIAL FOOD TEMPERATURE (T_{ih})											Equivalent	
		100	110	120	130	140	150	160	170	180	190	200	F_c^{18}	F_s^{18}
	12	54.2	53.0	51.6	50.2	48.6	46.9	45.0	42.9	40.6	38.0	34.9	5.15	5.67
45.31	14	52.1	50.8	49.5	48.0	46.5	44.7	42.9	40.8	38.5	35.8	32.8	3.88	4.40
	16	50.6	49.3	47.9	46.5	44.9	43.2	41.3	39.2	36.9	34.3	31.2	3.10	3.60
	18	49.0	47.7	46.4	44.9	43.3	41.6	39.7	37.7	35.3	32.7	29.7	2.44	2.93
	12	57.1	55.8	54.3	52.8	51.1	49.3	47.3	45.1	42.7	39.9	36.7	5.24	5.77
47.98	14	54.8	53.5	52.1	50.5	48.9	47.0	45.1	42.9	40.4	37.6	34.4	3.94	4.45
	16	53.2	51.8	50.4	48.8	47.2	45.3	43.4	41.2	38.7	35.9	32.7	3.11	3.61
	18	51.5	50.1	48.7	47.1	45.5	43.7	41.7	39.5	37.0	34.2	31.0	2.44	2.93
	12	59.9	58.5	57.0	55.4	53.6	51.7	49.6	47.3	44.7	41.8	38.4	5.32	5.85
50.64	14	57.6	56.2	54.7	53.0	51.3	49.4	47.3	44.9	42.3	39.4	36.0	4.00	4.52
	16	55.7	54.3	52.8	51.2	49.4	47.5	45.4	43.1	40.5	37.5	34.2	3.13	3.63
	18	54.0	52.5	51.0	49.4	47.6	45.7	43.6	41.3	38.7	35.8	32.4	2.44	2.92
	12	62.8	61.3	59.7	57.9	56.1	54.1	51.9	49.4	46.7	43.6	40.0	5.40	5.93
53.31	14	60.3	58.8	57.2	55.5	53.6	51.6	49.4	47.0	44.3	41.2	37.6	4.05	4.57
	16	58.3	56.8	55.2	53.5	51.6	49.6	47.4	45.0	42.3	39.2	35.6	3.14	3.65
	18	56.4	54.9	53.3	51.6	49.7	47.7	45.5	43.1	40.4	37.3	33.7	2.43	2.93
	12	65.6	64.0	62.4	60.6	58.6	56.5	54.2	51.6	48.8	45.5	41.8	5.49	6.03
55.97	14	63.0	61.4	59.8	58.0	56.0	53.9	51.6	49.0	46.1	42.9	39.2	4.10	4.62
	16	60.9	59.3	57.6	55.8	53.9	51.7	49.4	46.9	44.0	40.8	37.0	3.15	3.66
	18	58.9	57.3	55.6	53.8	51.9	49.8	47.4	44.9	42.0	38.8	35.0	2.43	2.93

TABLE 105

Process Times (B) at Retort Temperature of 230°F for Conduction-Heating Foods in 307 x 400 Can

f_h	z	INITIAL FOOD TEMPERATURE (T_{ih})											Equivalent	
		100	110	120	130	140	150	160	170	180	190	200	F_c^{18}	F_s^{18}
	12	217.6	215.9	213.9	211.8	209.5	206.9	204.0	200.6	196.6	191.6	185.3	10.49	10.82
50.79	14	158.2	156.5	154.6	152.5	150.1	147.5	144.6	141.2	137.2	132.2	125.9	6.01	6.33
	16	130.2	128.4	126.5	124.4	122.0	119.4	116.5	113.1	109.1	104.2	97.8	3.94	4.25
	18	113.5	111.7	109.8	107.7	105.4	102.8	99.8	96.4	92.4	87.5	81.1	2.63	2.94
	12	223.2	221.3	219.3	217.1	214.6	211.8	208.7	205.1	200.9	195.7	188.9	10.61	10.94
53.78	14	163.2	161.4	159.3	157.1	154.6	151.9	148.8	145.2	140.9	135.7	129.0	6.05	6.37
	16	135.2	133.3	131.3	129.0	126.6	123.8	120.7	117.1	112.9	107.6	100.9	3.93	4.25
	18	117.6	115.8	113.7	111.5	109.1	106.3	103.2	99.6	95.3	90.1	83.4	2.63	2.94
	12	228.1	226.2	224.0	221.7	219.1	216.2	212.9	209.1	204.6	199.1	102.0	10.62	10.96
56.77	14	167.9	166.0	163.8	161.5	158.9	156.0	152.7	148.9	144.4	138.9	131.8	6.05	6.38
	16	140.1	138.1	135.9	133.6	131.0	128.1	124.8	121.0	116.5	111.0	103.9	3.92	4.25
	18	121.7	119.7	117.6	115.2	112.6	109.7	106.4	102.6	98.1	92.6	85.5	2.63	2.94
	12	233.0	230.9	228.7	226.2	223.5	220.4	216.9	212.9	208.2	202.4	194.9	10.60	10.95
59.75	14	172.9	170.8	168.5	166.1	163.3	160.3	156.8	152.8	148.1	142.3	134.8	6.08	6.41
	16	144.9	142.8	140.5	138.1	135.3	132.3	128.8	124.8	120.1	114.3	106.8	3.91	4.25
	18	125.6	123.5	121.3	118.8	116.1	113.0	109.5	105.5	100.8	95.0	87.5	2.63	2.94
	12	237.4	235.2	232.9	230.3	227.4	224.2	220.5	216.3	211.4	205.3	197.5	10.58	10.93
62.74	14	177.7	175.5	173.1	170.5	167.6	164.4	160.8	156.6	151.6	145.5	137.7	6.10	6.44
	16	149.6	147.4	145.0	142.4	139.6	136.4	132.7	128.5	123.6	117.5	109.6	3.91	4.25
	18	129.4	127.2	124.8	122.2	119.4	116.2	112.5	108.3	103.4	97.3	89.4	2.63	2.94

TABLE 106

Process Times (B) at Retort Temperature of 240°F for Conduction-Heating Foods in 307 x 400 Can

f_h	z	INITIAL FOOD TEMPERATURE (T_{ih})											Equivalent	
		100	110	120	130	140	150	160	170	180	190	200	F_c^{18}	F_s^{18}
50.79	12	103.2	101.5	99.8	97.8	95.7	93.4	90.8	87.9	84.5	80.4	75.5	7.07	7.47
	14	92.8	91.2	89.4	87.5	85.4	83.1	80.5	77.5	74.1	70.1	65.2	4.85	5.26
	16	85.2	83.6	81.8	79.9	77.8	75.5	72.9	70.0	66.6	62.5	57.6	3.45	3.85
	18	79.6	78.0	76.2	74.3	72.2	69.9	67.3	64.3	60.9	56.9	52.0	2.55	2.94
53.78	12	107.7	106.0	104.1	102.1	99.9	97.4	94.6	91.5	87.9	83.7	78.5	7.11	7.52
	14	96.9	95.2	93.3	91.3	89.1	86.6	83.9	80.7	77.1	72.9	67.7	4.87	5.28
	16	89.1	87.3	85.5	83.4	81.2	78.7	76.0	72.9	69.3	65.0	59.8	3.44	3.85
	18	83.2	81.5	79.6	77.6	75.3	72.9	70.1	67.0	63.4	59.2	53.9	2.55	2.94
56.77	12	112.4	110.5	108.6	106.4	104.1	101.5	98.6	95.3	91.5	87.0	81.5	7.19	7.60
	14	101.1	99.2	97.3	95.1	92.8	90.2	87.3	84.0	80.2	75.7	70.2	4.89	5.31
	16	92.9	91.1	89.1	87.0	84.6	82.0	79.1	75.8	72.0	67.5	62.0	3.45	3.86
	18	86.8	85.0	83.0	80.8	78.5	75.9	73.0	69.7	65.9	61.4	55.9	2.54	2.94
59.75	12	117.0	115.0	113.0	110.7	108.2	105.5	102.4	99.0	95.0	90.2	84.4	7.26	7.68
	14	105.2	103.2	101.2	98.9	96.4	93.7	90.6	87.2	83.2	78.4	72.7	4.91	5.33
	16	96.7	94.8	92.7	90.4	88.0	85.2	82.2	78.7	74.7	70.0	64.2	3.46	3.87
	18	90.3	88.4	86.3	84.1	81.6	78.9	75.8	72.4	68.4	63.6	57.8	2.54	2.94
62.74	12	121.5	119.5	117.3	114.9	112.3	109.4	106.2	102.6	98.4	93.4	87.3	7.33	7.75
	14	109.2	107.2	105.0	102.6	100.0	97.2	93.9	90.3	86.1	81.1	75.1	4.93	5.35
	16	100.4	98.4	96.2	93.9	91.3	88.4	85.2	81.6	77.4	72.4	66.3	3.47	3.89
	18	93.9	91.8	89.7	87.3	84.7	81.8	78.6	75.0	70.8	65.8	59.7	2.54	2.94

TABLE 107

Process Times (B) at Retort Temperature of 250°F for Conduction-Heating Foods in 307 x 400 Can

f_h	z	INITIAL FOOD TEMPERATURE (T_{ih})											Equivalent	
		100	110	120	130	140	150	160	170	180	190	200	F_c^{18}	F_s^{18}
	12	73.2	71.7	70.0	68.3	66.3	64.2	61.9	59.3	56.4	53.0	48.9	5.53	6.01
50.79	14	69.8	58.3	66.6	64.9	62.9	60.8	58.5	55.9	53.0	49.6	45.5	4.22	4.70
	16	66.5	65.0	63.4	61.6	59.7	57.6	55.2	52.7	49.7	46.3	42.3	3.26	3.73
	18	63.6	62.0	60.4	58.6	56.7	54.6	52.3	49.7	46.7	43.3	39.3	2.49	2.94
	12	76.9	75.2	73.5	71.6	69.6	67.4	64.9	62.2	59.1	55.5	51.2	5.61	6.10
53.78	14	73.3	71.7	70.7	68.1	66.1	63.8	61.4	58.6	55.5	51.9	47.6	4.28	4.76
	16	69.8	68.2	66.5	64.6	62.6	60.4	57.9	55.2	52.0	48.4	44.2	3.28	3.75
	18	66.7	65.1	63.4	61.5	59.5	57.2	54.8	52.0	48.9	45.3	41.0	2.49	2.94
	12	80.5	78.8	77.0	75.0	72.8	70.5	67.9	65.0	61.7	57.9	53.4	5.68	6.18
56.77	14	76.8	75.1	73.3	71.3	69.1	66.8	64.2	61.3	58.0	54.2	49.7	4.33	4.82
	16	73.1	71.4	69.6	67.6	65.5	63.1	60.5	57.6	54.3	50.5	46.1	3.30	3.77
	18	69.8	68.1	66.3	64.3	62.2	59.8	57.2	54.3	51.0	47.2	42.7	2.49	2.94
	12	84.1	82.3	80.4	78.3	76.0	73.5	70.8	67.8	64.3	60.3	55.6	5.70	6.20
59.75	14	80.2	78.4	76.5	74.4	72.2	69.7	67.0	63.9	60.4	56.4	51.7	4.38	4.87
	16	76.4	74.6	72.7	70.6	68.3	65.9	63.1	60.1	56.6	52.6	47.9	3.31	3.78
	18	72.9	71.1	69.1	67.1	64.8	62.3	59.6	56.5	53.1	49.1	44.3	2.49	2.94
	12	87.6	85.7	83.7	81.5	79.2	76.6	73.7	70.5	66.9	62.7	57.7	5.73	6.23
62.74	14	83.6	81.7	79.7	77.5	75.2	72.6	69.7	66.5	62.9	58.7	53.7	4.44	4.93
	16	79.6	77.7	75.7	73.5	71.1	68.5	65.7	62.5	58.8	54.6	49.7	3.33	3.80
	18	75.9	74.0	72.0	69.8	67.4	64.8	52.0	58.8	55.1	50.9	46.0	2.49	2.94

TABLE 108

Process Times (B) at Retort Temperature of 260°F for Conduction-Heating F-ods in 307 x 400 Can

f_h	z	INITIAL FOOD TEMPERATURE (T_{ih})											Equivalent	
		100	110	120	130	140	150	160	170	180	190	200	F_c^{18}	F_s^{18}
	12	60.1	58.7	57.2	55.6	53.8	51.9	49.8	47.4	44.8	41.9	38.5	5.35	5.88
50.79	14	57.8	56.4	54.8	53.2	51.4	49.5	47.4	45.1	42.5	39.5	36.1	4.02	4.54
	16	55.9	54.5	53.0	51.3	49.6	47.7	45.6	43.2	40.6	37.7	34.3	3.15	3.65
	18	54.1	52.7	51.2	49.6	47.8	45.9	43.8	41.4	38.8	35.9	32.5	2.45	2.94
	12	63.3	61.8	60.2	58.4	56.6	54.5	52.3	49.9	47.1	44.0	40.4	5.44	5.97
53.78	14	60.8	59.3	57.7	56.0	54.1	52.1	49.8	47.4	44.6	41.5	37.9	4.08	4.60
	16	58.8	57.3	55.7	53.9	52.1	50.0	47.8	45.4	42.6	39.5	35.9	3.16	3.67
	18	56.9	55.4	53.8	52.0	50.2	48.1	45.9	43.4	40.7	37.6	34.0	2.45	2.94
	12	66.5	64.9	63.2	61.4	59.4	57.3	54.9	52.3	49.4	46.1	42.3	5.54	6.08
56.77	14	63.8	62.2	60.5	58.7	56.7	54.6	52.3	49.7	46.8	43.5	39.7	4.13	4.66
	16	61.7	60.1	58.4	56.5	54.6	52.4	50.1	47.5	44.6	41.3	37.5	3.17	3.68
	18	59.6	58.0	56.3	54.5	52.5	50.4	48.1	45.5	42.6	39.3	35.5	2.45	2.94
	12	69.7	68.0	66.2	64.3	62.2	59.9	57.5	54.7	51.7	48.2	44.2	5.64	6.18
59.75	14	66.8	65.1	63.4	61.4	59.4	57.1	54.6	51.9	48.8	45.4	41.4	4.16	4.69
	16	64.5	62.9	61.1	59.2	57.1	54.8	52.3	49.6	46.6	43.1	39.1	3.20	3.71
	18	62.4	60.7	58.9	57.0	54.9	52.6	50.2	47.4	44.4	40.9	36.9	2.45	2.94
	12	72.8	71.0	69.1	67.1	64.9	62.6	60.0	57.1	53.9	50.3	46.1	5.72	6.27
62.74	14	69.8	68.0	66.1	64.1	61.9	59.6	57.0	54.1	50.9	47.2	43.0	4.18	4.71
	16	67.4	65.7	63.8	61.8	59.6	57.2	54.6	51.7	48.5	44.9	40.7	3.24	3.75
	18	65.1	63.3	61.4	59.4	57.2	54.9	52.3	49.4	46.2	42.6	38.4	2.45	2.94

TABLE 109

Process Times (B) at Retort Temperature of 230°F for Conduction-Heating Foods in 307 x 409 Can

f_h	z	INITIAL FOOD TEMPERATURE (T_{ih}) 100	110	120	130	140	150	160	170	180	190	200	Equivalent F_c^{18}	F_s^{18}
	12	224.8	222.9	220.8	218.6	216.1	213.3	210.2	206.5	202.2	196.9	190.2	10.66	10.99
54.37	14	164.5	162.6	160.6	158.3	155.8	153.1	149.9	146.3	142.0	136.7	129.9	6.08	6.40
	16	136.4	134.5	132.4	130.2	127.7	124.9	121.8	118.1	113.8	108.5	101.7	3.94	4.27
	18	118.7	116.8	114.7	112.5	110.0	107.2	104.0	100.4	96.1	90.8	84.0	2.64	2.95
	12	230.0	228.0	225.9	223.5	220.9	217.9	214.6	210.7	206.2	200.6	103.4	10.66	11.00
57.57	14	169.6	167.6	165.4	163.0	160.4	157.4	154.1	150.2	145.7	140.1	132.9	6.08	6.41
	16	141.6	139.6	137.4	135.0	132.4	129.5	126.1	122.3	117.7	112.1	104.9	3.93	4.27
	18	123.0	121.0	118.8	116.4	113.8	110.8	107.5	103.6	99.1	93.5	86.3	2.64	2.95
	12	235.2	233.1	230.8	228.3	225.5	222.4	218.8	214.8	210.0	204.1	106.5	10.64	10.99
60.77	14	174.9	172.8	170.5	168.0	165.2	162.1	158.5	154.5	149.7	143.8	136.2	6.11	6.45
	16	146.7	144.6	142.3	139.8	137.0	133.9	130.4	126.3	121.5	115.6	108.0	3.93	4.27
	18	127.1	125.0	122.7	120.2	117.4	114.3	110.8	106.7	101.9	96.0	88.4	2.64	2.95
	12	240.1	237.9	235.5	232.9	229.9	226.7	222.9	218.7	213.6	207.4	199.4	20.64	10.99
63.97	14	179.9	177.7	175.3	172.6	169.7	166.4	162.7	158.4	153.4	147.2	139.2	6.13	6.47
	16	151.7	149.5	147.1	144.5	141.5	138.3	134.5	130.3	125.2	119.0	111.0	3.93	4.27
	18	131.1	128.9	126.5	123.9	120.9	117.7	114.0	109.7	104.6	98.4	90.4	2.64	2.95
	12	245.8	243.5	240.9	238.2	235.1	231.6	227.7	223.3	217.9	211.4	203.0	10.72	11.07
67.17	14	185.2	182.8	180.3	177.5	174.4	171.0	167.1	162.6	157.3	150.8	143.4	6.16	6.50
	16	156.7	154.3	151.8	149.0	145.9	142.5	138.6	134.1	128.8	122.3	113.9	3.92	4.27
	18	135.0	132.7	130.1	127.3	124.3	120.8	116.9	112.4	107.1	100.6	92.2	2.64	2.95

TABLE 110

Process Times (B) at Retort Temperature of 240°F for Conduction-Heating Foods in 307 x 409 Can

f_h	z	INITIAL FOOD TEMPERATURE (T_{ih})											Equivalent	
		100	110	120	130	140	150	160	170	180	190	200	F_c^{18}	F_s^{18}
54.37	12	108.8	107.0	105.1	103.1	100.8	98.3	95.5	92.4	88.7	84.4	79.2	7.15	7.56
	14	97.9	96.1	94.2	92.2	89.9	87.4	84.6	81.5	77.8	73.5	68.3	4.90	5.31
	16	89.9	88.2	86.3	84.2	82.0	79.5	76.7	73.5	69.9	65.6	60.3	3.46	3.86
	18	84.0	82.2	80.4	78.3	76.1	73.6	70.8	67.6	64.0	59.7	54.4	2.56	2.95
57.57	12	113.7	111.9	109.9	107.7	105.3	102.7	99.7	96.4	92.5	88.0	82.4	7.23	7.65
	14	102.3	100.4	98.4	96.3	93.9	91.2	88.3	85.0	81.1	76.5	71.0	4.92	5.33
	16	94.0	92.2	90.2	88.0	85.6	83.0	80.0	76.7	72.7	68.3	62.7	3.47	3.88
	18	87.8	86.0	84.0	81.8	79.4	76.8	73.8	70.5	66.7	62.1	56.5	2.55	2.95
60.77	12	118.6	116.7	114.6	112.3	109.7	107.0	103.9	100.3	96.3	91.4	85.6	7.31	7.73
	14	106.7	104.7	102.6	100.3	97.8	95.0	91.9	88.4	84.3	79.5	73.6	4.94	5.36
	16	98.1	96.1	94.0	91.7	89.2	86.4	83.3	79.8	75.7	70.9	65.0	3.48	3.89
	18	91.6	89.7	87.6	85.3	82.8	80.0	76.9	73.3	69.3	64.5	58.6	2.55	2.95
63.97	12	123.4	121.4	119.2	116.7	114.1	111.2	107.9	104.2	99.9	94.8	88.6	7.38	7.81
	14	111.0	108.9	106.7	104.3	101.6	98.7	95.4	91.7	87.4	82.4	76.2	4.96	5.38
	16	102.1	100.0	97.8	95.4	92.7	89.8	86.5	82.8	78.5	73.5	67.3	3.49	3.90
	18	95.4	93.3	91.1	88.7	86.0	83.1	79.8	76.1	71.9	66.8	60.6	2.55	2.95
67.17	12	128.2	126.0	123.7	121.2	118.4	115.3	111.9	108.0	103.5	98.2	91.7	7.45	7.89
	14	115.2	113.1	110.7	108.2	105.4	102.3	98.9	95.0	90.5	85.2	78.7	4.98	5.41
	16	106.1	103.9	101.6	99.0	96.3	93.2	89.8	85.9	81.4	76.0	69.5	3.49	3.91
	18	99.2	97.0	94.7	92.1	89.3	86.3	82.8	78.9	74.4	69.1	62.6	2.55	2.95

TABLE 111

Process Times (B) at Retort Temperature of 250°F for Conduction-Heating Foods in 307 x 409 Can

f_h	z	INITIAL FOOD TEMPERATURE (T_{ih})											Equivalent	
		100	110	120	130	140	150	160	170	180	190	200	F_c^{18}	F_s^{18}
	12	77.6	76.0	74.3	72.4	70.3	68.1	65.6	62.8	59.6	56.0	51.7	5.64	6.13
54.37	14	74.1	72.4	70.7	68.8	66.7	64.5	62.0	59.2	56.1	52.4	48.1	4.31	4.79
	16	70.6	68.9	67.2	65.3	63.2	61.0	58.5	55.7	52.6	48.9	44.6	3.30	3.77
	18	67.4	65.7	64.0	62.1	60.1	57.8	55.3	52.5	49.4	45.7	41.4	2.50	2.95
	12	81.5	79.8	77.9	75.9	73.8	71.4	68.7	65.8	62.5	58.6	54.0	5.71	6.21
57.57	14	77.8	76.0	74.2	72.2	70.0	67.6	65.0	62.1	58.7	54.9	50.3	4.36	4.85
	16	74.1	72.3	70.5	68.5	66.3	63.9	61.3	58.3	55.0	51.2	46.6	3.31	3.79
	18	70.7	69.0	67.1	65.1	62.9	60.5	57.9	55.0	51.6	47.8	43.2	2.50	2.95
	12	85.3	83.5	81.6	79.5	77.2	74.6	71.9	68.8	65.2	61.2	56.3	5.73	6.23
60.77	14	81.4	79.6	77.7	75.5	73.2	70.7	68.0	64.8	61.3	57.3	52.4	4.42	4.91
	16	77.5	75.7	73.8	71.6	69.3	66.8	64.0	60.9	57.4	53.3	48.5	3.33	3.80
	18	73.9	72.1	70.2	68.1	65.8	63.2	60.5	57.4	53.8	49.8	44.9	2.50	2.95
	12	89.2	87.2	85.2	83.0	80.5	77.9	75.0	71.7	68.0	63.7	58.6	5.77	6.28
63.97	14	85.1	83.2	81.1	78.9	76.5	73.8	70.9	67.6	63.9	59.6	54.6	4.48	4.97
	16	81.0	79.1	77.0	74.8	72.4	69.7	66.8	63.5	59.8	55.5	50.5	3.36	3.83
	18	77.2	75.3	73.2	71.0	68.6	65.9	63.0	59.7	56.0	51.8	46.7	2.50	2.95
	12	93.0	91.0	88.8	86.5	84.0	81.2	78.1	74.7	70.8	66.3	61.0	5.84	6.34
67.17	14	88.8	86.8	84.6	82.3	79.7	76.9	73.9	70.4	66.5	62.0	56.7	4.55	5.04
	16	84.4	82.4	80.3	77.9	75.4	72.6	69.5	66.1	62.2	57.7	52.4	3.39	3.87
	18	80.5	78.5	76.3	74.0	71.4	68.6	65.6	62.1	58.2	53.7	48.4	2.50	2.95

TABLE 112

Process Times (B) at Retort Temperature of 260°F for Conduction-Heating Foods in 307 x 409 Can

f_h	z	INITIAL FOOD TEMPERATURE (T_{ih})											Equivalent	
		100	110	120	130	140	150	160	170	180	190	200	F_c^{18}	F_s^{18}
	12	64.0	62.4	60.8	59.1	57.2	55.1	52.9	50.4	47.6	44.4	40.8	5.48	6.01
54.37	14	61.5	59.9	58.3	56.6	54.7	52.6	50.4	47.9	45.1	41.9	38.3	4.11	4.63
	16	59.4	57.9	56.3	54.5	52.6	50.6	48.3	45.8	43.0	39.9	36.2	3.18	3.69
	18	57.5	55.9	54.3	52.6	50.7	48.6	46.4	43.9	41.1	37.9	34.3	2.46	2.95
	12	67.4	65.8	64.0	62.2	60.2	58.0	55.6	53.0	50.0	46.7	42.9	5.58	6.13
57.57	14	64.7	63.1	61.3	59.5	57.5	55.3	52.9	50.3	47.3	44.0	40.2	4.16	4.69
	16	62.5	60.8	59.1	57.3	55.3	53.1	50.7	48.1	45.1	41.8	37.9	3.19	3.70
	18	60.4	58.8	57.1	55.2	53.2	51.0	48.7	46.0	43.1	39.7	35.9	2.46	2.95
	12	70.8	69.1	67.2	65.3	63.2	60.9	58.3	55.6	52.5	48.9	44.9	5.69	6.23
60.77	14	67.9	66.2	64.3	62.4	60.3	58.0	55.5	52.7	49.6	46.0	42.0	4.19	4.72
	16	65.6	63.9	62.0	60.1	58.0	55.7	53.2	50.4	47.3	43.7	39.7	3.22	3.74
	18	63.3	61.6	59.8	57.8	55.7	53.4	50.9	48.1	45.0	41.5	37.4	2.46	2.95
	12	74.1	72.3	70.4	68.3	66.1	63.7	61.0	58.1	54.8	51.1	46.9	5.78	6.32
63.97	14	71.0	69.2	67.3	65.2	63.0	60.6	58.0	55.0	51.8	48.0	43.8	4.21	4.74
	16	68.6	66.8	64.9	62.9	60.6	58.2	55.6	52.7	49.4	45.7	41.4	3.26	3.77
	18	66.2	64.4	62.5	60.5	58.2	55.8	53.2	50.2	47.0	43.3	39.0	2.46	2.95
	12	77.4	75.5	73.5	71.4	69.0	66.5	63.7	60.6	57.2	53.3	48.8	5.85	6.39
67.17	14	74.1	72.2	70.2	68.1	65.7	63.2	60.4	57.3	53.9	50.0	45.5	4.23	4.76
	16	71.7	69.8	67.8	65.6	63.3	60.8	58.0	54.9	51.5	47.6	43.1	3.28	3.79
	18	69.1	67.2	65.2	63.1	60.7	58.2	55.4	52.3	48.9	45.0	40.5	2.46	2.95

TABLE 113

Process Times (B) at Retort Temperature of 230°F for Conduction-Heating Foods in 307 x 510 Can

f_h	z	Initial Food Temperature (T_{ih}) 100	110	120	130	140	150	160	170	180	190	200	Equivalent F_c^{18}	F_s^{18}
58.89	12	233.2	231.1	228.9	226.5	223.8	220.8	217.4	213.4	208.8	203.0	195.7	10.73	11.08
	14	172.3	170.3	168.0	165.6	162.9	159.9	156.5	152.5	147.9	142.2	134.8	6.13	6.47
	16	144.1	142.0	139.8	137.4	134.7	131.6	128.2	124.3	119.6	113.9	106.6	3.96	4.30
	18	125.0	123.0	120.8	118.3	115.6	112.6	109.2	105.3	100.6	94.9	87.5	2.66	2.97
62.35	12	238.5	236.4	234.0	231.4	228.6	225.4	221.8	217.6	212.7	206.6	198.8	10.71	11.06
	14	178.0	175.8	173.4	170.9	168.0	164.8	161.2	157.0	152.1	146.1	138.3	6.17	6.50
	16	149.6	147.4	145.1	142.5	139.6	136.4	132.8	128.7	123.7	117.7	109.9	3.96	4.30
	18	129.5	127.3	125.0	122.4	119.5	116.4	112.7	108.6	103.6	97.6	89.8	2.66	2.97
65.82	12	244.3	242.0	239.6	236.8	233.8	230.5	226.6	222.2	217.0	210.6	202.4	10.75	11.10
	14	183.5	181.2	178.7	176.0	173.0	169.6	165.8	161.4	156.2	149.8	141.6	6.19	6.53
	16	155.0	152.7	150.2	147.5	144.5	141.1	137.3	132.9	127.7	121.3	113.1	3.95	4.30
	18	133.8	131.5	129.0	126.3	123.3	119.9	116.1	111.7	106.5	100.1	91.9	2.66	2.97
69.28	12	250.3	247.9	245.3	242.4	239.2	235.7	231.7	227.0	221.5	214.8	206.2	10.83	11.18
	14	189.1	186.7	184.1	181.2	178.1	174.5	170.5	165.9	160.4	153.7	145.0	6.21	6.56
	16	160.2	157.8	155.2	152.4	149.2	145.6	141.6	137.0	131.5	124.8	116.1	3.95	4.30
	18	138.1	135.6	133.0	130.2	127.0	123.4	119.4	114.8	109.3	102.6	93.9	2.66	2.97
72.75	12	255.8	253.3	250.5	247.5	244.2	240.5	236.3	231.4	225.6	218.5	209.5	10.82	11.17
	14	194.8	192.3	189.5	186.5	183.2	179.5	175.3	170.4	164.6	157.6	148.5	6.25	6.60
	16	165.4	162.8	160.1	157.1	153.8	150.0	145.8	140.9	135.2	128.1	119.0	3.95	4.30
	18	143.0	140.4	137.7	134.7	131.4	127.6	123.4	118.5	112.8	105.7	96.6	2.65	2.97

TABLE 114

Process Times (B) at Retort Temperature of 240°F for Conduction-Heating Foods in 307 x 510 Can

f_h	z	INITIAL FOOD TEMPERATURE (T_{ih})											Equivalent	
		100	110	120	130	140	150	160	170	180	190	200	F_c^{18}	F_s^{18}
	12	115.9	114.0	112.0	109.8	107.3	104.6	101.6	98.2	94.3	89.6	83.9	7.31	7.73
58.89	14	104.3	102.4	100.3	98.1	95.7	93.0	90.0	86.5	82.6	77.9	72.2	4.96	5.38
	16	95.9	94.0	91.9	89.7	87.3	84.6	81.5	78.1	74.2	69.5	63.8	3.50	3.91
	18	89.6	87.7	85.6	83.4	81.0	78.3	75.2	71.8	67.9	63.2	57.5	2.57	2.97
	12	121.2	119.2	117.0	114.7	112.1	109.3	106.1	102.4	98.3	93.3	87.3	7.39	7.82
62.35	14	109.0	107.0	104.8	102.4	99.9	97.0	93.8	90.2	86.0	81.1	75.0	4.98	5.40
	16	100.2	98.2	96.1	93.7	91.1	88.3	85.1	81.5	77.3	72.3	66.3	3.51	3.93
	18	93.7	91.6	89.5	87.1	84.5	81.7	78.5	74.9	70.7	65.8	59.7	2.57	2.97
	12	126.4	124.3	122.0	119.5	116.8	113.8	110.4	106.6	102.2	97.0	90.6	7.47	7.90
65.82	14	113.6	111.5	109.2	106.7	104.0	101.0	97.6	93.8	89.4	84.2	77.8	5.00	5.43
	16	104.5	102.4	100.1	97.7	94.9	91.9	88.5	84.7	80.3	75.1	68.7	3.51	3.93
	18	97.7	95.6	93.3	90.8	88.1	85.1	81.7	77.9	73.5	68.3	61.9	2.57	2.97
	12	131.5	129.3	126.9	124.3	121.4	118.2	114.7	110.7	106.0	100.6	93.8	7.54	7.98
69.28	14	118.3	116.0	113.6	111.0	108.2	105.0	101.4	97.4	92.8	87.3	80.6	5.04	5.47
	16	108.9	106.6	104.2	101.6	98.8	95.6	92.0	88.0	83.4	77.9	71.2	3.52	3.94
	18	101.8	99.5	97.1	94.5	91.6	88.5	84.9	80.9	76.3	70.8	64.1	2.56	2.97
	12	136.7	134.3	131.8	129.1	126.1	122.7	119.0	114.8	109.9	104.2	97.1	7.64	8.08
72.75	14	112.9	120.6	118.1	115.3	112.3	109.0	105.2	101.0	96.2	90.4	83.3	5.08	5.52
	16	113.2	110.8	108.3	105.5	102.5	99.2	95.5	91.3	86.4	80.6	73.6	3.53	3.95
	18	105.8	103.4	100.9	98.2	95.1	91.8	88.1	83.9	79.0	73.2	66.2	2.56	2.97

TABLE 115

Process Times (B) at Retort Temperature of 250°F for Conduction-Heating Foods in 307 x 510 Can

f_h	z	INITIAL FOOD TEMPERATURE (T_{ih})											Equivalent	
		100	110	120	130	140	150	160	170	180	190	200	F_c^{18}	F_s^{18}
58.89	12	83.2	81.4	79.5	77.5	75.3	72.8	70.1	67.1	63.7	59.8	55.1	5.76	6.26
	14	79.4	77.6	75.7	73.7	71.4	69.0	66.3	63.3	59.9	55.9	51.3	4.41	4.90
	16	75.9	73.8	71.9	69.9	67.7	65.2	62.5	59.5	56.1	52.2	47.5	3.34	3.82
	18	72.1	70.4	68.5	66.4	64.2	61.8	59.1	56.0	52.6	48.7	44.0	2.52	2.97
62.35	12	87.3	85.4	83.4	81.3	78.9	76.3	73.5	70.3	66.7	62.5	57.6	5.78	6.28
	14	83.3	81.5	79.5	77.3	74.9	72.3	69.5	66.3	62.7	58.5	53.6	4.47	4.96
	16	79.3	77.4	75.4	73.3	70.9	68.3	65.5	62.3	58.7	54.5	49.6	3.36	3.84
	18	75.6	73.8	71.8	69.6	67.2	64.7	61.8	58.6	55.0	50.8	45.9	2.52	2.97
65.82	12	91.5	89.5	87.4	85.1	82.6	79.9	76.9	73.5	69.7	65.3	60.1	5.84	6.35
	14	87.3	85.3	83.2	80.9	78.4	75.7	72.7	69.3	65.5	61.1	55.9	4.55	5.04
	16	83.1	81.1	79.0	76.7	74.2	71.5	68.5	65.1	61.3	56.9	51.7	3.40	3.87
	18	79.2	77.2	75.1	72.8	70.3	67.6	64.6	61.2	57.4	53.0	47.8	2.52	2.97
69.28	12	95.6	93.6	91.3	88.9	86.3	83.4	80.3	76.7	72.7	68.1	62.6	5.91	6.42
	14	91.3	89.2	87.0	84.6	81.9	79.1	75.9	72.4	68.3	63.7	58.2	4.62	5.11
	16	86.8	84.7	82.5	80.1	77.5	74.6	71.4	67.9	63.9	59.2	53.8	3.43	3.91
	18	82.7	80.6	78.4	76.0	73.4	70.5	67.3	63.8	59.8	55.1	49.7	2.51	2.97
72.75	12	99.7	97.5	95.2	92.7	89.9	86.9	83.6	79.9	75.6	70.8	65.0	5.97	6.48
	14	95.2	93.0	90.6	88.1	85.4	82.4	79.0	75.3	71.1	66.2	60.5	4.64	5.14
	16	90.5	88.3	86.0	83.4	80.7	77.7	74.3	70.6	66.4	61.5	55.8	3.43	3.91
	18	86.2	84.0	81.7	79.1	76.4	73.4	70.0	66.3	62.1	57.2	51.5	2.51	2.97

TABLE 116

Process Times (B) at Retort Temperature of 260°F for Conduction-Heating Foods in 307 x 510 Can

f_h	z	INITIAL FOOD TEMPERATURE (T_{ih})											Equivalent	
		100	110	120	130	140	150	160	170	180	190	200	F_c^{18}	F_s^{18}
58.89	12	68.8	67.2	65.4	63.5	61.5	59.2	56.8	54.1	51.1	47.7	43.7	5.66	6.20
	14	66.1	64.4	62.6	60.7	58.7	56.5	54.0	51.3	48.3	44.9	41.0	4.21	4.73
	16	63.8	62.1	60.4	58.5	56.4	54.2	51.8	49.1	46.1	42.6	38.7	3.22	3.73
	18	61.7	60.0	58.3	56.4	54.3	52.1	49.7	47.0	44.0	40.5	36.6	2.48	2.97
62.35	12	72.5	70.7	68.9	66.8	64.7	62.3	59.7	56.9	53.7	50.1	45.9	5.76	6.31
	14	69.5	67.7	65.9	63.9	61.7	59.3	56.8	53.9	50.7	47.1	42.9	4.23	4.76
	16	67.1	65.4	63.5	61.5	59.4	57.0	54.4	51.6	48.4	44.8	40.6	3.26	3.78
	18	64.8	63.1	61.2	59.2	57.0	54.7	52.1	49.2	46.1	42.4	38.3	2.48	2.97
65.82	12	76.1	74.2	72.3	70.1	67.9	65.4	62.6	59.6	56.3	52.5	48.0	5.86	6.40
	14	72.9	71.0	69.1	66.9	64.7	62.2	59.4	56.4	53.1	49.2	44.8	4.25	4.78
	16	70.5	68.6	66.6	64.5	62.2	59.8	57.0	54.0	50.7	46.8	42.4	3.29	3.81
	18	68.0	66.1	64.2	62.0	59.7	57.3	54.5	51.5	48.2	44.3	39.9	2.48	2.97
69.28	12	79.7	77.7	75.6	73.4	71.0	68.4	65.5	62.3	58.8	54.8	50.1	5.92	6.47
	14	76.2	74.3	72.2	70.0	67.6	65.0	62.1	58.9	55.4	51.4	46.7	4.28	4.81
	16	73.8	71.8	69.7	67.5	65.1	62.5	59.6	56.4	52.9	48.9	44.2	3.31	3.83
	18	71.1	69.2	67.1	64.8	62.4	59.8	57.0	53.8	50.2	46.2	41.6	2.47	2.97
72.75	12	83.2	81.2	79.0	76.7	74.1	71.4	68.4	65.1	61.3	57.1	52.2	6.00	6.55
	14	79.6	77.6	75.4	73.1	70.5	67.8	64.8	61.5	57.7	53.5	48.6	4.32	4.85
	16	77.0	75.0	72.8	70.4	67.9	65.2	62.2	58.8	55.1	50.9	46.0	3.33	3.85
	18	74.3	72.2	70.1	67.7	65.2	62.4	59.4	56.1	52.4	48.2	43.3	2.47	2.97

TABLE 117

Process Times (B) at Retort Temperature of 230°F for Conduction-Heating Foods in 307 x 512 Can

f_h	z	INITIAL FOOD TEMPERATURE (T_{ih}) 100	110	120	130	140	150	160	170	180	190	200	Equivalent F_c^{18}	Equivalent F_s^{18}
59.29	12	233.9	231.9	229.6	227.2	224.5	221.4	218.0	214.0	209.3	203.6	196.2	10.74	11.09
	14	173.0	171.0	168.7	166.3	163.6	160.5	157.1	153.1	148.4	142.7	135.3	6.14	6.48
	16	144.7	142.7	140.4	138.0	135.3	132.2	128.8	124.8	120.1	114.4	107.0	3.96	4.30
	18	125.6	123.5	121.3	118.8	116.1	113.1	109.7	105.7	101.0	95.3	87.8	2.66	2.98
62.77	12	239.3	237.1	234.7	232.1	229.2	226.0	222.4	218.2	213.2	207.1	199.3	10.71	11.06
	14	178.7	176.5	174.1	171.5	168.7	165.5	161.8	157.6	152.6	146.6	138.7	6.17	6.51
	16	150.3	148.1	145.7	143.1	140.3	137.1	133.4	129.2	124.2	118.2	110.3	3.96	4.31
	18	130.1	127.9	125.5	122.9	120.0	116.8	113.2	109.0	104.0	97.9	90.1	2.66	2.98
66.26	12	245.2	242.9	240.4	237.7	234.6	231.3	227.4	223.0	217.7	211.3	203.0	10.77	11.12
	14	184.3	182.0	179.5	176.7	173.7	170.3	166.5	162.0	156.8	150.4	142.1	6.19	6.53
	16	115.7	153.4	150.9	148.2	145.1	141.7	137.9	133.5	218.2	121.8	113.5	3.96	4.30
	18	134.4	132.1	129.6	126.8	123.8	120.4	116.6	112.1	106.9	100.5	92.2	2.66	2.98
69.75	12	251.1	248.7	246.1	243.2	240.0	236.4	232.4	227.7	222.2	215.4	206.7	10.84	11.19
	14	189.9	187.5	184.8	182.0	178.8	175.2	171.2	166.5	161.0	154.2	145.4	6.22	6.56
	16	161.0	158.6	155.9	153.0	149.9	146.3	142.2	137.6	132.0	125.3	116.6	3.96	4.30
	18	138.7	136.3	133.7	130.8	127.6	124.0	120.0	115.3	109.8	103.0	94.3	2.66	2.97
73.23	12	256.7	254.1	251.4	248.3	245.1	241.2	237.0	232.1	226.3	219.2	210.0	10.82	11.18
	14	195.7	193.2	190.4	187.4	184.0	180.3	176.1	171.2	165.4	158.3	149.1	6.27	6.62
	16	166.1	163.6	160.8	157.8	154.4	150.7	146.4	141.5	135.7	128.6	119.5	3.96	4.30
	18	143.7	141.1	138.4	135.3	132.0	128.2	124.0	119.1	113.3	106.2	97.0	2.65	2.98

TABLE 118

Process Times (B) at Retort Temperature of 240°F for Conduction-Heating Foods in 307 x 512 Can

f_h	z	INITIAL FOOD TEMPERATURE (T_{ih})											Equivalent	
		100	110	120	130	140	150	160	170	180	190	200	F_c^{18}	F_s^{18}
59.29	12	116.6	114.7	112.6	110.4	107.9	105.2	102.2	98.7	94.8	90.1	84.3	7.32	7.74
	14	104.8	102.9	100.9	98.6	96.2	93.5	90.4	87.0	83.0	78.3	72.6	4.97	5.38
	16	96.4	94.5	92.4	90.2	87.7	85.0	82.0	78.5	74.6	69.9	64.1	3.50	3.92
	18	90.0	88.1	86.1	83.8	81.4	78.7	75.6	72.2	68.2	63.5	57.8	2.57	2.98
62.77	12	121.9	119.9	117.7	115.3	112.7	109.8	106.6	103.0	98.8	93.8	87.7	7.40	7.83
	14	109.6	107.5	105.4	103.0	100.4	97.5	94.3	90.7	86.5	81.5	75.4	4.99	5.41
	16	100.8	98.7	96.6	94.2	91.6	88.7	85.5	81.9	77.7	72.7	66.6	3.51	3.93
	18	94.2	92.1	90.0	87.6	85.0	82.1	78.9	75.3	71.1	66.1	60.0	2.57	2.98
66.26	12	127.1	125.0	122.7	120.2	117.4	114.4	111.0	107.1	102.7	97.5	91.0	7.48	7.92
	14	114.2	112.1	109.8	107.3	104.5	101.5	98.1	94.3	89.8	84.6	78.2	5.01	5.44
	16	105.1	103.0	100.7	98.2	95.4	92.4	89.0	85.2	80.7	75.5	69.1	3.51	3.93
	18	98.3	96.1	93.8	91.3	88.6	85.5	82.2	78.3	73.9	68.6	62.2	2.57	2.98
69.75	12	132.2	130.0	127.6	124.9	122.0	118.9	115.3	111.2	106.6	101.1	94.3	7.56	8.00
	14	118.9	116.7	114.3	111.6	108.7	105.5	102.0	97.9	93.3	87.7	81.0	5.05	5.48
	16	109.5	107.2	104.8	102.2	99.3	96.1	92.5	88.5	83.8	78.3	71.5	3.52	3.94
	18	102.3	100.1	97.7	95.0	92.1	88.9	85.4	81.3	76.7	71.1	64.4	2.56	2.98
73.23	12	137.4	135.1	132.5	129.8	126.7	123.4	119.6	115.4	110.5	104.7	97.6	7.65	8.10
	14	123.6	121.2	118.7	115.9	112.9	109.5	105.8	101.5	96.6	90.8	83.8	5.09	5.53
	16	113.8	111.4	108.9	106.1	103.1	99.7	96.0	91.7	86.8	81.0	73.9	3.53	3.96
	18	106.3	104.0	101.4	98.7	95.6	92.3	88.5	84.3	79.4	73.6	66.5	2.56	2.98

TABLE 119

Process Times (B) at Retort Temperature of 250°F for Conduction-Heating Foods in 307 x 512 Can

f_h	z	INITIAL FOOD TEMPERATURE (T_{ih})											Equivalent	
		100	110	120	130	140	150	160	170	180	190	200	F_c^{18}	F_s^{18}
	12	83.7	81.9	80.0	77.9	75.7	73.2	70.5	67.5	64.1	60.1	55.4	5.77	6.27
59.29	14	79.8	78.1	76.2	74.1	71.9	69.4	66.7	63.7	60.2	56.2	51.6	4.42	4.91
	16	76.0	74.3	72.3	70.3	68.0	65.6	62.9	59.8	56.4	52.4	47.7	3.35	3.82
	18	72.5	70.8	68.9	66.8	64.6	62.1	59.4	56.4	52.9	48.9	44.3	2.52	2.98
	12	87.8	85.9	83.9	81.7	79.4	76.8	73.9	70.7	67.0	62.8	57.9	5.79	6.29
62.77	14	83.8	81.9	79.9	77.7	75.4	72.8	69.9	66.7	63.0	58.8	53.9	4.48	4.97
	16	79.8	77.9	75.9	73.7	71.3	68.7	65.8	62.6	59.0	54.8	49.8	3.37	3.84
	18	76.1	74.2	72.2	70.0	67.6	65.0	62.1	58.9	55.3	51.1	46.1	2.52	2.98
	12	92.0	90.0	87.9	85.6	83.1	80.4	77.3	73.9	70.1	65.7	60.4	5.86	6.36
66.26	14	87.8	85.8	83.7	81.4	78.9	76.2	73.1	69.7	65.9	61.5	56.2	4.56	5.05
	16	83.6	81.6	79.5	77.1	74.6	71.9	68.9	65.5	61.6	57.2	52.0	3.40	3.88
	18	79.7	77.7	75.5	73.2	70.7	68.0	65.0	61.6	57.7	53.3	48.0	2.52	2.98
	12	96.2	94.1	91.9	89.4	86.8	83.9	80.7	77.1	73.1	68.4	62.9	5.92	6.43
69.75	14	91.8	89.7	87.5	85.0	82.4	79.5	76.3	72.8	68.7	64.0	58.5	4.63	5.12
	16	87.3	85.2	83.0	80.6	77.9	75.0	71.8	68.3	64.2	59.6	54.0	3.43	3.91
	18	83.2	81.1	78.9	76.4	73.8	70.9	67.7	64.2	60.1	55.4	49.9	2.52	2.98
	12	100.3	98.1	95.7	93.2	90.4	87.4	84.1	80.3	76.1	71.2	65.4	5.98	6.49
73.23	14	95.7	93.5	91.2	88.6	85.9	82.8	79.5	75.7	71.5	66.6	60.8	4.65	5.14
	16	91.0	88.8	86.5	83.9	81.1	78.1	74.8	71.0	66.8	61.9	56.1	3.43	3.91
	18	86.7	84.5	82.1	79.6	76.8	73.8	70.4	66.7	62.4	57.5	51.7	2.51	2.98

TABLE 120

Process Times (B) at Retort Temperature of 260°F for Conduction-Heating Foods in 307 x 512 Can

f_h	z	INITIAL FOOD TEMPERATURE (T_{ih})											Equivalent	
		100	110	120	130	140	150	160	170	180	190	200	F_c^{18}	F_s^{18}
	12	69.2	67.6	65.8	63.9	61.8	59.6	57.1	54.4	51.4	48.0	44.0	5.67	6.22
59.29	14	66.5	64.8	63.0	61.1	59.0	56.8	54.4	51.6	48.6	45.2	41.2	4.21	4.74
	16	64.2	62.5	60.7	58.8	56.8	54.5	52.1	49.4	46.3	42.9	38.9	3.23	3.74
	18	62.0	60.4	58.6	56.7	54.6	52.4	49.9	47.2	44.2	40.8	36.8	2.48	2.98
	12	72.9	71.2	69.3	67.3	65.1	62.7	60.1	57.2	54.0	50.4	46.2	5.78	6.32
62.77	14	69.9	68.1	66.3	64.2	62.1	59.7	57.1	54.2	51.0	47.4	43.2	4.24	4.76
	16	67.6	65.8	63.9	61.9	59.7	57.3	54.7	51.9	48.7	45.0	40.8	3.27	3.78
	18	65.2	63.5	61.6	59.6	57.4	55.0	52.4	49.5	46.3	42.7	38.5	2.48	2.98
	12	76.5	74.7	72.7	70.6	68.3	65.8	63.0	60.0	56.6	52.8	48.3	5.87	6.42
66.26	14	73.3	71.5	69.5	67.3	65.0	62.5	59.8	56.8	53.4	49.5	45.1	4.26	4.79
	16	70.9	69.0	67.1	64.9	62.6	60.1	57.4	54.3	50.9	47.1	42.7	3.30	3.81
	18	68.4	66.5	64.5	62.4	60.1	57.6	54.9	51.8	48.4	44.6	40.2	2.48	2.98
	12	80.1	78.2	76.1	73.9	71.4	68.8	65.9	62.7	59.1	55.1	50.4	5.94	6.48
69.75	14	76.7	74.7	72.6	70.4	68.0	65.3	62.5	59.3	55.7	51.6	47.0	4.28	4.81
	16	74.2	72.2	70.2	67.9	65.5	62.8	60.0	56.8	53.2	49.2	44.5	3.32	3.83
	18	71.5	69.6	67.5	65.2	62.8	60.2	57.3	54.1	50.5	46.5	41.8	2.48	2.98
	12	83.7	81.7	79.5	77.1	74.6	71.8	68.8	65.4	61.7	57.4	52.5	6.02	6.57
73.23	14	80.1	78.1	75.9	73.5	71.0	68.2	65.2	61.8	58.1	53.8	48.9	4.33	4.87
	16	77.5	75.4	73.2	70.9	68.3	65.5	62.5	59.2	55.4	51.2	46.3	3.34	3.85
	18	74.7	72.7	70.5	68.1	65.6	62.8	59.8	56.4	52.7	48.4	43.5	2.47	2.98

TABLE 121

Process Times (B) at Retort Temperature of 230°F for Conduction-Heating Foods in 307 x 704 Can

f_h	z	INITIAL FOOD TEMPERATURE (T_{ih})											Equivalent	
		100	110	120	130	140	150	160	170	180	190	200	F_c^{18}	F_s^{18}
	12	240.3	238.1	235.7	233.1	230.2	227.0	223.4	219.2	214.2	208.2	200.3	10.80	11.15
62.69	14	179.2	177.0	174.6	172.0	169.2	165.9	162.3	158.1	153.2	147.1	139.2	6.22	6.56
	16	150.6	148.4	146.0	143.4	140.5	137.3	133.7	129.5	124.5	118.5	110.6	3.99	4.34
	18	130.4	128.2	125.8	123.2	120.3	117.1	113.5	109.3	104.3	98.3	90.4	2.68	3.00
	12	246.4	244.1	241.6	238.8	235.8	232.4	228.5	224.1	218.8	212.4	204.1	10.84	11.19
66.37	14	185.0	182.7	180.2	177.5	174.4	171.0	167.2	162.8	157.5	151.1	142.8	6.24	6.58
	16	156.3	154.0	151.5	148.7	145.7	142.3	138.5	134.0	128.8	122.3	114.0	3.99	4.34
	18	134.9	132.6	130.1	127.4	124.3	120.9	117.1	112.6	107.4	101.0	92.7	2.68	3.00
	12	252.7	250.3	247.6	244.7	241.5	237.9	233.9	229.2	223.6	216.8	208.1	10.92	11.27
70.06	14	191.0	188.6	185.9	183.0	179.8	176.3	172.2	167.5	162.0	155.2	146.4	6.27	6.61
	16	161.9	159.5	156.8	153.9	150.7	147.1	143.1	138.4	132.8	126.0	117.3	3.99	4.33
	18	139.5	137.1	134.4	131.5	128.3	124.7	120.7	116.0	110.4	103.6	94.9	2.68	2.99
	12	258.6	256.0	253.2	250.1	246.8	243.0	238.7	233.8	227.9	220.8	211.6	10.90	11.26
73.75	14	197.2	194.6	191.8	188.8	185.4	181.6	177.3	172.4	166.6	159.4	150.2	6.31	6.66
	16	167.3	164.8	162.0	158.9	155.6	151.8	147.5	142.6	136.7	129.6	120.4	3.99	4.33
	18	144.7	142.2	139.4	136.3	132.9	129.2	124.9	120.0	114.1	107.0	97.8	2.67	3.00
	12	264.4	261.7	258.8	255.6	252.1	248.1	243.6	238.4	232.3	224.8	215.1	10.90	11.27
77.44	14	203.8	201.1	198.2	195.0	191.4	187.5	183.0	177.8	171.7	164.2	154.5	6.39	6.74
	16	172.6	169.9	167.0	163.8	160.3	156.3	151.8	146.6	140.5	133.0	123.3	3.99	4.33
	18	149.8	147.1	144.2	141.0	137.5	133.5	129.0	123.8	117.7	110.2	100.5	2.67	3.00

TABLE 122

Process Times (B) at Retort Temperature of 240°F for Conduction-Heating Foods in 307 x 704 Can

f_h	z	INITIAL FOOD TEMPERATURE (T_{ih}) 100	110	120	130	140	150	160	170	180	190	200	Equivalent F_c^{18}	Equivalent F_s^{18}
62.69	12	122.0	119.9	117.8	115.4	112.8	109.9	106.7	103.1	98.9	93.9	87.9	7.45	7.88
	14	109.6	107.6	105.4	103.1	100.5	97.6	94.4	90.8	86.6	81.6	75.5	5.02	5.45
	16	100.8	98.8	96.6	94.3	91.7	88.8	85.6	82.0	77.8	72.8	66.7	3.54	3.96
	18	94.2	92.2	90.0	87.7	85.1	82.2	79.0	75.4	71.2	66.2	60.1	2.59	3.00
66.37	12	127.5	125.4	123.0	120.5	117.8	114.8	111.4	107.5	103.1	97.8	91.4	7.53	7.97
	14	114.6	112.4	110.1	107.6	104.9	101.8	98.5	94.6	90.2	84.9	78.5	5.05	5.47
	16	105.4	103.3	101.0	98.5	95.7	92.7	89.3	85.5	81.0	75.8	69.3	3.54	3.96
	18	98.6	96.4	94.1	91.6	88.9	85.8	82.4	78.6	74.1	68.9	62.4	2.59	3.00
70.06	12	132.9	130.7	128.2	125.6	122.7	119.5	115.9	111.8	107.2	101.6	94.8	7.61	8.05
	14	119.5	117.3	114.9	112.2	109.3	106.1	102.5	98.5	93.8	88.2	81.4	5.09	5.52
	16	110.0	107.8	105.4	102.7	99.8	96.6	93.0	89.0	84.3	78.7	71.9	3.55	3.97
	18	102.9	100.6	98.2	95.5	92.6	89.4	85.8	81.8	77.1	71.5	64.7	2.59	3.00
73.75	12	138.4	136.1	133.5	130.7	127.7	124.3	120.5	116.2	111.3	105.4	98.3	7.71	8.16
	14	124.5	122.1	119.5	116.8	113.7	110.3	106.6	102.3	97.3	91.5	84.4	5.13	5.57
	16	114.6	112.2	109.7	106.9	103.8	100.5	96.7	92.4	87.5	81.6	74.5	3.56	3.99
	18	107.1	104.7	102.2	99.4	96.3	93.0	89.2	84.9	80.0	74.1	67.0	2.58	3.00
77.44	12	143.9	141.4	138.7	135.8	132.6	129.0	125.1	120.6	115.4	109.3	101.8	7.82	8.27
	14	129.4	126.9	124.2	121.2	118.0	114.5	110.5	106.0	100.9	94.7	87.2	5.15	5.59
	16	119.1	116.6	113.9	111.0	107.8	104.3	100.3	95.8	90.6	84.5	77.0	3.57	4.00
	18	111.4	108.9	106.2	103.2	100.0	96.5	92.5	88.0	82.9	76.7	69.2	2.58	3.00

TABLE 123

Process Times (B) at Retort Temperature of 250°F for Conduction-Heating Foods in 307 x 704 Can

f_h	z	INITIAL FOOD TEMPERATURE (T_{ih})											Equivalent	
		100	110	120	130	140	150	160	170	180	190	200	F_c^{18}	F_s^{18}
	12	87.8	86.0	83.9	81.8	79.4	76.8	73.9	70.7	67.1	62.9	57.9	5.84	6.34
62.69	14	83.8	81.9	79.9	77.7	75.4	72.8	69.9	66.7	63.1	58.9	53.9	4.51	5.00
	16	79.8	77.9	75.9	73.7	71.3	68.7	65.9	62.7	59.0	54.8	49.9	3.39	3.87
	18	76.1	74.2	72.2	70.0	67.6	65.0	62.2	59.0	55.3	51.1	46.2	2.54	3.00
	12	92.3	90.3	88.1	85.8	83.3	80.6	77.5	74.1	70.3	65.9	60.6	5.90	6.40
66.37	14	88.1	86.1	83.9	81.6	79.1	76.4	73.3	69.9	66.1	61.6	56.4	4.59	5.08
	16	83.8	81.8	79.7	77.4	74.8	72.1	69.1	65.7	61.8	57.4	52.1	3.43	3.91
	18	79.9	77.9	75.7	73.4	70.9	68.2	65.1	61.7	57.9	53.5	48.2	2.54	3.00
	12	96.7	94.6	92.3	89.9	87.2	84.3	81.1	77.5	73.5	68.8	63.2	5.96	6.47
70.06	14	92.3	90.2	87.9	85.5	82.8	79.9	76.7	73.1	69.1	64.4	58.8	4.67	5.16
	16	87.8	85.7	83.4	81.0	78.3	75.4	72.2	68.6	64.6	59.9	54.3	3.46	3.94
	18	83.6	81.5	79.3	76.8	74.2	71.3	68.1	64.5	60.4	55.7	50.2	2.54	3.00
	12	101.0	98.8	96.4	93.9	91.1	88.0	84.7	80.9	76.6	71.7	65.8	6.03	6.54
73.75	14	96.4	94.2	91.8	89.3	86.5	83.4	80.1	76.3	72.0	67.1	61.2	4.68	5.18
	16	91.7	89.5	87.1	84.5	81.7	78.7	75.3	71.5	67.3	62.3	56.5	3.46	3.94
	18	87.3	85.1	82.7	80.2	77.4	74.3	70.9	67.2	62.9	58.0	52.1	2.54	3.00
	12	105.4	103.0	100.5	97.8	94.9	91.7	88.2	84.2	79.7	74.5	68.4	6.10	6.61
77.44	14	100.5	98.2	95.7	93.0	90.1	86.9	83.4	79.4	74.9	69.7	63.6	4.71	5.21
	16	95.6	93.2	90.7	88.1	85.1	81.9	78.4	74.4	69.9	64.7	58.6	3.47	3.95
	18	91.0	88.7	86.2	83.5	80.5	77.3	73.8	69.8	65.3	60.2	54.0	2.53	3.00

TABLE 124

Process Times (B) at Retort Temperature of 260°F for Conduction-Heating Foods in 307 x 704 Can

f_h	z	INITIAL FOOD TEMPERATURE (T_{ih})											Equivalent	
		100	110	120	130	140	150	160	170	180	190	200	F_c^{18}	F_s^{18}
	12	72.9	71.1	69.3	67.2	65.1	62.7	60.1	57.2	54.0	50.4	46.2	5.81	6.35
62.69	14	69.9	68.1	66.3	64.2	62.1	59.7	57.1	54.2	51.0	47.4	43.2	4.27	4.80
	16	67.5	65.8	63.9	61.9	59.7	57.3	54.7	51.9	48.7	45.0	40.8	3.29	3.80
	18	65.2	63.4	61.6	59.5	57.4	55.0	52.4	49.5	46.3	42.7	38.5	2.50	3.00
	12	76.7	74.9	72.9	70.7	68.4	65.9	63.2	60.1	56.8	52.9	48.5	5.91	6.46
66.37	14	73.5	71.6	69.7	67.5	65.2	62.7	60.0	56.9	53.5	49.7	45.2	4.29	4.82
	16	71.1	69.2	67.2	65.1	62.8	60.3	57.5	54.5	51.1	47.2	42.8	3.32	3.84
	18	68.6	66.7	64.7	62.6	60.3	57.8	55.0	52.0	48.6	44.7	40.3	2.50	3.00
	12	80.5	78.6	76.5	74.2	71.8	69.1	66.2	63.0	59.4	55.4	50.7	5.98	6.53
70.06	14	77.1	75.1	73.0	70.8	68.3	65.7	62.8	59.6	56.0	51.9	47.2	4.32	4.85
	16	74.6	72.6	70.5	68.2	65.8	63.2	60.3	57.1	53.5	49.4	44.7	3.34	3.86
	18	71.9	69.9	67.8	65.6	63.1	60.5	57.6	54.4	50.8	46.7	42.0	2.50	3.00
	12	84.3	82.3	80.1	77.7	75.1	72.3	69.3	65.9	62.1	57.9	52.9	6.07	6.62
73.75	14	80.7	78.6	76.4	74.0	71.5	68.7	65.6	62.3	58.5	54.2	49.3	4.37	4.90
	16	78.0	76.0	73.7	71.4	68.8	66.0	63.0	59.6	55.8	51.5	46.6	3.36	3.88
	18	75.3	73.2	71.0	68.6	66.0	63.3	60.2	56.8	53.1	48.8	43.8	2.49	3.00
	12	88.1	86.0	83.7	81.2	78.5	75.5	72.3	68.8	64.8	60.3	55.2	6.17	6.72
77.44	14	84.3	82.2	79.8	77.4	74.7	71.7	68.5	65.0	61.0	56.5	51.4	4.42	4.96
	16	81.4	79.3	76.9	74.5	71.8	68.8	65.6	62.1	58.1	53.6	48.5	3.37	3.89
	18	78.6	76.4	74.1	71.6	68.9	66.0	62.8	59.3	55.3	50.8	45.6	2.49	3.00

TABLE 125

Process Times (B) at Retort Temperature of 230°F for Conduction-Heating Foods in 401 x 205 Can

f_h	z	INITIAL FOOD TEMPERATURE (T_{ih})											Equivalent	
		100	110	120	130	140	150	160	170	180	190	200	F_c^{18}	F_s^{18}
35.23	12	192.2	191.0	189.6	188.2	186.6	184.8	182.7	180.4	177.6	174.2	169.8	10.34	10.64
	14	132.4	131.2	129.8	128.4	126.8	125.0	122.9	120.6	117.8	114.4	110.0	5.87	6.17
	16	104.9	103.7	102.4	100.9	99.3	97.5	95.5	93.1	90.3	86.9	82.5	3.81	4.10
	18	89.2	87.9	86.6	85.2	83.5	81.7	79.7	77.3	74.6	71.1	66.7	2.63	2.92
37.30	12	194.5	193.2	191.8	190.2	188.5	186.6	184.5	182.0	179.0	175.4	170.7	10.32	10.62
	14	135.8	134.5	133.1	131.5	129.8	127.9	125.8	123.3	120.3	116.7	112.0	5.90	6.20
	16	108.1	106.8	105.4	103.9	102.1	100.2	98.1	95.6	92.6	89.0	84.3	3.81	4.10
	18	92.6	91.3	89.9	88.3	86.6	84.7	82.6	80.1	77.1	73.5	68.8	2.62	2.92
39.38	12	198.1	196.8	195.3	193.6	191.8	189.8	187.5	184.9	181.8	178.0	173.0	10.42	10.72
	14	139.3	137.9	136.4	134.8	133.0	131.0	128.7	126.0	122.9	119.1	114.2	5.92	6.22
	16	111.4	110.0	108.5	106.9	105.1	103.1	100.8	98.2	95.1	91.2	86.3	3.82	4.12
	18	95.9	94.5	93.1	91.4	89.6	87.6	85.3	82.7	79.6	75.8	70.8	2.61	2.92
41.45	12	201.6	200.1	198.6	196.9	195.0	192.8	190.4	187.7	184.4	180.4	175.2	10.46	10.77
	14	142.5	141.1	139.5	137.8	135.9	133.8	131.4	128.6	125.3	121.3	116.1	5.91	6.22
	16	114.6	113.1	111.6	109.9	108.0	105.8	103.4	100.7	97.4	93.4	88.2	3.82	4.12
	18	99.2	97.7	96.2	94.5	92.6	90.4	88.0	85.3	82.0	78.0	72.8	2.61	2.92
43.52	12	205.4	203.8	202.2	200.4	198.4	196.2	193.7	190.7	187.3	183.1	177.6	10.44	10.77
	14	145.8	144.2	142.6	140.8	138.8	136.6	134.1	131.1	127.7	123.5	118.0	5.91	6.23
	16	117.8	116.3	114.7	112.9	110.9	108.6	106.1	103.2	99.8	95.5	90.1	3.83	4.13
	18	102.4	100.9	99.2	97.4	95.4	93.2	90.7	87.8	84.3	80.1	74.7	2.61	2.92

TABLE 126

Process Times (B) at Retort Temperature of 240°F for Conduction-Heating Foods in 401 x 205 Can

f_h	z	INITIAL FOOD TEMPERATURE (T_{ih}) 100	110	120	130	140	150	160	170	180	190	200	Equivalent F_c^{18}	F_s^{18}
	12	78.3	77.2	76.0	74.6	73.2	71.6	69.8	67.7	65.4	62.6	59.1	6.21	6.60
35.23	14	70.6	69.5	68.2	66.9	65.4	63.8	62.0	60.0	57.6	54.8	51.4	4.67	5.04
	16	64.6	63.4	62.2	60.9	59.4	57.8	56.0	53.9	51.6	48.8	45.4	3.39	3.77
	18	60.1	58.9	57.7	56.4	54.9	53.3	51.5	49.4	47.1	44.3	40.9	2.55	2.92
	12	81.8	80.6	79.3	77.9	76.3	74.6	72.7	70.5	68.1	65.1	61.5	6.34	6.72
37.30	14	73.5	72.3	71.0	69.6	68.1	66.4	64.5	62.3	59.8	56.8	53.2	4.65	5.03
	16	67.4	66.2	64.9	63.5	61.9	60.2	58.3	56.1	53.7	50.7	47.1	3.41	3.79
	18	62.7	61.5	60.2	58.8	57.2	55.5	53.6	51.4	48.9	46.0	42.4	2.54	2.92
	12	85.2	83.9	82.5	81.0	79.4	77.6	75.6	73.3	70.7	67.6	63.7	6.45	6.84
39.38	14	76.4	75.2	73.8	72.3	70.7	68.9	66.8	64.6	61.9	58.8	55.0	4.64	5.02
	16	70.1	68.9	67.5	66.0	64.4	62.6	60.6	58.3	55.7	52.5	48.7	3.40	3.78
	18	65.3	64.1	62.7	61.2	59.6	57.8	55.8	53.5	50.8	47.7	43.9	2.54	2.92
	12	88.5	87.2	85.7	84.2	82.4	80.6	78.4	76.0	73.3	70.0	66.0	6.56	6.96
41.45	14	79.4	78.1	76.7	75.1	73.4	71.5	69.4	67.0	64.2	60.9	56.9	4.67	5.06
	16	72.9	71.5	70.1	68.5	66.8	64.9	62.8	60.4	57.6	54.3	50.3	3.39	3.78
	18	67.9	66.6	65.2	63.6	61.9	60.0	57.9	55.4	52.7	49.4	45.4	2.53	2.92
	12	91.8	90.4	88.9	87.2	85.4	83.4	81.2	78.7	75.8	72.3	68.1	6.67	7.07
43.52	14	82.4	81.0	79.5	77.9	76.1	74.1	71.9	69.3	66.4	63.0	58.8	4.70	5.10
	16	75.6	74.2	72.7	71.0	69.2	67.2	65.0	62.5	59.6	56.1	51.9	3.39	3.78
	18	70.5	69.1	67.6	65.9	64.1	62.1	59.9	57.4	54.5	51.0	46.8	2.53	2.92

TABLE 127

Process Times (B) at Retort Temperature of 250°F for Conduction-Heating Foods in 401 x 205 Can

f_h	z	INITIAL FOOD TEMPERATURE (T_{ih})											Equivalent	
		100	110	120	130	140	150	160	170	180	190	200	F_c^{18}	F_s^{18}
	12	53.8	52.7	51.6	50.3	49.0	47.6	45.9	44.1	42.1	39.7	36.9	5.11	5.58
35.23	14	51.1	50.1	49.0	47.7	46.4	44.9	43.3	41.5	39.5	37.1	34.3	3.98	4.44
	16	48.9	47.8	46.7	45.5	44.1	42.7	41.1	39.3	37.2	34.9	32.1	3.10	3.55
	18	46.9	45.9	44.7	43.5	42.2	40.7	39.1	37.3	35.3	32.9	30.1	2.48	2.92
	12	56.3	55.2	54.0	52.7	51.3	49.8	48.0	46.1	44.0	41.5	3.85	5.14	5.61
37.30	14	53.6	52.5	51.3	50.0	48.6	47.0	45.3	43.4	41.3	38.8	35.8	4.00	4.46
	16	51.2	50.1	48.9	47.6	46.2	44.6	42.9	41.0	38.9	36.4	33.4	3.09	3.54
	18	49.1	48.0	46.8	45.5	44.1	42.5	40.8	38.9	36.8	34.3	31.3	2.48	2.92
	12	59.0	57.8	56.5	55.2	53.7	52.0	50.2	48.2	46.0	43.3	40.2	5.21	5.69
39.38	14	56.2	55.0	53.7	52.3	50.9	49.2	47.4	45.4	43.1	40.5	37.4	4.06	4.52
	16	53.6	52.4	51.2	49.8	48.3	46.7	44.9	42.9	40.6	38.0	34.8	3.12	3.57
	18	51.4	50.2	48.9	47.6	46.1	44.5	42.7	40.6	38.4	35.7	32.6	2.48	2.92
	12	61.6	60.4	59.0	57.6	56.0	54.3	52.4	50.3	47.9	45.1	41.8	5.28	5.76
41.45	14	58.7	57.4	56.1	54.7	53.1	51.4	49.5	47.4	45.0	42.2	38.9	4.11	4.57
	16	56.0	54.8	53.4	52.0	50.4	48.7	46.8	44.7	42.3	39.5	36.2	3.15	3.60
	18	53.6	52.4	51.1	49.6	48.1	46.3	44.4	42.3	39.9	37.1	33.9	2.47	2.92
	12	64.2	62.9	61.5	60.0	58.3	56.5	54.5	52.3	49.8	46.9	43.4	5.34	5.82
43.52	14	61.2	59.9	58.5	56.9	55.3	53.5	51.5	49.3	46.8	43.8	40.4	4.12	4.59
	16	58.4	57.1	55.7	54.1	52.5	50.7	48.7	46.5	44.0	41.0	37.6	3.18	3.63
	18	55.9	54.6	53.2	51.6	50.0	48.2	46.2	44.0	41.5	38.5	35.1	2.47	2.92

TABLE 128

Process Times (B) at Retort Temperature of 260°F for Conduction-Heating Foods in 401 x 205 Can

f_h	z	INITIAL FOOD TEMPERATURE (T_{ih})											Equivalent	
		100	110	120	130	140	150	160	170	180	190	200	F_c^{18}	F_s^{18}
	12	43.1	42.1	41.1	39.9	38.7	37.4	35.9	34.3	32.5	30.5	28.1	4.64	5.16
35.23	14	41.7	40.7	39.7	38.6	37.3	36.0	34.5	32.9	31.1	29.1	26.7	3.72	4.23
	16	40.6	39.6	38.5	37.4	36.2	34.8	33.4	31.8	30.0	27.9	25.6	3.04	3.53
	18	39.4	38.4	37.3	36.2	35.0	33.6	32.2	30.6	28.8	26.7	24.4	2.44	2.92
	12	45.4	44.4	43.3	42.1	40.8	39.4	37.8	36.1	34.2	32.0	29.5	4.76	5.28
37.30	14	43.9	42.8	41.7	40.5	39.2	37.8	36.3	34.6	32.6	30.5	28.0	3.75	4.26
	16	42.6	41.6	40.5	39.3	38.0	36.6	35.0	33.3	31.4	29.2	26.7	3.06	3.55
	18	41.4	40.3	39.2	38.0	36.7	35.3	33.7	32.0	30.1	28.0	25.5	2.44	2.92
	12	47.7	46.6	45.5	44.2	42.8	41.3	39.7	37.9	35.9	33.6	31.0	4.88	5.40
39.38	14	46.0	44.9	43.7	42.5	41.1	39.6	38.0	36.2	34.2	31.9	29.3	3.79	4.29
	16	44.7	43.6	42.4	41.1	39.8	38.3	36.7	34.9	32.8	30.6	27.9	3.07	3.56
	18	43.3	42.2	41.1	39.8	38.4	36.9	35.3	33.5	31.5	29.2	26.6	2.43	2.92
	12	50.0	48.9	47.6	46.3	44.8	43.3	41.6	39.7	37.5	35.1	32.4	4.99	5.51
41.45	14	48.1	47.0	45.7	44.4	43.0	41.4	39.7	37.8	35.7	33.3	30.5	3.82	4.33
	16	46.7	45.6	44.3	43.0	41.6	40.0	38.3	36.4	34.3	31.9	29.1	3.08	3.58
	18	45.3	44.1	42.9	41.6	40.1	38.6	36.8	34.9	32.8	30.4	27.7	2.43	2.92
	12	52.3	51.1	49.8	48.4	46.8	45.2	43.4	41.4	39.2	36.7	33.7	5.07	5.60
43.52	14	50.3	49.1	47.7	46.3	44.8	43.2	41.4	39.4	37.2	34.6	31.7	3.85	4.36
	16	48.8	47.6	46.3	44.9	43.3	41.7	39.9	37.9	35.7	33.2	30.2	3.09	3.59
	18	47.3	46.1	44.8	43.4	41.8	40.2	38.4	36.4	34.2	31.7	28.7	2.43	2.92

TABLE 129

Process Times (B) at Retort Temperature of 230°F for Conduction-Heating Foods in 401 x 211 Can

f_h	z	INITIAL FOOD TEMPERATURE (T_{ih})											Equivalent	
		100	110	120	130	140	150	160	170	180	190	200	F_c^{18}	F_s^{18}
	12	206.0	204.5	202.9	201.1	199.1	196.9	194.3	191.4	188.0	183.8	178.3	10.50	10.83
43.50	14	146.1	144.6	143.0	141.2	139.2	137.0	134.4	131.5	128.1	123.9	118.4	5.94	6.26
	16	118.1	116.5	114.9	113.1	111.1	108.9	106.4	103.5	100.0	95.8	90.4	3.85	4.15
	18	102.6	101.1	99.4	97.6	95.6	93.4	90.9	88.0	84.5	80.3	74.9	2.62	2.93
	12	210.4	208.8	207.1	205.2	203.1	200.7	198.1	195.0	191.3	186.9	181.1	10.50	10.82
46.06	14	150.5	148.9	147.1	145.2	143.1	140.8	138.1	135.0	131.4	126.9	121.1	5.99	6.30
	16	122.0	120.4	118.7	116.7	114.6	112.3	109.6	106.5	102.9	98.4	92.7	3.86	4.17
	18	106.4	104.8	103.1	101.2	99.1	96.7	94.1	91.0	87.3	82.9	77.1	2.62	2.93
	12	214.2	212.6	210.7	208.7	206.5	204.0	201.2	197.9	194.1	189.4	183.3	10.48	10.80
48.62	14	154.6	152.9	151.0	149.0	146.8	144.3	141.5	138.2	134.4	129.7	123.6	5.99	6.30
	16	126.3	124.6	122.7	120.7	118.5	116.0	113.2	110.0	106.1	101.4	95.3	3.89	4.20
	18	110.2	108.5	106.7	104.7	102.5	100.0	97.2	93.9	90.0	85.3	79.3	2.62	2.93
	12	218.0	216.2	214.3	212.2	209.8	207.2	204.2	200.8	196.8	191.8	185.4	10.48	10.81
51.18	14	158.7	156.9	155.0	152.8	150.5	147.9	144.9	141.5	137.4	132.5	126.1	6.00	6.32
	16	130.7	128.9	127.0	124.8	122.5	119.9	116.9	113.5	109.4	104.5	98.1	3.92	4.24
	18	113.9	112.1	110.2	108.1	105.7	103.1	100.1	96.7	92.6	87.7	81.3	2.62	2.93
	12	222.7	220.8	218.8	216.6	214.1	211.4	208.3	204.7	200.4	195.2	188.5	10.58	10.91
53.74	14	162.9	161.0	159.0	156.8	154.3	151.6	148.5	144.9	140.6	135.4	128.7	6.03	6.35
	16	135.0	133.1	131.1	128.8	126.4	123.6	120.5	116.9	112.7	107.5	100.7	3.91	4.24
	18	117.5	115.6	113.6	111.3	108.9	106.1	103.0	99.4	95.1	89.9	83.2	2.62	2.93

TABLE 130

Process Times (B) at Retort Temperature of 240°F for Conduction-Heating Foods in 401 x 211 Can

f_h	z	INITIAL FOOD TEMPERATURE (T_{ih})											Equivalent	
		100	110	120	130	140	150	160	170	180	190	200	F_c^{18}	F_s^{18}
	12	91.9	90.5	89.0	87.3	85.5	83.5	81.3	78.8	75.9	72.4	68.2	6.70	7.09
43.50	14	82.5	81.1	79.6	78.0	76.2	74.2	72.0	69.4	66.5	63.1	58.9	4.72	5.12
	16	75.7	74.3	72.7	71.1	69.3	67.3	65.1	62.6	59.6	56.2	52.0	3.41	3.80
	18	70.6	69.2	67.7	66.0	64.2	62.2	60.0	57.5	54.6	51.1	46.9	2.55	2.93
	12	95.9	94.4	92.8	91.1	89.2	87.0	84.7	82.0	78.9	75.3	70.8	6.83	7.22
46.06	14	86.2	84.7	83.1	81.4	79.4	77.3	75.0	72.3	69.2	65.6	61.1	4.76	5.17
	16	79.0	77.6	76.0	74.2	72.3	70.2	67.9	65.2	62.1	58.5	54.0	3.42	3.82
	18	73.7	72.2	70.6	68.9	67.0	64.9	62.5	59.9	56.8	53.1	48.7	2.54	2.93
	12	99.8	98.2	96.5	94.7	92.7	90.5	88.0	85.2	81.9	78.1	73.3	6.95	7.35
48.62	14	89.8	88.2	86.5	84.7	82.7	80.4	77.9	75.1	71.9	68.0	63.3	4.80	5.21
	16	82.4	80.8	79.1	77.3	75.3	73.1	70.6	67.8	64.5	60.6	55.9	3.44	3.83
	18	76.9	75.3	73.6	71.8	69.8	67.6	65.1	62.3	59.0	55.1	50.4	2.54	2.93
	12	103.6	102.0	100.2	98.3	96.2	93.8	91.2	88.2	84.8	80.8	75.8	7.05	7.45
51.18	14	93.3	91.6	89.9	87.9	85.8	83.5	80.8	77.9	74.5	70.4	65.4	4.84	5.25
	16	85.7	84.0	82.3	80.3	78.2	75.9	73.2	70.3	66.8	62.8	57.8	3.43	3.84
	18	80.0	78.4	76.6	74.7	72.5	70.2	67.6	64.6	61.2	57.1	52.2	2.54	2.93
	12	107.6	105.8	104.0	101.9	99.7	97.3	94.5	91.4	87.8	83.5	78.3	7.09	7.50
53.74	14	96.8	95.1	93.2	91.2	88.9	86.5	83.7	80.6	77.0	72.8	67.6	4.86	5.27
	16	88.9	87.2	85.3	83.3	81.1	78.6	75.9	72.8	69.2	64.9	59.7	3.43	3.83
	18	83.1	81.4	79.5	77.5	75.2	72.8	70.0	66.9	63.3	59.1	53.9	2.54	2.93

TABLE 131

Process Times (B) at Retort Temperature of 250°F for Conduction-Heating Foods in 401 x 211 Can

f_h	z	INITIAL FOOD TEMPERATURE (T_{ih})											Equivalent	
		100	110	120	130	140	150	160	170	180	190	200	F_c^{18}	F_s^{18}
43.50	12	64.2	62.9	61.5	60.0	58.4	56.6	54.6	52.4	49.8	46.9	43.5	5.36	5.84
	14	61.2	59.9	58.5	57.0	55.3	53.5	51.5	49.3	46.8	43.9	40.4	4.14	4.61
	16	58.4	57.1	55.7	54.2	52.5	50.7	48.7	46.5	44.0	41.1	37.6	3.19	3.65
	18	55.9	54.6	53.2	51.7	50.0	48.2	46.2	44.0	41.5	38.6	35.1	2.49	2.93
46.06	12	67.4	66.0	64.5	62.9	61.2	59.3	57.2	54.8	52.1	49.1	45.4	5.42	5.90
	14	64.2	62.8	61.4	59.8	58.0	56.1	54.0	51.6	49.0	45.9	42.2	4.16	4.64
	16	61.3	59.9	58.4	56.8	55.1	53.2	51.0	48.7	46.0	42.9	39.3	3.22	3.68
	18	58.6	57.2	55.7	54.1	52.4	50.5	48.4	46.0	43.4	40.3	36.6	2.48	2.93
48.62	12	70.5	69.0	67.5	65.8	63.9	61.9	59.7	57.2	54.4	51.1	47.3	5.46	5.95
	14	67.2	65.7	64.2	62.5	60.7	58.6	56.4	53.9	51.1	47.9	44.0	4.18	4.66
	16	64.1	62.6	61.1	59.4	57.5	55.5	53.3	50.8	48.0	44.7	40.9	3.25	3.71
	18	61.3	59.8	58.2	56.5	54.7	52.7	50.5	48.0	45.2	41.9	38.1	2.48	2.93
51.18	12	73.6	72.1	70.4	68.7	66.7	64.6	62.3	59.7	56.7	53.3	49.2	5.52	6.01
	14	70.2	68.7	67.0	65.3	63.3	61.2	58.9	56.2	53.3	49.8	45.8	4.22	4.70
	16	66.9	65.4	63.7	62.0	60.0	57.9	55.6	52.9	50.0	46.6	42.5	3.25	3.72
	18	63.9	62.4	60.8	59.0	57.0	54.9	52.6	50.0	47.0	43.6	39.5	2.48	2.93
53.74	12	76.8	75.2	73.4	71.6	69.5	67.3	64.8	62.1	59.0	55.4	51.1	5.59	6.08
	14	73.2	71.6	69.9	68.0	66.0	63.8	61.3	58.6	55.4	51.8	47.6	4.27	4.75
	16	69.8	68.2	66.4	64.6	62.5	60.3	57.8	55.1	52.0	48.4	44.1	3.27	3.74
	18	66.6	65.0	63.3	61.4	59.4	57.2	54.7	52.0	48.8	45.2	41.0	2.48	2.93

TABLE 132

Process Times (B) at Retort Temperature of 260°F for Conduction-Heating Foods in 401 x 211 Can

f_h	z	INITIAL FOOD TEMPERATURE (T_{ih})											Equivalent	
		100	110	120	130	140	150	160	170	180	190	200	F_c^{18}	F_s^{18}
43.50	12	52.3	51.1	49.8	48.4	46.9	45.2	43.4	41.4	39.2	36.7	33.8	5.09	5.62
	14	50.3	49.1	47.8	46.4	44.9	43.2	41.4	39.4	37.2	34.7	31.8	3.87	4.38
	16	48.8	47.6	46.3	44.9	43.4	41.7	39.9	37.9	35.7	33.2	30.3	3.11	3.61
	18	47.3	46.1	44.8	43.4	41.9	40.2	38.4	36.4	34.2	31.7	28.8	2.45	2.93
46.06	12	55.1	53.8	52.4	50.9	49.3	47.6	45.7	43.6	41.2	38.5	35.4	5.18	5.71
	14	52.9	51.6	50.2	48.7	47.1	45.4	43.5	41.4	39.0	36.4	33.3	3.90	4.42
	16	51.3	50.0	48.6	47.1	45.5	43.8	41.9	39.8	37.4	34.8	31.7	3.11	3.61
	18	49.7	48.4	47.0	45.5	43.9	42.2	40.3	38.2	35.8	33.2	30.1	2.45	2.93
48.62	12	57.8	56.4	55.0	53.4	51.7	49.9	47.9	45.7	43.2	40.4	37.1	5.27	5.80
	14	55.5	54.2	52.7	51.1	49.5	47.6	45.6	43.4	40.9	38.1	34.8	3.96	4.48
	16	53.8	52.4	51.0	49.4	47.7	45.9	43.9	41.6	39.2	36.3	33.1	3.12	3.63
	18	52.1	50.7	49.3	47.7	46.0	44.2	42.2	39.9	37.4	34.6	31.4	2.44	2.93
51.18	12	60.5	59.1	57.6	55.9	54.1	52.2	50.1	47.7	45.1	42.1	38.7	5.35	5.88
	14	58.2	56.7	55.2	53.5	51.8	49.8	47.7	45.4	42.8	39.8	36.4	4.02	4.54
	16	56.3	54.8	53.3	51.7	49.9	47.9	45.8	43.5	40.9	37.9	34.5	3.14	3.64
	18	54.5	53.0	51.5	49.9	48.1	46.1	44.0	41.7	39.1	36.1	32.7	2.44	2.93
53.74	12	63.2	61.7	60.1	58.4	56.5	54.5	52.3	49.8	47.1	43.9	40.3	5.42	5.96
	14	60.8	59.3	57.6	55.9	54.1	52.0	49.8	47.3	44.6	41.5	37.9	4.07	4.59
	16	58.7	57.2	55.6	53.9	52.0	50.0	47.8	45.3	42.6	39.4	35.8	3.15	3.66
	18	56.8	55.3	53.7	52.0	50.1	48.1	45.9	43.4	40.6	37.5	33.9	2.44	2.93

TABLE 133

Process Times (B) at Retort Temperature of 230°F for Conduction-Heating Foods in 401 x 411 Can

f_h	z	INITIAL FOOD TEMPERATURE (T_{ih}) 100	110	120	130	140	150	160	170	180	190	200	Equivalent F_c^{18}	F_s^{18}
71.80	12	255.0	252.5	249.8	246.8	243.5	239.9	235.7	230.9	225.2	218.3	209.3	10.88	11.23
	14	193.4	190.9	188.2	185.2	181.9	178.3	174.1	169.3	163.6	156.6	147.7	6.25	6.60
	16	164.3	161.8	159.1	156.1	152.8	149.1	145.0	140.2	134.5	127.5	118.5	3.97	4.32
	18	141.8	139.3	136.6	133.6	130.4	126.7	122.5	117.7	112.0	105.1	96.1	2.66	2.99
76.02	12	261.5	258.8	256.0	252.8	249.3	245.5	241.0	236.0	229.9	222.6	213.1	10.85	11.21
	14	201.0	198.4	195.5	192.4	188.9	185.0	180.6	175.5	169.5	162.1	152.6	6.34	6.69
	16	170.4	167.7	164.9	161.7	158.2	154.4	150.0	144.9	138.8	131.5	122.0	3.97	4.32
	18	147.7	145.1	142.2	139.1	135.6	131.7	127.3	122.2	116.2	108.8	99.3	2.66	2.99
80.24	12	268.8	266.0	263.0	259.7	256.0	251.9	247.3	241.9	235.5	227.8	217.7	10.91	11.28
	14	208.5	205.7	202.7	199.3	195.7	191.6	186.9	181.5	175.2	167.4	157.4	6.42	6.78
	16	176.3	173.5	170.5	167.2	163.5	159.4	154.8	149.4	143.0	135.3	125.2	3.97	4.32
	18	153.5	150.7	147.7	144.3	140.7	136.6	131.9	126.5	120.2	112.4	102.4	2.65	2.99
84.47	12	275.8	272.9	269.7	266.2	262.3	258.0	253.1	247.4	240.8	232.6	222.0	10.97	11.34
	14	215.8	212.9	209.7	206.2	202.3	198.0	193.1	187.4	180.7	172.5	162.0	6.49	6.85
	16	182.1	179.1	176.0	172.5	168.6	164.3	159.4	153.7	147.0	138.8	128.3	3.97	4.32
	18	159.1	156.2	153.0	149.5	145.6	141.3	136.4	130.8	124.1	115.9	105.3	2.64	2.99
88.69	12	282.4	279.3	276.0	272.3	268.3	263.7	258.6	252.6	245.6	237.0	225.9	10.96	11.33
	14	222.9	219.8	216.5	212.8	208.8	204.2	199.1	193.1	186.1	177.5	166.4	6.48	6.85
	16	187.7	184.6	181.2	177.6	173.5	169.0	163.8	157.9	150.9	142.3	131.2	3.97	4.32
	18	164.6	161.6	158.2	154.5	150.5	145.9	140.8	134.9	127.8	119.2	108.2	2.64	2.99

TABLE 134

Process Times (B) at Retort Temperature of 240°F for Conduction-Heating Foods in 401 x 411 Can

f_h	z	INITIAL FOOD TEMPERATURE (T_{ih}) 100	110	120	130	140	150	160	170	180	190	200	Equivalent F_c^{18}	F_s^{18}
71.80	12	135.4	133.1	130.6	127.9	124.9	121.6	118.0	113.8	109.0	103.3	96.3	7.64	8.08
	14	121.8	119.5	117.0	114.3	111.3	108.0	104.3	100.2	95.4	89.7	82.7	5.09	5.52
	16	112.1	109.8	107.3	104.6	101.6	98.3	94.7	90.5	85.7	80.0	73.0	3.54	3.97
	18	104.8	102.5	100.0	97.3	94.3	91.0	87.3	83.2	78.4	72.7	65.7	2.57	2.99
76.02	12	141.7	139.2	136.6	133.7	130.6	127.1	123.2	118.8	113.7	107.7	100.3	7.76	8.21
	14	127.4	124.9	122.3	119.4	116.3	112.8	108.9	104.5	99.4	93.4	86.0	5.12	5.56
	16	117.3	114.8	112.2	109.3	106.2	102.7	98.8	94.4	89.3	83.3	75.9	3.55	3.98
	18	109.6	107.2	104.6	101.7	98.5	95.1	91.2	86.8	81.7	75.7	68.3	2.57	2.99
80.24	12	147.9	145.3	142.5	139.5	136.1	132.5	128.4	123.7	118.3	112.0	104.2	7.87	8.33
	14	132.9	130.3	127.5	124.5	121.2	117.5	113.4	108.8	103.4	97.0	89.3	5.14	5.58
	16	122.5	119.9	117.1	114.1	110.7	107.1	103.0	98.3	92.9	86.6	78.8	3.56	3.99
	18	114.5	111.9	109.1	106.1	102.7	99.1	95.0	90.3	84.9	78.6	70.8	2.57	2.99
84.47	12	154.0	151.3	148.3	145.1	141.6	137.8	133.4	128.5	122.9	116.2	108.0	7.99	8.44
	14	138.5	135.8	132.8	129.6	126.1	122.3	117.9	113.0	107.4	100.7	92.5	5.17	5.62
	16	127.6	124.9	121.9	118.8	115.3	111.4	107.1	102.2	96.5	89.8	81.6	3.57	4.01
	18	119.2	116.5	113.6	110.4	106.9	103.0	98.7	93.8	88.2	81.5	73.3	2.57	2.99
88.69	12	160.0	157.2	154.1	150.7	147.1	143.0	138.5	133.3	127.4	120.4	111.8	8.07	8.53
	14	144.0	141.1	138.0	134.7	131.0	127.0	122.4	117.3	111.3	104.3	95.7	5.21	5.65
	16	132.7	129.8	126.8	123.4	119.7	115.7	111.1	106.0	100.1	93.0	84.4	3.59	4.02
	18	124.0	121.1	118.1	114.7	111.0	107.0	102.4	97.3	91.4	84.3	75.7	2.56	2.99

TABLE 135

Process Times (B) at Retort Temperature of 250°F for Conduction-Heating Foods in 401 x 411 Can

f_h	z	INITIAL FOOD TEMPERATURE (T_{ih})											Equivalent	
		100	110	120	130	140	150	160	170	180	190	200	F_c^{18}	F_s^{18}
71.80	12	98.7	96.5	94.2	91.7	89.0	86.0	82.7	79.1	74.9	70.1	64.4	5.98	6.48
	14	94.2	92.0	89.7	87.2	84.5	81.5	78.2	74.6	70.4	65.6	59.9	4.66	5.15
	16	89.5	87.4	85.1	82.6	79.9	76.9	73.9	69.9	65.8	61.0	55.3	3.45	3.93
	18	85.3	83.2	80.8	78.3	75.6	72.7	69.4	65.7	61.5	56.7	51.0	2.53	2.99
76.02	12	103.6	101.3	98.9	96.2	93.4	90.2	86.7	82.9	78.5	73.4	67.3	6.05	6.56
	14	98.9	96.6	94.2	91.5	88.7	85.5	82.0	78.1	73.7	68.6	62.6	4.68	5.18
	16	94.0	91.7	89.3	86.6	83.8	80.6	77.1	73.2	68.8	63.7	57.7	3.45	3.93
	18	89.5	87.2	84.8	82.1	79.3	76.1	72.6	68.7	64.3	59.2	53.2	2.52	2.99
80.24	12	108.6	106.2	103.6	100.8	97.8	94.5	90.8	86.7	82.1	76.7	70.3	6.15	6.66
	14	103.6	101.2	98.7	95.9	92.8	89.5	85.8	81.7	77.1	71.7	65.4	4.73	5.23
	16	98.5	96.1	93.5	90.7	87.7	84.4	80.7	76.6	71.9	66.5	60.2	3.47	3.96
	18	93.7	91.3	88.7	86.0	82.9	79.6	75.9	71.8	67.2	61.8	55.4	2.52	2.99
84.47	12	113.6	111.0	108.3	105.4	102.2	98.7	94.8	90.5	85.6	79.9	73.3	6.25	6.76
	14	108.3	105.8	103.1	100.1	97.0	93.5	89.6	85.3	80.4	74.7	68.0	4.77	5.28
	16	102.9	100.4	97.7	94.7	91.5	88.0	84.2	79.8	74.9	69.3	62.6	3.50	3.98
	18	97.9	95.4	92.7	89.7	86.5	83.0	79.2	74.8	69.9	64.3	57.6	2.52	2.99
88.69	12	118.5	115.8	112.9	109.9	106.5	102.8	98.8	94.2	89.1	83.2	76.1	6.34	6.86
	14	113.0	110.3	107.5	104.4	101.0	97.4	93.3	88.8	83.6	77.7	70.7	4.82	5.32
	16	107.3	104.6	101.8	98.7	95.3	91.7	87.6	83.1	77.9	72.0	65.0	3.51	4.00
	18	102.0	99.4	96.5	93.4	90.1	86.4	82.3	77.8	72.7	66.7	59.7	2.52	2.99

TABLE 136

Process Times (B) at Retort Temperature of 260 F° for Conduction-Heating Foods in 401 x 411 Can

f_h	z	INITIAL FOOD TEMPERATURE (T_{ih}) 100	110	120	130	140	150	160	170	180	190	200	Equivalent F_c^{18}	F_s^{18}
71.80	12	82.3	80.3	78.1	75.8	73.3	70.6	67.6	64.3	60.7	56.5	51.7	5.99	6.55
	14	78.7	76.7	74.6	72.2	69.7	67.0	64.1	60.8	57.1	52.9	48.1	4.32	4.85
	16	76.2	74.1	72.0	69.7	67.2	64.5	61.5	58 2	54.5	50.4	45.6	3.34	3.86
	18	73.4	71.4	69.3	67.0	64.5	61.8	58.8	55.5	51.8	47.7	42.9	2.49	2.99
76.02	12	86.7	84.5	82.2	79.8	77.2	74.3	71.1	67.7	63.8	59.4	54.3	6.11	6.67
	14	82.9	80.8	78.5	76.1	73.4	70.5	67.4	63.9	60.0	55.6	50.5	4.39	4.92
	16	80.1	78.0	75.7	73.2	70.6	67.7	64.6	61.1	57.2	52.8	47.7	3.36	3.87
	18	77.3	75.2	72.9	70.4	67.8	64.9	61.8	58.3	54.4	50.0	44.9	2.48	2.99
80.24	12	91.0	88.7	86.3	83.7	81.0	77.9	74.6	70.9	66.8	62.2	56.8	6.20	6.76
	14	87.1	84.8	82.4	79.8	77.0	74.0	70.7	67.0	62.9	58.2	52.9	4.44	4.98
	16	84.0	81.7	79.3	76.7	73.9	70.9	67.6	63.9	59.8	55.2	49.8	3.35	3.88
	18	81.1	78.8	76.4	73.8	71.1	68.0	64.7	61.0	56.9	52.3	46.9	2.48	2.99
84.47	12	95.3	92.9	90.4	87.7	84.7	81.5	78.0	74.2	69.8	64.9	59.3	6.28	6.84
	14	91.2	88.8	86.3	83.5	80.6	77.4	73.9	70.1	65.7	60.8	55.2	4.49	5.03
	16	87.8	85.4	82.9	80.2	77.3	74.1	70.6	66.7	62.4	57.5	51.8	3.35	3.88
	18	84.8	82.5	79.9	77.2	74.3	71.1	67.6	63.7	59.4	54.5	48.9	2.48	2.99
88.69	12	99.5	97.0	94.4	91.5	88.4	85.1	81.4	77.4	72.8	67.7	61.7	6.35	6.91
	14	95.2	92.7	90.1	87.2	84.1	80.8	77.1	73.1	68.5	63.4	57.4	4.54	5.08
	16	91.6	89.1	86.5	83.6	80.6	77.2	73.5	69.5	64.9	59.8	53.9	3.35	3.87
	18	88.5	86.1	83.4	80.5	77.5	74.1	70.4	66.4	61.8	56.7	50.8	2.48	2.99

TABLE 137

Process Times (B) at Retort Temperature of 230°F for Conduction-Heating Foods in 401 x 602 Can

f_h	z	INITIAL FOOD TEMPERATURE (T_{ih})											Equivalent	
		100	110	120	130	140	150	160	170	180	190	200	F_c^{18}	F_s^{18}
81.11	12	271.5	268.7	265.6	262.2	258.5	254.4	249.7	244.2	237.8	230.0	219.8	11.01	11.38
	14	210.6	207.8	204.7	201.4	197.7	193.5	188.8	183.4	177.0	169.1	159.0	6.48	6.84
	16	178.1	175.3	172.2	168.9	165.2	161.0	156.3	150.9	144.5	136.6	126.5	4.01	4.36
	18	155.1	152.2	149.2	145.8	142.1	138.0	133.3	127.8	121.4	113.5	103.4	2.67	3.01
85.88	12	279.3	276.3	273.1	269.5	265.6	261.2	256.2	250.5	243.7	235.4	224.6	11.08	11.44
	14	218.9	215.9	212.6	209.1	205.1	200.7	195.8	190.0	183.2	174.9	164.2	6.55	6.91
	16	184.6	181.6	178.4	174.8	170.9	166.5	161.5	155.8	149.0	140.6	129.9	4.01	4.36
	18	161.4	158.4	155.2	151.6	147.7	143.3	138.3	132.6	125.8	117.5	106.7	2.67	3.01
90.65	12	287.0	283.6	280.4	276.6	272.5	267.8	262.6	256.5	249.3	240.6	229.2	11.07	11.44
	14	226.9	223.7	220.3	216.5	212.4	207.8	202.5	196.4	189.3	180.5	169.1	6.53	6.90
	16	190.9	187.7	184.3	180.5	176.4	171.8	166.5	160.4	153.3	144.5	133.1	4.01	4.36
	18	167.6	164.5	161.1	157.3	153.2	148.5	143.3	137.2	130.0	121.2	109.9	2.66	3.01
95.43	12	295.0	291.7	288.1	284.2	279.8	274.9	269.4	263.0	255.4	246.2	234.3	11.12	11.50
	14	234.8	231.5	227.9	223.9	219.5	214.7	209.1	202.7	195.2	185.9	174.0	6.53	6.91
	16	196.9	193.6	190.0	186.1	181.7	176.8	171.3	164.9	157.3	148.1	136.2	4.01	4.36
	18	173.8	170.5	166.9	162.9	158.5	153.7	148.1	141.7	134.2	124.9	113.0	2.66	3.01
100.20	12	302.7	299.2	295.4	291.3	286.7	281.6	275.8	269.1	261.1	251.4	238.9	11.17	11.55
	14	242.5	239.1	235.3	231.1	226.5	221.4	215.6	208.9	201.0	191.2	178.7	6.53	6.91
	16	204.0	200.5	196.7	192.6	188.0	182.9	177.0	170.3	162.4	152.7	140.2	4.06	4.41
	18	179.8	176.3	172.5	168.4	163.8	158.7	152.9	146.2	138.2	128.5	116.0	2.66	3.01

TABLE 138

Process Times (B) at Retort Temperature of 240°F for Conduction-Heating Foods in 401 x 602 Can

f_h	z	INITIAL FOOD TEMPERATURE (T_{ih})											Equivalent	
		100	110	120	130	140	150	160	170	180	190	200	F_c^{18}	F_s^{18}
81.11	12	149.4	146.8	144.0	140.9	137.6	133.9	129.7	125.0	119.6	113.2	105.3	7.95	8.40
	14	134.3	131.7	128.9	125.8	122.5	118.7	114.6	109.9	104.5	98.0	90.2	5.19	5.63
	16	123.8	121.2	118.3	115.3	111.9	108.2	104.1	99.3	93.9	87.5	79.6	3.60	4.03
	18	115.7	113.1	110.2	107.2	103.8	100.1	96.0	91.3	85.8	79.4	71.5	2.59	3.01
85.88	12	156.3	153.5	150.6	147.3	143.8	139.8	135.4	130.5	124.7	117.9	109.6	8.08	8.53
	14	140.6	137.8	134.8	131.6	128.0	124.1	119.7	114.7	109.0	102.2	93.9	5.23	5.67
	16	129.6	126.8	123.8	120.6	117.0	113.1	108.7	103.7	97.9	91.1	82.8	3.61	4.04
	18	121.1	118.3	115.3	112.1	108.5	104.6	100.2	95.2	89.5	82.7	74.3	2.59	3.01
90.65	12	163.2	160.2	157.1	153.7	149.9	145.8	141.1	135.9	129.8	122.6	113.8	8.16	8.62
	14	146.8	143.9	140.7	137.3	133.5	129.4	124.8	119.5	113.4	106.3	97.5	5.27	5.71
	16	135.3	132.4	129.2	125.8	122.1	117.9	113.3	108.0	101.9	94.8	86.0	3.63	4.06
	18	126.4	123.5	120.4	116.9	113.2	109.0	104.4	99.1	93.1	85.9	77.1	2.59	3.01
95.43	12	170.0	166.9	163.6	160.0	156.1	151.7	146.8	141.3	134.9	127.3	118.1	8.24	8.70
	14	152.9	149.9	146.5	142.9	139.0	134.6	129.7	124.2	117.8	110.3	101.0	5.31	5.76
	16	141.0	138.0	134.6	131.0	127.1	122.7	117.8	112.3	105.9	98.4	89.1	3.64	4.08
	18	131.8	128.7	125.4	121.8	117.8	113.5	108.6	103.1	96.7	89.1	79.9	2.59	3.01
100.20	12	176.8	173.6	170.1	166.3	162.1	157.6	152.4	146.6	139.9	132.0	122.3	8.32	8.78
	14	159.1	155.9	152.4	148.6	144.5	139.9	134.7	128.9	122.2	114.3	104.6	5.34	5.79
	16	146.7	143.5	140.0	136.2	132.1	127.5	122.3	116.5	109.8	101.9	92.2	3.65	4.09
	18	137.1	133.9	130.4	126.6	122.5	117.9	112.8	107.0	100.3	92.3	82.6	2.58	3.01

TABLE 139

Process Times (B) at Retort Temperature of 250°F for Conduction-Heating Foods in 401 x 602 Can

f_h	z	INITIAL FOOD TEMPERATURE (T_{ih})											Equivalent	
		100	110	120	130	140	150	160	170	180	190	200	F_c^{18}	F_s^{18}
81.11	12	109.8	107.3	104.7	101.9	98.9	95.5	91.8	87.6	82.9	77.5	71.1	6.21	6.73
	14	104.7	102.3	99.7	96.9	93.8	90.5	86.8	82.6	77.9	72.5	66.0	4.78	5.28
	16	99.5	97.1	94.5	91.7	88.6	85.2	81.5	77.4	72.7	67.3	60.8	3.51	3.99
	18	94.7	92.3	89.7	86.9	83.8	80.4	76.7	72.6	67.9	62.5	56.0	2.55	3.01
85.88	12	115.4	112.8	110.0	107.0	103.8	100.2	96.3	91.9	86.9	81.2	74.4	6.32	6.84
	14	110.0	107.5	104.7	101.7	98.5	94.9	91.0	86.6	81.6	75.9	69.1	4.83	5.33
	16	104.5	101.9	99.2	96.2	92.9	89.4	85.5	81.1	76.1	70.3	63.5	3.53	4.02
	18	99.4	96.9	94.1	91.1	87.9	84.3	80.4	76.0	71.0	65.3	58.5	2.54	3.01
90.65	12	120.9	118.2	115.3	112.1	108.7	104.9	100.8	96.1	90.9	84.8	77.6	6.43	6.95
	14	115.3	112.6	109.7	106.5	103.1	99.3	95.2	90.5	85.3	79.2	72.0	4.88	5.39
	16	109.5	106.7	103.8	100.7	97.3	93.5	89.4	84.7	79.5	73.4	66.2	3.55	4.04
	18	104.1	101.4	98.5	95.3	91.9	88.1	84.0	79.4	74.1	68.0	60.9	2.54	3.01
95.43	12	126.5	123.6	120.5	117.2	113.6	109.7	105.3	100.4	94.9	88.5	80.9	6.56	7.08
	14	120.5	117.7	114.6	111.3	107.7	103.7	99.4	94.5	89.0	82.6	75.0	4.95	5.46
	16	114.4	111.5	108.5	105.2	101.6	97.6	93.2	88.4	82.8	76.4	68.9	3.56	4.05
	18	108.8	105.9	102.8	99.5	95.9	92.0	87.6	82.7	77.2	70.8	63.2	2.54	3.01
100.20	12	132.0	129.0	125.7	122.3	118.5	114.3	109.7	104.6	98.8	92.1	84.2	6.68	7.20
	14	125.7	122.7	119.5	116.0	112.2	108.1	103.5	98.4	92.6	85.9	77.9	5.01	5.52
	16	119.3	116.3	113.1	109.6	105.8	101.6	97.1	91.9	86.1	79.4	71.5	3.57	4.06
	18	113.4	110.4	107.2	103.7	99.9	95.7	91.2	86.0	80.2	73.5	65.6	2.54	3.01

TABLE 140

Process Times (B) at Retort Temperature of 260°F for Conduction-Heating Foods in 401 x 602 Can

f_h	z	INITIAL FOOD TEMPERATURE (T_{ih})											Equivalent	
		100	110	120	130	140	150	160	170	180	190	200	F_c^{18}	F_s^{18}
81.11	12	92.0	89.7	87.3	84.6	81.8	78.8	75.4	71.7	67.5	62.8	57.4	6.26	6.82
	14	88.0	85.7	83.3	80.7	77.9	74.8	71.4	67.7	63.6	58.9	53.4	4.49	5.03
	16	84.9	82.6	80.2	77.6	74.7	71.7	68.3	64.6	60.5	55.7	50.3	3.39	3.91
	18	81.9	79.7	77.2	74.6	71.8	68.8	65.4	61.7	57.5	52.8	47.4	2.50	3.01
85.88	12	96.8	94.4	91.8	89.1	86.1	82.8	79.3	75.3	70.9	66.0	60.2	6.35	6.91
	14	92.6	90.2	87.6	84.9	81.9	78.6	75.1	71.2	66.8	61.8	56.0	4.55	5.09
	16	89.2	86.8	84.2	81.5	78.5	75.2	71.7	67.7	63.3	58.4	52.6	3.38	3.91
	18	86.2	83.8	81.2	78.4	75.5	72.2	68.7	64.7	60.3	55.4	49.6	2.50	3.01
90.65	12	101.6	99.1	96.3	93.4	90.3	86.8	83.1	78.9	74.3	69.0	63.0	6.43	6.99
	14	97.2	94.7	91.9	89.0	85.9	82.5	78.7	74.6	69.9	64.7	58.6	4.59	5.14
	16	93.5	91.0	88.3	85.4	82.2	78.8	75.0	70.9	66.3	61.0	54.9	3.39	3.91
	18	90.4	87.8	85.1	82.2	79.0	75.6	71.9	67.7	63.1	57.8	51.8	2.50	3.01
95.43	12	106.4	103.7	100.9	97.8	94.5	90.9	86.9	82.6	77.7	72.1	65.8	6.50	7.07
	14	101.7	99.1	96.2	93.1	89.8	86.2	82.3	77.9	73.0	67.5	61.1	4.62	5.16
	16	98.0	95.3	92.4	89.3	86.0	82.4	78.5	74.1	69.2	63.7	57.3	3.42	3.94
	18	94.5	91.8	89.0	85.9	82.6	79.0	75.0	70.6	65.8	60.2	53.8	2.50	3.01
100.20	12	111.2	108.4	105.4	102.1	98.7	94.9	90.7	86.1	81.0	75.2	68.5	6.57	7.14
	14	106.3	103.5	100.5	97.3	93.8	90.0	85.9	81.3	76.2	70.4	63.7	4.68	5.23
	16	102.3	99.5	96.5	93.3	89.8	86.0	81.9	77.3	72.1	66.3	59.6	3.41	3.94
	18	98.6	95.8	92.8	89.5	86.1	82.3	78.1	73.5	68.4	62.6	55.9	2.50	3.01

TABLE 141

Process Times (B) at Retort Temperature of 230°F for Conduction-Heating Foods in 404 x 200 Can

f_h	z	INITIAL FOOD TEMPERATURE (T_{ih})											Equivalent	
		100	110	120	130	140	150	160	170	180	190	200	F_c^{18}	F_s^{18}
	12	179.6	178.6	177.5	176.3	175.0	173.6	171.9	170.0	167.8	165.0	161.4	10.30	10.59
28.49	14	121.4	120.4	119.3	118.1	116.8	115.3	113.7	111.8	109.5	106.8	103.2	5.84	6.11
	16	94.1	93.1	92.1	90.9	89.6	88.1	86.5	84.6	82.3	79.5	76.0	3.78	4.05
	18	79.0	78.0	76.9	75.7	74.4	72.9	71.3	69.4	67.1	64.4	60.8	2.64	2.91
	12	183.2	182.1	181.0	179.8	178.4	176.8	175.1	173.1	170.7	167.7	164.0	10.30	10.59
30.16	14	124.2	123.1	122.0	120.8	119.4	117.8	116.1	114.1	111.7	108.8	105.0	5.88	6.16
	16	96.9	95.8	94.7	93.5	92.1	90.5	88.8	86.8	84.4	81.5	77.7	3.79	4.07
	18	81.4	80.4	79.2	78.0	76.6	75.1	73.3	71.3	68.9	66.0	62.2	2.64	2.91
	12	186.4	185.3	184.1	182.8	181.3	179.7	177.9	175.7	173.2	170.1	166.1	10.31	10.60
31.84	14	126.9	125.8	124.6	123.3	121.9	120.2	118.4	116.3	113.7	110.6	106.7	5.87	6.16
	16	99.5	98.4	97.2	95.9	94.4	92.8	90.9	88.8	86.3	83.2	79.2	3.79	4.07
	18	83.9	82.8	81.6	80.3	78.8	77.2	75.3	73.2	70.7	67.6	63.6	2.63	2.91
	12	189.3	188.1	186.8	185.5	183.9	182.2	180.3	178.0	175.4	172.1	167.9	10.31	10.61
33.51	14	129.6	128.5	127.2	125.8	124.3	122.6	120.6	118.4	115.7	112.5	108.3	5.86	6.16
	16	102.1	100.9	99.6	98.2	96.7	95.0	93.0	90.8	88.2	84.9	80.7	3.79	4.08
	18	86.3	85.1	83.9	82.5	81.0	79.2	77.3	75.1	72.4	69.2	65.0	2.63	2.91
	12	191.8	190.5	189.2	187.8	186.1	184.3	182.3	179.9	177.2	173.7	169.4	10.32	10.61
35.19	14	132.1	130.9	129.6	128.1	126.5	124.7	122.7	120.3	117.5	114.1	109.7	5.86	6.15
	16	104.7	103.5	102.2	100.7	99.1	97.3	95.3	92.9	90.1	86.7	82.3	3.80	4.09
	18	89.0	87.8	86.5	85.0	83.4	81.6	79.6	77.2	74.4	71.0	66.6	2.62	2.91

TABLE 142

Process Times (B) at Retort Temperature of 240°F for Conduction-Heating Foods in 404 x 200 Can

f_h	z	INITIAL FOOD TEMPERATURE (T_{ih})											Equivalent	
		100	110	120	130	140	150	160	170	180	190	200	F_c^{18}	F_s^{18}
	12	68.1	67.1	66.1	65.1	63.9	62.6	61.1	59.5	57.6	55.3	52.6	6.17	6.55
28.49	14	60.5	59.6	58.6	57.5	56.3	55.0	53.6	51.9	50.0	47.8	45.0	4.45	4.81
	16	55.3	54.4	53.4	52.3	51.1	49.8	48.4	46.7	44.8	42.6	39.8	3.36	3.72
	18	51.2	50.3	49.3	48.2	47.0	45.7	44.3	42.6	40.7	38.5	35.7	2.55	2.91
	12	70.7	69.7	68.7	67.5	66.3	64.9	63.4	61.6	59.6	57.2	54.3	6.17	6.56
30.16	14	63.1	62.1	61.1	59.9	58.7	57.3	55.7	54.0	52.0	49.6	46.7	4.52	4.89
	16	57.6	56.6	55.6	54.4	53.2	51.8	50.2	48.5	46.5	44.1	41.2	3.35	3.71
	18	53.5	52.5	51.4	50.3	49.0	47.7	46.1	44.4	42.4	40.0	37.0	2.55	2.91
	12	73.3	72.2	71.1	69.9	68.6	67.1	65.5	63.7	61.5	59.0	55.9	6.18	6.57
31.84	14	65.6	64.6	63.5	62.3	60.9	59.5	57.9	56.0	53.9	51.4	48.3	4.60	4.96
	16	59.8	58.8	57.7	56.5	55.2	53.7	52.1	50.2	48.1	45.6	42.5	3.34	3.71
	18	55.7	54.6	53.5	52.3	51.0	49.6	47.9	46.1	43.9	41.4	38.3	2.55	2.91
	12	75.7	74.7	73.5	72.2	70.9	69.3	67.6	65.7	63.4	60.8	57.5	6.19	6.58
33.51	14	68.1	67.0	65.8	64.5	63.2	61.6	59.9	58.0	55.7	53.1	49.8	4.67	5.03
	16	62.1	61.1	59.9	58.6	57.2	55.7	54.0	52.0	49.8	47.1	43.9	3.36	3.73
	18	57.8	56.7	55.6	54.3	52.9	51.4	49.7	47.7	45.5	42.8	39.6	2.54	2.91
	12	78.2	77.1	75.8	74.5	73.0	71.4	69.6	67.6	65.2	62.5	59.0	6.20	6.59
35.19	14	70.5	69.3	68.1	66.8	65.3	63.7	61.9	59.9	57.5	54.7	51.3	4.65	5.02
	16	64.5	63.3	62.1	60.8	59.3	57.7	55.9	53.9	51.5	48.7	45.3	3.38	3.76
	18	60.0	58.8	57.6	56.3	54.8	53.2	51.4	49.4	47.0	44.2	40.8	2.54	2.91

TABLE 143

Process Times (B) at Retort Temperature of 250°F for Conduction-Heating Foods in 404 x 200 Can

f_h	z	INITIAL FOOD TEMPERATURE (T_{ih}) 100	110	120	130	140	150	160	170	180	190	200	Equivalent F_c^{18}	F_s^{18}
28.49	12	45.1	44.2	43.3	42.3	41.2	40.0	38.7	37.3	35.6	33.7	31.5	4.91	5.37
	14	42.8	42.0	41.1	40.1	39.0	37.8	36.5	35.1	33.4	31.5	29.2	3.84	4.29
	16	41.0	40.2	39.2	38.2	37.2	36.0	34.7	33.2	31.6	29.7	27.4	3.09	3.52
	18	39.5	38.6	37.7	36.7	35.6	34.4	33.1	31.7	30.0	28.1	25.9	2.48	2.91
30.16	12	47.3	46.4	45.4	44.3	43.2	42.0	40.6	39.0	37.3	35.3	32.9	4.98	5.44
	14	44.9	44.0	43.1	42.0	40.9	39.6	38.2	36.7	35.0	32.9	30.5	3.89	4.34
	16	43.0	42.1	41.1	40.1	38.9	37.7	36.3	34.8	33.0	31.0	28.6	3.11	3.55
	18	41.4	40.4	39.5	38.4	37.3	36.0	34.7	33.1	31.4	29.3	27.0	2.48	2.91
31.84	12	49.4	48.5	47.5	46.3	45.1	43.8	42.4	40.7	38.9	36.8	34.2	5.02	5.48
	14	47.0	46.1	45.0	43.9	42.7	41.4	39.9	38.3	36.5	34.3	31.8	3.93	4.38
	16	45.0	44.0	43.0	41.9	40.7	39.4	37.9	36.3	34.4	32.3	29.8	3.11	3.56
	18	43.2	42.3	41.2	40.1	38.9	37.6	36.1	34.5	32.7	30.5	28.0	2.48	2.91
33.51	12	51.6	50.6	49.5	48.3	47.1	45.7	44.1	42.4	40.5	38.2	35.6	5.06	5.53
	14	49.1	48.0	47.0	45.8	44.5	43.2	41.6	39.9	38.0	35.7	33.1	3.95	4.41
	16	46.9	45.9	44.8	43.7	42.4	41.0	39.5	37.8	35.8	33.6	30.9	3.10	3.55
	18	45.0	44.0	43.0	41.8	40.5	39.1	37.6	35.9	33.9	31.7	29.1	2.47	2.91
35.19	12	53.7	52.6	51.5	50.3	48.9	47.5	45.9	44.1	42.0	39.7	36.9	5.10	5.57
	14	51.1	50.0	48.9	47.7	46.3	44.9	43.3	41.5	39.4	37.1	34.3	3.97	4.43
	16	48.8	47.8	46.6	45.4	44.1	42.6	41.0	39.2	37.2	34.8	32.0	3.09	3.54
	18	46.8	45.8	44.7	43.4	42.1	40.6	39.0	37.2	35.2	32.8	30.1	2.47	2.91

TABLE 144

Process Times (B) at Retort Temperature of 260°F for Conduction-Heating Foods in 404 x 200 Can

f_h	z	INITIAL FOOD TEMPERATURE (T_{ih})											Equivalent	
		100	110	120	130	140	150	160	170	180	190	200	F_c^{18}	F_s^{18}
28.49	12	35.6	34.8	33.9	33.0	32.0	30.9	29.7	28.4	27.0	25.3	23.4	4.28	4.79
	14	34.6	33.8	33.0	32.0	31.1	30.0	28.8	27.5	26.0	24.4	22.5	3.58	4.07
	16	33.7	32.9	32.0	31.1	30.1	29.1	27.9	26.6	25.1	23.5	21.6	2.99	3.47
	18	32.8	32.0	31.1	30.2	29.2	28.1	26.9	25.6	24.2	22.5	20.6	2.44	2.91
30.16	12	37.5	36.6	35.7	34.7	33.7	32.5	31.3	29.9	28.4	26.6	24.6	4.39	4.89
	14	36.4	35.6	34.7	33.7	32.6	31.5	30.2	28.9	27.3	25.6	23.6	3.63	4.12
	16	35.4	34.6	33.7	32.7	31.7	30.5	29.3	27.9	26.3	24.6	22.6	3.00	3.49
	18	34.4	33.6	32.7	31.7	30.6	29.5	28.2	26.9	25.3	23.6	21.6	2.44	2.91
31.84	12	39.3	38.4	37.5	36.3	35.3	34.1	32.8	31.4	29.7	27.9	25.8	4.47	4.98
	14	38.2	37.3	36.3	35.3	34.2	33.0	31.7	30.2	28.6	26.7	24.6	3.65	4.15
	16	37.1	36.2	35.3	34.3	33.2	32.0	30.6	29.2	27.5	25.7	23.6	3.02	3.50
	18	36.0	35.2	34.2	33.2	32.1	30.9	29.5	28.1	26.5	24.6	22.5	2.44	2.91
33.51	12	41.2	40.3	39.3	38.2	37.0	35.7	34.4	32.8	31.1	29.2	26.9	4.55	5.06
	14	39.9	39.0	38.0	36.9	35.7	34.5	33.1	31.6	29.8	27.9	25.6	3.68	4.18
	16	38.8	37.9	36.9	35.8	34.6	33.4	32.0	30.4	28.7	26.8	24.5	3.03	3.51
	18	37.7	36.7	35.7	34.7	33.5	32.2	30.8	29.3	27.6	25.6	23.4	2.43	2.91
35.19	12	43.1	42.1	41.0	39.9	38.7	37.3	35.9	34.3	32.5	30.4	28.1	4.63	5.14
	14	41.7	40.7	39.6	38.5	37.3	35.9	34.5	32.9	31.1	29.0	26.7	3.71	4.22
	16	40.5	39.5	38.5	37.3	36.1	34.8	33.3	31.7	29.9	27.9	25.5	3.03	3.52
	18	39.3	38.3	37.3	36.1	34.9	33.6	32.1	30.5	28.7	26.7	24.3	2.43	2.91

TABLE 145

Process Times (B) at Retort Temperature of 230°F for Conduction-Heating Foods in 404 x 211 Can

f_h	z	INITIAL FOOD TEMPERATURE (T_{ih})											Equivalent	
		100	110	120	130	140	150	160	170	180	190	200	F_c^{18}	f_s^{18}
	12	209.5	208.0	206.3	204.4	202.3	200.0	197.4	194.3	190.8	186.4	180.7	10.53	10.86
45.30	14	149.4	147.8	146.1	144.3	142.2	139.9	137.2	134.2	130.6	126.2	120.6	5.99	6.30
	16	121.0	119.4	117.7	115.9	113.8	111.5	108.8	105.8	102.2	97.8	92.2	3.87	4.18
	18	105.4	103.8	102.1	100.3	98.2	95.9	93.2	90.2	86.6	82.2	76.6	2.63	2.94
	12	213.8	212.1	210.3	208.3	206.1	203.6	200.9	197.6	193.8	189.2	183.2	10.51	10.84
47.97	14	153.8	152.1	150.3	148.4	146.1	143.7	140.9	137.7	133.9	129.2	123.2	6.01	6.32
	16	125.3	123.6	121.8	119.8	117.6	115.1	112.4	109.1	105.4	100.7	94.7	3.88	4.20
	18	109.4	107.7	105.9	103.9	101.7	99.1	96.5	93.3	89.5	84.8	78.8	2.63	2.94
	12	217.3	215.6	213.6	211.5	209.2	206.6	203.7	200.3	196.3	191.4	185.1	10.49	10.82
50.63	14	158.0	156.2	154.3	152.2	149.9	147.3	144.3	141.0	136.9	132.0	125.7	6.00	6.33
	16	129.9	128.1	126.2	124.1	121.8	119.2	116.3	112.9	108.9	104.0	97.6	3.93	4.25
	18	113.2	111.5	109.6	107.5	105.1	102.6	99.6	96.2	92.2	87.3	81.0	2.63	2.94
	12	222.3	220.5	218.5	216.2	213.8	211.1	208.8	204.4	200.2	195.0	188.4	10.59	10.92
53.30	14	162.4	160.6	158.5	156.3	153.9	151.2	148.1	144.5	140.3	135.1	128.5	6.04	6.37
	16	134.4	132.5	130.5	128.3	125.8	123.1	120.0	116.5	112.2	107.1	100.4	3.93	4.25
	18	117.0	115.1	113.1	110.9	108.5	105.7	102.6	99.1	94.9	89.7	83.0	2.63	2.94
	12	226.8	224.8	222.7	220.4	217.8	215.0	211.7	208.0	203.6	198.1	191.1	10.63	10.96
55.96	14	166.6	164.7	162.2	160.3	157.7	154.8	151.6	147.9	143.4	138.0	131.0	6.05	6.38
	16	138.7	136.8	134.7	132.4	129.8	126.9	123.7	120.0	115.5	110.1	103.1	3.92	4.25
	18	120.6	118.7	116.5	114.2	111.7	108.8	105.6	101.8	97.4	92.0	85.0	2.63	2.94

TABLE 146

Process Times (B) at Retort Temperature of 240°F for Conduction-Heating Foods in 404 x 211 Can

f_h	z	INITIAL FOOD TEMPERATURE (T_{ih})											Equivalent	
		100	110	120	130	140	150	160	170	180	190	200	F_c^{18}	F_s^{18}
45.30	12	94.8	93.3	91.7	90.0	88.2	86.1	83.8	81.1	78.1	74.5	70.1	6.80	7.20
	14	85.2	83.7	82.1	80.4	78.5	76.5	74.2	71.5	68.5	64.9	60.5	4.76	5.17
	16	78.1	76.6	75.1	73.4	71.5	69.4	67.1	64.5	61.4	57.8	53.5	3.43	3.82
	18	72.8	71.4	69.8	68.1	66.2	64.1	61.8	59.2	56.2	52.6	48.2	2.55	2.94
47.97	12	98.9	97.3	95.7	93.9	91.9	89.7	87.2	84.4	81.2	77.4	72.8	6.94	7.33
	14	88.9	87.4	85.7	83.9	81.9	79.7	77.3	74.5	71.3	67.5	62.8	4.80	5.21
	16	81.6	80.1	78.4	76.6	74.6	72.4	69.9	67.2	63.9	60.1	55.5	3.44	3.84
	18	76.1	74.6	72.9	71.1	69.1	66.9	64.5	61.7	58.5	54.7	50.0	2.55	2.94
50.63	12	102.9	101.3	99.5	97.6	95.5	93.2	90.6	87.7	84.3	80.3	75.4	7.06	7.46
	14	92.6	91.0	89.2	87.3	85.2	82.9	80.3	77.4	74.0	70.0	65.1	4.84	5.25
	16	85.0	83.4	81.6	79.7	77.6	75.3	72.7	69.8	66.4	62.4	57.5	3.45	3.85
	18	79.4	77.8	76.0	74.1	72.0	69.7	67.1	64.2	60.8	56.8	51.9	2.55	2.94
53.30	12	106.9	105.2	103.4	101.4	99.2	96.7	94.0	90.9	87.3	83.1	77.9	7.10	7.50
	14	96.2	94.5	92.7	90.7	88.5	86.0	83.3	80.2	76.6	72.4	67.2	4.87	5.28
	16	88.4	86.7	84.9	82.9	80.6	78.2	75.5	72.4	68.8	64.6	59.4	3.44	3.85
	18	82.6	80.9	79.0	77.0	74.8	72.4	69.7	66.6	63.0	58.8	53.6	2.54	2.94
55.96	12	111.1	109.3	107.4	105.2	102.9	100.4	97.5	94.3	90.5	86.1	80.7	7.16	7.58
	14	100.0	98.2	96.2	94.1	91.8	89.2	86.4	83.1	79.4	74.9	69.5	4.88	5.30
	16	91.9	90.1	88.1	86.0	83.7	81.1	78.3	75.0	71.3	66.8	61.4	3.45	3.86
	18	85.8	84.0	82.1	80.0	77.6	75.1	72.2	69.0	65.2	60.8	55.4	2.54	2.94

TABLE 147

Process Times (B) at Retort Temperature of 250°F for Conduction-Heating Foods in 404 x 211 Can

f_h	z	INITIAL FOOD TEMPERATURE (T_{ih})											Equivalent	
		100	110	120	130	140	150	160	170	180	190	200	F_c^{18}	F_s^{18}
45.30	12	66.5	65.1	63.7	62.1	60.4	58.5	56.4	54.1	51.5	48.5	44.9	5.42	5.90
	14	63.4	62.0	60.5	59.0	57.3	55.4	53.3	51.0	48.4	45.3	41.7	4.17	4.64
	16	60.4	59.1	57.6	56.1	54.3	52.5	50.4	48.1	45.5	42.4	38.8	3.22	3.68
	18	57.8	56.5	55.0	53.4	51.7	49.9	47.8	45.5	42.8	39.8	36.2	2.49	2.94
47.97	12	69.7	68.3	66.8	65.1	63.3	61.3	59.1	56.6	53.9	50.7	46.9	5.47	5.95
	14	66.5	65.0	63.5	61.8	60.0	58.0	55.8	53.4	50.6	47.4	43.6	4.19	4.66
	16	63.4	62.0	60.4	58.7	56.9	55.0	52.8	50.3	47.5	44.3	40.5	3.25	3.71
	18	60.6	59.2	57.6	56.0	54.2	52.2	50.0	47.5	44.7	41.5	37.7	2.49	2.94
50.63	12	73.0	71.5	69.8	68.1	66.2	64.1	61.7	59.2	56.2	52.8	48.8	5.52	6.01
	14	69.6	68.1	66.4	64.7	62.8	60.7	58.4	55.8	52.8	49.4	45.4	4.22	4.69
	16	66.3	64.8	63.2	61.4	59.5	57.4	55.1	52.5	49.6	46.2	42.2	3.26	3.73
	18	63.4	61.9	60.2	58.5	56.6	54.5	52.2	49.6	46.6	43.2	39.2	2.49	2.94
53.30	12	76.3	74.7	73.0	71.1	69.1	66.9	64.4	61.7	58.6	55.1	50.8	5.59	6.08
	14	72.7	71.1	69.4	67.6	65.6	63.4	60.9	58.2	55.1	51.5	47.3	4.27	4.75
	16	69.3	67.7	66.0	64.1	62.1	59.9	57.5	54.8	51.7	48.1	43.9	3.28	3.74
	18	66.2	64.6	62.9	61.0	59.0	56.8	54.4	51.6	48.6	45.0	40.8	2.49	2.94
55.96	12	79.5	77.8	76.0	74.1	72.0	69.7	67.1	64.2	61.0	57.2	52.8	5.66	6.15
	14	75.8	74.2	72.4	70.4	68.3	66.0	63.4	60.6	57.3	53.6	49.1	4.32	4.80
	16	72.3	70.6	68.8	66.8	64.7	62.4	59.8	57.0	53.7	50.0	45.5	3.29	3.76
	18	69.0	67.3	65.6	63.5	61.4	59.1	56.6	53.7	50.4	46.7	42.3	2.49	2.94

TABLE 148

Process Times (B) at Retort Temperature of 260°F for Conduction-Heating Foods in 404 x 211 Can

f_h	z	INITIAL FOOD TEMPERATURE (T_{ih})											Equivalent	
		100	110	120	130	140	150	160	170	180	190	200	F_c^{18}	F_s^{18}
	12	54.3	53.0	51.6	50.2	48.6	46.9	45.0	42.9	40.6	38.0	35.0	5.17	5.70
45.30	14	52.1	50.9	49.5	48.1	46.5	44.8	42.9	40.8	38.5	35.9	32.8	3.90	4.42
	16	50.6	49.3	48.0	46.5	44.9	43.2	41.3	39.3	36.9	34.3	31.3	3.12	3.62
	18	49.0	47.7	46.4	44.9	43.4	41.6	39.8	37.7	35.4	32.7	29.7	2.45	2.94
	12	57.1	55.8	54.3	52.8	51.1	49.3	47.3	45.1	42.7	39.9	36.7	5.26	5.79
47.97	14	54.9	53.5	52.1	50.5	48.9	47.1	45.1	42.9	40.4	37.6	34.4	3.95	4.47
	16	53.2	51.8	50.4	48.9	47.2	45.4	43.4	41.2	38.7	36.0	32.7	3.13	3.63
	18	51.5	50.1	48.7	47.2	45.5	43.7	41.7	39.5	37.1	34.3	31.1	2.45	2.94
	12	60.0	58.5	57.0	55.4	53.6	51.7	49.6	47.3	44.7	41.8	38.4	5.34	5.88
50.63	14	57.6	56.2	54.7	53.1	51.3	49.4	47.3	45.0	42.4	39.4	36.0	4.02	4.54
	16	55.8	54.3	52.8	51.2	49.4	47.5	45.4	43.1	40.5	37.6	34.2	3.14	3.65
	18	54.0	52.6	51.0	49.4	47.7	45.7	43.6	41.3	38.7	35.8	32.4	2.45	2.94
	12	62.8	61.3	59.7	58.0	56.1	54.1	51.9	49.5	46.7	43.6	40.1	5.42	5.95
53.30	14	60.3	58.8	57.2	55.5	53.7	51.7	49.5	47.0	44.3	41.2	37.6	4.07	4.59
	16	58.3	56.8	55.2	53.5	51.7	49.7	47.5	45.0	42.3	39.2	35.6	3.16	3.67
	18	56.4	54.9	53.4	51.6	49.8	47.8	45.6	43.1	40.4	37.3	33.7	2.45	2.94
	12	65.6	64.1	62.4	60.6	58.6	56.5	54.2	51.6	48.8	45.5	41.8	5.51	6.05
55.96	14	63.0	61.5	59.8	58.0	56.0	53.9	51.6	49.0	46.2	42.9	39.2	4.12	4.64
	16	60.9	59.3	57.6	55.8	53.9	51.8	49.5	46.9	44.0	40.8	37.0	3.17	3.68
	18	58.9	57.3	55.7	53.8	51.9	49.8	47.5	44.9	42.0	38.8	35.1	2.45	2.94

TABLE 149

Process Times (B) at Retort Temperature of 230°F for Conduction-Heating Foods in 404 x 307 Can

f_h	z	INITIAL FOOD TEMPERATURE (T_{ih}) 100	110	120	130	140	150	160	170	180	190	200	Equivalent F_c^{18}	F_s^{18}
60.21	12	234.9	232.8	230.5	228.0	225.3	222.2	218.7	214.7	209.9	204.1	196.5	10.69	11.04
	14	174.3	172.2	169.9	167.4	164.6	161.6	158.1	154.0	149.3	143.4	135.9	6.13	6.46
	16	146.0	143.9	141.7	139.2	136.4	133.3	129.8	125.8	121.0	115.2	107.7	3.94	4.29
	18	126.6	124.5	122.2	119.7	117.0	113.9	110.4	106.4	101.6	95.8	88.3	2.65	2.97
63.75	12	240.2	238.0	235.6	233.0	230.0	226.8	223.1	218.8	213.8	207.6	199.6	10.67	11.02
	14	179.9	177.7	175.3	172.6	169.7	166.5	162.8	158.5	153.5	147.3	139.3	6.16	6.50
	16	151.6	149.4	147.0	144.4	141.4	138.2	134.5	130.2	125.2	119.0	111.0	3.94	4.29
	18	131.1	128.9	126.5	123.8	120.9	117.6	113.9	109.7	104.6	98.5	90.5	2.65	2.97
67.29	12	246.5	244.2	241.6	238.9	235.8	232.3	228.4	223.9	218.6	212.1	203.7	10.76	11.11
	14	185.7	183.3	180.8	178.0	174.9	171.5	167.6	163.1	157.7	151.2	142.8	6.18	6.52
	16	157.1	154.7	152.2	149.4	146.3	142.9	139.0	134.5	129.1	122.6	114.2	3.94	4.29
	18	135.4	133.0	130.5	127.7	124.6	121.2	117.3	112.8	107.5	100.9	92.5	2.65	2.96
70.83	12	252.4	249.9	247.3	244.3	241.1	237.5	233.3	228.6	223.0	216.1	207.3	10.80	11.15
	14	191.3	188.8	186.1	183.2	180.0	176.3	172.2	167.5	161.9	155.0	146.2	6.20	6.55
	16	162.4	159.9	157.2	154.3	151.1	147.4	143.3	138.6	133.0	126.1	117.3	3.94	4.29
	18	140.1	137.7	135.0	132.1	128.8	125.2	121.1	116.4	110.7	103.9	95.0	2.64	2.96
74.37	12	257.9	255.3	252.5	249.4	246.0	242.2	237.9	232.9	227.0	219.8	210.5	10.77	11.13
	14	197.6	195.0	192.2	189.1	185.7	181.9	177.6	172.6	166.7	159.5	150.2	6.27	6.62
	16	167.5	165.0	162.1	159.1	155.7	151.9	147.5	142.6	136.7	129.5	120.2	3.94	4.29
	18	145.1	142.5	139.7	136.6	133.2	129.4	125.1	120.1	114.3	107.0	97.8	2.64	2.97

TABLE 150

Process Times (B) at Retort Temperature of 240°F for Conduction-Heating Foods in 404 x 307 Can

f_h	z	INITIAL FOOD TEMPERATURE (T_{ih})											Equivalent	
		100	110	120	130	140	150	160	170	180	190	200	F_c^{18}	F_s^{18}
	12	117.9	115.9	113.8	111.6	109.1	106.3	103.2	99.7	95.7	91.0	85.1	7.32	7.74
60.21	14	106.0	104.1	102.0	99.7	97.2	94.4	91.4	87.9	83.8	79.1	73.2	4.95	5.37
	16	97.5	95.5	93.4	91.2	88.7	85.9	82.8	79.3	75.3	70.5	64.7	3.49	3.91
	18	91.1	89.1	87.0	84.8	82.3	79.5	76.4	72.9	68.9	64.1	58.3	2.56	2.97
	12	123.2	121.2	119.0	116.6	113.9	111.0	107.7	104.0	99.8	94.7	88.5	7.40	7.83
63.75	14	110.8	108.7	106.5	104.1	101.5	98.5	95.3	91.6	87.3	82.3	76.1	4.97	5.40
	16	101.9	99.8	97.6	95.2	92.6	89.7	86.4	82.7	78.4	73.4	67.2	3.50	3.92
	18	95.2	93.2	91.0	88.5	85.9	83.0	79.7	76.0	71.8	66.7	60.5	2.56	2.97
	12	128.5	126.3	124.0	121.5	118.7	115.6	112.2	108.3	103.7	98.4	91.9	7.48	7.92
67.29	14	115.5	113.3	111.0	108.5	105.7	102.6	99.2	95.2	90.7	85.4	78.9	5.00	5.43
	16	106.3	104.2	101.8	99.3	96.5	93.4	90.0	86.1	81.6	76.2	69.7	3.50	3.92
	18	99.4	97.2	94.9	92.3	89.5	86.5	83.0	79.1	74.6	69.3	62.8	2.56	2.97
	12	133.7	131.5	129.0	126.3	123.4	120.1	116.5	112.4	107.7	102.1	95.2	7.56	8.00
70.83	14	120.3	118.0	115.5	112.9	109.9	106.7	103.1	99.0	94.2	88.6	81.7	5.05	5.48
	16	110.7	108.4	106.0	103.3	100.4	97.1	93.5	89.4	84.7	79.1	72.2	3.51	3.93
	18	103.5	101.2	98.8	96.1	93.1	89.9	86.3	82.2	77.4	71.8	65.0	2.55	2.97
	12	139.0	136.6	134.0	131.2	128.1	124.7	120.9	116.6	111.6	105.8	98.5	7.67	8.11
74.37	14	125.0	122.6	120.0	117.2	114.1	110.7	106.9	102.6	97.6	91.7	84.5	5.08	5.51
	16	115.1	112.7	110.1	107.3	104.2	100.8	97.0	92.7	87.7	81.8	74.6	3.52	3.95
	18	107.6	105.2	102.6	99.8	96.7	93.3	89.5	85.2	80.2	74.3	67.1	2.55	2.97

TABLE 151

Process Times (B) at Retort Temperature of 250°F for Conduction-Heating Foods in 404 x 307 Can

f_h	z	INITIAL FOOD TEMPERATURE (T_{ih})											Equivalent	
		100	110	120	130	140	150	160	170	180	190	200	F_c^{18}	F_s^{18}
60.21	12	84.7	82.9	81.0	78.9	76.6	74.1	71.4	68.3	64.8	60.8	56.0	5.75	6.25
	14	80.8	79.0	77.1	75.0	72.7	70.2	67.5	64.4	60.9	56.9	52.1	4.42	4.91
	16	77.0	75.2	73.2	71.1	68.9	66.4	63.6	60.5	57.0	53.0	48.2	3.34	3.81
	18	73.4	71.6	69.7	67.6	65.3	62.8	60.1	57.0	53.5	49.5	44.7	2.51	2.96
63.75	12	88.9	87.0	85.0	82.8	80.4	77.7	74.8	71.5	67.8	63.6	58.5	5.79	6.29
	14	84.9	83.0	80.9	78.7	76.3	73.7	70.7	67.5	63.8	59.5	54.5	4.49	4.98
	16	80.8	78.9	76.8	74.6	72.2	69.6	66.7	63.4	59.7	55.4	50.4	3.37	3.84
	18	77.0	75.1	73.1	70.9	68.4	65.8	62.9	59.6	55.9	51.7	46.6	2.51	2.97
67.29	12	93.2	91.2	89.0	86.7	84.1	81.4	78.3	74.8	70.9	66.4	61.1	5.86	6.36
	14	89.0	86.9	84.8	82.4	79.9	77.1	74.0	70.6	66.7	62.2	56.9	4.57	5.06
	16	84.6	82.6	80.4	78.1	75.6	72.8	69.7	66.3	62.4	57.9	52.5	3.41	3.88
	18	80.7	78.6	76.5	74.1	71.6	68.8	65.7	62.3	58.4	53.9	48.5	2.51	2.97
70.83	12	97.4	95.3	93.0	90.6	87.9	84.9	81.7	78.1	74.0	69.2	63.6	5.92	6.43
	14	93.0	90.9	88.6	86.1	83.4	80.5	77.3	73.6	69.5	64.8	59.2	4.62	5.11
	16	88.4	86.3	84.0	81.6	78.9	75.9	72.7	69.1	65.0	60.2	54.6	3.42	3.90
	18	84.2	82.1	79.8	77.4	74.7	71.8	68.6	64.9	60.8	56.0	50.4	2.51	2.97
74.37	12	101.6	99.3	96.9	94.4	91.6	88.5	85.1	81.3	77.0	72.0	66.1	5.98	6.49
	14	96.9	94.7	92.3	89.7	86.9	83.8	80.4	76.6	72.3	67.3	61.5	4.63	5.13
	16	92.1	89.9	87.5	84.9	82.1	79.1	75.6	71.8	67.5	62.6	56.7	3.42	3.90
	18	87.7	85.5	83.1	80.5	77.7	74.7	71.2	67.4	63.1	58.2	52.3	2.50	2.97

TABLE 152

Process Times (B) at Retort Temperature of 260°F for Conduction-Heating Foods in 404 x 307 Can

f_h	z	INITIAL FOOD TEMPERATURE (T_{ih})											Equivalent	
		100	110	120	130	140	150	160	170	180	190	200	F_c^{18}	F_s^{18}
	12	70.2	68.5	66.7	64.8	62.7	60.4	57.9	55.1	52.1	48.6	44.5	5.68	6.23
60.21	14	67.3	65.7	63.8	61.9	59.8	57.5	55.0	52.3	49.2	45.7	41.7	4.20	4.73
	16	65.0	63.4	61.6	59.6	57.5	55.2	52.8	50.0	46.9	43.4	39.4	3.23	3.74
	18	62.9	61.2	59.4	57.4	55.3	53.1	50.6	47.8	44.7	41.2	37.2	2.47	2.97
	12	73.9	72.1	70.2	68.2	65.9	63.5	60.9	58.0	54.7	51.0	46.7	5.79	6.34
63.75	14	70.8	69.0	67.1	65.1	62.9	60.5	57.8	54.9	51.6	47.9	43.7	4.23	4.76
	16	68.5	66.7	64.8	62.7	60.5	58.1	55.4	52.5	49.3	45.6	41.3	3.27	3.78
	18	66.1	64.3	62.4	60.3	58.1	55.7	53.1	50.1	46.9	43.2	38.9	2.47	2.97
	12	77.6	75.7	73.7	71.5	69.2	66.6	63.8	60.8	57.3	53.4	48.9	5.87	6.42
67.29	14	74.3	72.4	70.4	68.2	65.9	63.3	60.5	57.5	54.0	50.1	45.6	4.25	4.78
	16	71.8	70.0	67.9	65.8	63.4	60.9	58.1	55.0	51.6	47.7	43.2	3.29	3.81
	18	69.3	67.4	65.4	63.2	60.9	58.3	55.5	52.5	49.0	45.1	40.6	2.47	2.96
	12	81.2	79.2	77.1	74.8	72.4	69.7	66.8	63.5	59.9	55.8	51.0	5.94	6.49
70.83	14	77.7	75.7	73.6	71.3	68.8	66.2	63.2	60.0	56.4	52.3	47.5	4.28	4.81
	16	75.2	73.2	71.1	68.8	66.3	63.7	60.7	57.5	53.9	49.8	45.0	3.31	3.83
	18	72.5	70.5	68.4	66.1	63.6	61.0	58.0	54.8	51.2	47.1	42.3	2.46	2.97
	12	84.9	82.8	80.6	78.2	75.6	72.8	69.7	66.3	62.5	58.2	53.2	6.03	6.59
74.37	14	81.2	79.1	76.9	74.5	71.9	69.1	66.0	62.6	58.8	54.5	49.5	4.34	4.87
	16	78.5	76.4	74.2	71.8	69.2	66.4	63.3	59.9	56.1	51.8	46.8	3.33	3.85
	18	75.7	73.6	71.4	69.0	66.4	63.6	60.5	57.1	53.3	49.0	44.0	2.46	2.97

TABLE 153

Process Times (B) at Retort Temperature of 230°F for Conduction-Heating Foods in 404 x 309 Can

f_h	z	INITIAL FOOD TEMPERATURE (T_{ih})											Equivalent	
		100	110	120	130	140	150	160	170	180	190	200	F_c^{18}	F_s^{18}
	12	238.2	236.0	233.7	231.1	228.2	225.1	221.4	217.3	212.3	206.3	198.5	10.69	11.04
62.30	14	177.7	175.6	173.2	170.6	167.8	164.6	161.0	156.8	151.9	145.8	138.1	6.16	6.49
	16	149.4	147.2	144.9	142.3	139.5	136.3	132.7	128.5	123.6	117.5	109.7	3.95	4.29
	18	129.3	127.2	124.8	122.2	119.4	116.2	112.6	108.4	103.5	97.4	89.7	2.66	2.97
	12	244.4	242.1	239.6	236.8	233.8	230.5	226.6	222.2	217.0	210.6	202.4	10.74	11.09
65.96	14	183.6	181.3	178.8	176.1	173.1	169.7	165.9	161.4	156.2	149.8	141.6	6.18	6.52
	16	155.1	152.8	150.3	147.6	144.6	141.2	137.4	133.0	127.7	121.3	113.1	3.95	4.29
	18	133.9	131.6	129.1	126.4	123.3	120.0	116.1	111.7	106.5	100.1	91.9	2.65	2.97
	12	250.6	248.2	245.5	242.7	239.5	235.9	231.9	227.2	221.7	215.0	206.3	10.82	11.17
69.63	14	189.5	187.1	184.5	181.6	178.4	174.8	170.8	166.1	160.6	153.9	145.2	6.20	6.55
	16	160.7	158.2	155.6	152.7	149.5	146.0	141.9	137.3	131.8	125.0	116.3	3.95	4.29
	18	138.5	136.1	133.4	130.5	127.4	123.8	119.8	115.1	109.6	102.8	94.1	2.65	2.97
	12	256.4	253.8	251.1	248.0	244.7	240.9	236.7	231.8	226.0	218.9	209.7	10.79	11.15
73.29	14	195.7	193.1	190.4	187.3	184.0	180.2	176.0	171.1	165.3	158.2	149.0	6.26	6.60
	16	166.1	163.5	160.7	157.7	154.4	150.6	146.4	141.4	135.6	128.5	199.4	3.95	4.29
	18	143.7	141.1	138.3	135.3	132.0	128.2	124.0	119.0	113.2	106.1	97.00	2.64	2.97
	12	262.3	259.6	256.7	253.5	250.0	246.1	241.6	236.5	230.4	222.9	213.3	10.80	11.16
76.96	14	202.3	199.6	196.7	193.5	190.0	186.0	181.6	176.4	170.3	162.9	153.3	6.33	6.68
	16	171.3	168.6	165.7	162.5	159.0	155.1	150.6	145.5	139.4	131.9	122.3	3.94	4.29
	18	148.7	146.0	143.1	140.0	136.4	132.5	128.0	122.9	116.8	109.3	99.7	2.64	2.97

TABLE 154

Process Times (B) at Retort Temperature of 240°F for Conduction-Heating Foods in 404 x 309 Can

f_h	z	INITIAL FOOD TEMPERATURE (T_{ih}) 100	110	120	130	140	150	160	170	180	190	200	Equivalent F_c^{18}	F_s^{18}
62.30	12	121.1	119.1	116.9	114.6	112.0	109.1	105.9	102.3	98.2	93.2	87.2	7.38	7.80
	14	108.8	106.8	104.7	102.3	99.7	96.9	93.7	90.1	85.9	81.0	75.0	4.97	5.39
	16	100.1	98.1	95.9	93.6	91.0	88.2	85.0	81.4	77.2	72.3	66.2	3.50	3.92
	18	93.5	91.5	89.4	87.0	84.4	81.6	78.4	74.8	70.6	65.7	59.7	2.56	2.97
65.96	12	126.6	124.5	122.2	119.7	116.9	113.9	110.5	106.7	102.3	97.1	90.7	7.46	7.89
	14	113.8	111.6	109.3	106.8	104.1	101.1	97.7	93.9	89.5	84.3	77.9	5.00	5.42
	16	104.7	102.6	100.3	97.8	95.0	92.0	88.7	84.8	80.4	75.2	68.8	3.50	3.92
	18	97.9	95.7	93.4	90.9	88.2	85.2	81.8	78.0	73.6	68.4	62.0	2.56	2.97
69.63	12	132.0	129.7	127.3	124.7	121.8	118.6	115.1	111.0	106.4	100.8	94.1	7.54	7.98
	14	118.7	116.5	114.0	111.4	108.5	105.3	101.8	97.7	93.1	87.6	80.8	5.04	5.47
	16	109.3	107.0	104.6	102.0	99.1	95.9	92.3	88.3	83.6	78.1	71.4	3.51	3.94
	18	102.1	99.9	97.5	94.8	92.0	88.8	85.2	81.2	76.5	71.0	64.2	2.56	2.97
73.29	12	137.4	135.1	132.5	129.8	126.7	123.4	119.6	115.4	110.5	104.7	97.6	7.64	8.09
	14	123.6	121.2	118.7	115.9	112.9	109.5	105.8	101.5	96.6	90.8	83.7	5.08	5.51
	16	113.8	111.4	108.9	106.1	103.1	99.7	96.0	91.7	86.8	81.0	73.9	3.52	3.95
	18	106.4	104.0	101.4	98.7	95.6	92.3	88.5	84.3	79.4	73.6	66.5	2.56	2.97
76.96	12	142.9	140.4	137.7	134.8	131.6	128.1	124.2	119.7	114.5	108.4	101.0	7.75	8.19
	14	128.4	126.0	123.3	120.4	117.2	113.7	109.7	105.3	100.1	94.0	86.6	5.10	5.53
	16	118.3	115.8	113.1	110.2	107.0	103.5	99.6	95.1	90.0	83.9	76.4	3.53	3.96
	18	110.6	108.1	105.4	102.5	99.3	95.8	91.9	87.4	82.2	76.2	68.7	2.55	2.97

TABLE 155

Process Times (B) at Retort Temperature of 250°F for Conduction-Heating Foods in 404 x 309 Can

f_h	z	INITIAL FOOD TEMPERATURE (T_{ih})											Equivalent	
		100	110	120	130	140	150	160	170	180	190	200	F_c^{18}	F_s^{18}
	12	87.2	85.4	83.4	81.2	78.8	76.3	73.4	70.2	66.6	62.4	57.5	5.77	6.27
62.30	14	83.2	81.4	79.4	77.2	74.8	72.3	69.4	66.2	62.6	58.4	53.5	4.46	4.95
	16	79.2	77.4	75.4	73.2	70.8	68.3	65.4	62.2	58.6	54.4	49.5	3.36	3.83
	18	75.6	73.7	71.7	69.5	67.2	64.6	61.7	58.5	54.9	50.8	45.8	2.51	2.97
	12	91.6	89.7	87.5	85.2	82.8	80.0	77.0	73.6	69.8	65.4	60.2	5.84	6.34
65.96	14	87.5	85.5	83.4	81.1	78.6	75.8	72.8	69.4	65.6	61.2	56.0	4.54	5.03
	16	83.2	81.2	79.1	76.8	74.3	71.6	68.6	65.2	61.4	57.0	51.7	3.39	3.87
	18	79.3	77.3	75.2	72.9	70.4	67.7	64.7	61.3	57.5	53.1	47.8	2.51	2.97
	12	96.0	93.9	91.7	89.3	86.6	83.7	80.6	77.0	73.0	68.3	62.8	5.91	6.41
69.63	14	91.6	89.5	87.3	84.9	82.3	79.4	76.2	72.6	68.6	63.9	58.4	4.62	5.11
	16	87.2	85.1	82.8	80.4	77.8	74.9	71.7	68.1	64.1	59.4	53.9	3.42	3.90
	18	83.0	80.9	78.7	76.3	73.7	70.8	67.6	64.0	60.0	55.3	49.8	2.51	2.97
	12	100.3	98.1	95.8	93.2	90.5	87.4	84.1	80.3	76.1	71.2	65.4	5.97	6.48
73.29	14	95.7	93.6	91.2	88.6	85.9	82.8	79.5	75.7	71.5	66.6	60.8	4.64	5.13
	16	91.0	88.8	86.5	83.9	81.2	78.1	74.8	71.0	66.8	61.9	56.1	3.42	3.90
	18	86.7	84.5	82.1	79.6	76.8	73.8	70.4	66.7	62.4	57.5	51.7	2.51	2.97
	12	104.6	102.3	99.9	97.2	94.3	91.1	87.6	83.6	79.2	74.0	67.9	6.04	6.55
76.96	14	99.9	97.6	95.1	92.4	89.5	86.3	82.8	78.9	74.4	69.2	63.1	4.67	5.17
	16	94.9	92.6	90.1	87.5	84.5	81.4	77.8	73.9	69.4	64.3	58.2	3.43	3.92
	18	90.4	88.0	85.6	82.9	80.0	76.8	73.3	69.3	64.9	59.7	53.6	2.51	2.97

TABLE 156

Process Times (B) at Retort Temperature of 260°F for Conduction-Heating Foods in 404 x 309 Can

f_h	z	INITIAL FOOD TEMPERATURE (T_{ih})											Equivalent	
		100	110	120	130	140	150	160	170	180	190	200	F_c^{18}	F_s^{18}
	12	72.4	70.7	68.8	66.8	64.6	62.3	59.7	56.8	53.6	50.0	45.9	5.75	6.30
62.30	14	69.4	67.7	65.8	63.8	61.6	59.3	56.7	53.8	50.7	47.1	42.9	4.22	4.75
	16	67.1	65.3	63.5	61.5	59.3	56.9	54.4	51.5	48.3	44.7	40.5	3.26	3.77
	18	64.8	63.0	61.1	59.1	57.0	54.6	52.0	49.2	46.0	42.4	38.2	2.47	2.97
	12	76.2	74.4	72.4	70.3	68.0	65.5	62.8	59.7	56.4	52.5	48.1	5.85	6.40
65.96	14	73.0	71.2	69.2	67.1	64.8	62.3	59.5	56.5	53.1	49.3	44.9	4.25	4.78
	16	70.6	68.7	66.8	64.6	62.3	59.9	57.1	54.1	50.7	46.9	42.5	3.29	3.80
	18	68.1	66.2	64.3	62.1	59.8	57.4	54.6	51.6	48.2	44.4	40.0	2.47	2.97
	12	80.0	78.0	76.0	73.7	71.3	68.7	65.8	62.6	59.0	55.0	50.3	5.92	6.47
69.63	14	76.5	74.6	72.5	70.3	67.8	65.2	62.3	59.1	55.6	51.5	46.9	4.27	4.80
	16	74.1	72.1	70.0	67.8	65.4	62.7	59.8	56.7	53.1	49.1	44.4	3.31	3.83
	18	71.4	69.4	67.4	65.1	62.7	60.1	57.2	54.0	50.4	46.4	41.7	2.47	2.97
	12	83.8	81.7	79.5	77.2	74.6	71.9	68.8	65.5	61.7	57.5	52.6	6.01	6.56
73.29	14	80.2	78.1	75.9	73.5	71.0	68.2	65.2	61.8	58.1	53.8	48.9	4.32	4.86
	16	77.5	75.4	73.2	70.9	68.3	65.6	62.5	59.2	55.4	51.2	46.3	3.33	3.85
	18	74.8	72.7	70.5	68.1	65.6	62.8	59.8	56.4	52.7	48.4	43.5	2.47	2.97
	12	87.6	85.4	83.1	80.6	77.9	75.0	71.9	68.3	64.4	59.9	54.8	6.10	6.66
76.96	14	83.8	81.6	79.3	76.8	74.2	71.3	68.1	64.5	60.6	56.1	51.0	4.38	4.91
	16	80.9	78.7	76.4	73.9	71.3	68.4	65.2	61.7	57.7	53.3	48.1	3.33	3.85
	18	78.1	75.9	73.6	71.1	68.5	65.5	62.4	58.8	54.9	50.4	45.3	2.46	2.97

TABLE 157

Process Times (B) at Retort Temperature of 230°F for Conduction-Heating Foods in 404 x 700 Can

f_h	z	INITIAL FOOD TEMPERATURE (T_{ih})											Equivalent	
		100	110	120	130	140	150	160	170	180	190	200	F_c^{18}	F_s^{18}
	12	289.7	286.5	283.0	279.2	275.0	270.3	265.0	258.9	251.6	242.7	231.3	11.15	11.52
91.67	14	229.1	225.9	222.5	218.7	214.5	209.8	204.5	198.3	191.1	182.2	170.7	6.58	6.95
	16	192.7	189.5	186.1	182.3	178.1	173.4	168.1	162.0	154.7	145.8	134.4	4.04	4.39
	18	169.3	166.1	162.7	158.9	154.7	150.0	144.7	138.5	131.3	122.4	111.0	2.68	3.03
	12	298.7	295.3	291.7	287.7	283.2	278.3	272.6	266.1	258.4	249.0	236.9	11.21	11.59
97.06	14	238.0	234.7	231.0	227.0	222.5	217.6	211.9	205.5	197.8	188.4	176.2	6.58	6.96
	16	199.8	196.4	102.7	188.7	184.3	179.3	173.7	167.2	159.5	150.1	138.0	4.05	4.40
	18	176.2	172.9	169.2	165.2	160.7	155.8	150.2	143.7	136.0	126.6	114.4	2.68	3.03
	12	307.3	303.8	299.9	295.7	291.0	285.7	279.8	272.9	264.8	254.9	242.1	11.26	11.64
102.45	14	246.8	243.2	239.3	235.1	230.4	225.1	219.2	212.3	204.2	104.3	181.5	6.57	6.96
	16	207.7	204.1	200.3	196.0	191.3	186.1	180.2	173.3	165.2	155.3	142.5	4.11	4.46
	18	183.0	179.5	175.6	171.4	166.7	161.4	155.5	148.6	140.5	130.6	117.8	2.67	3.03
	12	316.5	312.7	308.6	304.2	299.2	293.7	287.5	280.2	271.7	261.3	247.8	11.30	11.69
107.85	14	255.3	251.5	247.4	243.0	238.0	232.5	226.3	219.0	210.5	200.1	186.6	6.58	6.97
	16	215.4	211.7	207.6	203.2	198.2	192.7	186.4	179.2	170.7	160.2	146.8	4.17	4.53
	18	190.1	186.3	182.3	177.8	172.9	167.3	161.1	153.9	145.3	134.9	121.4	2.67	3.03
	12	325.2	321.3	317.0	312.3	307.1	301.3	294.7	287.2	278.2	267.2	253.1	11.34	11.73
113.24	14	263.6	259.6	255.3	250.6	245.5	239.7	233.1	225.5	216.6	205.6	191.4	6.58	6.97
	16	223.0	219.1	214.8	210.1	204.9	199.2	192.6	185.0	176.0	165.1	150.9	4.16	4.52
	18	197.1	193.2	188.9	184.2	179.0	173.3	166.7	159.1	150.1	139.2	125.0	2.67	3.03

TABLE 158

Process Times (B) at Retort Temperature of 240°F for Conduction-Heating Foods in 404 x 700 Can

f_h	z	INITIAL FOOD TEMPERATURE (T_{ih})											Equivalent	
		100	110	120	130	140	150	160	170	180	190	200	F_c^{18}	F_s^{18}
	12	164.9	161.9	158.7	155.3	151.5	147.3	142.6	137.3	131.1	123.9	115.0	8.23	8.69
91.67	14	148.3	145.4	142.2	138.7	134.9	139.7	126.0	120.7	114.6	107.3	98.4	5.31	5.76
	16	136.7	133.8	130.6	127.1	123.3	119.1	114.4	109.1	103.0	95.7	86.9	3.65	4.09
	18	127.8	124.8	121.6	118.2	114.4	110.2	105.5	100.2	94.0	86.8	77.9	2.61	3.03
	12	172.6	169.5	166.1	162.4	158.4	154.0	149.0	143.4	136.9	129.2	119.8	8.32	8.78
97.06	14	155.3	152.2	148.8	145.1	141.1	136.7	131.7	126.1	119.6	111.9	102.5	5.35	5.80
	16	143.2	140.1	136.7	133.0	129.0	124.6	119.6	114.0	107.5	99.8	90.4	3.67	4.11
	18	133.8	130.7	127.3	123.6	119.6	115.2	110.2	104.6	98.1	90.4	81.0	2.60	3.03
	12	180.2	176.9	173.4	169.5	165.3	160.6	155.3	149.4	142.5	134.4	124.5	8.40	8.87
102.45	14	162.2	158.9	155.4	151.5	147.2	142.6	137.3	131.4	124.5	116.4	106.5	5.39	5.84
	16	149.6	146.3	142.7	138.9	134.6	129.9	124.7	118.8	111.9	103.8	93.9	3.68	4.12
	18	139.8	136.6	133.0	129.1	124.9	120.2	114.9	109.0	102.1	94.0	84.1	2.60	3.03
	12	187.8	184.3	180.6	176.5	172.0	167.1	161.6	155.3	148.1	139.6	129.1	8.49	8.96
107.85	14	169.1	165.6	161.9	157.8	153.3	148.4	142.9	136.6	129.4	120.8	110.4	5.42	5.88
	16	156.0	152.5	148.7	144.7	140.2	135.3	129.7	123.5	116.3	107.7	97.3	3.70	4.14
	18	145.8	142.3	138.6	134.5	130.0	125.1	119.6	113.3	106.1	97.6	87.1	2.60	3.03
	12	195.3	191.7	187.8	183.5	178.8	173.6	167.8	161.3	153.7	144.7	133.7	8.59	9.06
113.24	14	175.9	172.3	168.3	164.1	159.4	154.2	148.4	141.8	134.3	125.3	114.3	5.46	5.92
	16	162.3	158.7	154.8	150.5	145.8	140.6	134.8	128.2	120.7	111.7	100.7	3.72	4.16
	18	151.7	148.1	144.1	139.8	135.2	130.0	124.2	117.6	110.0	101.1	90.1	2.60	3.03

TABLE 159

Process Times (B) at Retort Temperature of 250°F for Conduction-Heating Foods in 404 x 700 Can

f_h	z	INITIAL FOOD TEMPERATURE (T_{ih})											Equivalent	
		100	110	120	130	140	150	160	170	180	190	200	F_c^{18}	F_s^{18}
91.67	12	122.2	119.5	116.5	113.3	109.9	106.1	101.9	97.2	91.9	85.7	78.5	6.49	7.01
	14	116.5	113.8	110.8	107.7	104.2	100.4	96.2	91.5	86.2	80.1	72.8	4.92	5.43
	16	110.6	107.9	104.9	101.8	98.3	94.5	90.3	85.6	80.3	74.2	66.9	3.58	4.07
	18	105.2	102.5	99.5	96.3	92.9	89.1	84.9	80.2	74.9	68.7	61.5	2.56	3.03
97.06	12	128.5	125.6	122.4	119.1	115.4	111.4	106.9	102.0	96.4	89.9	82.2	6.63	7.15
	14	122.5	119.5	116.4	113.1	109.4	105.4	100.9	96.0	90.3	83.8	76.1	5.00	5.51
	16	116.2	113.3	110.2	106.8	103.1	99.1	94.7	89.7	84.1	77.6	69.9	3.59	4.08
	18	110.5	107.6	104.5	101.1	97.4	93.4	89.0	84.0	78.4	71.9	64.2	2.56	3.03
102.45	12	134.7	131.6	128.3	124.8	120.9	116.6	112.0	106.7	100.8	93.9	85.8	6.74	7.27
	14	128.3	125.2	121.9	118.4	114.5	110.3	105.6	100.3	94.4	87.5	79.4	5.05	5.56
	16	121.7	118.6	115.3	111.8	107.9	103.7	99.0	93.7	87.8	80.9	72.8	3.60	4.09
	18	115.7	112.6	109.3	105.8	101.9	97.6	93.0	87.7	81.8	74.9	66.8	2.56	3.03
107.85	12	140.9	137.7	134.2	130.5	126.4	121.9	117.0	111.5	105.2	98.0	89.5	6.83	7.36
	14	134.2	130.9	127.5	123.7	119.6	115.2	110.2	104.7	98.5	91.3	82.7	5.09	5.60
	16	127.2	124.0	120.5	116.8	112.7	108.3	103.3	97.8	91.6	84.3	75.8	3.63	4.13
	18	120.9	117.7	114.2	110.5	106.4	101.9	97.0	91.5	85.2	78.0	69.5	2.56	3.03
113.24	12	147.1	143.7	140.1	136.1	131.9	127.2	122.0	116.2	109.6	102.0	93.1	6.91	7.45
	14	140.0	136.6	132.9	129.0	124.7	120.0	114.8	109.0	102.5	94.9	85.9	5.12	5.64
	16	132.7	129.3	125.7	121.7	117.4	112.8	107.6	101.8	95.2	87.6	78.7	3.64	4.14
	18	126.1	122.7	119.0	115.1	110.8	106.1	100.9	95.2	88.6	81.0	72.0	2.55	3.03

TABLE 160

Process Times (B) at Retort Temperature of 260°F for Conduction-Heating Foods in 404 x 700 Can

f_h	z	INITIAL FOOD TEMPERATURE (T_{ih})											Equivalent	
		100	110	120	130	140	150	160	170	180	190	200	F_c^{18}	F_s^{18}
	12	102.7	100.1	97.4	94.4	91.2	87.8	84.0	79.8	75.1	69.8	63.7	6.48	7.05
91.67	14	98.3	95.7	92.9	90.0	86.8	83.3	79.5	75.4	70.7	65.3	59.2	4.63	5.17
	16	94.6	92.0	89.2	86.3	83.1	79.6	75.9	71.7	67.0	61.7	55.5	3.42	3.94
	18	91.3	88.8	86.0	83.1	79.9	76.4	72.6	68.4	63.7	58.4	52.3	2.52	3.03
	12	108.1	105.4	102.5	99.4	96.0	92.3	88.3	83.9	78.9	73.3	66.8	6.57	7.13
97.06	14	103.4	100.7	97.8	94.6	91.3	87.6	83.6	79.1	74.2	68.5	62.1	4.67	5.21
	16	99.5	96.8	93.9	90.8	87.4	83.7	79.7	75.3	70.3	64.7	58.2	3.44	3.97
	18	96.0	93.3	90.4	87.2	83.9	80.2	76.2	71.7	66.8	61.2	54.7	2.52	3.03
	12	113.5	110.6	107.6	104.3	100.7	96.8	92.6	87.9	82.7	76.7	69.9	6.65	7.21
102.45	14	108.6	105.7	102.7	99.4	95.8	91.9	87.7	83.0	77.8	71.8	65.0	4.74	5.29
	16	104.4	101.6	98.5	95.2	91.6	87.8	83.5	78.8	73.6	67.7	60.8	3.43	3.96
	18	100.6	97.7	94.6	91.4	87.8	83.9	79.7	75.0	69.7	63.8	56.9	2.52	3.03
	12	118.8	115.8	112.6	109.1	105.3	101.3	96.8	91.9	86.4	80.1	72.9	6.72	7.29
107.85	14	113.7	110.7	107.5	104.0	100.3	96.2	91.7	86.8	81.3	75.0	67.8	4.80	5.35
	16	109.3	106.3	103.0	99.6	95.8	91.7	87.3	82.4	76.8	70.6	63.4	3.42	3.96
	18	105.2	102.2	99.0	95.5	91.8	87.7	83.2	78.3	72.8	66.5	59.3	2.52	3.03
	12	124.1	121.0	117.6	113.9	110.0	105.7	101.0	95.8	90.1	83.5	75.9	6.81	7.38
113.24	14	118.8	115.7	112.3	108.6	104.7	100.4	95.7	90.5	84.7	78.2	70.6	4.84	5.39
	16	114.1	110.9	107.5	103.9	100.0	95.7	91.0	85.8	80.0	73.4	65.9	3.41	3.95
	18	109.9	106.8	103.4	99.7	95.8	91.5	86.8	81.6	75.8	69.3	61.7	2.52	3.03

TABLE 161

Process Times (B) at Retort Temperature of 230°F for Conduction-Heating Foods in 603 x 700 Can

f_h	z	INITIAL FOOD TEMPERATURE (T_{ih})											Equivalent	
		100	110	120	130	140	150	160	170	180	190	200	F_c^{18}	F_s^{18}
170.00	12	427.8	421.9	415.5	408.5	400.7	392.0	382.1	370.7	357.3	340.8	319.6	12.46	12.89
	14	348.6	342.6	336.2	329.2	321.4	312.7	302.8	291.5	278.0	261.5	240.3	7.02	7.42
	16	300.7	294.8	288.4	281.4	273.6	264.9	255.0	243.7	230.2	213.7	192.5	4.28	4.68
	18	268.8	262.9	256.5	249.5	241.7	233.0	223.1	211.8	198.3	181.8	160.6	2.71	3.10
180.00	12	444.8	438.5	431.7	424.3	416.0	406.8	396.4	383.3	370.1	352.6	330.1	12.47	12.91
	14	363.2	356.9	350.1	342.6	334.4	325.2	314.8	302.7	288.5	271.0	248.5	7.14	7.54
	16	313.7	307.5	300.7	293.2	285.0	275.8	265.3	253.3	239.0	221.6	199.1	4.26	4.67
	18	280.9	274.6	267.8	260.4	252.1	242.9	232.5	220.4	206.2	188.7	166.2	2.70	3.10
190.00	12	461.3	454.7	447.6	439.7	431.0	421.3	410.3	397.5	382.5	364.1	340.3	12.49	12.93
	14	377.5	370.8	363.7	355.8	347.1	337.4	326.4	313.7	298.6	280.2	256.5	7.20	7.61
	16	326.5	319.9	312.7	304.8	296.1	286.4	275.4	262.7	247.6	229.2	205.5	4.25	4.66
	18	292.9	286.3	279.1	271.2	262.5	252.8	241.8	229.1	214.0	195.6	171.9	2.70	3.10
200.00	12	477.5	470.5	463.0	454.7	445.6	435.3	423.7	410.3	394.5	375.1	350.1	12.51	12.95
	14	391.5	384.5	376.9	368.7	359.7	349.3	337.7	324.3	308.5	289.1	264.1	7.18	7.59
	16	339.4	332.4	324.8	316.6	307.4	297.2	285.6	272.2	256.4	237.0	212.0	4.26	4.67
	18	304.7	297.7	290.1	281.9	272.7	262.5	250.9	237.5	221.7	202.3	177.3	2.70	3.10
210.00	12	493.3	486.0	478.0	469.3	459.7	449.0	436.8	422.7	406.1	385.8	359.5	12.52	12.97
	14	405.2	397.9	389.9	381.2	371.6	360.9	348.7	334.7	318.0	297.7	271.4	7.15	7.57
	16	352.2	344.9	337.0	328.3	318.7	307.9	295.8	281.7	265.1	244.7	218.5	4.27	4.69
	18	316.3	309.0	301.1	292.4	282.8	272.0	259.9	245.8	229.2	208.8	182.6	2.70	3.10

TABLE 162

Process Times (B) at Retort Temperature of 240°F for Conduction-Heating Foods in 603 x 700 Can

f_h	z	INITIAL FOOD TEMPERATURE (T_{ih})											Equivalent	
		100	110	120	130	140	150	160	170	180	190	200	F_c^{18}	F_s^{18}
170.00	12	273.0	267.5	261.6	255.2	248.1	240.3	231.6	221.8	210.4	196.9	180.5	9.53	10.03
	14	247.3	241.8	235.9	229.5	222.4	214.6	205.9	196.1	184.7	171.2	154.8	6.00	6.48
	16	227.9	222.5	216.6	210.1	203.1	195.3	186.6	176.8	165.4	151.9	135.5	3.92	4.39
	18	212.4	206.9	201.0	194.6	187.5	179.8	171.1	161.2	149.8	136.4	119.9	2.65	3.10
180.00	12	286.1	280.3	274.0	267.2	259.8	251.5	242.3	231.9	219.8	205.6	188.1	9.62	10.13
	14	259.3	253.5	247.3	240.5	233.0	224.8	215.6	205.1	193.1	178.8	161.4	6.05	6.54
	16	239.2	233.4	227.1	220.3	212.9	212.9	195.4	185.0	172.9	158.7	141.2	3.95	4.42
	18	222.6	216.8	210.6	203.8	196.3	188.1	178.9	168.4	156.4	142.1	124.7	2.65	3.10
190.00	12	299.2	293.1	286.5	279.3	271.4	262.7	253.0	242.0	229.3	214.2	195.8	9.74	10.25
	14	271.2	265.1	258.5	251.3	243.5	234.8	225.0	214.0	201.3	186.3	167.9	6.10	6.60
	16	250.3	244.1	237.5	230.4	222.5	213.8	204.1	193.1	180.3	165.3	146.9	3.98	4.45
	18	232.7	226.6	220.0	212.8	205.0	196.3	186.6	175.5	162.8	147.8	129.4	2.64	3.10
200.00	12	312.2	305.8	298.8	291.3	283.0	273.8	263.6	252.0	238.6	222.8	203.4	9.86	10.37
	14	283.0	276.6	269.6	262.1	253.8	244.6	234.4	222.8	209.4	193.6	174.2	6.15	6.65
	16	261.3	254.8	247.9	240.3	232.0	222.9	212.6	201.0	187.7	171.8	152.4	4.01	4.49
	18	243.0	236.5	229.6	222.0	213.7	204.6	194.3	182.8	169.4	153.5	134.1	2.64	3.10
210.00	12	325.1	318.4	311.1	303.1	294.4	284.8	274.1	261.9	247.8	231.2	210.9	9.97	10.48
	14	294.8	288.0	280.7	272.8	264.1	254.5	243.8	231.6	217.5	200.9	180.5	6.20	6.70
	16	272.1	265.4	258.1	250.1	241.5	231.8	221.1	208.9	194.9	178.2	157.9	4.04	4.52
	18	253.1	246.3	239.0	231.1	222.4	212.8	202.0	189.9	175.8	159.2	138.8	2.64	3.10

TABLE 163

Process Times (B) at Retort Temperature of 250°F for Conduction-Heating Foods in 603 x 700 Can

f_h	z	INITIAL FOOD TEMPERATURE (T_{ih}) 100	110	120	130	140	150	160	170	180	190	200	Equivalent F_c^{18}	F_s^{18}
170.00	12	211.9	206.8	201.3	195.4	189.0	181.9	174.1	165.4	155.6	144.2	130.7	8.11	8.67
	14	200.1	195.0	189.5	183.6	177.2	170.2	162.4	153.7	143.8	132.5	119.0	5.64	6.17
	16	189.4	184.3	178.8	172.9	166.5	159.4	151.6	143.0	133.1	121.7	108.3	3.85	4.36
	18	179.6	174.5	169.0	163.1	156.7	149.6	141.9	133.2	123.3	111.9	98.5	2.61	3.10
180.00	12	223.0	217.6	211.8	205.5	198.7	191.3	183.0	173.8	163.4	151.3	137.1	8.26	8.81
	14	210.3	204.9	199.1	192.9	186.1	178.6	170.4	161.2	150.8	138.7	124.5	5.67	6.21
	16	199.0	193.6	187.8	181.5	174.7	167.3	159.0	149.8	139.4	127.3	113.1	3.86	4.37
	18	188.6	183.2	177.4	171.2	164.4	156.9	148.7	139.5	129.1	117.0	102.7	2.61	3.10
190.00	12	234.1	228.4	222.3	215.7	208.5	200.6	191.9	182.2	171.2	158.5	143.4	8.43	8.99
	14	220.6	214.9	208.8	202.1	195.0	187.1	178.4	168.7	157.7	145.0	129.9	5.73	6.26
	16	208.6	202.9	196.8	190.2	183.0	175.1	166.4	156.7	145.7	133.0	117.9	3.88	4.40
	18	197.7	192.0	185.9	179.3	172.1	164.2	155.5	145.8	134.8	122.1	107.0	2.60	3.10
200.0	12	245.2	239.2	232.7	225.8	218.2	209.9	200.8	190.6	179.0	165.6	149.7	8.59	9.16
	14	230.7	224.7	218.3	211.3	203.7	195.5	186.3	176.1	164.5	151.1	135.3	5.78	6.32
	16	218.1	212.1	205.7	198.7	191.2	182.9	173.8	163.5	151.9	138.5	122.7	3.89	4.41
	18	206.7	200.7	194.3	187.3	179.7	171.5	162.3	152.1	140.5	127.1	111.3	2.60	3.10
210.00	12	256.1	249.8	243.1	235.8	227.9	219.2	209.6	198.8	186.6	172.6	155.9	8.76	9.32
	14	240.7	234.4	227.7	220.4	212.4	203.8	194.1	183.4	171.2	157.2	140.5	5.81	6.36
	16	227.6	221.3	214.5	207.2	199.3	190.6	181.0	170.3	158.1	144.0	127.4	3.89	4.41
	18	215.6	209.3	202.5	195.2	187.3	178.6	169.0	158.3	146.1	132.0	115.4	2.60	3.10

TABLE 164

Process Times (B) at Retort Temperature of 260°F for Conduction-Heating Foods in 603 x 700 Can

f_h	z	INITIAL FOOD TEMPERATURE (T_{ih})											Equivalent	
		100	110	120	130	140	150	160	170	180	190	200	F_c^{18}	F_s^{18}
170.00	12	179.1	174.3	169.2	163.8	157.9	151.4	144.4	136.6	127.9	118.1	106.7	7.50	8.09
	14	171.8	167.0	161.9	156.4	150.5	144.1	137.1	129.3	120.6	110.7	99.4	5.25	5.83
	16	164.3	159.5	154.5	149.0	143.1	136.6	129.6	121.8	113.1	103.3	91.9	3.63	4.18
	18	158.0	153.2	148.1	142.7	136.8	130.3	123.3	115.5	106.8	97.0	85.6	2.57	3.10
180.00	12	188.5	183.5	178.1	172.3	166.0	159.2	151.8	143.5	134.3	123.9	111.8	7.57	8.16
	14	180.9	175.8	170.4	164.7	158.4	151.6	144.1	135.9	126.7	116.3	104.2	5.30	5.88
	16	172.9	167.8	162.4	156.6	150.4	143.6	136.1	127.9	118.7	108.2	96.2	3.63	4.18
	18	166.2	161.1	155.7	149.9	143.7	136.9	129.4	121.2	112.0	101.5	89.5	2.56	3.10
190.00	12	197.9	192.6	186.9	180.8	174.2	167.0	159.1	150.4	140.7	129.7	117.0	7.66	8.25
	14	189.9	184.6	178.9	172.8	166.2	159.0	151.1	142.4	132.7	121.7	109.0	5.35	5.93
	16	181.5	176.1	170.4	164.3	157.7	150.5	142.7	134.0	124.3	113.2	100.5	3.66	4.21
	18	174.4	169.1	163.4	157.3	150.7	143.5	135.6	126.9	117.2	106.2	93.5	2.56	3.10
200.00	12	207.3	201.7	195.7	189.2	182.3	174.7	166.5	157.3	147.1	135.5	122.1	7.74	8.34
	14	198.9	193.3	187.3	180.8	173.9	166.3	158.0	148.9	138.7	127.1	113.7	5.41	5.99
	16	190.0	184.4	178.4	171.9	165.0	157.4	149.2	140.0	129.8	118.2	104.8	3.68	4.24
	18	182.6	177.0	171.0	164.5	157.6	150.0	141.7	132.6	122.4	110.8	97.4	2.56	3.10
210.00	12	216.6	210.7	204.4	197.6	190.3	182.4	173.7	164.1	153.3	141.2	127.1	7.81	8.40
	14	207.8	201.9	195.6	188.9	181.6	173.6	165.0	155.3	144.6	132.4	118.4	5.47	6.05
	16	198.4	192.5	186.2	179.5	172.2	164.2	155.5	145.9	135.2	123.0	109.0	3.69	4.25
	18	190.6	184.7	178.4	171.7	164.4	156.5	147.8	138.1	127.4	115.2	101.2	2.56	3.10

SECTION II: SAFE THERMAL PROCESSES WITH z VALUES FROM 18 TO 24; TABLES 165 TO 328

Hypothetical Processing Criteria to Achieve Safety in Conduction-Heating Products

Thermobacteriological considerations

Organism of concern	: *C. botulinum*
Initial population	: One per gram of food
Extent of reduction	: 12 log cycles
D_{250} Value	: 0.20 min
z Values	: 18, 20, 22, and 24F°

Processing conditions

Initial food temperatures (T_{ih})	: 100 to 200°F
Retort temperatures (T_r)	: 230 to 260°F
Heating rate function (f_h)	: Based on 5 values for No. 10 can
Heating lag factor (j_{ch})	: 2.00
Cooling lag factor (j_{cc})	: 2.00

TABLE 165

Process Times (B) at Retort Temperature of 230°F for Conduction-Heating Foods in 202 x 204 Can

f_h	z	INITIAL FOOD TEMPERATURE (T_{ih})											Equivalent	
		100	110	120	130	140	150	160	170	180	190	200	F_c^{18}	F_s^{18}
16.91	18	60.1	59.5	58.9	58.2	57.4	56.5	55.5	54.4	53.1	51.4	49.3	2.57	2.79
	20	51.4	50.9	50.2	49.5	48.7	47.9	46.9	45.8	44.4	42.8	40.7	1.91	2.14
	22	45.5	44.9	44.2	43.5	42.8	41.9	40.9	39.8	38.5	36.8	34.7	1.47	1.69
	24	41.2	40.6	40.0	39.3	38.5	37.7	36.7	35.5	34.2	32.6	30.5	1.13	1.36
17.90	18	61.7	61.1	60.4	59.6	58.8	57.9	56.9	55.7	54.3	52.5	50.3	2.56	2.80
	20	52.8	52.2	51.5	50.8	50.0	49.0	48.0	46.8	45.4	43.6	41.4	1.90	2.13
	22	46.9	46.2	45.6	44.8	44.0	43.1	42.0	40.8	39.4	37.7	35.5	1.46	1.68
	24	42.7	42.1	41.4	40.7	39.8	38.9	37.9	36.7	35.3	33.5	31.3	1.12	1.35
18.89	18	63.1	62.5	61.8	61.0	60.1	59.2	58.1	56.8	55.3	53.5	51.1	2.56	2.80
	20	54.3	53.6	52.9	52.2	51.3	50.3	49.2	48.0	46.5	44.6	42.3	1.90	2.13
	22	48.2	47.6	46.9	46.1	45.2	44.3	43.2	41.9	40.3	38.6	36.2	1.45	1.68
	24	44.2	43.5	42.8	42.0	41.2	40.2	39.1	37.9	36.4	34.5	32.2	1.11	1.35
19.89	18	64.5	63.9	63.1	62.3	61.4	60.4	59.2	57.9	56.3	54.4	51.9	2.55	2.79
	20	55.7	55.0	54.3	53.5	52.5	51.5	50.4	49.0	47.5	45.5	43.1	1.89	2.13
	22	49.6	48.9	48.2	47.3	46.4	45.4	44.3	42.9	41.4	39.4	36.9	1.42	1.66
	24	45.6	45.0	44.2	43.4	42.5	41.5	40.3	39.0	37.4	35.5	33.0	1.11	1.35
20.88	18	66.1	65.4	64.6	63.8	62.8	61.7	60.5	59.1	57.5	55.4	52.8	2.55	2.80
	20	57.2	56.4	55.6	54.8	53.8	52.8	51.5	50.1	48.5	46.5	43.9	1.88	2.12
	22	51.1	50.4	49.6	48.7	47.7	46.7	45.5	44.1	42.4	40.4	37.8	1.40	1.65
	24	47.1	46.3	45.6	44.7	43.7	42.7	41.5	40.1	38.4	36.4	33.8	1.11	1.35

TABLE 166

Process Times (B) at Retort Temperature of 240°F for Conduction-Heating Foods in 202 x 204 Can

f_h	z	INITIAL FOOD TEMPERATURE (T_{ih})											Equivalent	
		100	110	120	130	140	150	160	170	180	190	200	F_c^{18}	F_s^{18}
	18	35.1	34.6	34.0	33.3	32.6	31.9	31.0	30.0	28.9	27.5	25.9	2.49	2.80
16.91	20	32.8	32.3	31.7	31.0	30.3	29.6	28.7	27.7	26.6	25.2	23.6	1.99	2.30
	22	31.0	30.5	29.9	29.2	28.5	27.8	26.9	25.9	24.8	23.4	21.8	1.63	1.95
	24	29.4	28.9	28.3	27.6	26.9	26.2	25.3	24.3	23.2	21.9	20.2	1.33	1.63
	18	36.3	35.7	35.1	34.4	33.7	32.9	32.0	30.9	29.7	28.3	26.6	2.48	2.79
17.90	20	34.1	33.6	32.9	32.3	31.5	30.7	29.8	28.8	27.6	26.1	24.4	1.98	2.30
	22	32.2	31.7	31.0	30.4	29.6	28.8	27.9	26.8	25.6	24.2	22.5	1.62	1.93
	24	30.6	30.0	29.4	28.7	28.0	27.1	26.2	25.2	24.0	22.6	20.8	1.31	1.62
	18	37.8	37.2	36.5	35.8	35.0	34.1	33.2	32.1	30.8	29.3	27.5	2.48	2.80
18.89	20	35.4	34.8	34.2	33.5	32.7	31.8	30.9	29.8	28.5	27.0	25.2	1.97	2.30
	22	33.4	32.8	32.2	31.5	30.7	29.8	28.8	27.8	26.5	25.0	23.2	1.59	1.91
	24	31.7	31.1	30.4	29.7	28.9	28.1	27.1	26.0	24.8	23.3	21.4	1.28	1.60
	18	39.2	38.5	37.8	37.1	36.3	35.4	34.3	33.2	31.9	30.3	28.4	2.47	2.80
19.89	20	36.7	36.1	35.4	34.6	33.8	32.9	31.9	30.7	29.4	27.8	25.9	1.97	2.30
	22	34.6	34.0	33.3	32.6	31.7	30.8	29.8	28.6	27.3	25.7	23.8	1.57	1.89
	24	32.9	32.2	31.6	30.8	30.0	29.1	28.1	26.9	25.6	24.0	22.1	1.26	1.58
	18	40.6	39.9	39.2	38.4	37.5	36.5	35.5	34.3	32.9	31.2	29.2	2.47	2.80
20.88	20	38.0	37.3	36.6	35.8	34.9	34.0	32.9	31.7	30.3	28.6	26.6	1.96	2.29
	22	35.8	35.1	34.4	33.6	32.7	31.8	30.7	29.5	28.1	26.5	24.4	1.54	1.87
	24	34.1	33.4	32.7	31.9	31.0	30.1	29.0	27.8	26.4	24.7	22.7	1.25	1.58

TABLE 167

Process Times (B) at Retort Temperature of 250°F for Conduction-Heating Foods in 202 x 204 Can

f_h	z	INITIAL FOOD TEMPERATURE (T_{ih})											Equivalent	
		100	110	120	130	140	150	160	170	180	190	200	F_c^{18}	F_s^{18}
	18	25.7	25.2	24.6	24.0	23.4	22.7	21.9	21.0	20.1	18.9	17.6	2.39	2.80
16.91	20	24.7	24.2	23.7	23.1	22.5	21.8	21.0	20.1	19.1	18.0	16.7	1.99	2.39
	22	23.9	23.4	22.9	22.3	21.7	21.0	20.2	19.3	18.3	17.2	15.9	1.68	2.06
	24	23.2	22.7	22.2	21.6	20.9	20.2	19.5	18.6	17.6	16.5	15.2	1.42	1.80
	18	26.9	26.3	25.7	25.1	24.4	23.7	22.9	22.0	20.9	19.7	18.3	2.39	2.80
17.90	20	25.9	25.4	24.8	24.2	23.5	22.7	21.9	21.0	20.0	18.8	17.3	1.99	2.39
	22	25.0	24.5	23.9	23.3	22.6	21.9	21.1	20.1	19.1	17.9	16.5	1.66	2.05
	24	24.3	23.7	23.2	22.5	21.9	21.1	20.3	19.4	18.4	17.2	15.7	1.40	1.78
	18	28.0	27.5	26.9	26.2	25.5	24.7	23.8	22.9	21.8	20.5	19.0	2.39	2.80
18.89	20	27.0	26.5	25.8	25.2	24.5	23.7	22.8	21.9	20.8	19.5	18.0	1.98	2.38
	22	26.1	25.6	24.9	24.3	23.6	22.8	21.9	21.0	19.9	18.6	17.1	1.64	2.03
	24	25.3	24.8	24.1	23.5	22.8	22.0	21.1	20.2	19.1	17.8	16.3	1.38	1.77
	18	29.2	28.6	28.0	27.3	26.5	25.7	24.8	23.8	22.6	21.3	19.7	2.39	2.80
19.89	20	28.1	27.5	26.9	26.2	25.5	24.6	23.7	22.7	21.6	20.2	18.7	1.97	2.37
	22	27.2	26.6	26.0	25.3	24.5	23.7	22.8	21.8	20.6	19.3	17.7	1.63	2.02
	24	26.4	25.8	25.1	24.4	23.7	22.9	21.9	20.9	19.8	18.4	16.9	1.37	1.76
	18	30.4	29.7	29.1	28.3	27.6	26.7	25.7	24.7	23.5	22.1	20.4	2.38	2.80
20.88	20	29.3	28.6	28.0	27.2	26.4	25.6	24.6	23.6	22.3	20.9	19.3	1.95	2.36
	22	28.3	27.6	27.0	26.2	25.5	24.6	23.6	22.6	21.4	20.0	18.3	1.61	2.01
	24	27.4	26.8	26.1	25.4	24.6	23.7	22.8	21.7	20.5	19.1	17.4	1.36	1.74

TABLE 168

Process Times (B) at Retort Temperature of 260°F for Conduction-Heating Foods in 202 x 204 Can

f_h	z	INITIAL FOOD TEMPERATURE (T_{ih})											Equivalent	
		100	110	120	130	140	150	160	170	180	190	200	F_c^{18}	F_s^{18}
16.91	18	20.8	20.4	19.9	19.3	18.7	18.1	17.4	16.6	15.7	14.8	13.6	2.34	2.80
	20	20.4	19.9	19.4	18.9	18.3	17.7	17.0	16.2	15.3	14.4	13.2	2.05	2.49
	22	20.0	19.5	19.0	18.5	17.9	17.3	16.6	15.8	14.9	13.9	12.8	1.78	2.22
	24	19.6	19.1	18.6	18.1	17.5	16.8	16.1	15.4	14.5	13.5	12.4	1.52	1.95
17.90	18	21.9	21.4	20.8	20.3	19.6	19.0	18.2	17.4	16.5	15.4	14.2	2.34	2.80
	20	21.4	20.9	20.4	19.8	19.2	18.5	17.8	16.9	16.0	15.0	13.8	2.03	2.48
	22	21.0	20.5	19.9	19.4	18.7	18.1	17.3	16.5	15.6	14.6	13.4	1.76	2.20
	24	20.4	20.0	19.5	18.9	18.3	17.6	16.9	16.0	15.1	14.1	12.9	1.49	1.92
18.89	18	22.9	22.4	21.8	21.2	20.5	19.8	19.0	18.2	17.2	16.1	14.9	2.34	2.80
	20	22.4	21.9	21.3	20.7	20.1	19.3	18.6	17.7	16.7	15.6	14.4	2.02	2.47
	22	21.9	21.4	20.8	20.2	19.6	18.9	18.1	17.2	16.3	15.2	13.9	1.74	2.18
	24	21.4	20.9	20.3	19.7	19.1	18.4	17.6	16.7	15.8	14.7	13.4	1.47	1.90
19.89	18	23.9	23.4	22.8	22.1	21.4	20.7	19.9	19.0	17.9	16.8	15.4	2.34	2.80
	20	23.4	22.8	22.3	21.6	20.9	20.2	19.3	18.4	17.4	16.3	14.9	2.01	2.46
	22	22.9	22.3	21.7	21.1	20.4	19.7	18.8	17.9	16.9	15.8	14.4	1.72	2.16
	24	22.4	21.8	21.2	20.6	19.9	19.1	18.3	17.4	16.4	15.2	13.9	1.45	1.88
20.88	18	24.9	24.4	23.7	23.1	22.3	21.5	20.7	19.7	18.7	17.4	16.0	2.34	2.80
	20	24.4	23.8	23.2	22.5	21.8	21.0	20.1	19.2	18.1	16.9	15.5	2.00	2.45
	22	23.8	23.3	22.6	22.0	21.2	20.4	19.6	18.6	17.6	16.3	14.9	1.70	2.14
	24	23.3	22.7	22.1	21.4	20.7	19.9	19.0	18.1	17.0	15.8	14.4	1.43	1.86

TABLE 169

Process Times (B) at Retort Temperature of 230°F for Conduction-Heating Foods in 202 x 214 Can

f_h	z	INITIAL FOOD TEMPERATURE (T_{ih})											Equivalent	
		100	110	120	130	140	150	160	170	180	190	200	F_c^{18}	F_s^{18}
	18	64.6	64.0	63.2	62.4	61.5	60.5	59.3	58.0	56.5	54.6	52.1	2.58	2.82
19.73	20	55.8	55.1	54.3	53.5	52.6	51.6	50.5	49.1	47.6	45.7	43.2	1.91	2.15
	22	49.6	48.9	48.2	47.4	46.5	45.5	44.3	43.0	41.4	39.5	37.1	1.44	1.68
	24	45.6	44.9	44.1	43.3	42.4	41.4	40.3	39.0	37.4	35.5	33.0	1.12	1.36
	18	66.5	65.7	64.9	64.1	63.1	62.1	60.8	59.4	57.8	55.8	53.2	2.58	2.82
20.89	20	57.4	56.7	55.9	55.0	54.1	53.0	51.8	50.4	48.7	46.7	44.1	1.90	2.14
	22	51.3	50.5	49.7	48.9	47.9	46.9	45.6	44.2	42.6	40.6	38.0	1.42	1.67
	24	47.2	46.5	45.7	44.9	43.9	42.8	41.6	40.2	38.6	36.6	33.9	1.12	1.36
	18	68.2	67.5	66.6	65.7	64.7	63.6	62.3	60.8	59.1	56.9	54.2	2.57	2.82
22.05	20	59.1	58.3	57.5	56.6	55.6	54.4	53.2	51.7	49.9	47.8	45.1	1.90	2.14
	22	53.1	52.3	51.5	50.6	49.6	48.4	47.2	45.7	43.9	41.8	39.0	1.41	1.67
	24	48.9	48.1	47.3	46.4	45.4	44.2	43.0	41.5	39.7	37.6	34.8	1.12	1.36
	18	69.9	69.0	68.2	67.2	66.1	65.0	63.6	62.1	60.2	58.0	55.1	2.57	2.82
23.21	20	60.7	59.9	59.1	58.1	57.0	55.8	54.5	52.9	51.1	48.9	46.0	1.89	2.14
	22	54.9	54.1	53.2	52.2	51.2	50.0	48.6	47.1	45.2	43.0	40.1	1.41	1.67
	24	50.5	49.7	48.8	47.8	46.8	45.6	44.2	42.7	40.9	38.6	35.7	1.12	1.36
	18	71.1	70.8	69.9	68.9	67.8	66.5	65.1	63.5	61.5	59.2	56.1	2.57	2.82
24.37	20	62.4	61.6	60.6	59.6	58.5	57.3	55.9	54.2	52.3	49.9	46.9	1.89	2.14
	22	56.6	55.7	54.8	53.8	52.7	51.4	50.0	48.4	46.5	44.1	41.1	1.41	1.66
	24	52.0	51.2	50.3	49.3	48.1	46.9	45.5	43.9	41.9	39.6	36.5	1.12	1.36

TABLE 170

Process Times (B) at Retort Temperature of 240°F for Conduction-Heating Foods in 202 x 214 Can

f_h	z	INITIAL FOOD TEMPERATURE (T_{ih})											Equivalent	
		100	110	120	130	140	150	160	170	180	190	200	F_c^{18}	F_s^{18}
19.73	18	39.1	38.4	37.7	37.0	36.2	35.3	34.3	33.1	31.8	30.2	28.3	2.50	2.82
	20	36.6	36.0	35.3	34.6	33.8	32.8	31.8	30.7	29.4	27.8	25.9	1.99	2.32
	22	34.5	33.9	33.2	32.5	31.7	30.8	29.8	28.6	27.3	25.7	23.8	1.59	1.91
	24	32.8	32.1	31.5	30.7	29.9	29.0	28.0	26.8	25.5	24.0	22.0	1.28	1.60
20.89	18	40.7	40.0	39.3	38.5	37.6	36.7	35.6	34.4	33.0	31.3	29.3	2.49	2.82
	20	38.1	37.4	36.7	35.9	35.1	34.1	33.0	31.8	30.4	28.8	26.7	1.98	2.31
	22	35.9	35.2	34.5	33.7	32.9	31.9	30.8	29.6	28.2	26.6	24.6	1.56	1.89
	24	34.2	33.5	32.8	32.0	31.1	30.2	29.1	27.9	26.5	24.8	22.8	1.27	1.59
22.05	18	42.3	41.6	40.8	40.0	39.0	38.0	36.9	35.6	34.2	32.4	30.3	2.48	2.82
	20	39.6	38.9	38.1	37.3	36.3	35.3	34.2	32.9	31.4	29.7	27.6	1.96	2.30
	22	37.3	36.6	35.9	35.0	34.1	33.1	32.0	30.7	29.2	27.5	25.3	1.55	1.88
	24	35.5	34.8	34.0	33.2	32.3	31.2	30.2	28.9	27.4	25.7	23.5	1.25	1.58
23.21	18	43.8	43.1	42.3	41.1	40.4	39.4	38.2	36.8	35.3	33.4	31.2	2.48	2.82
	20	41.0	40.2	39.4	38.6	37.6	36.5	35.3	34.0	32.4	30.6	28.4	1.93	2.27
	22	38.8	38.0	37.2	36.3	35.4	34.3	33.1	31.8	30.2	28.4	26.1	1.54	1.87
	24	36.9	36.1	35.3	34.4	33.5	32.4	31.2	29.9	28.3	26.5	24.2	1.24	1.56
24.37	18	45.3	44.6	43.7	42.8	41.8	40.7	39.4	38.0	36.4	34.5	32.1	2.47	2.82
	20	42.5	41.7	40.8	39.9	38.9	37.8	36.6	35.1	33.5	31.6	29.2	1.93	2.27
	22	40.2	39.4	38.5	37.6	36.6	35.5	34.2	32.8	31.2	29.3	26.9	1.53	1.86
	24	38.2	37.4	36.5	35.6	34.6	33.5	32.2	30.8	29.2	27.3	24.9	1.22	1.55

TABLE 171

Process Times (B) at Retort Temperature of 250°F for Conduction-Heating Foods in 202 x 214 Can

f_h	z	INITIAL FOOD TEMPERATURE (T_{ih})											Equivalent	
		100	110	120	130	140	150	160	170	180	190	200	F_c^{18}	F_s^{18}
19.73	18	29.1	28.5	27.9	27.2	26.4	25.6	24.7	23.7	22.5	21.2	19.7	2.41	2.82
	20	28.0	27.4	26.8	26.1	25.4	24.5	23.6	22.6	21.5	20.9	18.6	1.99	2.39
	22	27.1	26.5	25.9	25.2	24.4	23.6	22.7	21.7	20.5	19.2	17.7	1.65	2.04
	24	26.2	25.7	25.0	24.3	23.6	22.8	21.9	20.9	19.7	18.4	16.8	1.39	1.78
20.89	18	30.4	29.8	29.1	28.4	27.6	26.8	25.8	24.7	23.5	22.1	20.5	2.41	2.82
	20	29.3	28.7	28.0	27.3	26.5	25.6	24.7	23.6	22.4	21.0	19.4	1.97	2.38
	22	28.3	27.7	27.0	26.3	25.5	24.7	23.7	22.6	21.4	20.0	18.4	1.63	2.03
	24	27.4	26.8	26.2	25.4	24.6	23.8	22.8	21.7	20.5	19.1	17.5	1.37	1.76
22.05	18	31.8	31.1	30.4	29.6	28.8	27.9	26.9	25.8	24.5	23.0	21.3	2.41	2.82
	20	30.6	30.0	29.2	28.5	27.6	26.7	25.7	24.6	23.3	21.8	20.1	1.96	2.37
	22	29.6	28.9	28.2	27.4	26.6	25.7	24.7	23.6	22.3	20.8	19.1	1.62	2.02
	24	28.6	28.0	27.3	26.5	25.7	24.8	23.7	22.6	21.3	19.9	18.1	1.35	1.74
23.21	18	33.1	32.4	31.7	30.9	30.0	29.0	28.0	26.8	25.4	23.9	22.1	2.40	2.82
	20	31.9	31.2	30.5	39.6	28.8	27.8	26.7	25.6	24.2	22.7	20.8	1.95	2.36
	22	30.8	30.1	29.4	28.6	27.7	26.7	25.7	24.5	23.1	21.6	19.7	1.62	2.02
	24	29.8	29.1	28.4	27.6	26.7	25.7	24.7	23.5	22.1	20.6	18.8	1.33	1.73
24.37	18	34.5	33.7	32.9	32.1	31.2	30.2	29.1	27.8	26.4	24.8	22.8	2.40	2.82
	20	33.2	32.4	3-.7	30.8	29.9	28.9	27.8	26.5	25.1	23.5	21.5	1.94	2.35
	22	32.0	31.3	30.5	29.7	28.8	27.8	26.6	25.4	24.0	22.4	20.4	1.61	2.01
	24	31.0	30.3	29.5	28.6	27.7	26.7	25.6	24.3	22.9	21.3	19.4	1.32	1.71

TABLE 172

Process Times (B) at Retort Temperature of 260°F for Conduction-Heating Foods in 202 x 214 Can

f_h	z	INITIAL FOOD TEMPERATURE (T_{ih})											Equivalent	
		100	110	120	130	140	150	160	170	180	190	200	F_c^{18}	F_s^{18}
19.73	18	23.8	23.2	22.6	22.0	21.3	20.6	19.8	18.9	17.9	16.7	15.4	2.36	2.82
	20	23.3	22.7	22.1	21.5	20.8	20.1	19.3	18.4	17.3	16.2	14.9	2.04	2.49
	22	22.8	22.2	21.6	21.0	20.3	19.6	18.8	17.9	16.8	15.7	14.4	1.74	2.19
	24	22.3	21.7	21.1	20.5	19.8	19.0	18.2	17.3	16.3	15.2	13.9	1.47	1.90
20.89	18	25.0	24.4	23.8	23.1	22.4	21.6	20.7	19.8	18.7	17.5	16.1	2.36	2.82
	20	24.4	23.8	23.2	22.5	21.8	21.0	20.2	19.2	18.1	16.9	15.5	2.02	2.47
	22	23.9	23.3	22.7	22.0	21.3	20.5	19.6	18.7	17.6	16.4	15.0	1.72	2.16
	24	23.3	22.7	22.1	21.4	20.7	19.9	19.1	18.1	17.0	15.8	14.4	1.45	1.88
22.05	18	26.2	25.5	24.9	24.2	23.4	22.6	21.7	20.7	19.5	18.2	16.8	2.36	2.82
	20	25.6	24.9	24.3	23.6	22.8	22.0	21.1	20.1	18.9	17.7	16.2	2.01	2.46
	22	25.0	24.4	23.7	23.0	22.2	21.4	20.5	19.5	18.3	17.1	15.6	1.70	2.14
	24	24.4	23.8	23.1	22.4	21.6	20.8	19.9	18.9	17.8	16.5	15.0	1.42	1.85
23.21	18	27.3	26.7	26.0	25.2	24.4	23.6	22.6	21.5	20.3	19.0	17.4	2.36	2.82
	20	26.7	26.0	25.4	24.6	23.8	22.9	22.9	20.9	19.7	18.4	16.8	2.00	2.45
	22	26.1	25.4	24.7	24.0	23.2	22.3	21.3	20.3	19.1	17.7	16.2	1.68	2.12
	24	25.4	24.8	24.1	23.4	22.5	21.7	20.7	19.7	18.5	17.1	15.6	1.40	1.83
24.37	18	28.5	27.8	27.1	26.3	25.5	24.5	23.5	22.4	21.2	19.8	18.1	2.36	2.82
	20	27.8	27.1	26.4	25.6	24.8	23.9	22.9	21.7	20.5	19.1	17.4	1.98	2.44
	22	27.2	26.5	25.7	25.0	24.1	23.2	22.2	21.1	19.8	18.4	16.8	1.66	2.10
	24	26.5	25.8	25.1	24.3	23.5	22.5	21.5	20.4	19.2	17.8	16.1	1.38	1.81

TABLE 173

Process Times (B) at Retort Temperature of 230°F for Conduction-Heating Foods in 202 x 308 Can

f_h	z	INITIAL FOOD TEMPERATURE (T_{ih}) 100	110	120	130	140	150	160	170	180	190	200	Equivalent F_c^{18}	F_s^{18}
21.38	18	67.5	66.7	65.9	65.0	64.1	63.0	61.7	60.3	58.6	56.5	53.9	2.59	2.84
	20	58.3	57.6	56.8	55.9	54.9	53.8	52.6	51.2	49.5	47.4	44.7	1.92	2.16
	22	52.2	51.4	50.6	49.7	48.8	47.7	46.4	45.0	43.3	41.2	38.6	1.43	1.68
	24	48.1	47.3	46.5	45.6	44.7	43.6	42.3	40.9	39.2	37.1	34.5	1.13	1.37
22.64	18	69.3	68.5	67.7	66.8	65.7	64.6	63.2	61.7	59.9	57.7	54.9	2.59	2.84
	20	60.1	59.3	58.5	57.5	56.5	55.4	54.0	52.5	50.7	48.5	45.7	1.91	2.16
	22	54.1	53.4	52.5	51.6	50.5	49.4	48.1	46.5	44.7	42.6	39.7	1.42	1.68
	24	49.8	49.1	48.2	47.3	46.2	45.1	43.8	42.2	40.4	38.3	35.4	1.13	1.37
23.89	18	71.2	70.3	69.4	68.4	67.4	66.1	64.7	63.1	61.3	58.9	56.0	2.59	2.84
	20	61.9	61.1	60.2	69.2	58.1	56.9	55.5	53.9	52.0	49.7	46.7	1.90	2.15
	22	56.0	55.2	54.3	53.3	52.2	51.0	49.6	48.0	46.1	43.8	40.8	1.42	1.68
	24	51.6	50.7	49.8	48.8	47.7	46.5	45.1	43.5	41.6	39.3	36.3	1.13	1.36
25.15	18	73.1	72.2	71.3	70.2	69.1	67.8	66.3	64.7	62.7	60.2	57.1	2.58	2.84
	20	63.7	62.8	61.9	60.8	59.7	58.4	56.9	55.3	53.3	50.8	47.7	1.88	2.14
	22	57.9	57.0	56.1	55.0	53.9	52.6	51.1	49.4	47.5	45.0	41.9	1.42	1.67
	24	53.2	52.3	51.4	50.4	49.2	47.9	46.5	44.8	42.8	40.3	37.2	1.13	1.37
26.41	18	74.9	74.0	73.0	71.9	70.7	69.3	67.8	66.0	64.0	61.4	58.1	2.58	2.84
	20	65.7	64.7	63.7	62.6	61.4	60.1	58.6	56.8	54.7	52.1	48.8	1.86	2.13
	22	59.7	58.8	57.8	56.7	55.5	54.2	52.6	50.9	48.8	46.2	42.9	1.41	1.67
	24	54.8	53.9	52.9	51.8	50.6	49.3	47.7	46.0	43.9	41.3	38.0	1.13	1.37

TABLE 174

Process Times (B) at Retort Temperature of 240°F for Conduction-Heating Foods in 202 x 308 Can

f_h	z	INITIAL FOOD TEMPERATURE (T_{ih}) 100	110	120	130	140	150	160	170	180	190	200	Equivalent F_c^{18}	F_s^{18}
21.38	18	41.4	40.8	40.0	39.2	38.3	37.3	36.2	35.0	33.6	31.9	29.8	2.51	2.84
	20	38.8	38.1	37.4	36.6	35.7	34.7	33.6	32.4	30.9	29.3	27.2	1.99	2.33
	22	36.6	35.9	35.1	34.3	33.5	32.5	31.4	30.1	28.7	27.0	24.9	1.57	1.90
	24	34.8	34.1	33.4	32.6	31.7	30.7	29.6	28.4	27.0	25.3	23.2	1.27	1.60
22.64	18	43.2	42.4	41.6	40.8	39.8	38.8	37.7	36.3	34.8	33.0	30.8	2.50	2.84
	20	40.4	39.7	38.9	38.0	37.1	36.0	34.9	33.6	32.1	30.3	28.1	1.97	2.30
	22	38.1	37.4	36.6	35.8	34.8	33.8	32.6	31.3	29.8	28.0	25.8	1.56	1.89
	24	36.3	35.6	34.8	33.9	33.0	31.9	30.8	29.5	28.0	26.2	24.0	1.26	1.59
23.89	18	44.8	44.1	43.2	42.3	41.3	40.2	39.0	37.6	36.0	34.1	31.8	2.49	2.84
	20	41.9	41.2	40.3	39.4	38.4	37.4	36.1	34.7	33.1	31.3	38.9	1.94	2.28
	22	39.7	38.9	38.1	37.2	36.2	35.1	33.9	32.5	30.9	29.0	26.7	1.55	1.88
	24	37.7	36.9	36.1	35.2	34.2	33.1	31.9	30.5	28.9	27.0	24.7	1.24	1.57
25.15	18	46.5	45.7	44.8	43.8	42.8	41.7	40.4	38.9	37.2	35.2	32.8	2.49	2.84
	20	43.6	42.8	41.9	40.9	39.9	38.7	37.5	36.0	34.3	32.3	29.9	1.94	2.28
	22	41.2	40.4	39.5	38.5	37.5	36.3	35.1	33.6	31.9	29.9	27.5	1.53	1.87
	24	39.1	38.3	37.4	36.5	35.4	34.3	33.0	31.5	29.9	27.9	25.4	1.22	1.55
26.41	18	48.1	47.2	46.3	45.3	44.2	43.0	41.7	40.1	38.4	36.3	33.7	2.49	2.84
	20	45.2	44.3	43.4	42.4	41.3	40.1	38.7	37.2	35.4	33.4	30.8	1.93	2.28
	22	42.6	41.8	40.9	39.9	38.8	37.6	36.2	34.7	32.9	30.8	28.3	1.52	1.86
	24	40.5	39.7	38.7	37.7	36.7	35.4	34.1	32.6	30.8	28.7	26.1	1.20	1.54

TABLE 175

Process Times (B) at Retort Temperature of 250°F for Conduction-Heating Foods in 202 x 308 Can

f_h	z	INITIAL FOOD TEMPERATURE (T_{ih})											Equivalent	
		100	110	120	130	140	150	160	170	180	190	200	F_c^{18}	F_s^{18}
	18	31.1	30.4	29.7	29.0	28.2	27.3	26.3	25.2	24.0	22.5	20.9	2.43	2.84
21.38	20	29.9	29.3	28.6	27.8	27.0	26.1	25.2	24.1	22.8	21.4	19.7	1.98	2.39
	22	28.9	28.3	27.6	26.8	26.0	25.1	24.2	23.1	21.8	20.4	18.7	1.64	2.04
	24	28.0	27.4	26.7	25.9	25.1	24.2	23.3	22.2	20.9	19.5	17.8	1.38	1.77
	18	32.5	31.8	31.1	30.3	29.5	28.5	27.5	26.3	25.0	23.5	21.7	2.42	2.84
22.64	20	31.3	30.6	29.9	29.1	28.3	27.3	26.3	25.1	23.8	22.3	20.5	1.97	2.38
	22	30.3	29.6	28.8	28.1	27.2	26.3	25.2	24.1	22.8	21.2	19.5	1.63	2.03
	24	29.3	28.6	27.9	27.1	26.2	25.3	24.3	23.1	21.8	20.3	18.5	1.36	1.75
	18	34.0	33.2	32.5	31.6	30.7	29.8	28.7	27.4	26.1	24.5	22.6	2.42	2.84
23.89	20	32.7	32.0	31.2	30.4	29.5	28.5	27.4	26.2	24.8	23.2	21.3	1.96	2.37
	22	31.6	30.9	30.1	29.3	28.4	27.4	26.3	25.1	23.7	22.1	20.2	1.63	2.03
	24	30.6	29.8	29.1	28.2	27.3	26.4	25.3	24.0	22.7	21.1	19.2	1.34	1.73
	18	35.4	34.7	33.9	33.0	32.0	31.0	29.8	28.5	27.1	25.4	23.4	2.42	2.84
25.15	20	34.1	33.3	32.5	31.7	30.7	29.7	28.5	27.2	25.8	24.1	22.1	1.96	2.37
	22	32.9	32.2	31.4	30.5	29.5	28.5	27.4	26.1	24.6	22.9	20.9	1.62	2.02
	24	31.8	31.1	30.3	29.4	28.5	27.4	26.3	25.0	23.5	21.8	19.8	1.32	1.72
	18	36.9	36.1	35.2	34.3	33.3	32.2	31.0	29.6	28.1	26.3	24.3	2.42	2.84
26.41	20	35.5	34.7	33.8	32.9	31.9	30.8	29.6	28.3	26.7	25.0	22.9	1.96	2.37
	22	34.3	33.5	32.6	31.7	30.7	29.6	28.4	27.1	25.5	23.8	21.7	1.61	2.01
	24	33.1	32.3	31.5	30.6	29.6	28.5	27.3	25.9	24.4	22.6	20.5	1.31	1.71

TABLE 176

Process Times (B) at Retort Temperature of 260°F for Conduction-Heating Foods in 202 x 308 Can

f_h	z	INITIAL FOOD TEMPERATURE (T_{ih})											Equivalent	
		100	110	120	130	140	150	160	170	180	190	200	F_c^{18}	F_s^{18}
21.38	18	25.5	24.9	24.3	23.6	22.8	22.0	21.1	20.2	19.1	17.8	16.4	2.38	2.84
	20	24.9	24.3	23.7	23.0	22.3	21.5	20.6	19.6	18.5	17.3	15.8	2.03	2.49
	22	24.4	23.8	23.1	22.5	21.7	20.9	20.0	19.0	17.9	16.7	15.3	1.73	2.17
	24	23.8	23.2	22.6	21.9	21.1	20.3	19.5	18.5	17.4	16.1	14.7	1.45	1.88
22.64	18	26.8	26.2	25.5	24.7	24.0	23.1	22.2	21.1	20.0	18.7	17.1	2.38	2.84
	20	26.2	25.5	24.9	24.1	23.3	22.5	21.6	20.5	19.4	18.0	16.5	2.02	2.47
	22	25.6	24.9	24.3	23.5	22.7	21.9	21.0	19.9	18.8	17.4	15.9	1.70	2.15
	24	25.0	24.3	23.7	22.9	22.1	21.3	20.3	19.3	18.1	16.8	15.3	1.42	1.86
23.89	18	28.1	27.4	26.7	25.9	25.1	24.2	23.2	22.1	20.9	19.5	17.9	2.38	2.84
	20	27.4	26.7	26.0	25.2	24.4	23.5	22.5	21.4	20.2	18.8	17.2	2.01	2.46
	22	26.7	26.1	25.4	24.6	23.8	22.9	21.9	20.8	19.6	18.2	16.6	1.68	2.13
	24	26.1	25.4	24.7	24.0	23.1	22.2	21.2	20.1	18.9	17.5	15.9	1.40	1.84
25.15	18	29.3	28.6	27.9	27.0	26.2	25.2	24.2	23.0	21.7	20.3	18.6	2.37	2.84
	20	28.6	27.9	27.2	26.3	25.5	24.5	23.5	22.3	21.0	19.6	17.9	1.99	2.45
	22	27.9	27.2	26.5	25.6	24.8	23.8	22.8	21.6	20.3	18.9	17.2	1.66	2.10
	24	27.2	26.5	25.8	25.0	24.1	23.1	22.1	21.0	19.7	18.2	16.5	1.38	1.81
26.41	18	30.6	29.8	29.0	28.2	27.3	26.3	25.2	24.0	22.6	21.1	19.3	2.37	2.84
	20	29.8	29.1	28.3	27.4	26.5	25.5	24.4	23.2	21.9	20.3	18.6	1.98	2.44
	22	29.1	28.3	27.5	26.7	25.8	24.8	23.7	22.5	21.1	19.6	17.8	1.64	2.09
	24	28.4	27.6	26.8	26.0	25.1	24.1	23.0	21.8	20.4	18.9	17.1	1.36	1.79

TABLE 177

Process Times (B) at Retort Temperature of 230°F for Conduction-Heating Foods in 202 x 314 Can

f_h	z	INITIAL FOOD TEMPERATURE (T_{ih})											Equivalent	
		100	110	120	130	140	150	160	170	180	190	200	F^{18}_c	F^{18}_s
22.04	18	68.6	67.8	67.0	66.1	65.1	64.0	62.7	61.2	59.5	57.3	54.6	2.60	2.85
	20	59.4	58.6	57.8	56.9	55.9	54.8	53.5	52.0	50.3	48.1	45.4	1.92	2.17
	22	53.3	52.5	51.7	50.8	49.8	48.6	47.4	45.9	44.1	42.0	39.3	1.43	1.69
	24	49.1	48.3	47.5	46.6	45.6	44.4	43.2	41.7	39.9	37.8	35.0	1.13	1.37
23.34	18	70.5	69.6	68.8	67.8	66.7	65.5	64.2	62.6	60.8	58.5	55.6	2.60	2.85
	20	61.2	60.4	59.5	58.6	57.5	56.3	54.9	53.4	51.5	49.3	46.4	1.91	2.16
	22	55.3	54.5	53.6	52.6	51.6	50.4	49.0	47.4	45.6	43.3	40.4	1.43	1.68
	24	50.9	50.0	49.2	48.2	47.1	46.0	44.6	43.0	41.2	38.9	36.0	1.13	1.37
24.64	18	72.4	71.6	70.7	69.6	68.5	67.3	65.8	64.2	62.2	59.8	56.8	2.59	2.85
	20	63.1	62.2	61.3	60.3	59.2	57.9	56.5	54.8	52.9	50.5	47.4	1.91	2.16
	22	57.2	56.4	55.4	54.4	53.3	52.0	50.6	48.9	47.0	44.6	41.5	1.42	1.68
	24	52.6	51.8	50.8	49.8	48.7	47.4	46.0	44.3	42.4	40.0	36.9	1.13	1.37
25.93	18	74.4	73.5	72.5	71.4	70.2	68.9	67.4	65.7	63.6	61.1	57.9	2.59	2.85
	20	65.0	64.1	63.1	62.0	60.8	59.5	58.0	56.2	54.2	51.7	48.4	1.87	2.14
	22	59.1	58.2	57.2	56.2	55.0	53.7	52.1	5014	48.4	45.8	42.6	1.42	1.68
	24	54.3	53.4	52.4	51.4	50.2	48.8	47.3	45.6	43.5	41.0	37.8	1.13	1.37
27.23	18	76.3	75.3	74.3	73.2	71.9	70.5	69.0	67.1	65.0	62.3	58.9	2.59	2.85
	20	67.1	66.1	65.1	64.0	62.7	61.3	59.8	57.9	55.8	53.1	49.7	1.87	2.14
	22	61.0	60.0	59.0	57.9	56.6	55.2	53.7	51.8	49.7	47.0	43.6	1.42	1.68
	24	55.9	55.0	54.0	52.8	51.6	50.2	48.6	46.8	44.6	42.0	38.6	1.13	1.37

TABLE 178

Process Times (B) at Retort Temperature of 240°F for Conduction-Heating Foods in 202 x 314 Can

f_h	z	INITIAL FOOD TEMPERATURE (T_{ih})											Equivalent	
		100	110	120	130	140	150	160	170	180	190	200	F_c^{18}	F_s^{18}
22.04	18	42.4	41.7	40.9	40.1	39.2	38.2	37.0	35.8	34.3	32.5	30.4	2.51	2.85
	20	39.7	39.0	38.2	37.4	36.5	35.5	34.3	33.1	31.6	29.8	27.7	1.99	2.32
	22	37.4	36.7	36.0	35.1	34.2	33.2	32.1	30.8	29.3	27.6	35.5	1.57	1.90
	24	35.6	34.9	34.2	33.3	32.4	31.4	30.3	29.0	27.5	25.8	23.6	1.27	1.60
23.34	18	44.1	43.4	42.6	41.7	40.7	39.7	38.5	37.1	35.6	33.7	31.4	2.51	2.85
	20	41.3	40.5	39.7	38.9	37.9	36.8	35.6	43.3	32.7	30.9	28.6	1.96	2.30
	22	39.0	38.3	37.5	36.6	35.6	34.6	33.4	32.0	30.5	38.6	26.3	1.56	1.89
	24	37.1	36.4	35.6	34.7	33.7	32.6	31.5	30.1	28.5	26.7	24.4	1.25	1.58
24.64	18	45.9	45.1	44.2	43.3	42.3	41.1	39.9	38.4	36.8	34.8	32.5	2.50	2.85
	20	42.9	42.2	41.3	40.4	39.3	38.2	37.0	35.5	33.9	31.9	29.5	1.95	2.29
	22	40.6	39.8	39.0	38.0	37.0	35.9	34.6	33.2	31.5	29.6	27.2	1.54	1.88
	24	38.6	37.8	36.9	36.0	35.0	33.9	32.6	31.2	29.5	27.6	25.2	1.23	1.56
25.93	18	47.5	46.7	45.8	44.8	43.8	42.6	41.2	39.7	38.0	35.9	33.4	2.50	2.85
	20	44.6	43.8	42.9	41.9	40.8	39.6	38.3	36.8	35.1	33.0	30.5	1.94	2.29
	22	42.1	41.3	40.4	39.4	38.3	37.2	35.8	34.3	32.6	30.5	28.0	1.53	1.87
	24	40.0	39.2	38.3	37.3	36.2	35.0	33.7	32.2	30.4	28.4	25.9	1.21	1.55
27.23	18	49.2	48.3	47.4	46.4	45.2	44.0	42.6	41.0	39.2	37.0	34.4	2.50	2.85
	20	46.2	45.4	44.4	43.4	42.3	41.0	39.6	38.0	36.2	34.1	31,4	1.94	2.29
	22	43.6	42.8	41.8	40.8	39.7	38.4	37.0	35.4	33.6	31.5	28.8	1.51	1.86
	24	41.5	40.6	39.7	38.6	37.5	36.3	34.9	33.3	31.5	29.3	26.7	1.20	1.54

TABLE 179

Process Times (B) at Retort Temperature of 250°F for Conduction-Heating Foods in 202 x 314 Can

f_h	z	INITIAL FOOD TEMPERATURE (T_{ih})											Equivalent	
		100	110	120	130	140	150	160	170	180	190	200	F_c^{18}	F_s^{18}
	18	31.9	31.2	30.5	29.7	28.9	28.0	27.0	25.8	24.6	23.1	21.3	2.44	2.85
22.04	20	30.7	30.0	29.3	28.5	27.7	26.8	25.8	24.7	23.4	21.9	20.2	1.98	2.39
	22	29.6	29.0	28.3	27.5	26.7	25.8	24.8	23.6	22.3	20.9	19.1	1.64	2.04
	24	28.7	28.0	27.3	26.6	25.7	24.8	23.8	22.7	21.4	19.9	18.2	1.37	1.76
	18	33.4	32.7	31.9	31.1	30.2	29.2	28.2	27.0	25.6	24.1	22.2	2.43	2.85
23.34	20	32.1	31.4	30.7	29.9	29.0	28.0	26.9	25.7	24.4	22.8	21.0	1.97	2.38
	22	31.0	30.3	29.6	28.8	27.9	26.9	25.9	24.7	23.3	21.7	19.9	1.64	2.04
	24	30.0	29.3	28.6	27.8	26.9	25.9	24.9	23.7	22.3	20.7	18.9	1.35	1.74
	18	34.8	34.1	33.3	32.5	31.5	30.5	29.4	28.1	26.7	25.0	23.1	2.43	2.85
24.64	20	33.5	32.8	32.0	31.2	30.2	29.2	28.1	26.8	25.4	23.7	21.8	1.96	2.38
	22	32.4	31.7	30.9	30.0	29.1	28.1	26.9	25.7	24.3	22.6	20.6	1.63	2.03
	24	31.3	30.6	29.8	29.0	28.0	27.0	25.9	24.6	23.2	21.5	19.6	1.33	1.73
	18	36.3	35.6	34.7	33.8	32.8	31.8	30.6	29.3	27.8	26.0	24.0	2.43	2.85
25.93	20	35.0	34.2	33.4	32.5	31.5	30.4	29.2	27.9	26.4	24.7	22.6	1.96	2.38
	22	33.8	33.0	32.2	31.3	30.3	29.2	28.0	26.7	25.2	23.5	21.4	1.62	2.02
	24	32.7	31.9	31.1	30.2	29.2	28.1	26.9	25.6	24.1	22.3	20.3	1.32	1.72
	18	37.8	37.0	36.1	35.2	34.2	33.0	31.8	30.4	28.8	27.0	24.8	2.43	2.85
27.23	20	36.4	35.6	34.7	33.8	32.7	31.6	30.4	29.0	27.4	25.6	23.4	1.96	2.38
	22	35.2	34.2	33.5	32.5	31.5	30.4	29.1	27.1	26.1	24.3	22.2	1.61	2.01
	24	34.0	33.2	32.3	31.3	30.3	29.2	27.9	26.5	25.0	23.1	21.0	1.31	1.71

TABLE 180

Process Times (B) at Retort Temperature of 260°F for Conduction-Heating Foods in 202 x 314 Can

f_h	z	INITIAL FOOD TEMPERATURE (T_{ih})											Equivalent	
		100	110	120	130	140	150	160	170	180	190	200	F_c^{18}	F_s^{18}
	18	26.2	25.6	24.9	24.2	23.4	22.6	21.7	20.7	19.6	18.3	16.8	2.39	2.85
22.04	20	25.6	25.0	24.3	23.6	22.9	22.0	21.1	20.1	19.0	17.7	16.2	2.03	2.49
	22	25.0	24.4	23.8	23.0	22.3	21.4	20.5	19.5	18.4	17.1	15.6	1.72	2.17
	24	24.4	23.8	23.2	22.5	21.7	20.9	19.9	18.9	17.8	16.5	15.1	1.44	1.88
	18	27.5	26.9	26.2	25.4	24.6	23.7	22.7	21.7	20.5	19.1	17.6	2.39	2.85
23.34	20	26.9	26.2	25.5	24.8	24.0	23.1	22.1	21.0	19.9	18.5	16.9	2.02	2.48
	22	26.2	25.6	24.9	24.1	23.3	22.5	21.5	20.4	19.2	17.9	16.3	1.70	2.15
	24	25.6	25.0	24.3	23.5	22.7	21.8	20.9	19.8	18.6	17.2	15.7	1.42	1.85
	18	28.8	28.1	27.4	26.6	25.7	24.8	23.8	22.7	21.4	20.0	18.3	2.38	2.85
24.64	20	28.1	27.4	26.7	25.9	25.1	24.1	23.1	22.0	20.7	19.3	17.6	2.01	2.46
	22	27.5	26.8	26.0	25.2	24.4	23.4	22.4	21.3	20.0	18.6	17.0	1.68	2.12
	24	26.8	26.1	25.4	24.6	23.7	22.8	21.8	20.6	19.4	18.0	16.3	1.39	1.83
	18	30.1	29.4	28.6	27.8	26.9	25.9	24.8	23.6	22.3	20.8	19.1	2.38	2.85
25.93	20	29.4	28.7	27.9	27.0	26.1	25.2	24.1	22.9	21.6	20.1	18.3	1.99	2.45
	22	28.7	27.9	27.2	26.3	25.4	24.4	23.4	22.2	20.8	19.3	17.6	1.65	2.10
	24	28.0	27.2	26.5	25.6	24.7	23.7	22.7	21.5	20.2	18.7	16.9	1.37	1.81
	18	31.4	30.6	29.8	28.9	28.0	27.0	25.8	24.6	23.2	21.6	19.8	2.38	2.85
27.23	20	30.6	29.9	29.0	28.2	27.2	26.2	25.1	23.8	22.4	20.8	19.0	1.98	2.44
	22	29.8	29.1	28.3	27.4	26.4	25.4	24.3	23.0	21.7	20.1	18.2	1.64	2.08
	24	29.1	28.4	27.5	26.7	25.7	24.7	23.6	22.3	20.9	19.3	17.5	1.35	1.79

TABLE 181

Process Times (B) at Retort Temperature of 230°F for Conduction-Heating Foods in 211 x 200 Can

f_h	z	INITIAL FOOD TEMPERATURE (T_{ih}) 100	110	120	130	140	150	160	170	180	190	200	Equivalent F_c^{18}	F_s^{18}
20.00	18	65.1	64.4	63.7	62.8	61.9	60.9	59.7	58.4	56.8	54.9	52.4	2.58	2.82
	20	56.2	55.5	54.7	53.9	53.0	52.0	50.8	49.5	47.9	46.0	43.5	1.91	2.15
	22	50.0	49.3	48.6	47.8	46.8	45.8	44.7	43.3	41.7	39.8	37.3	1.44	1.68
	24	46.0	45.3	44.6	43.7	42.8	41.8	40.6	39.3	37.7	35.8	33.3	1.12	1.36
21.18	18	67.0	66.2	65.4	64.6	63.6	62.5	61.3	59.9	58.2	56.1	53.5	2.58	2.83
	20	57.9	57.2	56.4	55.5	54.5	53.4	52.2	50.8	49.1	47.1	44.4	1.91	2.15
	22	51.8	51.0	50.2	49.3	48.4	47.3	46.1	44.6	43.0	40.9	38.3	1.42	1.67
	24	47.7	47.0	46.2	45.3	44.3	43.2	42.0	40.6	38.9	36.9	34.2	1.12	1.36
22.35	18	68.7	68.0	67.1	66.2	65.2	64.0	62.7	61.2	59.5	57.3	54.5	2.58	2.83
	20	59.6	58.8	58.0	57.0	56.0	54.9	53.6	52.1	50.3	48.1	45.3	1.90	2.15
	22	53.6	52.8	52.0	51.1	50.0	48.9	47.6	46.1	44.3	42.2	39.4	1.42	1.67
	24	49.4	48.6	47.7	46.8	45.8	44.6	43.3	41.8	40.1	37.9	35.1	1.12	1.36
23.53	18	70.4	69.6	68.7	67.7	66.7	65.5	64.1	62.5	60.7	58.4	55.4	2.57	2.83
	20	61.3	60.4	59.6	58.6	57.5	56.3	54.9	53.4	51.5	49.2	46.3	1.89	2.14
	22	55.4	54.6	53.7	52.7	51.6	50.4	49.1	47.5	45.6	43.3	40.4	1.41	1.67
	24	51.0	50.1	49.3	48.3	47.2	46.0	44.6	43.1	41.2	38.9	36.0	1.12	1.36
24.71	18	72.2	71.4	70.5	69.4	68.3	67.0	65.6	64.0	62.0	59.6	56.5	2.57	2.83
	20	62.9	62.1	61.1	60.1	59.0	57.7	56.3	54.6	52.7	50.3	47.2	1.88	2.14
	22	57.1	56.3	55.3	54.3	53.2	51.9	50.5	48.8	46.9	44.5	41.4	1.41	1.67
	24	52.5	51.7	50.7	49.7	48.6	47.3	45.9	44.2	42.3	39.3	36.8	1.12	1.36

TABLE 182

Process Times (B) at Retort Temperature of 240°F for Conduction-Heating Foods in 211 x 200 Can

f_h	z	INITIAL FOOD TEMPERATURE (T_{ih})											Equivalent	
		100	110	120	130	140	150	160	170	180	190	200	F_c^{18}	F_s^{18}
	18	29.5	38.8	38.1	37.4	36.5	35.6	34.6	33.4	32.1	30.5	28.6	2.50	2.83
20.00	20	37.0	36.4	35.7	34.9	34.1	33.2	32.1	31.0	29.7	28.1	26.1	1.99	2.32
	22	34.9	34.3	33.6	32.8	32.0	31.1	30.0	28.9	27.5	26.0	24.0	1.59	1.91
	24	33.1	32.5	31.8	31.0	30.2	29.3	28.3	27.1	25.8	24.2	22.2	1.28	1.60
	18	41.1	40.4	39.7	38.9	38.0	37.0	36.0	34.7	33.3	31.6	29.6	2.50	2.83
21.81	20	38.5	37.8	37.1	36.3	35.4	34.4	33.3	32.1	30.7	29.0	27.0	1.98	2.32
	22	36.3	35.6	34.9	34.1	33.2	32.2	31.1	29.9	28.5	26.8	24.8	1.56	1.89
	24	34.5	33.8	33.1	32.3	31.4	30.5	29.4	28.2	26.7	25.1	23.0	1.27	1.59
	18	42.7	42.0	41.2	40.0	39.4	38.4	37.3	36.0	34.5	32.7	30.5	2.49	2.83
23.35	20	40.0	39.2	38.5	37.6	36.7	35.7	34.5	33.2	31.7	30.0	27.8	1.96	2.29
	22	37.7	37.0	36.2	35.4	34.5	33.5	32.3	31.0	29.5	27.7	25.6	1.56	1.89
	24	35.9	35.2	34.4	33.6	32.6	31.6	30.5	29.2	27.7	25.9	23.7	1.25	1.58
	18	44.3	43.5	42.7	41.8	40.8	39.8	38.6	37.2	35.6	33.8	31.5	2.48	2.83
23.53	20	41.4	40.7	39.8	38.9	38.0	36.9	35.7	34.3	32.7	30.9	28.6	1.93	2.27
	22	39.2	38.4	37.6	36.7	35.7	34.7	33.5	32.1	30.5	28.7	26.4	1.54	1.88
	24	37.2	36.5	35.7	34.8	33.8	32.7	31.5	30.2	28.6	26.7	24.4	1.24	1.56
	18	45.8	45.0	44.2	43.2	42.2	41.1	39.8	38.4	36.7	34.8	32.4	2.48	2.83
24.71	20	42.9	42.1	41.3	40.3	39.3	38.2	36.9	35.5	33.8	31.9	29.5	1.93	2.27
	22	40.6	39.8	38.9	38.0	37.0	35.8	34.6	33.1	31.5	29.5	27.1	1.53	1.86
	24	38.6	37.8	36.9	36.0	34.9	33.8	32.6	31.1	29.5	27.5	25.1	1.22	1.55

TABLE 183

Process Times (B) at Retort Temperature of 250°F for Conduction-Heating Foods in 211 x 200 Can

f_h	z	INITIAL FOOD TEMPERATURE (T_{ih})											Equivalent	
		100	110	120	130	140	150	160	170	180	190	200	F_c^{18}	F_s^{18}
20.00	18	29.4	28.8	28.2	27.5	26.7	25.9	25.0	24.0	22.8	21.5	19.9	2.42	2.83
	20	28.3	27.7	27.1	26.4	25.6	24.8	23.9	22.9	21.7	20.4	18.8	1.99	2.40
	22	27.4	26.8	26.1	25.5	24.7	23.9	23.0	21.9	20.8	19.4	17.8	1.65	2.04
	24	26.5	25.9	25.3	24.6	23.9	23.0	22.1	21.1	19.9	18.6	17.0	1.39	1.78
21.18	18	30.8	30.2	29.5	28.7	27.9	27.1	26.1	25.0	23.8	22.4	20.7	2.41	2.83
	20	29.7	29.0	28.3	27.6	26.8	25.9	25.0	23.9	22.6	21.2	19.6	1.98	2.38
	22	28.7	28.0	27.3	26.6	25.8	24.9	24.0	22.9	21.7	20.2	18.6	1.63	2.03
	24	27.8	27.1	26.4	25.7	24.9	24.0	23.1	22.0	20.8	19.3	17.7	1.37	1.76
22.35	18	32.2	31.5	30.8	30.0	29.1	28.2	27.2	26.1	24.8	23.3	21.5	2.41	2.83
	20	31.0	30.3	29.6	28.8	28.0	27.0	26.0	24.9	23.6	22.1	20.3	1.96	2.37
	22	29.9	29.3	28.5	27.8	26.9	26.0	25.0	23.8	22.5	21.0	19.3	1.62	2.02
	24	29.0	28.3	27.6	26.8	26.0	25.0	24.0	22.9	21.6	20.1	18.3	1.35	1.74
23.53	18	33.5	32.8	32.0	31.2	30.3	29.4	28.3	27.1	25.7	24.1	22.3	2.41	2.83
	20	32.3	31.6	30.8	30.0	29.1	28.1	27.0	25.8	24.5	22.9	21.0	1.95	2.36
	22	31.2	30.5	29.7	28.9	28.0	27.0	26.0	24.7	23.4	21.8	19.9	1.62	2.02
	24	30.2	29.5	28.7	27.9	27.0	26.0	24.9	23.7	22.4	20.8	18.9	1.33	1.72
24.71	18	34.9	34.1	33.3	32.5	31.5	30.5	29.4	28.1	26.7	25.0	23.1	2.41	2.83
	20	33.6	32.8	32.0	31.2	30.2	29.2	28.1	26.8	25.4	23.7	21.8	1.95	2.36
	22	32.4	31.7	30.9	30.0	29.1	28.1	26.9	25.7	23.2	22.6	20.6	1.61	2.01
	24	31.4	30.6	29.8	29.0	28.0	27.0	25.9	24.6	23.2	21.5	19.6	1.32	1.71

TABLE 184

Process Times (B) at Retort Temperature of 260°F for Conduction-Heating Foods in 211 x 200 Can

f_h	z	INITIAL FOOD TEMPERATURE (T_{ih})											Equivalent	
		100	110	120	130	140	150	160	170	180	190	200	F_c^{18}	F_s^{18}
	18	24.1	23.5	22.9	22.3	21.6	20.8	20.0	19.1	18.1	16.9	15.6	2.37	2.83
20.00	20	23.6	23.0	22.4	21.8	21.1	20.3	19.5	18.6	17.5	16.4	15.0	2.04	2.49
	22	23.1	22.5	21.9	21.2	20.6	19.8	19.0	18.1	17.0	15.9	14.5	1.74	2.18
	24	22.5	22.0	21.4	20.7	20.0	19.3	18.4	17.5	16.5	15.3	14.0	1.47	1.90
	18	25.3	24.7	24.1	23.4	22.6	21.8	21.0	20.0	18.9	17.7	16.3	2.37	2.83
21.18	20	24.7	24.1	23.5	22.8	22.1	21.3	20.4	19.4	18.3	17.1	15.7	2.02	2.48
	22	24.2	23.6	22.9	22.3	21.5	20.7	19.8	18.9	17.8	16.6	15.1	1.72	2.16
	24	23.6	23.0	22.4	21.7	21.0	20.2	19.3	18.3	17.2	16.0	14.6	1.44	1.88
	18	26.5	25.9	25.2	24.5	23.7	22.8	21.9	20.9	19.7	18.5	17.0	2.36	2.83
22.35	20	25.9	25.2	24.6	23.9	23.1	22.2	21.3	20.3	19.1	17.8	16.4	2.01	2.46
	22	25.3	24.7	24.0	23.3	22.5	21.6	20.7	19.7	18.6	17.3	15.8	1.70	2.14
	24	24.7	24.1	23.4	22.7	21.9	21.0	20.1	19.1	18.0	16.7	15.2	1.42	1.85
	18	27.7	27.0	26.3	25.5	24.7	23.8	22.9	21.8	20.6	19.2	17.6	2.36	2.83
23.53	20	27.0	26.4	25.7	24.9	24.1	23.2	22.2	21.1	19.9	18.6	17.0	2.00	2.45
	22	26.4	25.7	25.0	24.3	23.4	22.6	21.6	20.5	19.3	17.9	16.4	1.68	2.12
	24	25.8	25.1	24.4	23.6	22.8	21.9	20.9	19.9	18.7	17.3	15.7	1.40	1.83
	18	28.8	28.2	27.4	26.6	25.8	24.8	23.8	22.7	21.4	20.0	18.3	2.36	2.83
24.71	20	28.2	27.5	26.7	25.9	25.1	24.1	23.1	22.0	20.7	19.3	17.6	1.99	2.44
	22	27.5	26.8	26.0	25.2	24.4	23.5	22.4	21.3	20.0	18.6	17.0	1.65	2.10
	24	26.8	26.1	25.4	24.6	23.7	22.8	21.8	20.6	19.4	17.9	16.3	1.38	1.81

TABLE 185

Process Times (B) at Retort Temperature of 230°F for Conduction-Heating Foods in 211 x 210 Can

f_h	z	INITIAL FOOD TEMPERATURE (T_{ih})											Equivalent	
		100	110	120	130	140	150	160	170	180	190	200	F_c^{18}	F_s^{18}
	18	75.3	74.4	73.4	72.3	71.1	69.7	68.2	66.4	64.3	61.7	58.4	2.59	2.86
26.54	20	66.0	65.1	64.1	63.0	61.7	60.4	58.9	57.1	55.0	52.4	49.1	1.87	2.14
	22	60.0	59.1	58.1	57.0	55.8	54.4	52.9	51.1	49.0	46.4	43.1	1.42	1.68
	24	55.1	54.2	53.2	52.1	50.9	49.5	48.0	46.2	44.1	41.5	38.2	1.13	1.37
	18	77.6	76.7	75.6	74.4	73.2	71.7	70.1	68.2	66.0	63.3	59.8	2.59	2.86
28.10	20	68.5	67.5	66.5	65.3	64.0	62.6	60.9	59.1	56.8	54.1	50.6	1.87	2.14
	22	62.2	61.3	60.2	59.0	57.8	56.3	54.7	52.8	50.6	47.9	44.4	1.42	1.68
	24	57.1	56.1	55.0	53.8	52.6	51.1	49.5	47.6	45.4	42.7	39.2	1.13	1.37
	18	79.9	78.9	77.8	76.5	75.2	73.7	72.0	70.0	67.6	64.7	61.0	2.59	2.86
29.66	20	70.9	69.9	68.8	67.5	66.2	64.7	62.9	61.0	58.6	55.7	52.0	1.86	2.14
	22	64.4	63.4	62.3	61.0	59.7	58.2	56.4	54.4	52.1	49.2	45.5	1.42	1.68
	24	58.9	57.9	56.8	55.5	54.2	52.7	50.9	49.0	46.6	43.7	40.0	1.12	1.37
	18	82.3	81.2	80.0	78.7	77.3	75.7	73.9	71.8	69.3	66.3	62.4	2.58	2.86
31.22	20	73.3	72.2	71.0	69.7	68.3	66.7	64.9	62.8	60.3	57.3	53.4	1.86	2.14
	22	66.5	65.4	64.2	62.9	61.5	59.9	58.1	56.0	53.5	50.5	46.6	1.42	1.68
	24	60.7	59.6	58.5	57.2	55.7	54.1	52.3	50.2	47.8	44.7	40.8	1.09	1.35
	18	84.5	83.4	82.1	80.8	79.3	77.6	75.7	73.5	70.9	67.7	63.6	2.58	2.85
32.78	20	75.6	74.5	73.3	71.9	70.4	68.7	66.8	64.6	62.0	58.9	54.8	1.86	2.14
	22	68.5	67.4	66.1	64.8	63.3	61.6	59.7	57.5	54.9	51.7	47.6	1.42	1.68
	24	62.5	61.3	60.1	58.7	57.2	55.5	53.6	51.4	48.9	45.7	41.6	1.07	1.33

TABLE 186

Process Times (B) at Retort Temperature of 240°F for Conduction-Heating Foods in 211 x 210 Can

f_h	z	INITIAL FOOD TEMPERATURE (T_{ih})											Equivalent	
		100	110	120	130	140	150	160	170	180	190	200	F_c^{18}	F_s^{18}
	18	48.3	47.5	46.6	45.6	44.5	43.3	41.9	40.4	38.6	36.5	33.9	2.50	2.86
26.54	20	45.4	44.5	43.6	42.6	41.5	40.3	38.9	37.4	35.6	33.5	31.0	1.95	2.29
	22	42.9	42.0	41.1	40.1	39.0	37.8	36.4	34.9	33.1	31.0	28.4	1.52	1.87
	24	40.7	39.9	38.9	37.9	36.8	35.6	34.3	32.7	31.0	28.9	26.3	1.21	1.54
	18	50.4	49.5	48.5	47.5	46.3	45.0	43.6	42.0	40.1	37.9	35.1	2.50	2.86
28.10	20	47.3	46.4	45.5	44.4	43.2	41.9	40.5	38.9	37.0	34.8	32.0	1.94	2.29
	22	44.6	43.7	42.8	41.7	40.5	39.3	37.8	36.2	34.3	32.1	29.4	1.50	1.85
	24	42.5	41.6	40.6	39.5	38.4	37.1	35.6	34.0	32.1	29.9	27.2	1.19	1.53
	18	52.5	51.6	50.5	49.4	48.2	46.8	45.3	43.6	41.6	39.3	36.4	2.50	2.86
29.66	20	49.2	48.3	47.3	46.1	44.9	43.5	42.0	40.3	38.3	36.0	33.1	1.92	2.27
	22	46.5	45.5	44.5	43.4	42.1	40.8	39.3	37.5	35.6	33.2	30.3	1.49	1.83
	24	44.2	43.3	42.2	41.1	39.9	38.5	37.0	35.3	33.3	30.9	28.1	1.18	1.52
	18	54.6	53.6	52.5	51.3	50.0	48.6	47.0	45.2	43.1	40.6	37.6	2.49	2.86
31.22	20	51.1	50.1	49.0	47.8	46.5	45.1	43.5	41.7	39.6	37.1	34.1	1.90	2.26
	22	48.3	47.3	46.2	45.0	43.7	42.3	40.7	38.9	36.8	34.3	31.3	1.47	1.82
	24	45.9	44.9	43.8	42.6	41.4	39.9	38.3	36.5	34.4	32.0	28.9	1.16	1.50
	18	56.6	55.5	54.4	53.1	51.8	50.3	48.6	46.7	44.5	41.9	38.7	2.49	2.86
32.78	20	53.0	52.0	50.8	49.6	48.2	46.7	45.0	43.1	40.9	38.4	35.2	1.89	2.25
	22	50.1	49.0	47.9	46.6	45.3	43.8	42.1	40.2	38.0	35.4	32.2	1.46	1.81
	24	47.6	46.5	45.4	44.2	42.8	41.3	39.6	37.7	35.5	32.9	29.8	1.15	1.49

TABLE 187

Process Times (B) at Retort Temperature of 250°F for Conduction-Heating Foods in 211 x 210 Can

f_h	z	INITIAL FOOD TEMPERATURE (T_{ih})											Equivalent	
		100	110	120	130	140	150	160	170	180	190	200	F_c^{18}	F_s^{18}
	18	37.0	36.2	35.4	34.5	33.5	32.4	31.2	29.8	28.3	26.5	24.4	2.43	2.86
26.54	20	35.7	34.9	34.0	33.1	32.1	31.0	29.8	28.4	26.9	25.1	23.0	1.97	2.38
	22	34.4	33.6	32.8	31.9	30.9	29.8	28.5	27.2	25.7	23.9	21.8	1.62	2.02
	24	33.3	32.5	31.6	30.7	29.7	28.6	27.4	26.0	24.5	22.7	20.6	1.32	1.72
	18	38.8	38.0	37.1	36.1	35.0	33.9	32.6	31.1	29.5	27.6	25.4	2.43	2.86
28.10	20	37.4	36.5	35.6	34.6	33.6	32.4	31.1	29.7	28.1	26.2	23.9	1.97	2.39
	22	36.1	35.2	34.3	33.3	32.3	31.1	29.8	28.4	26.8	24.9	22.7	1.61	2.01
	24	34.8	34.0	33.1	32.1	31.1	29.9	28.6	27.2	25.5	23.7	21.4	1.30	1.70
	18	40.6	39.7	38.7	37.7	36.6	35.3	34.0	32.5	30.8	28.8	26.4	2.43	2.86
29.66	20	39.0	38.1	37.2	36.2	35.0	33.8	32.5	30.9	29.2	27.2	24.9	1.97	2.39
	22	37.7	36.8	35.8	34.8	33.7	32.5	31.1	29.6	27.9	25.9	23.5	1.59	2.00
	24	36.4	35.5	34.5	33.5	32.4	31.2	29.8	28.3	26.6	24.6	22.2	1.29	1.68
	18	42.3	41.4	40.4	39.3	38.1	36.8	35.4	33.8	32.0	29.9	27.4	2.42	2.86
31.22	20	40.7	39.8	38.8	37.7	36.5	35.2	33.8	32.2	30.4	28.3	25.8	1.95	2.38
	22	39.3	38.3	37.3	36.3	35.1	33.8	32.4	30.8	28.9	26.9	24.4	1.58	2.00
	24	37.9	37.0	36.0	34.9	33.7	32.4	31.0	29.4	27.6	25.5	23.0	1.27	1.67
	18	44.0	43.0	42.0	40.8	39.6	38.2	36.7	35.1	33.2	31.0	28.4	2.42	2.86
32.78	20	42.3	41.4	40.3	39.2	37.9	36.6	35.1	33.4	31.5	29.3	26.7	1.94	2.36
	22	40.9	39.9	38.8	37.7	36.4	35.1	33.6	31.9	30.0	27.8	25.2	1.57	1.98
	24	39.4	38.4	37.4	36.2	35.0	33.6	32.1	30.5	28.6	26.4	23.8	1.25	1.65

TABLE 188

Process Times (B) at Retort Temperature of 260°F for Conduction-Heating Foods in 211 x 210 Can

f_h	z	INITIAL FOOD TEMPERATURE (T_{ih})											Equivalent	
		100	110	120	130	140	150	160	170	180	190	200	F_c^{18}	F_s^{18}
	18	30.7	30.0	29.2	28.3	27.4	26.4	25.3	24.1	22.7	21.2	19.4	2.39	2.86
26.54	20	30.0	29.2	28.4	27.6	26.7	25.6	24.6	23.3	22.0	20.4	18.7	1.99	2.45
	22	29.2	28.5	27.7	26.8	25.9	24.9	23.8	22.6	21.2	19.7	17.9	1.65	2.10
	24	28.5	27.8	27.0	26.1	25.2	24.2	23.1	21.9	20.5	19.0	17.2	1.37	1.80
	18	32.3	31.5	30.6	29.7	28.8	27.7	26.5	25.2	23.8	22.2	20.3	2.38	2.86
28.10	20	31.5	30.7	29.8	28.9	27.9	26.9	25.7	24.4	23.0	21.4	19.5	1.98	2.44
	22	30.6	29.9	29.0	28.1	27.1	26.1	24.9	23.6	22.2	20.6	18.7	1.63	2.07
	24	29.9	29.1	28.3	27.4	26.4	25.3	24.2	22.9	21.4	19.8	17.9	1.34	1.78
	18	33.8	33.0	32.1	31.1	30.1	29.0	27.8	26.4	24.9	23.2	21.2	2.38	2.86
29.66	20	32.9	32.1	31.2	30.3	29.2	28.1	26.9	25.5	24.0	22.3	20.3	1.97	2.43
	22	32.1	31.2	30.3	29.4	28.4	27.2	26.0	24.7	23.1	21.4	19.4	1.60	2.05
	24	31.3	30.4	29.6	28.6	27.6	26.5	25.2	23.9	22.3	20.6	18.6	1.32	1.76
	18	35.3	34.5	33.5	32.5	31.4	30.3	29.0	27.5	25.9	24.1	22.0	2.38	2.86
31.22	20	34.4	33.5	32.6	31.6	30.5	29.3	28.0	26.6	25.0	23.2	21.1	1.95	2.42
	22	33.5	32.6	31.7	30.7	29.6	28.4	27.1	25.7	24.1	22.3	20.2	1.58	2.03
	24	32.6	31.8	30.8	29.8	28.7	27.6	26.3	24.8	23.2	21.4	19.3	1.30	1.74
	18	36.8	35.9	34.9	33.9	32.8	31.5	30.2	28.7	27.0	25.1	22.9	2.38	2.86
32.78	20	35.9	35.0	34.0	32.9	31.8	30.5	29.2	27.7	26.0	24.1	21.9	1.94	2.41
	22	34.9	34.0	33.0	31.9	30.8	29.5	28.2	26.7	25.0	23.1	20.9	1.56	2.02
	24	34.0	33.1	32.1	31.0	29.9	28.7	27.3	25.8	24.1	22.2	20.0	1.28	1.72

TABLE 189

Process Times (B) at Retort Temperature of 230°F for Conduction-Heating Foods in 211 x 212 Can

f_h	z	INITIAL FOOD TEMPERATURE (T_{ih})											Equivalent	
		100	110	120	130	140	150	160	170	180	190	200	F_c^{18}	F_s^{18}
	18	76.9	75.9	74.9	73.7	72.5	71.1	69.5	67.6	65.4	62.8	59.3	2.60	2.86
27.54	20	67.7	66.7	65.7	64.5	63.3	61.8	60.3	58.4	56.2	53.6	50.1	1.88	2.15
	22	61.5	60.6	59.5	58.4	57.1	55.7	54.1	52.3	50.1	47.4	44.0	1.42	1.68
	24	56.4	55.5	54.4	53.3	52.0	50.6	49.0	47.2	45.0	42.3	38.9	1.13	1.37
	18	79.3	78.3	77.2	76.0	74.6	73.1	71.4	69.5	67.2	64.4	60.7	2.59	2.86
29.16	20	70.2	69.2	68.1	66.9	65.6	64.1	62.4	60.4	58.1	55.3	51.6	1.87	2.15
	22	63.8	62.8	61.7	60.4	59.1	57.6	54.0	54.0	51.7	48.8	45.2	1.42	1.68
	24	58.4	57.4	56.3	55.1	53.7	52.2	50.5	48.6	46.3	43.4	39.8	1.13	1.37
	18	81.7	80.6	79.4	78.2	76.7	75.2	73.4	71.3	68.9	65.9	62.1	2.59	2.86
30.78	20	72.7	71.6	70.4	69.2	67.8	66.2	64.4	62.3	59.9	56.9	53.1	1.86	2.14
	22	66.0	64.9	63.7	62.5	61.0	59.5	57.7	55.6	53.2	50.2	46.4	1.42	1.68
	24	60.3	59.2	58.0	56.8	55.3	53.8	52.0	49.9	47.5	44.5	40.7	1.11	1.36
	18	84.0	82.9	81.7	80.3	78.9	77.2	75.3	73.2	70.6	67.4	63.4	2.58	2.86
32.40	20	75.1	74.0	72.8	71.4	70.0	68.3	66.4	64.2	61.6	58.5	54.5	1.86	2.14
	22	68.1	67.0	65.7	64.4	62.9	61.3	59.4	57.2	54.6	51.5	47.5	1.42	1.68
	24	62.1	61.0	59.7	58.4	56.9	55.3	53.4	51.2	48.6	45.5	41.5	1.08	1.33
	18	86.5	85.3	84.0	82.6	81.1	79.3	77.4	75.1	72.4	69.1	64.8	2.58	2.86
34.02	20	77.5	76.3	75.0	73.6	72.1	70.3	68.4	66.1	63.4	60.1	55.8	1.86	2.14
	22	70.1	69.0	67.7	66.3	64.7	63.0	61.0	58.7	56.0	52.7	48.5	1.42	1.68
	24	63.8	62.6	61.4	59.9	58.4	56.7	54.7	52.4	49.7	46.4	42.2	1.05	1.31

TABLE 190

Process Times (B) at Retort Temperature of 240°F for Conduction-Heating Foods in 211 x 212 Can

f_h	z	INITIAL FOOD TEMPERATURE (T_{ih})											Equivalent	
		100	110	120	130	140	150	160	170	180	190	200	F_c^{18}	F_s^{18}
	18	49.7	48.8	47.8	46.8	45.7	44.4	43.0	41.4	39.6	37.4	34.7	2.51	2.86
27.54	20	46.7	45.8	44.8	43.8	42.6	41.4	40.0	38.4	36.5	34.4	31.7	1.95	2.29
	22	44.0	43.2	42.2	41.2	40.0	38.8	37.3	35.7	33.9	31.7	29.1	1.51	1.86
	24	41.9	41.0	40.0	39.0	37.9	36.6	35.2	33.6	31.7	29.6	26.9	1.20	1.54
	18	51.9	50.9	49.9	48.8	47.6	46.3	44.8	43.1	41.1	38.8	36.0	2.50	2.86
29.16	20	48.7	47.7	46.7	45.6	44.4	43.1	41.6	39.9	37.9	35.6	32.8	1.93	2.28
	22	45.9	45.0	44.0	42.9	41.6	40.3	38.8	37.1	35.2	32.9	30.0	1.49	1.84
	24	43.7	42.7	41.7	40.6	39.4	38.1	36.6	34.9	33.0	30.6	27.8	1.19	1.53
	18	54.0	53.0	52.0	50.8	49.5	48.1	46.5	44.8	42.7	40.3	37.3	2.50	2.86
30.78	20	50.6	49.6	48.6	47.4	46.1	44.7	43.1	41.3	39.3	36.8	33.9	1.91	2.27
	22	47.8	46.8	45.7	44.6	43.3	41.9	40.3	38.5	36.5	34.0	31.0	1.48	1.83
	24	45.5	44.5	43.4	42.2	41.0	39.6	38.0	36.2	34.1	31.7	28.7	1.17	1.51
	18	56.1	55.1	54.0	52.7	51.4	49.9	48.2	46.4	44.2	41.6	38.5	2.50	2.86
32.40	20	52.6	51.5	50.4	49.2	47.8	46.4	44.7	42.8	40.6	38.1	34.9	1.90	2.26
	22	49.7	48.6	47.5	46.3	44.9	43.4	41.8	39.9	37.7	35.2	32.0	1.47	1.82
	24	47.2	46.2	45.0	43.8	42.5	41.0	39.3	37.5	35.3	32.7	29.6	1.15	1.50
	18	58.2	57.1	55.9	54.6	53.2	51.7	49.9	47.9	45.7	43.0	39.7	2.49	2.86
34.02	20	54.5	53.4	52.3	51.0	49.6	48.0	46.3	44.3	42.0	39.3	36.0	1.89	2.26
	22	51.5	50.4	49.2	47.9	46.5	45.0	43.2	41.2	39.0	36.3	33.0	1.45	1.81
	24	49.0	47.9	46.7	45.4	44.0	42.5	40.7	38.7	36.5	33.8	30.5	1.14	1.49

TABLE 191

Process Times (B) at Retort Temperature of 250°F for Conduction-Heating Foods in 211 x 212 Can

f_h	z	INITIAL FOOD TEMPERATURE (T_{ih})											Equivalent	
		100	110	120	130	140	150	160	170	180	190	200	F_c^{18}	F_s^{18}
27.54	18	38.2	37.4	36.5	35.5	34.5	33.4	32.1	30.7	29.1	27.2	25.1	2.43	2.86
	20	36.8	35.9	35.1	34.1	33.1	31.9	30.7	29.2	27.6	25.8	23.6	1.97	2.39
	22	35.5	34.7	33.8	32.8	31.8	30.7	29.4	28.0	26.4	24.5	22.4	1.61	2.02
	24	34.3	33.5	32.6	31.6	30.6	29.5	28.2	26.8	25.2	23.3	21.2	1.31	1.71
29.16	18	40.0	39.2	38.2	37.2	36.1	34.9	33.6	32.1	30.4	28.4	26.1	2.43	2.86
	20	38.5	37.6	36.7	35.7	34.6	33.4	32.0	30.6	28.9	26.9	24.6	1.97	2.39
	22	37.2	36.3	35.4	34.4	33.3	32.1	30.7	29.2	27.5	25.6	23.3	1.60	2.01
	24	35.9	35.0	34.1	33.1	32.0	30.8	29.4	28.0	26.3	24.3	22.0	1.29	1.69
30.78	18	41.8	40.9	39.9	38.8	37.7	36.4	35.0	33.4	31.6	29.6	27.1	2.43	2.86
	20	40.2	39.3	38.3	37.3	36.1	34.8	33.4	31.8	30.1	28.0	25.6	1.96	2.38
	22	38.9	37.9	36.9	35.9	34.7	33.4	32.0	30.4	28.7	26.6	24.2	1.59	2.00
	24	37.5	36.6	35.6	34.5	33.4	32.1	30.7	29.1	27.3	25.3	22.8	1.28	1.68
32.40	18	43.6	42.6	41.6	40.5	39.3	37.9	36.4	34.8	32.9	30.7	28.2	2.43	2.86
	20	42.0	41.0	39.9	38.8	37.6	36.2	34.8	33.1	31.2	29.1	26.5	1.95	2.37
	22	40.5	39.5	38.5	37.4	36.1	34.8	33.3	31.6	29.8	27.6	25.0	1.58	1.99
	24	39.1	38.1	37.1	35.9	34.7	33.4	31.9	30.2	28.3	26.2	23.6	1.26	1.66
34.02	18	45.4	44.4	43.3	42.1	40.8	39.4	37.8	36.1	34.1	31.8	29.1	2.43	2.86
	20	43.6	42.6	41.5	40.3	39.1	37.7	36.1	34.4	32.4	30.1	27.4	1.94	2.36
	22	42.1	41.1	40.0	38.8	37.5	36.1	34.6	32.8	30.9	28.6	25.9	1.56	1.97
	24	40.6	39.6	38.5	37.3	36.0	34.6	33.1	31.3	29.4	27.1	24.4	1.24	1.64

TABLE 192

Process Times (B) at Retort Temperature of 260°F for Conduction-Heating Foods in 211 x 212 Can

f_h	z	INITIAL FOOD TEMPERATURE (T_{ih})											Equivalent	
		100	110	120	130	140	150	160	170	180	190	200	F_c^{18}	F_s^{18}
	18	31.7	31.0	30.1	29.2	28.3	27.2	26.1	24.8	23.4	21.8	20.0	2.39	2.86
27.54	20	30.9	30.2	29.3	28.5	27.5	26.5	25.3	24.1	22.6	21.1	19.2	1.99	2.45
	22	30.2	29.4	28.6	27.7	26.7	25.7	24.5	23.3	21.9	20.3	18.4	1.64	2.09
	24	29.4	28.6	27.8	26.9	26.0	24.9	23.8	22.5	21.1	19.5	17.7	1.35	1.79
	18	33.3	32.5	31.6	30.7	29.7	28.6	27.4	26.0	24.5	22.9	20.9	2.39	2.86
29.16	20	32.5	31.7	30.8	29.8	28.8	27.7	26.5	25.2	23.7	22.0	20.1	1.97	2.44
	22	31.6	30.8	29.9	29.0	28.0	26.9	25.7	24.3	22.8	21.2	19.2	1.61	2.06
	24	30.8	30.0	29.2	28.2	27.2	26.1	24.9	23.6	22.1	20.4	18.4	1.33	1.77
	18	34.9	34.1	33.1	32.1	31.1	29.9	28.6	27.2	25.6	23.9	21.8	2.39	2.86
30.78	20	34.0	33.1	32.2	31.2	30.2	29.0	27.7	26.3	24.7	23.0	20.9	1.96	2.42
	22	33.1	32.2	31.3	30.3	29.2	28.1	26.8	25.4	23.8	22.0	20.0	1.59	2.04
	24	32.3	31.4	30.5	29.5	28.4	27.3	26.0	24.6	23.0	21.2	19.2	1.31	1.75
	18	36.5	35.6	34.6	33.6	32.4	31.2	29.9	28.4	26.7	24.9	22.7	2.39	2.86
32.40	20	35.5	34.6	33.6	32.6	31.5	30.3	28.9	27.4	25.8	23.9	21.7	1.95	2.41
	22	34.6	33.6	32.7	31.6	30.5	29.3	27.9	26.5	24.8	22.9	20.8	1.57	2.02
	24	33.7	32.8	31.8	30.8	29.6	28.4	27.1	25.6	23.9	22.1	19.9	1.29	1.73
	18	38.1	37.1	36.1	35.0	33.8	32.5	31.1	29.6	27.8	25.9	23.6	2.38	2.86
34.02	20	37.0	36.1	35.1	34.0	32.8	31.5	30.1	28.5	26.8	24.8	22.5	1.94	2.40
	22	36.0	35.0	34.0	32.9	31.8	30.5	29.1	27.5	25.8	23.8	21.5	1.55	2.01
	24	35.1	34.1	33.1	32.0	30.8	29.6	28.1	26.6	24.9	22.9	20.6	1.27	1.71

TABLE 193

Process Times (B) at Retort Temperature of 230°F for Conduction-Heating Foods in 211 x 214 Can

f_h	z	INITIAL FOOD TEMPERATURE (T_{ih}) 100	110	120	130	140	150	160	170	180	190	200	Equivalent F_c^{18}	F_s^{18}
28.46	18	78.3	77.3	76.3	75.1	73.8	72.3	70.7	68.8	66.5	63.7	60.2	2.60	2.86
	20	69.2	68.2	67.1	65.9	64.6	63.2	61.5	59.6	57.3	54.6	51.0	1.87	2.15
	22	62.8	61.8	60.8	59.6	58.3	56.8	55.2	53.3	51.0	48.3	44.7	1.43	1.69
	24	57.6	56.6	55.5	54.3	53.0	51.6	49.9	48.0	45.8	43.0	39.4	1.14	1.38
30.14	18	80.7	79.7	78.6	77.3	75.9	74.4	72.6	70.6	68.2	65.3	61.5	2.59	2.86
	20	71.7	70.7	69.6	68.3	66.9	65.4	63.6	61.6	59.2	56.3	52.5	1.87	2.15
	22	65.1	64.1	63.0	61.7	60.3	58.8	57.0	55.0	52.6	49.7	45.9	1.43	1.69
	24	59.6	58.5	57.4	56.1	54.7	53.2	51.5	49.4	47.1	44.1	40.4	1.12	1.37
31.81	18	83.3	82.2	81.0	79.6	78.2	76.6	74.7	72.6	70.1	67.0	63.0	2.59	2.87
	20	74.3	73.2	72.0	70.7	69.2	67.6	65.7	63.6	61.1	58.0	54.0	1.87	2.15
	22	67.4	66.3	65.1	63.7	62.3	60.7	58.8	56.7	54.2	51.1	47.1	1.43	1.69
	24	61.5	60.4	59.2	57.8	56.4	54.8	52.9	50.8	48.3	45.2	41.2	1.09	1.34
33.49	18	85.6	84.5	83.2	81.8	80.3	78.6	76.6	74.4	71.8	68.5	64.3	2.58	2.86
	20	76.8	75.6	74.3	73.0	71.4	69.7	67.8	65.5	62.9	59.6	55.5	1.86	2.15
	22	69.5	68.4	67.1	65.7	64.2	62.5	60.5	58.3	55.6	52.4	48.2	1.43	1.69
	24	63.3	62.2	60.9	59.5	58.0	56.3	54.3	52.1	49.4	46.2	42.0	1.06	1.32
35.16	18	88.5	87.3	85.9	84.5	82.9	81.1	79.0	76.7	73.9	70.5	66.1	2.58	2.87
	20	79.2	78.0	76.7	75.2	73.6	71.8	69.8	67.4	64.6	61.2	56.8	1.86	2.15
	22	71.6	70.4	69.1	67.6	66.0	64.2	62.1	59.8	57.0	53.6	49.2	1.43	1.69
	24	65.2	63.9	62.6	61.1	59.5	57.7	55.7	53.3	50.6	47.2	42.8	1.04	1.31

TABLE 194

Process Times (B) at Retort Temperature of 240°F for Conduction-Heating Foods in 211 x 214 Can

f_h	z	INITIAL FOOD TEMPERATURE (T_{ih})											Equivalent	
		100	110	120	130	140	150	160	170	180	190	200	F_c^{18}	F_s^{18}
28.46	18	51.0	50.0	49.1	48.0	46.8	45.5	44.0	42.4	40.5	38.2	35.5	2.51	2.86
	20	47.8	46.9	45.9	44.8	43.7	42.4	40.9	39.3	37.4	35.1	32.3	1.94	2.29
	22	45.1	44.2	43.2	42.1	40.9	39.6	38.2	36.5	34.6	32.4	29.6	1.50	1.85
	24	42.9	42.0	41.0	39.9	38.8	37.5	36.0	34.4	32.5	30.2	27.4	1.19	1.53
30.14	18	53.2	52.2	51.2	50.0	48.8	47.4	45.9	44.1	42.1	39.7	36.8	2.51	2.87
	20	49.9	48.9	47.8	46.7	45.5	44.1	42.5	40.8	38.8	36.4	33.5	1.92	2.28
	22	47.1	46.1	45.1	43.9	42.7	41.3	39.7	38.0	36.0	33.6	30.7	1.49	1.84
	24	44.8	43.8	42.8	41.6	40.4	39.0	37.5	35.7	33.7	31.3	28.4	1.18	1.52
31.81	18	55.4	54.4	53.3	52.1	50.7	49.3	47.7	45.8	43.7	41.2	38.1	2.50	2.87
	20	51.9	50.8	49.7	48.5	47.2	45.8	44.1	42.3	40.2	37.6	34.6	1.90	2.26
	22	49.0	48.0	46.9	45.7	44.4	42.9	41.3	39.4	37.3	34.8	31.7	1.48	1.83
	24	46.6	45.6	44.5	43.3	41.9	40.5	38.9	37.0	34.9	32.4	29.3	1.16	1.50
33.49	18	57.5	56.5	55.3	54.0	52.6	51.1	49.4	47.5	45.2	42.6	39.3	2.50	2.87
	20	53.9	52.8	51.7	50.4	49.0	47.5	45.8	43.8	41.6	38.9	35.7	1.90	2.26
	22	50.9	49.8	48.7	47.4	46.0	44.5	42.8	40.8	38.6	35.9	32.7	1.46	1.81
	24	48.4	47.3	46.2	44.9	43.5	42.0	40.3	38.3	36.1	33.4	30.2	1.15	1.49
35.16	18	59.6	58.5	57.3	56.0	54.5	52.9	51.1	49.1	46.7	43.9	40.5	2.50	2.87
	20	55.9	54-8	53.6	52.3	50.8	49.2	47.4	45.4	43.0	40.2	36.8	1.89	2.25
	22	52.8	51.7	50.4	49.1	47.6	46.0	44.2	42.2	39.8	37.1	33.7	1.44	1.80
	24	50.2	49.1	47.9	46.6	45.1	43.5	41.7	39.7	37.3	34.5	31.1	1.13	1.48

TABLE 195

Process Times (B) at Retort Temperature of 250°F for Conduction-Heating Foods in 211 x 214 Can

f_h	z	INITIAL FOOD TEMPERATURE (T_{ih})											Equivalent	
		100	110	120	130	140	150	160	170	180	190	200	F_c^{18}	F_s^{18}
28.46	18	39.3	38.4	37.5	36.5	35.4	34.2	32.9	31.5	29.8	27.9	25.7	2.44	2.86
	20	37.8	36.9	36.0	35.0	33.9	32.8	31.5	30.0	28.4	26.4	24.2	1.98	2.39
	22	36.5	35.6	34.7	33.7	32.6	31.5	30.2	28.7	27.1	25.1	22.9	1.61	2.02
	24	35.2	34.4	33.5	32.5	31.4	30.2	28.9	27.5	25.8	23.9	21.7	1.31	1.70
30.14	18	41.1	40.2	39.3	38.2	37.1	35.8	34.4	32.9	31.2	29.1	26.7	2.43	2.86
	20	39.6	38.7	37.7	36.7	35.5	34.3	32.9	31.3	29.6	27.6	25.2	1.97	2.39
	22	38.2	37.3	36.3	35.3	34.1	32.9	31.5	30.0	28.2	26.2	23.8	1.60	2.01
	24	36.9	36.0	35.0	34.0	32.8	31.6	30.2	28.7	26.9	24.9	22.5	1.29	1.68
31.81	18	43.0	42.0	41.0	39.9	38.7	37.4	35.9	34.3	32.5	30.3	27.8	2.43	2.86
	20	41.3	40.4	39.4	38.3	37.1	35.7	34.3	32.7	30.8	28.7	26.2	1.96	2.38
	22	39.9	39.0	37.9	36.8	35.6	34.3	32.9	31.2	29.4	27.3	24.7	1.59	2.00
	24	38.5	37.6	36.5	35.4	34.2	32.9	31.5	29.8	28.0	25.9	23.3	1.27	1.67
33.49	18	44.8	43.8	42.7	41.6	40.3	38.9	37.4	35.7	33.7	31.5	28.8	2.43	2.86
	20	43.1	42.1	41.0	39.9	38.6	37.2	35.7	34.0	32.0	29.8	27.1	1.94	2.37
	22	41.6	40.6	39.5	38.3	37.1	35.7	34.2	32.5	30.5	28.3	25.6	1.57	1.98
	24	40.1	39.1	38.0	36.9	35.6	34.2	32.7	31.0	29.0	26.8	24.1	1.25	1.65
35.16	18	46.6	45.6	44.4	43.2	41.9	40.4	38.8	37.0	35.0	32.6	29.8	2.43	2.86
	20	44.8	43.8	42.7	41.4	40.1	38.6	37.0	35.2	33.2	30.8	28.1	1.93	2.36
	22	43.3	42.2	41.1	39.9	38.5	37.1	35.5	33.7	31.6	29.3	26.5	1.55	1.96
	24	41.7	40.7	39.5	38.3	37.0	35.5	33.9	32.1	30.1	27.7	24.9	1.23	1.63

TABLE 196

Process Times (B) at Retort Temperature of 260°F for Conduction-Heating Foods in 211 x 214 Can

f_h	z	INITIAL FOOD TEMPERATURE (T_{ih})											Equivalent	
		100	110	120	130	140	150	160	170	180	190	200	F_c^{18}	F_s^{18}
	18	32.6	31.8	31.0	30.1	29.1	28.0	26.8	25.5	24.1	22.4	20.5	2.39	2.86
28.46	20	31.8	31.0	30.2	29.3	28.3	27.2	26.0	24.7	23.3	21.6	19.7	1.98	2.45
	22	31.0	30.2	29.4	28.4	27.4	26.4	25.2	23.9	22.4	29.8	18.9	1.63	2.08
	24	30.2	29.4	28.6	27.7	26.7	25.6	24.4	23.1	21.7	20.0	18.1	1.34	1.78
	18	34.3	33.4	32.5	31.6	30.5	29.4	28.1	26.8	25.2	23.5	21.5	2.39	2.86
30.14	20	33.4	32.6	31.7	30.7	29.6	28.5	27.3	25.9	24.3	22.6	20.6	1.97	2.43
	22	32.5	31.7	30.8	29.8	28.8	27.6	26.4	25.0	23.4	21.7	19.7	1.60	2.05
	24	31.7	30.9	30.0	29.0	28.0	26.8	25.6	24.2	22.6	20.9	18.9	1.32	1.76
	18	35.9	35.0	34.1	33.1	32.0	30.8	29.4	28.0	26.4	24.5	22.4	2.39	2.86
31.81	20	35.0	34.1	33.1	32.1	31.0	29.8	28.5	27.0	25.4	23.6	21.4	1.96	2.42
	22	34.0	33.1	32.2	31.2	30.1	28.9	27.5	26.1	24.5	22.6	20.5	1.58	2.03
	24	33.2	32.3	31.3	30.3	29.2	28.0	26.7	25.2	23.6	21.8	19.6	1.30	1.74
	18	37.6	36.6	35.6	34.5	33.4	32.1	30.7	29.2	27.5	25.5	23.3	2.39	2.86
33.49	20	36.5	35.6	34.6	33.5	32.4	31.1	29.7	28.2	26.5	24.5	22.3	1.95	2.41
	22	35.5	34.6	33.6	32.5	31.3	30.1	28.7	27.2	25.5	23.5	21.3	1.56	2.02
	24	34.6	33.7	32.7	31.6	30.5	29.2	27.8	26.3	24.6	22.6	20.4	1.28	1.72
	18	39.2	38.2	37.1	36.0	34.8	33.5	32.0	30.4	28.6	26.6	24.2	2.39	2.87
35.16	20	38.1	37.1	36.1	34.9	33.7	32.4	30.9	29.3	27.5	25.5	23.1	1.93	2.40
	22	37.0	36.0	35.0	33.9	32.6	31.3	29.8	28.2	26.4	24.4	22.0	1.55	2.00
	24	36.1	35.1	34.0	32.9	31.7	30.4	28.9	27.3	25.5	23.5	21.1	1.26	1.70

TABLE 197

Process Times (B) at Retort Temperature of 230°F for Conduction-Heating Foods in 211 x 300 Can

f_h	z	INITIAL FOOD TEMPERATURE (T_{ih})											Equivalent	
		100	110	120	130	140	150	160	170	180	190	200	F_c^{18}	F_s^{18}
29.31	18	79.6	78.6	77.5	76.3	74.9	73.4	71.7	69.8	67.4	64.6	60.9	2.60	2.87
	20	70.5	69.5	68.4	67.2	65.8	64.3	62.6	60.7	58.3	55.5	51.8	1.87	2.15
	22	64.0	63.0	61.9	60.7	59.4	57.9	56.2	54.2	51.9	49.0	45.4	1.43	1.69
	24	58.6	57.6	56.5	55.3	53.9	52.4	50.7	48.8	46.5	43.6	40.0	1.14	1.38
31.03	18	82.2	81.1	79.9	78.6	77.2	75.6	73.8	71.7	69.3	66.3	62.4	2.60	2.87
	20	73.1	72.1	70.9	69.6	68.2	66.6	64.8	62.7	60.3	57.3	53.4	1.87	2.15
	22	66.4	65.3	64.1	62.8	61.4	59.8	58.0	56.0	53.5	50.5	46.6	1.43	1.69
	24	60.6	59.6	58.4	57.1	55.7	54.1	52.3	50.2	47.8	44.7	40.9	1.11	1.36
32.76	18	84.7	83.5	82.3	80.9	79.4	77.7	75.8	73.7	71.1	67.9	63.8	2.59	2.87
	20	75.7	74.6	73.4	72.0	70.5	68.8	66.9	64.7	62.1	59.0	54.9	1.87	2.15
	22	68.6	67.5	66.3	64.9	63.4	61.7	59.8	57.6	55.0	51.9	47.8	1.43	1.69
	24	62.6	61.4	60.2	58.8	57.3	55.7	53.8	51.6	49.0	45.8	41.7	1.08	1.34
34.48	18	87.4	86.2	84.9	83.4	81.9	80.1	78.1	75.8	73.1	69.7	65.4	2.58	2.87
	20	78.3	77.1	75.8	74.3	72.8	71.0	69.0	66.7	64.0	60.6	56.3	1.87	2.15
	22	70.8	69.6	68.3	66.9	65.3	63.5	61.5	59.2	56.5	53.2	48.8	1.43	1.69
	24	64.4	63.2	61.9	60.5	58.9	57.1	55.1	52.8	50.1	46.7	42.4	1.05	1.31
36.20	18	90.2	89.0	87.6	86.1	84.5	82.6	80.5	78.1	75.2	71.7	67.2	2.58	2.87
	20	80.7	79.5	78.1	76.6	75.0	73.1	71.0	68.6	65.7	62.2	57.7	1.87	2.15
	22	72.9	71.7	70.3	68.8	67.1	65.3	63.2	60.8	57.9	54.4	49.9	1.43	1.69
	24	66.5	65.3	63.9	62.4	60.7	58.9	56.8	54.4	51.5	48.0	43.5	1.04	1.31

TABLE 198

Process Times (B) at Retort Temperature of 240°F for Conduction-Heating Foods in 211 x 300 Can

f_h	z	INITIAL FOOD TEMPERATURE (T_{ih})											Equivalent	
		100	110	120	130	140	150	160	170	180	190	200	F_c^{18}	F_s^{18}
	18	52.1	51.2	50.2	49.0	47.8	46.5	45.0	43.3	41.3	39.0	36.2	2.51	2.87
29.31	20	48.9	47.9	46.9	45.8	44.6	43.3	41.8	40.1	38.1	35.8	32.9	1.94	2.29
	22	46.1	45.2	44.2	43.0	41.8	40.5	39.0	37.3	35.3	33.0	30.2	1.50	1.84
	24	43.9	42.9	41.9	40.8	39.6	38.3	36.8	35.1	33.1	30.8	27.9	1.19	1.53
	18	54.4	53.4	52.3	51.1	49.9	48.4	46.8	45.0	43.0	40.5	37.5	2.51	2.87
31.03	20	51.0	50.0	48.9	47.7	46.4	45.0	43.4	41.6	39.5	37.1	34.1	1.91	2.27
	22	48.1	47.1	46.0	44.9	43.6	42.2	40.6	38.8	36.7	34.2	31.2	1.48	1.83
	24	45.8	44.8	43.7	42.5	41.2	39.8	38.2	36.4	34.4	31.9	28.9	1.17	1.51
	18	56.6	55.6	54.4	53.2	51.8	50.3	48.7	46.8	44.6	42.0	38.8	2.50	2.87
32.76	20	53.0	52.0	50.9	49.6	48.3	46.8	45.1	43.2	41.0	38.4	35.2	1.90	2.26
	22	50.1	49.0	47.9	46.7	45.3	43.8	42.1	40.2	38.0	35.5	32.3	1.47	1.82
	24	47.6	46.6	45.4	44.2	42.8	41.4	39.7	37.8	35.6	33.0	29.8	1.15	1.50
	18	58.8	57.7	56.5	55.2	53.8	52.2	50.4	48.4	46.1	43.4	40.1	2.50	2.87
34.48	20	55.1	54.0	52.8	51.5	50.1	48.5	46.8	44.8	42.5	39.7	36.4	1.90	2.26
	22	52.0	50.9	49.7	48.4	47.0	45.4	43.7	41.7	39.4	36.6	33.3	1.45	1.81
	24	49.5	48.4	47.2	45.9	44.5	42.9	41.1	39.1	36.8	34.1	30.8	1.14	1.49
	18	61.0	59.8	58.6	57.2	55.7	54.0	52.2	50.1	47.7	44.8	41.3	2.50	2.87
36.20	20	57.2	56.0	54.8	53.4	51.9	50.3	48.4	46.3	43.9	41.0	37.5	1.89	2.25
	22	54.0	52.8	51.6	50.2	48.7	47.0	45.2	43.1	40.7	37.8	34.3	1.44	1.80
	24	51.4	50.2	48.9	47.6	46.1	44.4	42.6	40.5	38.1	35.2	31.7	1.13	1.48

TABLE 199

Process Times (B) at Retort Temperature of 250°F for Conduction-Heating Foods in 211 x 300 Can

f_h	z	INITIAL FOOD TEMPERATURE (T_{ih})											Equivalent	
		100	110	120	130	140	150	160	170	180	190	200	F_c^{18}	F_s^{18}
29.31	18	40.2	39.3	38.4	37.4	36.3	35.1	33.7	32.2	30.5	28.6	26.2	2.44	2.87
	20	38.7	37.8	36.9	35.9	34.7	33.5	32.2	30.7	29.0	27.0	24.7	1.98	2.40
	22	37.4	36.5	35.5	34.5	33.4	32.2	30.9	29.4	27.7	25.7	23.4	1.61	2.02
	24	36.1	35.2	34.3	33.2	32.1	30.9	29.6	28.1	26.4	24.4	22.1	1.30	1.70
31.03	18	42.1	41.2	40.2	39.1	38.0	36.7	35.2	33.7	31.9	29.8	27.3	2.44	2.87
	20	40.5	39.6	38.6	37.5	36.4	35.1	33.7	32.1	30.3	28.2	25.7	1.97	2.39
	22	39.1	38.2	37.2	36.1	34.9	33.7	32.2	30.7	28.9	26.8	24.3	1.60	2.01
	24	37.8	36.8	35.8	34.8	33.6	32.3	30.9	29.3	27.5	25.4	23.0	1.28	1.68
32.76	18	44.0	43.0	42.0	40.9	39.6	38.3	36.8	35.1	33.2	31.0	28.4	2.44	2.87
	20	42.4	41.4	40.3	39.2	37.9	37.9	35.1	33.4	31.5	29.3	26.7	1.95	2.38
	22	40.9	39.9	38.8	37.7	36.5	35.1	33.6	31.9	30.0	27.8	25.2	1.58	1.99
	24	39.4	38.5	37.4	36.3	35.0	33.7	32.2	30.5	28.6	26.4	23.8	1.26	1.66
34.48	18	45.9	44.9	43.8	42.6	41.3	39.8	38.3	36.5	34.5	32.2	29.4	2.43	2.87
	20	44.1	43.1	42.0	40.8	39.5	38.1	36.5	34.7	32.7	30.4	27.7	1.94	2.36
	22	42.6	41.6	40.5	39.3	38.0	36.5	34.9	33.2	31.2	28.9	26.1	1.56	1.97
	24	41.1	40.0	38.9	37.7	36.4	35.0	33.4	31.7	29.7	27.4	24.6	1.24	1.64
36.20	18	47.8	46.7	45.5	44.2	42.9	41.4	39.7	37.9	35.8	33.3	30.5	2.43	2.87
	20	45.9	44.8	43.7	42.4	41.0	39.5	37.9	36.0	33.9	31.5	28.6	1.93	2.35
	22	44.3	43.2	42.1	40.8	39.4	37.9	36.3	34.4	32.3	29.9	27.0	1.54	1.96
	24	42.7	41.6	40.4	39.2	37.8	36.3	34.7	32.8	30.7	28.3	25.4	1.22	1.62

TABLE 200

Process Times (B) at Retort Temperature of 260°F for Conduction-Heating Foods in 211 x 300 Can

f_h	z	INITIAL FOOD TEMPERATURE (T_{ih})											Equivalent	
		100	110	120	130	140	150	160	170	180	190	200	F_c^{18}	F_s^{18}
	18	33.5	32.7	31.8	30.8	29.8	28.7	27.5	26.2	24.7	23.0	21.0	2.40	2.87
29.31	20	32.6	31.8	30.9	30.0	29.0	27.9	26.7	25.3	23.8	22.1	20.1	1.98	2.44
	22	31.8	31.0	30.1	29.1	28.1	27.0	25.8	24.5	23.0	21.3	19.3	1.62	2.07
	24	31.0	30.2	29.3	28.4	27.3	26.2	25.0	23.7	22.2	20.5	18.5	1.33	1.77
	18	35.2	34.3	33.4	32.4	31.3	30.1	28.8	27.4	25.8	24.0	22.0	2.40	2.87
31.03	20	34.3	33.4	32.5	31.5	30.4	29.2	27.9	26.5	24.9	23.1	21.0	1.97	2.43
	22	33.3	32.5	31.5	30.5	29.5	28.3	27.0	25.6	24.0	22.2	20.1	1.60	2.05
	24	32.5	31.6	30.7	29.7	28.6	27.5	26.2	24.8	23.2	21.4	19.3	1.31	1.75
	18	36.9	35.9	35.0	33.9	32.8	31.5	30.2	28.7	27.0	25.1	22.9	2.39	2.87
32.76	20	35.9	35.0	34.0	32.9	31.8	30.5	29.2	27.7	26.0	24.1	21.9	1.96	2.42
	22	34.9	34.0	33.0	31.9	30.8	29.6	28.2	26.7	25.0	23.1	20.9	1.58	2.03
	24	34.0	33.1	32.1	31.1	29.9	28.7	27.3	25.8	24.1	22.3	20.1	1.29	1.73
	18	38.5	37.6	36.5	35.4	34.2	32.9	31.5	29.9	28.1	26.1	23.8	2.39	2.87
34.48	20	37.5	36.5	35.5	34.4	33.2	31.9	30.4	28.9	27.1	25.1	22.8	1.94	2.41
	22	36.4	35.5	34.4	33.3	32.1	30.8	29.4	27.8	26.0	24.0	21.7	1.56	2.01
	24	35.5	34.5	33.5	32.4	31.2	29.9	28.5	26.9	25.1	23.1	20.8	1.27	1.71
	18	40.2	39.2	38.1	36.9	35.7	34.3	32.8	31.1	29.3	27.2	24.8	2.39	2.87
36.20	20	39.1	38.1	37.0	35.8	34.6	33.2	31.7	30.0	28.2	26.1	23.7	1.93	2.40
	22	38.0	36.9	35.9	34.7	33.4	32.1	30.6	28.9	27.1	25.0	22.5	1.54	1.99
	24	37.0	36.0	34.9	33.7	32.5	31.1	29.6	27.9	26.1	24.0	21.6	1.25	1.69

TABLE 201

Process Times (B) at Retort Temperature of 230°F for Conduction-Heating Foods in 211 x 304 Can

f_h	z	INITIAL FOOD TEMPERATURE (T_{ih})											Equivalent	
		100	110	120	130	140	150	160	170	180	190	200	F_c	F_s
	18	81.9	80.8	79.7	78.4	77.0	75.4	73.6	71.6	69.1	66.1	62.3	2.60	2.88
30.79	20	72.8	71.8	70.6	69.3	67.9	66.4	64.6	62.5	60.1	57.1	53.2	1.88	2.16
	22	66.1	65.1	63.9	62.6	61.2	59.6	57.8	55.8	53.3	50.4	46.5	1.43	1.69
	24	60.4	59.4	58.2	56.9	55.5	53.9	52.2	50.1	47.7	44.7	40.8	1.12	1.37
	18	84.5	83.4	82.2	80.8	79.3	77.7	75.8	73.6	71.0	67.9	63.8	2.60	2.88
32.60	20	75.6	74.5	73.2	71.9	70.4	68.7	66.8	64.6	62.1	58.9	54.8	1.87	2.16
	22	68.5	67.4	66.1	64.8	63.3	61.6	59.7	57.6	55.0	51.8	47.7	1.43	1.69
	24	62.5	61.3	60.1	58.8	57.3	55.6	53.7	51.5	48.9	45.8	41.7	1.08	1.34
	18	87.3	86.2	84.9	83.4	81.9	80.1	78.1	75.8	73.1	69.7	65.4	2.59	2.88
34.41	20	78.3	77.1	75.8	74.3	72.8	71.0	69.0	66.7	64.0	60.6	56.3	1.87	2.15
	22	70.8	69.6	68.3	66.9	65.3	63.5	61.6	59.2	56.5	53.2	48.9	1.43	1.69
	24	64.4	63.2	61.9	60.5	58.9	57.2	55.2	52.9	50.1	46.8	42.5	1.05	1.32
	18	90.4	89.1	87.7	86.2	84.6	82.7	80.6	78.2	75.3	71.8	67.3	2.58	2.88
36.22	20	80.9	79.6	78.2	76.7	75.1	73.2	71.1	68.7	65.8	62.3	57.8	1.87	2.15
	22	73.0	71.8	70.4	68.9	67.2	65.4	63.3	60.9	58.0	54.5	50.0	1.43	1.69
	24	66.6	65.3	64.0	62.5	60.8	59.0	56.9	54.4	51.6	48.1	43.5	1.04	1.31
	18	93.3	92.0	90.5	88.9	87.2	85.3	83.1	80.5	77.5	73.8	69.1	2.58	2.88
38.03	20	83.4	82.1	80.6	79.1	77.3	75.4	73.2	70.6	67.6	63.9	59.2	1.87	2.15
	22	75.2	73.9	72.4	70.8	69.1	67.2	64.9	62.4	59.4	55.7	51.0	1.41	1.68
	24	68.9	67.5	66.1	64.5	62.8	60.9	58.6	56.1	53.1	49.4	44.7	1.04	1.31

TABLE 202

Process Times (B) at Retort Temperature of 240°F for Conduction-Heating Foods in 211 x 304 Can

f_h	z	INITIAL FOOD TEMPERATURE (T_{ih})											Equivalent	
		100	110	120	130	140	150	160	170	180	190	200	F_c^{18}	F_s^{18}
30.79	18	54.1	53.1	52.1	50.9	49.6	48.2	46.6	44.8	42.8	40.3	37.4	2.52	2.88
	20	50.7	49.7	48.6	47.5	46.2	44.8	43.2	41.4	39.4	36.9	34.0	1.92	2.28
	22	47.9	46.9	45.8	44.7	43.4	42.0	40.4	38.6	36.6	34.1	31.1	1.49	1.84
	24	45.5	44.6	43.5	42.3	41.0	39.6	38.1	36.3	34.2	31.8	28.8	1.18	1.52
32.60	18	56.5	55.4	54.3	53.1	51.7	50.2	48.5	46.7	44.5	41.9	38.7	2.51	2.88
	20	52.9	51.8	50.7	49.5	48.1	46.6	45.0	43.1	40.9	38.3	35.2	1.91	2.27
	22	50.0	48.9	47.8	46.5	45.2	43.7	42.0	40.2	38.0	35.4	32.2	1.48	1.83
	24	47.5	46.5	45.3	44.1	42.7	41.2	39.6	37.7	35.5	32.9	29.8	1.16	1.50
34.41	18	58.8	57.7	56.5	55.2	53.7	52.2	50.4	48.4	46.1	43.4	40.1	2.51	2.88
	20	55.1	54.0	52.8	51.5	50.1	48.5	46.7	44.7	42.4	39.7	36.4	1.91	2.27
	22	52.0	50.9	49.7	48.4	47.0	45.4	43.6	41.7	39.3	36.6	33.3	1.46	1.81
	24	49.5	48.4	47.2	45.9	44.5	42.9	41.1	39.1	36.8	34.1	30.8	1.15	1.49
36.22	18	61.1	59.9	58.6	57.3	55.8	54.1	52.3	50.2	47.7	44.9	41.3	2.51	2.88
	20	57.3	56.1	54.8	53.5	52.0	50.3	48.5	46.4	43.9	41.1	37.6	1.89	2.26
	22	54.0	52.9	51.6	50.2	48.7	47.1	45.2	43.1	40.7	37.8	34.3	1.45	1.80
	24	51.4	50.3	49.0	47.6	46.1	44.5	42.6	40.5	38.1	35.2	31.7	1.13	1.48
38.03	18	63.4	62.2	60.8	59.4	57.8	56.1	54.1	51.9	49.4	46.4	42.7	2.50	2.88
	20	59.4	58.2	56.9	55.4	53.9	52.1	50.2	48.0	45.4	42.4	38.7	1.88	2.25
	22	56.1	54.9	53.5	52.1	50.5	48.8	46.8	44.6	42.1	39.1	35.4	1.43	1.79
	24	53.4	52.1	50.8	49.4	47.8	46.1	44.1	41.9	39.4	36.3	32.7	1.12	1.47

TABLE 203

Process Times (B) at Retort Temperature of 250°F for Conduction-Heating Foods in 211 x 304 Can

f_h	z	INITIAL FOOD TEMPERATURE (T_{ih}) 100	110	120	130	140	150	160	170	180	190	200	Equivalent F_c^{18}	F_s^{18}
30.79	18	41.9	41.0	40.0	38.9	37.7	36.5	35.1	33.5	31.7	29.6	27.2	2.45	2.88
	20	40.3	39.4	38.4	37.3	36.2	34.9	33.5	31.9	30.1	28.1	25.6	1.98	2.40
	22	38.9	38.0	37.0	35.9	34.8	33.5	32.1	30.5	28.7	26.7	24.2	1.60	2.01
	24	37.6	36.6	35.6	34.6	33.4	32.1	30.7	29.2	27.4	25.3	22.9	1.29	1.69
32.60	18	43.9	42.9	41.9	40.7	39.5	38.1	36.7	35.0	33.1	30.9	28.3	2.44	2.88
	20	42.2	41.2	40.2	39.1	37.8	36.5	35.0	33.3	31.4	29.2	26.7	1.96	2.38
	22	40.7	39.8	38.7	37.6	36.4	35.0	33.5	31.8	30.0	27.8	25.2	1.59	2.00
	24	39.3	38.3	37.3	36.2	34.9	33.6	32.1	30.4	28.5	26.3	23.8	1.27	1.67
34.41	18	45.9	44.8	43.7	42.5	41.2	39.8	38.2	36.5	34.5	32.2	29.4	2.44	2.88
	20	44.1	43.1	42.0	40.8	39.5	38.0	36.5	34.7	32.7	30.4	27.7	1.95	2.37
	22	42.6	41.5	40.4	39.2	37.9	36.5	34.9	33.2	31.2	28.9	26.1	1.57	1.98
	24	41.0	40.0	38.9	37.7	36.4	35.0	33.4	31.6	29.6	27.3	24.6	1.24	1.64
36.22	18	27.8	46.7	45.5	44.3	42.9	41.4	39.8	37.9	35.8	33.4	30.5	2.44	2.88
	20	46.0	44.9	43.7	42.5	41.1	39.6	37.9	36.1	34.0	31.6	28.7	1.93	2.36
	22	44.3	43.3	42.1	40.8	39.5	38.0	36.3	34.5	32.4	29.9	27.1	1.55	1.96
	24	42.7	41.7	40.5	39.2	37.9	36.4	34.7	32.9	30.8	28.3	25.5	1.22	1.62
38.03	18	49.8	48.6	47.4	46.1	44.6	43.1	41.3	39.4	37.2	34.6	31.6	2.44	2.88
	20	47.9	46.7	45.5	44.2	42.7	41.2	39.4	37.5	35.3	32.7	29.7	1.93	2.36
	22	46.2	45.0	43.8	42.5	41.0	39.5	37.7	35.8	33.6	31.0	28.0	1.54	1.95
	24	44.5	43.3	42.1	40.8	39.3	37.8	36.0	34.1	31.9	29.3	26.3	1.20	1.61

TABLE 204

Process Times (B) at Retort Temperature of 260°F for Conduction-Heating Foods in 211 x 304 Can

f_h	z	INITIAL FOOD TEMPERATURE (T_{ih})											Equivalent	
		100	110	120	130	140	150	160	170	180	190	200	F_c^{18}	F_s^{18}
30.79	18	35.0	34.1	33.2	32.2	31.1	29.9	28.7	27.3	25.7	23.9	21.8	2.40	2.88
	20	34.0	33.2	32.3	31.3	30.2	29.0	27.8	26.4	24.8	23.0	20.9	1.98	2.44
	22	33.1	32.3	31.3	30.4	29.3	28.1	26.8	25.4	23.9	22.1	20.0	1.61	2.06
	24	32.3	31.5	30.5	29.5	28.5	27.3	26.0	24.6	23.0	21.3	19.2	1.32	1.76
32.60	18	36.7	35.8	34.8	33.8	32.6	31.4	30.1	28.6	26.9	25.0	22.8	2.40	2.88
	20	35.7	34.8	33.9	32.8	31.7	30.4	29.1	27.6	25.9	24.0	21.9	1.96	2.43
	22	34.8	33.9	32.9	31.8	30.7	29.5	28.1	26.6	25.0	23.1	20.9	1.58	2.04
	24	33.9	33.0	32.0	31.0	29.8	28.6	27.2	25.7	24.1	22.2	20.0	1.30	1.74
34.41	18	38.5	37.5	36.5	35.4	34.2	32.9	31.5	29.9	28.1	26.1	23.8	2.40	2.88
	20	37.4	36.5	35.4	34.3	33.1	31.8	30.4	28.8	27.1	25.1	22.8	1.95	2.41
	22	36.4	35.4	34.4	33.3	32.1	30.8	29.4	27.8	26.0	24.0	21.7	1.56	2.02
	24	35.5	34.5	33.5	32.4	31.2	29.9	28.4	26.9	25.1	23.1	20.8	1.27	1.72
36.22	18	40.2	39.2	38.1	37.0	35.7	34.3	32.8	31.2	29.3	27.2	24.8	2.40	2.88
	20	39.1	38.1	37.0	35.8	34.6	33.2	31.7	30.1	28.2	26.1	23.7	1.94	2.40
	22	38.0	37.0	35.9	34.7	33.5	32.1	30.6	28.9	27.1	25.0	22.6	1.55	2.00
	24	37.0	36.0	34.9	33.8	32.5	31.1	29.6	28.0	26.1	24.0	21.6	1.25	1.69
38.03	18	42.0	40.9	39.8	38.5	37.2	35.8	34.2	32.5	30.5	28.3	25.8	2.40	2.88
	20	40.8	39.7	38.6	37.3	36.0	34.6	33.0	31.3	29.3	27.1	24.6	1.93	2.39
	22	39.6	38.5	37.4	36.2	34.8	33.4	31.8	30.1	28.1	25.9	23.4	1.53	1.98
	24	38.6	37.5	36.4	35.1	33.8	32.4	30.8	29.1	27.1	24.9	22.4	1.23	1.67

TABLE 205

Process Times (B) at Retort Temperature of 230°F for Conduction-Heating Foods in 211 x 306 Can

f_h	z	INITIAL FOOD TEMPERATURE (T_{ih}) 100	110	120	130	140	150	160	170	180	190	200	Equivalent F_c^{18}	F_s^{18}
31.44	18	82.9	81.8	80.6	79.3	77.9	76.3	74.5	72.4	69.9	66.8	62.9	2.61	2.88
	20	73.9	72.8	71.6	70.3	68.9	67.2	65.4	63.3	60.8	57.8	53.9	1.88	2.16
	22	67.0	65.9	64.7	63.4	62.0	60.4	58.6	56.5	54.0	50.9	47.0	1.44	1.70
	24	61.2	60.1	58.9	57.6	56.2	54.6	52.8	50.6	48.2	45.1	41.2	1.11	1.36
33.29	18	85.6	84.4	83.1	81.8	80.2	78.5	76.6	74.4	71.8	68.5	64.4	2.60	2.88
	20	76.7	75.5	74.2	72.9	71.3	69.6	67.7	65.5	62.8	59.6	55.5	1.88	2.16
	22	69.4	68.3	67.0	65.6	64.1	62.4	60.5	58.2	55.6	52.4	48.2	1.44	1.70
	24	63.3	62.1	60.8	59.5	57.9	56.2	54.3	52.1	49.4	46.2	42.1	1.07	1.34
35.14	18	88.6	87.4	86.1	84.6	83.0	81.2	79.2	76.8	74.0	70.6	66.2	2.59	2.88
	20	79.3	78.1	76.8	75.3	73.7	71.9	69.9	67.5	64.8	61.4	57.0	1.87	2.16
	22	71.7	70.5	69.2	67.7	66.1	64.3	62.3	59.9	57.2	53.8	49.4	1.44	1.70
	24	65.2	64.0	62.7	61.2	59.6	57.8	55.8	53.4	50.7	47.3	42.9	1.05	1.31
36.99	18	91.6	90.4	89.0	87.4	85.7	83.8	81.7	79.2	76.3	72.7	68.1	2.59	2.88
	20	82.0	80.7	79.3	77.8	76.1	74.2	72.0	69.6	66.6	63.0	58.4	1.87	2.16
	22	74.0	72.7	71.3	69.8	68.1	66.2	64.0	61.6	58.6	55.0	50.4	1.44	1.70
	24	67.6	66.3	64.9	63.4	61.7	59.8	57.7	55.2	52.2	48.7	44.0	1.04	1.32
38.84	18	94.6	93.2	91.8	90.2	88.4	86.4	84.2	81.6	78.5	74.7	69.9	2.58	2.88
	20	84.5	83.2	81.7	80.1	78.3	76.3	74.1	71.5	68.4	64.7	59.8	1.87	2.16
	22	76.1	74.8	73.3	71.7	69.9	68.0	65.7	63.1	60.0	56.3	51.4	1.40	1.67
	24	69.9	68.5	67.1	65.5	63.7	61.7	59.4	56.8	53.8	50.0	45.2	1.04	1.31

TABLE 206

Process Times (B) at Retort Temperature of 240°F for Conduction-Heating Foods in 211 x 306 Can

f_h	z	INITIAL FOOD TEMPERATURE (T_{ih})											Equivalent	
		100	110	120	130	140	150	610	170	180	190	200	F_c^{18}	F_s^{18}
31.44	18	55.0	54.0	52.9	51.7	50.4	49.0	47.3	45.5	43.4	40.9	37.9	2.52	2.88
	20	51.5	50.5	49.4	48.2	46.9	45.5	43.9	42.0	39.9	37.4	34.4	1.92	2.28
	22	48.6	47.6	46.5	45.4	44.1	42.6	41.0	39.2	37.1	34.6	31.5	1.49	1.84
	24	46.3	45.3	44.2	43.0	41.7	40.2	38.6	36.8	34.7	32.2	29.2	1.17	1.52
33.29	18	57.4	56.3	55.1	53.9	52.5	51.0	49.3	47.4	45.1	42.5	39.3	2.51	2.88
	20	53.8	52.7	51.5	50.3	48.9	47.4	45.7	43.7	41.5	38.9	35.6	1.91	2.27
	22	50.8	49.7	48.5	47.3	45.9	44.4	42.7	40.7	38.5	35.9	32.7	1.47	1.83
	24	48.3	47.2	46.0	44.8	43.4	41.9	40.2	38.3	36.0	33.4	30.2	1.16	1.50
35.14	18	59.7	58.6	57.4	56.0	54.6	53.0	51.2	49.1	46.8	44.0	40.6	2.51	2.88
	20	56.0	54.9	53.6	52.3	50.9	49.2	47.5	45.4	43.1	40.3	36.9	1.90	2.27
	22	52.8	51.7	50.5	49.2	47.7	46.1	44.3	42.3	39.9	37.1	33.7	1.46	1.81
	24	50.3	49.2	47.9	46.6	45.2	43.5	41.7	39.7	37.4	34.6	31.2	1.14	1.49
36.99	18	62.1	60.9	59.6	58.2	56.7	55.0	53.1	50.9	48.5	45.5	41.9	2.51	2.88
	20	58.2	57.0	55.7	54.3	52.8	51.1	49.2	47.1	44.6	41.7	38.1	1.89	2.26
	22	54.9	53.7	52.5	51.1	49.5	47.8	45.9	43.8	41.3	38.4	34.8	1.44	1.80
	24	52.3	51.1	49.8	48.4	46.9	45.2	43.3	41.1	38.7	35.7	32.1	1.13	1.48
38.84	18	64.4	63.2	61.8	60.4	58.7	57.0	55.0	52.7	50.1	47.1	43.3	2.50	2.88
	20	60.4	59.1	57.8	56.3	54.7	52.9	50.9	48.7	46.1	43.0	39.2	1.88	2.25
	22	57.0	55.8	54.4	52.9	51.3	49.6	47.6	45.3	42.7	39.6	35.9	1.43	1.79
	24	54.2	53.0	51.6	50.1	48.5	46.8	44.8	42.5	39.9	36.8	33.1	1.11	1.46

TABLE 207

Process Times (B) at Retort Temperature of 250°F for Conduction-Heating Foods in 211 x 306 Can

f_h	z	INITIAL FOOD TEMPERATURE (T_{ih})											Equivalent	
		100	110	120	130	140	150	160	170	180	190	200	F_c^{18}	F_s^{18}
	18	42.6	41.7	40.7	39.6	38.4	37.1	35.6	34.0	32.2	30.1	27.6	2.45	2.88
31.44	20	41.0	40.1	39.0	38.0	36.8	35.5	34.0	32.4	30.6	28.5	26.0	1.97	2.40
	22	39.6	38.6	37.6	36.5	35.3	34.0	32.6	31.0	29.2	27.1	24.6	1.60	2.01
	24	38.2	37.3	36.2	35.2	34.0	32.7	31.2	29.6	27.8	25.7	23.2	1.28	1.68
	18	44.6	43.6	42.6	41.4	40.2	38.8	37.3	35.6	33.6	31.4	28.8	2.45	2.88
33.29	20	42.9	41.9	40.9	39.7	38.5	37.1	35.6	33.9	31.9	29.7	27.1	1.96	2.38
	22	41.4	40.4	39.4	38.2	37.0	35.6	34.1	32.4	30.4	28.2	25.6	1.58	2.00
	24	40.0	39.0	37.9	36.8	35.5	34.1	32.6	30.9	29.0	26.7	24.1	1.26	1.66
	18	46.6	45.6	44.5	43.2	41.9	40.5	38.9	37.1	35.0	32.7	29.9	2.44	2.88
35.14	20	44.9	43.8	42.7	41.5	40.1	38.7	37.1	35.3	33.2	30.9	28.1	1.94	2.37
	22	43.3	42.2	41.1	39.9	38.6	37.1	35.5	33.7	31.7	29.3	26.5	1.56	1.98
	24	41.7	40.7	39.6	38.3	37.0	35.5	33.9	32.1	30.1	27.8	25.0	1.24	1.64
	18	48.6	47.3	46.3	45.1	43.7	42.1	40.4	38.5	36.4	33.9	31.0	2.44	2.88
36.99	20	46.8	45.7	44.5	43.2	41.8	40.3	38.6	36.7	34.5	32.1	29.1	1.93	2.36
	22	45.1	44.0	42.8	41.5	40.1	38.6	36.9	35.0	32.9	30.4	27.5	1.55	1.96
	24	43.5	42.4	41.2	39.9	38.5	37.0	35.3	33.4	31.2	28.8	25.8	1.22	1.62
	18	50.7	49.5	48.2	46.9	45.4	43.8	42.0	40.1	37.8	35.2	32.1	2.44	2.88
38.84	20	48.7	47.5	46.3	44.9	43.5	41.9	40.1	38.1	35.8	33.2	30.2	1.93	2.36
	22	47.0	45.8	44.5	43.2	41.7	40.1	38.3	36.4	34.1	31.5	28.4	1.54	1.95
	24	45.2	44.1	42.8	41.5	40.0	38.4	36.6	34.6	32.4	29.8	26.7	1.20	1.60

TABLE 208

Process Times (B) at Retort Temperature of 260°F for Conduction-Heating Foods in 211 x 306 Can

f_h	z	INITIAL FOOD TEMPERATURE (T_{ih})											Equivalent	
		100	110	120	130	140	150	160	170	180	190	200	F_c^{18}	F_s^{18}
31.44	18	35.6	34.7	33.8	32.8	31.7	30.5	29.2	27.7	26.1	24.3	22.2	2.41	2.88
	20	34.7	33.8	32.8	31.8	30.7	29.6	28.2	26.8	25.2	23.4	21.3	1.97	2.44
	22	33.7	32.8	31.9	30.9	29.8	28.6	27.3	25.9	24.3	22.4	20.3	1.60	2.05
	24	32.9	32.0	31.1	30.1	29.0	27.8	26.5	25.0	23.4	21.6	19.5	1.31	1.75
33.29	18	37.4	36.5	35.5	34.4	33.2	32.0	30.6	29.1	27.4	25.4	23.2	2.40	2.88
	20	36.4	35.5	34.5	33.4	32.2	31.0	29.6	28.1	26.4	24.4	22.2	1.96	2.43
	22	35.4	34.5	33.5	32.4	31.2	30.0	28.6	27.1	25.4	23.4	21.2	1.58	2.03
	24	34.5	33.6	32.6	31.5	30.3	29.1	27.7	26.2	24.5	22.5	20.3	1.29	1.73
35.14	18	39.2	38.2	37.1	36.0	34.8	33.5	32.0	30.4	28.6	26.6	24.2	2.40	2.88
	20	38.1	37.1	36.1	34.9	33.7	32.4	30.9	29.3	27.5	25.5	23.1	1.95	2.41
	22	37.0	36.1	35.0	33.9	32.7	31.3	29.9	28.3	26.5	24.4	22.1	1.56	2.01
	24	36.1	35.1	34.1	32.9	31.7	30.4	28.9	27.3	25.5	23.5	21.1	1.27	1.71
36.99	18	41.0	39.9	38.8	37.6	36.3	34.9	33.4	31.7	29.8	27.7	25.2	2.40	2.88
	20	39.8	38.8	37.7	36.5	35.2	33.8	32.3	30.6	28.7	26.5	24.1	1.94	2.40
	22	38.7	37.6	36.5	35.3	34.1	32.7	31.1	29.4	27.5	25.4	22.9	1.54	1.99
	24	37.7	36.6	35.5	34.4	33.1	31.7	30.1	28.4	26.6	24.4	21.9	1.24	1.69
38.84	18	42.7	41.6	40.5	39.2	37.9	36.4	34.8	33.0	31.0	28.8	2.62	2.40	2.88
	20	41.5	40.4	39.3	38.0	36.7	35.2	33.6	31.8	29.8	27.6	25.0	1.93	2.39
	22	40.3	39.2	38.1	36.8	35.5	34.0	32.4	30.6	28.6	26.4	23.8	1.52	1.98
	24	39.3	38.2	37.0	35.8	34.4	33.0	31.3	29.6	27.6	25.3	22.7	1.22	1.67

TABLE 209

Process Times (B) at Retort Temperature of 230°F for Conduction-Heating Foods in 211 x 400 Can

f_h	z	INITIAL FOOD TEMPERATURE (T_{ih})											Equivalent	
		100	110	120	130	140	150	160	170	180	190	200	F_c^{18}	F_s^{18}
33.98	18	86.8	85.7	84.4	83.0	81.4	79.7	77.7	75.4	72.7	69.4	65.2	2.61	2.89
	20	77.8	76.7	75.4	74.0	72.4	70.7	68.7	66.4	63.7	60.4	56.2	1.89	2.17
	22	70.5	69.3	68.0	66.6	65.0	63.3	61.3	59.1	56.4	53.1	48.8	1.44	1.71
	24	64.2	63.0	61.7	60.3	58.8	57.0	55.0	52.8	50.1	46.8	42.5	1.07	1.34
35.98	18	90.2	88.9	87.6	86.1	84.5	82.6	80.5	78.1	75.3	71.8	67.3	2.61	2.90
	20	80.7	79.5	78.1	76.6	75.0	73.2	71.1	68.7	65.8	62.3	57.8	1.89	2.17
	22	73.0	71.7	70.3	68.9	67.2	65.4	63.3	60.9	58.0	54.5	50.0	1.44	1.71
	24	66.4	65.2	63.8	62.3	60.7	58.9	56.8	54.4	51.5	48.0	43.5	1.05	1.32
37.98	18	93.4	92.1	90.7	89.1	87.4	85.4	83.2	80.7	77.7	74.0	69.3	2.60	2.90
	20	83.6	82.2	80.8	79.2	77.5	75.5	73.3	70.8	67.8	64.1	59.4	1.89	2.17
	22	75.3	74.0	72.6	71.0	69.3	67.3	65.1	62.6	59.6	55.9	51.2	1.43	1.70
	24	69.0	67.7	66.2	64.6	62.9	61.0	58.8	56.2	53.2	49.5	44.8	1.05	1.32
39.98	18	96.6	95.2	93.7	92.1	90.2	88.2	85.9	83.2	80.0	76.1	71.2	2.59	2.90
	20	86.3	84.9	83.4	81.7	79.9	77.9	75.5	72.9	69.7	65.8	60.8	1.89	2.17
	22	77.6	76.3	74.7	73.1	71.3	69.2	66.9	64.2	61.1	57.2	52.2	1.40	1.67
	24	71.4	70.0	68.5	66.9	65.0	63.0	60.7	58.0	54.8	51.0	46.0	1.04	1.32
41.98	18	99.8	98.3	96.7	95.0	93.0	90.9	88.5	85.7	82.3	78.3	73.0	2.59	2.90
	20	88.9	87.5	85.9	84.1	82.2	80.1	77.6	74.8	71.5	67.4	62.2	1.89	2.17
	22	79.9	78.4	76.8	75.1	73.2	71.0	68.6	65.8	62.4	58.4	53.1	1.36	1.64
	24	73.8	72.4	70.8	69.0	67.1	65.0	62.5	59.7	56.4	52.3	47.1	1.03	1.31

TABLE 210

Process Times (B) at Retort Temperature of 240°F for Conduction-Heating Foods in 211 x 400 Can

f_h	z	INITIAL FOOD TEMPERATURE (T_{ih}) 100	110	120	130	140	150	160	170	180	190	200	Equivalent F_c^{18}	F_s^{18}
	18	58.4	57.3	56.1	54.8	53.4	51.8	50.1	48.1	45.8	43.2	39.9	2.53	2.90
33.98	20	54.7	53.6	52.4	51.1	49.7	48.2	46.4	44.5	42.2	39.5	36.2	1.92	2.29
	22	51.6	50.5	49.4	48.1	46.7	45.1	43.4	41.4	39.1	36.4	33.1	1.48	1.83
	24	49.1	48.0	46.8	45.5	44.1	42.6	40.8	38.9	36.6	33.9	30.6	1.16	1.51
	18	60.9	59.7	58.5	57.1	55.6	54.0	52.1	50.0	47.6	44.8	41.3	2.53	2.90
35.98	20	57.1	55.9	54.7	53.3	51.8	50.2	48.3	46.3	43.8	41.0	37.5	1.91	2.28
	22	53.9	52.7	51.5	50.1	48.6	47.0	45.1	43.0	40.6	37.8	34.3	1.46	1.82
	24	51.3	50.1	48.9	47.5	46.0	44.4	42.5	40.4	38.0	35.2	31.7	1.15	1.49
	18	63.4	62.2	60.9	59.4	57.9	56.1	54.2	52.0	49.5	46.4	42.8	2.52	2.90
37.98	20	59.5	58.2	56.9	55.5	53.9	52.2	50.2	48.0	45.5	42.5	38.8	1.90	2.26
	22	56.1	54.9	53.6	52.2	50.6	48.8	46.9	44.7	42.2	39.2	35.5	1.45	1.81
	24	53.4	52.2	50.9	49.4	47.8	46.1	44.2	42.0	39.4	36.4	32.7	1.13	1.48
	18	66.0	64.7	63.3	61.8	60.1	58.3	56.2	53.9	51.2	48.1	44.2	2.52	2.90
39.98	20	61.8	60.5	59.1	57.6	56.0	54.1	52.1	49.8	47.1	43.9	40.0	1.89	2.26
	22	58.4	57.1	55.7	54.2	52.5	50.7	48.7	46.3	43.7	40.5	36.6	1.44	1.80
	24	55.5	54.2	52.8	51.3	49.7	47.8	45.8	43.5	40.8	37.6	33.8	1.12	1.47
	18	68.5	67.1	65.6	64.1	62.3	60.4	58.3	55.8	53.0	49.7	45.6	2.51	2.90
41.98	20	64.2	62.8	61.4	59.8	58.0	56.1	54.0	51.5	48.7	45.4	41.3	1.88	2.25
	22	60.6	59.2	57.8	56.2	54.4	52.5	50.4	47.9	45.1	41.8	37.7	1.42	1.79
	24	57.6	56.3	54.8	53.2	51.5	49.6	47.4	45.0	42.2	38.8	34.8	1.10	1.45

TABLE 211

Process Times (B) at Retort Temperature of 250°F for Conduction-Heating Foods in 211 x 400 Can

f_h	z	INITIAL FOOD TEMPERATURE (T_{ih})											Equivalent	
		100	110	120	130	140	150	160	170	180	190	200	F_c^{18}	F_s^{18}
33.98	18	45.5	44.4	43.3	42.2	40.9	39.5	37.9	36.2	34.2	31.9	29.2	2.46	2.90
	20	43.7	42.7	41.6	40.4	39.1	37.7	36.2	34.4	32.5	30.2	27.5	1.97	2.39
	22	42.2	41.2	40.1	38.9	37.6	36.2	34.7	32.9	30.9	28.7	26.0	1.59	2.00
	24	40.7	39.7	38.6	37.4	36.1	34.7	33.2	31.4	29.4	27.2	24.5	1.26	1.66
35.98	18	47.6	46.5	45.4	44.1	42.8	41.3	39.6	37.8	35.7	33.3	30.4	2.46	2.90
	20	45.8	44.7	43.6	42.3	40.9	39.5	37.8	36.0	33.9	31.5	28.6	1.95	2.38
	22	44.2	43.1	41.9	40.7	39.3	37.8	36.2	34.4	32.3	29.9	27.0	1.57	1.98
	24	42.6	41.5	40.4	39.1	37.7	36.3	34.6	32.8	30.7	28.3	25.4	1.24	1.64
37.98	18	49.8	48.6	47.4	46.1	44.7	43.1	41.4	39.4	37.2	34.7	31.7	2.46	2.90
	20	47.9	46.7	45.5	44.2	42.7	41.2	39.4	37.5	35.3	32.7	29.7	1.95	2.37
	22	46.2	45.0	43.8	42.5	41.0	39.5	37.7	35.8	33.6	31.0	28.0	1.55	1.97
	24	44.5	43.3	42.1	40.8	39.4	37.8	36.1	34.1	31.9	29.4	26.4	1.22	1.62
39.98	18	51.9	50.8	49.5	48.1	46.6	44.9	43.1	41.0	38.7	36.0	32.9	2.46	2.90
	20	49.9	48.7	47.5	46.1	44.6	42.9	41.1	39.0	36.7	34.0	30.9	1.94	2.37
	22	48.1	46.9	45.7	44.3	42.8	41.4	39.3	37.2	34.9	32.2	29.1	1.54	1.96
	24	46.4	45.2	43.9	42.5	41.0	39.3	37.5	35.5	33.1	30.5	27.3	1.20	1.60
41.98	18	54.1	52.8	51.5	50.0	48.4	46.7	44.8	42.6	40.2	37.4	34.1	2.45	2.90
	20	52.0	50.7	49.4	47.9	46.3	44.6	42.7	40.5	38.1	35.3	32.0	1.93	2.36
	22	50.1	48.9	47.5	46.0	44.5	42.7	40.8	38.7	36.2	33.4	30.1	1.53	1.94
	24	48.2	47.0	45.6	44.2	42.6	40.9	38.9	36.8	34.4	31.5	28.2	1.18	1.59

TABLE 212

Process Times at Retort Temperature of 260°F for Conduction-Heating Foods in 211 x 400 Can

f_h	z	INITIAL FOOD TEMPERATURE (T_{ih})											Equivalent	
		100	110	120	130	140	150	160	170	180	190	200	F_c^{18}	F_s^{18}
	18	38.1	37.1	36.1	35.0	33.9	32.6	31.2	29.6	27.9	25.9	23.6	2.42	2.90
33.98	20	37.1	36.1	35.1	34.0	32.8	31.5	30.1	28.6	26.8	24.9	22.6	1.97	2.44
	22	36.0	35.1	34.1	33.0	31.8	30.5	29.1	27.6	25.8	23.8	21.6	1.58	2.04
	24	35.1	34.2	33.2	32.1	30.9	29.6	28.2	26.6	24.9	22.9	20.7	1.29	1.73
	18	40.0	39.0	37.9	36.8	35.5	34.2	32.7	31.0	29.2	27.1	24.7	2.42	2.90
35.98	20	38.9	37.9	36.8	35.7	34.4	33.1	31.6	29.9	28.1	26.0	23.6	1.96	2.42
	22	37.8	36.8	35.7	34.6	33.3	32.0	30.5	28.8	27.0	24.9	22.5	1.56	2.02
	24	36.9	35.9	34.8	33.6	32.4	31.0	29.5	27.9	26.0	23.9	21.5	1.27	1.71
	18	42.0	40.9	39.7	38.5	37.2	35.8	34.2	32.5	30.5	28.3	25.8	2.42	2.90
37.98	20	40.8	39.7	38.6	37.4	36.0	34.6	33.0	31.3	29.3	27.1	24.6	1.94	2.41
	22	39.6	38.5	37.4	36.2	34.8	33.4	31.8	30.1	28.2	26.0	23.4	1.54	2.00
	24	38.6	37.5	36.4	35.2	33.8	32.4	30.8	29.1	27.1	24.9	22.4	1.24	1.69
	18	43.9	42.7	41.5	40.2	38.9	37.3	35.7	33.9	31.8	29.5	26.8	2.41	2.90
39.98	20	42.6	41.5	40.3	39.0	37.6	36.1	34.5	32.6	30.6	28.3	25.6	1.93	2.40
	22	41.4	40.2	39.0	37.7	36.4	34.8	33.2	31.4	29.3	27.0	24.3	1.52	1.98
	24	40.3	39.2	38.0	36.7	35.3	33.8	32.1	30.3	28.2	25.9	23.3	1.22	1.67
	18	45.8	44.6	43.3	42.0	40.5	38.9	37.2	35.3	33.1	30.7	27.9	2.41	2.90
41.98	20	44.4	43.3	42.0	40.7	39.2	37.6	35.9	33.9	31.8	29.4	26.6	1.92	2.39
	22	43.1	41.9	40.7	39.3	37.9	36.3	34.5	32.6	30.5	28.0	25.2	1.51	1.96
	24	42.0	40.8	39.5	38.2	36.7	35.1	33.4	31.5	29.3	26.9	24.1	1.20	1.65

TABLE 213

Process Times (B) at Retort Temperature of 230°F for Conduction-Heating Foods in 211 x 413 Can

f_h	z	INITIAL FOOD TEMPERATURE (T_{ih})											Equivalent	
		100	110	120	130	140	150	160	170	180	190	200	F_c^{18}	F_s^{18}
36.09	18	90.6	89.3	88.0	86.5	84.8	83.0	80.9	78.5	75.6	72.1	67.6	2.62	2.92
	20	81.1	79.8	78.5	77.0	75.3	73.5	71.4	69.0	66.1	62.6	58.1	1.90	2.18
	22	73.3	72.0	70.7	69.2	67.5	65.7	63.6	61.2	58.3	54.8	50.3	1.45	1.72
	24	66.7	65.5	64.1	62.6	61.0	59.1	57.0	54.6	51.7	48.3	43.7	1.06	1.33
38.22	18	94.0	92.7	91.3	89.7	87.9	86.0	83.8	81.2	78.2	74.5	69.7	2.61	2.92
	20	84.1	82.8	81.3	79.7	78.0	76.0	73.8	71.3	68.2	64.5	59.7	1.90	2.18
	22	75.8	74.5	73.1	71.5	69.7	67.8	65.5	63.0	60.0	56.3	51.5	1.44	1.71
	24	69.4	68.1	66.6	65.1	63.3	61.4	59.1	56.6	53.5	49.8	45.1	1.05	1.33
40.34	18	97.4	96.0	94.5	92.8	91.0	88.9	86.6	83.9	80.7	76.8	71.7	2.61	2.92
	20	87.0	85.6	84.1	82.4	80.5	78.5	76.1	73.4	70.2	66.3	61.3	1.90	2.18
	22	78.3	76.9	75.3	73.7	71.8	69.8	67.4	64.7	61.5	57.6	52.6	1.40	1.68
	24	72.0	70.6	69.1	67.4	65.6	63.5	61.2	58.5	55.3	51.4	46.3	1.05	1.33
42.46	18	100.7	99.3	97.6	95.9	93.9	91.8	89.3	86.5	83.1	79.0	73.7	2.61	2.92
	20	89.8	88.3	86.7	84.9	83.0	80.8	78.4	75.5	72.2	68.1	62.7	1.90	2.18
	22	80.7	79.2	77.6	75.8	73.9	71.7	69.3	66.4	63.1	58.9	53.6	1.37	1.65
	24	74.5	73.1	71.5	69.7	67.8	65.6	63.1	60.3	56.9	52.8	47.5	1.04	1.31
44.59	18	104.0	102.4	100.7	98.9	96.9	94.6	92.0	89.0	85.5	81.2	75.6	2.60	2.91
	20	92.5	91.0	89.3	87.4	85.4	83.1	80.5	77.5	74.0	69.7	64.1	1.90	2.18
	22	83.5	81.9	80.2	78.4	76.3	74.1	71.5	68.5	65.0	60.6	55.1	1.36	1.65
	24	77.0	75.5	73.8	71.9	69.9	67.6	65.0	62.1	58.5	54.2	48.6	1.02	1.30

TABLE 214

Process Times (B) at Retort Temperature of 240°F for Conduction-Heating Foods in 211 x 413 Can

f_h	z	INITIAL FOOD TEMPERATURE (T_{ih})											Equivalent	
		100	110	120	130	140	150	160	170	180	190	200	F_c^{18}	F_s^{18}
	18	61.1	60.0	58.7	57.3	55.8	54.2	52.3	50.3	47.8	45.0	41.5	2.54	2.91
36.09	20	57.3	56.2	54.9	53.5	52.0	50.4	48.5	46.5	44.0	41.2	37.7	1.92	2.29
	22	54.1	52.9	51.7	50.3	48.8	47.2	45.3	43.2	40.8	37.9	34.4	1.47	1.83
	24	51.5	50.3	49.1	47.7	46.2	44.6	42.7	40.6	38.2	35.3	31.8	1.15	1.50
	18	63.8	62.6	61.3	59.8	58.2	56.5	54.5	52.3	49.8	46.7	43.0	2.54	2.91
38.22	20	59.8	58.6	57.3	55.8	54.3	52.5	50.6	48.3	45.8	42.8	39.0	1.91	2.28
	22	56.5	55.3	53.9	52.5	50.9	49.2	47.2	45.0	42.4	39.4	35.7	1.46	1.82
	24	53.7	52.5	51.2	49.7	48.2	46.4	44.4	42.2	39.7	36.6	32.9	1.14	1.49
	18	66.5	65.2	63.8	62.3	60.6	58.8	56.7	54.4	51.7	48.5	44.6	2.53	2.91
40.34	20	62.3	61.0	59.6	58.1	56.4	54.6	52.5	50.2	47.5	44.3	40.4	1.90	2.27
	22	58.9	57.6	56.2	54.6	53.0	51.1	49.1	46.7	44.0	40.8	36.9	1.44	1.81
	24	56.0	54.7	53.3	51.7	50.1	48.2	46.2	43.8	41.1	37.9	34.0	1.12	1.48
	18	69.2	67.8	66.3	64.7	63.0	61.0	58.9	56.4	53.5	50.2	46.1	2.53	2.92
42.46	20	64.8	63.5	62.0	60.4	58.6	56.7	54.5	52.1	49.2	45.8	41.7	1.89	2.26
	22	61.2	59.8	58.4	56.7	55.0	53.0	50.9	48.4	45.6	42.2	38.1	1.43	1.80
	24	58.2	56.9	55.4	53.8	52.0	50.1	47.9	45.4	42.6	39.2	35.1	1.10	1.46
	18	71.8	70.4	68.8	67.1	65.3	63.2	61.0	58.4	55.4	51.9	47.5	2.53	2.91
44.59	20	67.3	65.9	64.3	62.6	60.8	58.8	56.5	53.9	50.9	47.4	43.1	1.88	2.26
	22	63.5	62.1	60.5	58.9	57.0	55.0	52.7	50.1	47.1	43.6	39.3	1.42	1.79
	24	60.4	59.0	57.4	55.8	53.9	51.9	49.6	47.0	44.0	40.5	36.2	1.09	1.45

TABLE 215

Process Times (B) at Retort Temperature of 250°F for Concuction-Heating Foods in 211 x 413 Can

f_h	z	INITIAL FOOD TEMPERATURE (T_{ih})											Equivalent	
		100	110	120	130	140	150	160	170	180	190	200	F_c^{18}	F_s^{18}
	18	47.8	46.7	45.6	44.3	42.9	41.4	39.8	37.9	35.8	33.4	30.6	2.48	2.91
36.09	20	46.0	44.9	43.7	42.5	41.1	39.6	38.0	36.1	34.0	31.6	28.7	1.97	2.39
	22	44.3	43.3	42.1	40.9	39.5	38.0	36.3	34.5	32.4	30.0	27.1	1.58	1.99
	24	42.8	41.7	40.5	39.3	37.9	36.4	34.7	32.9	30.8	28.4	25.5	1.25	1.65
	18	50.1	49.0	47.7	46.4	44.9	43.4	41.6	39.7	37.4	34.9	31.9	2.47	2.91
38.22	20	48.2	47.0	45.8	44.5	43.0	41.4	39.7	37.7	35.5	33.0	29.9	1.96	2.39
	22	46.5	45.3	44.1	42.8	41.3	39.7	38.0	36.0	33.8	31.2	28.2	1.56	1.98
	24	44.8	43.6	42.4	41.1	39.6	38.0	36.3	34.3	32.1	29.6	26.5	1.23	1.63
	18	52.4	51.2	49.9	48.5	47.0	45.3	43.4	41.4	39.0	36.3	33.2	2.47	2.91
40.34	20	50.4	49.2	47.9	46.5	44.9	43.3	41.4	39.4	37.0	34.3	31.1	1.95	2.38
	22	48.6	47.4	46.1	44.7	43.1	41.5	39.6	37.6	35.2	32.5	29.3	1.55	1.97
	24	46.8	45.6	44.3	42.9	41.3	39.7	37.8	35.8	33.4	30.7	27.5	1.21	1.61
	18	54.7	53.4	52.0	50.6	49.0	47.2	45.3	43.1	40.6	37.8	34.4	2.47	2.91
42.46	20	52.5	51.3	49.9	48.4	46.8	45.1	43.1	41.0	38.5	35.7	32.3	1.94	2.37
	22	50.6	49.4	48.0	46.5	44.9	43.2	41.2	39.1	36.6	33.8	30.4	1.54	1.95
	24	48.8	47.5	46.1	44.6	43.0	41.3	39.3	37.2	34.7	31.9	28.5	1.19	1.60
	18	56.9	55.6	54.2	52.6	50.9	49.1	47.0	44.8	42.2	39.2	35.7	2.47	2.91
44.59	20	54.7	53.4	51.9	50.4	48.7	46.9	44.8	42.5	39.9	37.0	33.4	1.93	2.37
	22	52.7	51.4	49.9	48.4	46.7	44.9	42.8	40.5	38.0	35.0	31.4	1.52	1.94
	24	50.7	49.4	48.0	46.4	44.7	42.9	40.8	38.6	36.0	33.0	29.5	1.17	1.58

TABLE 216

Process Times (B) at Retort Temperature of 260°F for Conduction-Heating Foods in 211 x 413 Can

f_h	z	100	110	120	130	140	150	160	170	180	190	200	Equivalent F_c^{18}	Equivalent F_s^{18}
		INITIAL FOOD TEMPERATURE (T_{ih})												
36.09	18	40.2	39.2	38.1	36.9	35.7	34.3	32.8	31.2	29.3	27.2	24.8	2.43	2.91
	20	39.1	38.1	37.0	35.8	34.6	33.2	31.7	30.1	28.2	26.1	23.7	1.97	2.44
	22	38.0	37.0	35.9	34.7	33.5	32.1	30.6	29.0	27.1	25.0	22.6	1.58	2.03
	24	37.0	36.0	34.9	33.7	32.5	31.1	29.6	28.0	26.1	24.0	21.6	1.28	1.72
38.22	18	42.2	41.1	40.0	38.8	37.4	36.0	34.4	32.7	30.7	28.5	25.9	2.43	2.91
	20	41.0	40.0	38.8	37.6	36.3	34.8	33.2	31.5	29.5	27.3	24.8	1.96	2.43
	22	39.8	38.8	37.6	36.4	35.1	33.6	32.0	30.3	28.3	26.1	23.6	1.55	2.01
	24	38.8	37.8	36.6	35.4	34.0	32.6	31.0	29.3	27.3	25.1	22.5	1.25	1.70
40.34	18	44.2	43.1	41.9	40.6	39.2	37.7	36.0	34.2	32.1	29.8	27.1	2.43	2.91
	20	43.0	41.9	40.6	39.3	37.9	36.4	34.8	32.9	30.8	28.5	25.8	1.95	2.42
	22	41.7	40.6	39.4	38.1	36.7	35.2	33.5	31.6	29.6	27.2	24.5	1.53	1.99
	24	40.6	39.5	38.3	37.0	35.6	34.1	32.4	30.6	28.5	26.2	23.5	1.23	1.68
42.46	18	46.3	45.1	43.8	42.4	40.9	39.3	37.6	35.6	33.5	31.0	28.2	2.43	2.91
	20	44.9	43.7	42.5	41.1	39.6	38.0	36.3	34.3	32.1	29.7	26.8	1.94	2.41
	22	43.6	42.4	41.1	39.7	38.3	36.7	34.9	33.0	30.8	28.3	25.5	1.52	1.97
	24	42.4	41.2	40.0	38.6	37.1	35.5	33.8	31.8	29.6	27.2	24.3	1.21	1.66
44.59	18	48.3	47.0	45.7	44.2	42.7	41.0	39.2	37.1	34.8	32.3	29.3	2.43	2.91
	20	46.8	45.6	44.3	42.8	41.3	39.6	37.7	35.7	33.4	30.8	27.8	1.93	2.40
	22	45.4	44.2	42.8	41.4	39.8	38.2	36.3	34.3	32.0	29.4	26.4	1.50	1.95
	24	44.2	43.0	41.6	40.2	38.6	37.0	35.1	33.1	30.8	28.2	25.2	1.19	1.64

TABLE 217

Process Times (B) at Retort Temperature of 230°F for Conduction-Heating Foods in 211 x 414 Can

f_h	z	INITIAL FOOD TEMPERATURE (T_{ih})											Equivalent	
		100	110	120	130	140	150	160	170	180	190	200	F_c^{18}	F_s^{18}
	18	90.8	89.5	88.2	86.7	85.0	83.2	81.1	78.6	75.8	72.3	67.7	2.62	2.92
36.22	20	81.3	80.0	78.7	77.2	75.5	73.6	71.5	69.1	66.3	62.7	58.2	1.90	2.18
	22	73.4	72.2	70.8	69.3	67.7	65.8	63.7	61.3	58.4	54.9	50.4	1.45	1.72
	24	66.9	65.6	64.3	62.8	61.1	59.3	57.2	54.7	51.9	48.4	43.8	1.06	1.33
	18	94.3	92.9	91.5	89.9	88.1	86.2	83.9	81.4	78.3	74.6	69.8	2.62	2.92
38.35	20	84.3	82.9	81.5	79.9	78.2	76.2	74.0	71.4	68.4	64.7	59.9	1.90	2.18
	22	76.0	74.7	73.2	71.6	69.9	67.9	65.7	63.1	60.1	56.4	51.6	1.44	1.71
	24	69.6	68.2	66.8	65.2	63.5	61.5	59.3	56.7	53.7	50.0	45.2	1.05	1.33
	18	97.6	96.2	94.7	93.0	91.2	89.1	86.8	84.0	80.8	76.9	71.9	2.61	2.92
40.48	20	87.2	85.8	84.2	82.6	80.7	78.6	76.3	73.6	70.4	66.5	61.4	1.90	2.18
	22	78.4	77.0	75.5	73.8	72.0	69.9	67.6	64.8	61.6	57.7	52.7	1.40	1.68
	24	72.2	70.8	69.3	67.6	65.7	63.7	61.3	58.6	55.4	51.5	46.4	1.05	1.33
	18	101.0	99.5	97.9	96.1	94.2	92.0	89.5	86.7	83.3	79.2	73.8	2.61	2.92
42.61	20	90.0	88.5	86.9	85.1	83.2	81.0	78.5	75.7	72.3	68.2	62.9	1.90	2.18
	22	80.9	79.4	77.8	76.0	74.1	71.9	69.4	66.6	63.2	59.1	53.7	1.37	1.65
	24	74.7	73.3	71.6	69.9	67.9	65.7	63.3	60.4	57.1	52.9	47.6	1.03	1.31
	18	104.2	102.7	101.0	99.1	97.1	94.8	92.2	89.2	85.7	81.3	75.7	2.61	2.92
44.74	20	92.7	91.2	89.5	87.6	85.6	83.3	80.7	77.7	74.2	69.8	64.2	1.90	2.18
	22	83.7	82.1	80.4	78.6	76.5	74.2	71.6	68.6	65.1	60.8	55.2	1.37	1.65
	24	77.2	75.7	74.0	72.1	70.1	67.8	65.2	62.2	58.7	54.3	48.7	1.02	1.30

TABLE 218

Process Times (B) at Retort Temperature of 240°F for Conduction-Heating Foods in 211 x 414 Can

f_h	z	INITIAL FOOD TEMPERATURE (T_{ih}) 100	110	120	130	140	150	160	170	180	190	200	Equivalent F_c^{18}	F_s^{18}
36.22	18	61.3	60.1	58.9	57.5	56.0	54.3	52.5	50.4	48.0	45.1	41.6	2.54	2.92
	20	57.5	56.3	55.0	53.7	52.2	50.5	48.7	46.6	44.1	41.3	37.8	1.92	2.29
	22	54.2	53.1	51.8	50.4	48.9	47.3	45.4	43.3	40.9	38.0	34.5	1.47	1.83
	24	51.6	50.5	49.2	47.8	46.3	44.7	42.8	40.7	38.3	35.4	31.9	1.15	1.50
38.35	18	64.0	62.8	61.4	60.0	58.4	56.6	54.7	52.5	49.9	46.9	43.1	2.54	2.92
	20	60.0	58.8	57.4	56.0	54.4	52.6	50.7	48.5	45.9	42.9	39.1	1.91	2.28
	22	56.6	55.4	54.1	52.6	51.0	49.3	47.3	45.1	42.5	39.5	35.8	1.46	1.82
	24	53.9	52.6	51.3	49.9	48.3	46.5	44.6	42.3	39.8	36.7	33.0	1.14	1.49
40.48	18	66.7	65.4	64.0	62.5	60.8	58.9	56.9	54.5	51.8	48.6	44.7	2.54	2.92
	20	62.5	61.2	59.8	58.3	56.6	54.7	52.7	50.3	47.6	44.4	40.5	1.90	2.27
	22	59.0	57.7	56.3	54.8	53.1	51.3	49.2	46.8	44.1	40.9	37.0	1.44	1.81
	24	56.1	54.8	53.4	51.9	50.2	48.4	46.3	43.9	41.2	38.0	34.1	1.12	1.47
42.61	18	69.4	68.0	66.5	64.9	63.1	61.2	59.0	56.5	53.7	50.3	46.2	2.53	2.92
	20	65.0	63.6	62.2	60.6	58.8	56.8	54.7	52.2	49.3	46.0	41.8	1.89	2.27
	22	61.4	60.0	58.5	56.9	55.1	53.2	51.0	48.5	45.7	42.3	38.2	1.43	1.80
	24	58.4	57.0	55.5	53.9	52.2	50.2	48.0	45.6	42.7	39.3	35.2	1.10	1.46
44.74	18	72.0	70.5	69.0	67.3	65.4	63.4	61.1	58.5	55.5	52.0	47.6	2.53	2.92
	20	67.5	66.1	64.5	62.8	61.0	58.9	56.6	54.0	51.0	47.5	43.2	1.88	2.26
	22	63.7	62.3	60.7	59.0	57.2	55.1	52.8	50.2	47.2	43.7	39.4	1.42	1.79
	24	60.6	59.2	57.6	55.9	54.1	52.0	49.7	47.1	44.1	40.6	36.3	1.09	1.45

TABLE 219

Process Times (B) at Retort Temperature of 250°F for Conduction-Heating Foods in 211 x 414 Can

f_h	z	INITIAL FOOD TEMPERATURE (T_{ih})											Equivalent	
		100	110	120	130	140	150	160	170	180	190	200	F_c^{18}	F_s^{18}
36.22	18	47.9	46.8	45.7	44.4	43.1	41.6	39.9	38.0	35.9	33.5	30.7	2.48	2.92
	20	46.1	45.0	43.8	42.6	41.2	39.7	38.1	36.2	34.1	31.7	28.8	1.97	2.39
	22	44.5	43.4	42.2	41.0	39.6	38.1	36.4	34.6	32.5	30.1	27.2	1.58	1.99
	24	42.9	41.8	40.6	39.4	38.0	36.5	34.8	33.0	30.9	28.5	25.6	1.25	1.65
38.35	18	50.2	49.1	47.9	46.5	45.1	43.5	41.7	39.8	37.6	35.0	31.9	2.48	2.92
	20	48.3	47.2	45.9	44.6	43.1	41.6	39.8	37.8	35.6	33.0	30.0	1.96	2.39
	22	46.6	45.4	44.2	42.9	41.4	39.8	38.1	36.1	33.9	31.3	28.3	1.56	1.98
	24	44.9	43.7	42.5	41.2	39.7	38.1	36.4	34.4	32.2	29.6	26.6	1.22	1.63
40.48	18	52.6	51.3	50.0	48.6	47.1	45.4	43.6	41.5	39.2	36.4	33.2	2.47	2.92
	20	50.5	49.3	48.0	46.6	45.1	43.4	41.5	39.5	37.1	34.4	31.2	1.95	2.38
	22	48.7	47.5	46.2	44.8	43.3	41.6	39.7	37.7	35.3	32.6	29.4	1.55	1.97
	24	46.9	45.7	44.4	43.0	41.5	39.8	37.9	35.9	33.5	30.8	27.6	1.21	1.61
42.61	18	54.8	53.6	52.2	50.7	49.1	47.3	45.4	43.2	40.7	37.9	34.5	2.47	2.92
	20	52.7	51.4	50.1	48.6	47.0	45.2	43.2	41.1	38.6	35.7	32.4	1.94	2.38
	22	50.8	49.5	48.1	46.7	45.1	43.3	41.3	39.2	36.7	33.8	30.5	1.54	1.95
	24	48.9	47.6	46.3	44.8	43.2	41.4	39.5	37.3	34.8	31.9	28.6	1.19	1.60
44.74	18	57.1	55.8	54.3	52.8	51.1	49.2	47.2	44.9	42.3	39.3	35.8	2.47	2.92
	20	54.9	53.5	52.1	50.5	48.8	47.0	44.9	42.7	40.1	37.1	33.5	1.93	2.37
	22	52.9	51.5	50.1	48.5	46.8	45.0	42.9	40.6	38.1	35.1	31.5	1.52	1.94
	24	50.9	49.5	48.1	46.5	44.9	43.0	41.0	38.7	36.1	33.1	29.5	1.17	1.58

TABLE 220

Process Times (B) at Retort Temperature of 260°F for Conduction-Heating Foods in 211 x 414 Can

f_h	z	INITIAL FOOD TEMPERATURE (T_{ih}) 100	110	120	130	140	150	160	170	180	190	200	Equivalent F_c^{18}	F_s^{18}
	18	40.3	39.3	38.2	37.0	35.8	34.4	32.9	31.3	29.4	27.3	24.9	2.44	2.92
36.22	20	39.2	38.2	37.1	35.9	34.7	33.3	31.8	30.1	28.3	26.2	23.8	1.97	2.44
	22	38.1	37.1	36.0	34.8	33.6	32.2	30.7	29.0	27.2	25.1	22.7	1.58	2.03
	24	37.1	36.1	35.0	33.8	32.6	31.2	29.7	28.1	26.2	24.1	21.7	1.28	1.72
	18	42.3	41.3	40.1	38.9	37.6	36.1	34.5	32.8	30.8	28.6	26.0	2.43	2.92
38.35	20	41.2	40.1	38.9	37.7	36.4	34.9	33.3	31.6	29.6	27.4	24.8	1.96	2.43
	22	40.0	38.9	37.7	36.5	35.2	33.7	32.1	30.4	28.4	26.2	23.6	1.55	2.01
	24	38.9	37.9	36.7	35.5	34.1	32.7	31.1	29.4	27.4	25.2	22.6	1.25	1.70
	18	44.4	43.2	42.0	40.7	39.3	37.8	36.1	34.3	32.2	29.8	27.1	2.43	2.92
40.48	20	43.1	42.0	40.8	39.5	38.1	36.5	34.9	33.0	30.9	28.6	25.9	1.95	2.42
	22	41.8	40.7	39.5	38.2	36.8	35.3	33.6	31.7	29.7	27.3	24.6	1.53	1.99
	24	40.8	39.6	38.4	37.1	35.7	34.2	32.5	30.6	28.6	26.2	23.5	1.23	1.68
	18	46.4	45.2	43.9	42.6	41.1	39.5	37.7	35.7	33.6	31.1	28.2	2.43	2.92
42.61	20	45.1	43.9	42.6	41.2	39.7	38.1	36.4	34.4	32.2	29.8	26.9	1.94	2.41
	22	43.7	42.5	41.2	39.9	38.4	36.8	35.0	33.1	30.9	28.4	25.5	1.51	1.97
	24	42.6	41.4	40.1	38.7	37.2	35.6	33.9	31.9	29.7	27.3	24.4	1.21	1.66
	18	48.4	47.2	45.8	44.4	42.8	41.1	39.3	37.2	34.9	32.3	29.3	2.43	2.92
44.74	20	47.0	45.7	44.4	42.9	41.4	39.7	37.9	35.8	33.5	30.9	27.9	1.93	2.40
	22	45.5	44.3	43.0	41.5	40.0	38.3	36.4	34.4	32.1	29.5	26.5	1.49	1.95
	24	44.3	43.1	41.8	40.3	38.8	37.1	35.2	33.2	30.9	28.3	25.3	1.19	1.64

TABLE 221

Process Times (B) at Retort Temperature of 230°F for Conduction-Heating Foods in 211 x 600 Can

f_h	z	Initial food temperature (T_{ih}) 100	110	120	130	140	150	160	170	180	190	200	Equivalent F_c^{18}	F_s^{18}
	18	93.7	92.4	91.0	89.4	87.7	85.7	83.6	81.0	78.0	74.3	69.6	2.64	2.94
37.88	20	83.8	82.5	81.1	79.5	77.8	75.9	73.7	71.1	68.1	64.5	59.7	1.91	2.20
	22	75.7	74.3	72.9	71.3	69.6	67.7	65.5	62.9	59.9	56.3	51.5	1.47	1.73
	24	69.1	67.8	66.4	64.8	63.1	61.2	59.0	56.4	53.4	49.8	45.0	1.06	1.34
	18	97.3	95.9	94.4	92.7	90.9	88.8	86.5	83.8	80.6	76.8	71.7	2.63	2.94
40.10	20	86.9	85.5	84.0	82.3	80.5	78.5	76.1	73.4	70.3	66.4	61.4	1.91	2.20
	22	78.3	76.9	75.3	73.7	71.8	69.8	67.5	64.8	61.6	57.7	52.7	1.42	1.70
	24	71.9	70.5	69.0	67.3	65.5	63.4	61.1	58.4	55.3	51.4	46.4	1.06	1.34
	18	100.8	99.3	97.7	96.0	94.0	91.9	89.4	86.6	83.2	79.1	73.8	2.63	2.94
42.33	20	89.9	88.4	86.8	85.1	83.1	81.0	78.5	75.7	72.3	68.2	62.9	1.91	2.20
	22	80.7	79.2	77.6	75.9	73.9	71.8	69.3	66.5	63.1	59.0	53.7	1.38	1.66
	24	74.6	73.1	71.5	69.8	67.8	65.7	63.2	60.4	57.0	52.9	47.6	1.05	1.33
	18	104.2	102.7	101.0	99.1	97.1	94.8	92.2	89.3	85.7	81.4	75.8	2.62	2.94
44.56	20	92.8	91.2	89.5	87.7	85.6	83.4	80.8	77.8	74.3	69.9	64.4	1.91	2.20
	22	83.6	82.1	80.4	78.5	76.5	74.2	71.6	68.7	65.1	60.8	55.2	1.38	1.66
	24	77.2	75.6	74.0	72.1	70.1	67.8	65.2	62.2	58.7	54.4	48.8	1.03	1.31
	18	107.6	105.9	104.2	102.2	100.1	97.7	95.0	91.9	88.1	83.6	77.8	2.62	2.94
46.79	20	95.5	93.9	92.1	90.2	88.1	85.7	83.0	79.8	76.1	71.6	65.7	1.91	2.20
	22	86.5	84.9	83.1	81.2	79.0	76.6	73.9	70.8	67.1	62.5	56.7	1.37	1.67
	24	79.8	78.1	76.4	74.4	72.3	69.9	67.2	64.0	60.3	55.8	50.0	1.01	1.30

TABLE 222

Process Times (B) at Retort Temperature of 240°F for Conduction-Heating Foods in 211 x 600 Can

f_h	z	INITIAL FOOD TEMPERATURE (T_{ih})											Equivalent	
		100	110	120	130	140	150	160	170	180	190	200	F_c^{18}	F_s^{18}
37.88	18	63.5	62.3	61.0	59.5	58.0	56.2	54.3	52.1	49.6	46.6	42.9	2.56	2.94
	20	59.6	58.3	57.0	55.6	54.0	52.3	50.3	48.2	45.6	42.6	38.9	1.93	2.30
	22	56.2	55.0	53.7	52.2	50.7	48.9	47.0	44.8	42.3	39.3	35.6	1.47	1.83
	24	53.5	52.3	50.9	49.5	47.9	46.2	44.3	42.1	39.5	36.5	32.9	1.15	1.50
40.10	18	66.3	65.1	63.7	62.1	60.5	58.7	56.6	54.3	51.6	48.4	44.5	2.56	2.94
	20	62.2	60.9	59.5	58.0	56.3	54.5	52.4	50.1	47.4	44.2	40.3	1.91	2.29
	22	58.7	57.4	56.0	54.5	52.9	51.0	49.0	46.6	44.0	40.8	36.9	1.46	1.82
	24	55.8	54.5	53.1	51.6	50.0	48.1	46.1	43.8	41.1	37.9	34.0	1.13	1.49
42.33	18	69.1	67.8	66.3	64.7	63.0	61.0	58.8	56.4	53.6	50.2	46.1	2.55	2.94
	20	64.8	63.4	62.0	60.4	58.6	56.7	54.5	52.1	49.2	45.9	41.8	1.91	2.28
	22	61.2	59.8	58.3	56.7	55.0	53.0	50.9	48.4	45.6	42.2	38.1	1.45	1.81
	24	58.2	56.8	55.4	53.8	52.0	50.1	47.9	45.4	42.6	39.3	35.2	1.12	1.47
44.56	18	71.9	70.5	68.9	67.2	65.4	63.3	61.1	58.5	55.5	52.0	47.7	2.55	2.94
	20	67.4	66.0	64.4	62.7	60.9	58.9	56.6	54.0	51.0	47.5	43.2	1.90	2.27
	22	63.6	62.2	60.6	58.9	57.1	55.1	52.8	50.2	47.2	43.7	39.4	1.43	1.80
	24	60.5	59.1	57.5	55.8	54.0	52.0	49.7	47.1	44.1	40.6	36.3	1.10	1.46
46.79	18	74.6	73.1	71.5	69.7	67.8	65.7	63.3	60.6	57.4	53.7	49.2	2.55	2.94
	20	70.0	68.5	66.8	65.1	63.1	61.0	58.6	55.9	52.7	49.0	44.5	1.89	2.27
	22	66.1	64.6	62.9	61.2	59.2	57.1	54.7	52.0	48.8	45.1	40.6	1.42	1.79
	24	62.8	61.3	59.7	57.9	56.0	53.8	51.4	48.7	45.6	41.9	37.4	1.09	1.44

TABLE 223

Process Times (B) at Retort Temperature of 250°F for Conduction-Heating Foods in 211 x 600 Can

f_h	z	INITIAL FOOD TEMPERATURE (T_{ih})											Equivalent	
		100	110	120	130	140	150	160	170	180	190	200	F_c^{18}	F_s^{18}
	18	49.8	48.7	47.4	46.1	44.7	43.1	41.4	39.5	37.3	34.7	31.7	2.50	2.94
37.88	20	47.9	46.7	45.5	44.2	42.8	41.2	39.5	37.5	35.3	32.8	29.8	1.97	2.40
	22	46.2	45.0	43.8	42.5	41.1	39.5	37.8	35.8	33.6	31.1	28.1	1.58	2.00
	24	44.5	43.4	42.1	40.8	39.4	37.8	36.1	34.2	32.0	29.4	26.4	1.24	1.64
	18	52.2	51.0	49.7	48.3	46.8	45.2	43.3	41.3	38.9	36.3	33.1	2.49	2.94
40.10	20	50.2	49.0	47.7	46.3	44.8	43.1	41.3	39.2	36.9	34.2	31.1	1.97	2.40
	22	48.4	47.2	45.9	44.5	43.0	41.3	39.5	37.5	35.1	32.4	29.3	1.57	1.98
	24	46.6	45.4	44.1	42.7	41.2	39.6	37.7	35.7	33.3	30.7	27.5	1.22	1.63
	18	54.6	53.3	52.0	50.5	48.9	47.2	45.2	43.1	40.6	37.8	34.4	2.49	2.94
42.33	20	52.5	51.2	49.9	48.4	46.8	45.0	43.1	40.9	38.5	35.6	32.3	1.96	2.39
	22	50.6	49.3	48.0	46.5	44.9	43.1	41.2	39.0	36.6	33.7	30.4	1.55	1.97
	24	48.7	47.4	46.1	44.6	43.0	41.3	39.3	37.2	34.7	31.9	28.5	1.21	1.61
	18	57.0	55.6	54.2	52.7	51.0	49.1	47.1	44.8	42.2	39.3	35.7	2.49	2.94
44.56	20	54.8	53.4	52.0	50.4	48.8	46.9	44.9	42.6	40.0	37.0	33.5	1.95	2.38
	22	52.8	51.4	50.0	48.4	46.8	44.9	42.9	40.6	38.0	35.0	31.5	1.54	1.96
	24	50.8	49.4	48.0	46.5	44.8	42.9	40.9	38.6	36.0	33.1	29.5	1.19	1.59
	18	59.3	57.9	56.4	54.8	53.0	51.1	49.0	46.6	43.8	40.7	37.0	2.49	2.94
46.79	20	57.0	55.6	54.1	52.5	50.7	48.8	46.6	44.2	41.5	38.4	34.7	1.94	2.38
	22	54.9	53.5	52.0	50.4	48.6	46.7	44.5	42.1	39.4	36.3	32.6	1.52	1.94
	24	52.8	51.4	49.9	48.3	46.5	44.6	42.5	40.1	37.3	34.2	30.5	1.17	1.57

TABLE 224

Process Times (B) at Retort Temperature of 260°F for Conduction-Heating Foods in 211 x 600 Can

f_h	z	INITIAL FOOD TEMPERATURE (T_{ih})											Equivalent	
		100	110	120	130	140	150	160	170	180	190	200	F_c^{18}	F_s^{18}
	18	41.9	40.9	39.7	38.5	37.2	35.8	34.2	32.5	30.5	28.3	25.8	2.45	2.94
37.88	20	40.8	39.7	38.6	37.4	36.0	34.6	33.0	31.3	29.4	27.2	24.6	1.98	2.45
	22	39.6	38.5	37.4	36.2	34.9	33.4	31.9	30.1	28.2	26.0	23.5	1.57	2.03
	24	38.6	37.5	36.4	35.2	33.8	32.4	30.8	29.1	27.2	25.0	22.4	1.27	1.71
	18	44.1	42.9	41.7	40.4	39.1	37.5	35.9	34.0	32.0	29.7	27.0	2.45	2.94
40.10	20	42.8	41.7	40.5	39.2	37.8	36.3	34.6	32.8	30.7	28.4	25.7	1.97	2.44
	22	41.6	40.4	39.2	37.9	36.5	35.0	33.4	31.5	29.5	27.2	24.5	1.55	2.01
	24	40.5	39.4	38.2	36.9	35.5	34.0	32.3	30.5	28.4	26.1	23.4	1.25	1.69
	18	46.2	45.0	43.7	42.4	40.9	39.3	37.5	35.6	33.4	31.0	28.1	2.45	2.94
42.33	20	44.9	43.7	42.4	41.0	39.6	38.0	36.2	34.3	32.1	29.7	26.8	1.95	2.43
	22	43.5	42.3	41.1	39.7	38.2	36.6	34.9	32.9	30.8	28.3	25.5	1.53	1.99
	24	42.4	41.2	39.9	38.6	37.1	35.5	33.7	31.8	29.6	27.2	24.3	1.23	1.67
	18	48.3	47.0	45.7	44.3	42.7	41.0	39.2	37.2	34.9	32.3	29.3	2.45	2.94
44.56	20	46.9	45.6	44.3	42.9	41.3	39.6	37.8	35.7	33.5	30.9	27.9	1.94	2.42
	22	45.4	44.2	42.9	41.4	39.9	38.2	36.4	34.3	32.0	29.4	26.5	1.51	1.97
	24	44.3	43.0	41.7	40.2	38.7	37.0	35.2	33.1	30.8	28.3	25.3	1.21	1.65
	18	50.4	49.1	47.7	46.2	44.5	42.8	40.8	38.7	36.3	33.6	30.4	2.45	2.94
46.79	20	48.9	47.6	46.2	44.7	43.0	41.3	39.3	37.2	34.8	32.1	28.9	1.93	2.41
	22	47.4	46.1	44.7	43.2	41.5	39.8	37.8	35.7	33.3	30.6	27.4	1.49	1.95
	24	46.1	44.8	43.4	41.9	40.3	38.5	36.6	34.4	32.0	29.3	26.2	1.19	1.64

TABLE 225

Process Times (B) at Retort Temperature of 230°F for Conduction-Heating Foods in 300 x 206 Can

f_h	z	INITIAL FOOD TEMPERATURE (T_{ih})											Equivalent	
		100	110	120	130	140	150	160	170	180	190	200	F_c^{18}	F_s^{18}
	18	77.0	76.0	75.0	73.8	72.6	71.2	69.6	67.7	65.5	62.9	59.4	2.60	2.87
27.58	20	67.8	66.8	65.8	64.6	63.3	61.9	60.3	58.5	56.3	53.6	50.2	1.88	2.15
	22	61.6	60.6	59.6	58.5	57.2	55.8	54.2	52.3	50.2	47.5	44.0	1.43	1.69
	24	56.5	55.5	54.5	53.4	52.1	50.7	49.1	47.2	45.1	42.4	38.9	1.14	1.38
	18	79.4	78.4	77.3	76.1	74.7	73.2	71.5	69.6	67.3	64.5	60.8	2.60	2.87
29.20	20	70.3	69.3	68.2	67.0	65.6	64.1	62.5	60.5	58.2	55.4	51.7	1.87	2.15
	22	63.9	62.8	61.7	60.5	59.2	57.7	56.0	54.1	51.7	48.9	45.3	1.43	1.69
	24	58.5	57.4	56.3	55.1	53.8	52.3	50.6	48.7	46.3	43.5	39.9	1.14	1.38
	18	81.8	80.7	79.5	78.3	76.9	75.3	73.5	71.4	69.0	66.0	62.2	2.59	2.87
30.82	20	72.8	71.7	70.5	69.3	67.9	66.3	64.5	62.4	60.0	57.0	53.2	1.87	2.15
	22	66.1	65.0	63.8	62.5	61.1	59.6	57.8	55.7	53.3	50.3	46.4	1.43	1.69
	24	60.4	59.3	58.1	56.8	55.4	53.9	52.1	50.0	47.6	44.6	40.7	1.11	1.36
	18	84.2	83.0	81.8	80.5	79.0	77.3	75.4	73.3	70.7	67.6	63.5	2.59	2.86
32.44	20	75.2	74.1	72.9	71.5	70.1	68.4	66.5	64.3	61.8	58.6	54.6	1.87	2.15
	22	68.2	67.1	65.8	64.5	63.0	61.3	59.5	57.3	54.7	51.6	47.5	1.43	1.69
	24	62.2	61.1	59.8	58.5	57.0	55.3	53.5	51.3	48.7	45.6	41.5	1.08	1.34
	18	86.6	85.4	84.2	82.8	81.2	79.5	77.5	75.2	72.5	69.2	64.9	2.58	2.86
34.06	20	77.6	76.4	75.2	73.7	72.2	70.4	68.5	66.2	63.5	60.2	55.9	1.86	2.15
	22	70.2	69.1	67.8	66.4	64.8	63.1	61.1	58.8	56.1	52.8	48.6	1.43	1.69
	24	63.9	62.7	61.5	60.0	58.5	56.7	54.8	52.5	49.8	46.5	42.2	1.05	1.32

TABLE 226

Process Times (B) at Retort Temperature of 240°F for Conduction-Heating Foods in 300 x 206 Can

f_h	z	INITIAL FOOD TEMPERATURE (T_{ih})											Equivalent	
		100	110	120	130	140	150	160	170	180	190	200	F_c^{18}	F_s^{18}
	18	49.8	48.9	47.9	46.9	45.7	44.5	43.1	41.5	39.6	37.4	34.8	2.51	2.86
27.58	20	46.7	45.8	44.9	43.8	42.7	41.4	40.0	38.4	36.6	34.4	31.7	1.95	2.30
	22	44.1	43.2	42.3	41.2	40.1	38.8	37.4	35.8	34.0	31.8	29.1	1.52	1.86
	24	41.9	41.0	40.1	39.0	37.9	36.6	35.2	33.6	31.8	29.6	26.9	1.20	1.54
	18	51.9	51.0	50.0	48.9	47.7	46.3	44.9	43.2	41.2	38.9	36.1	2.51	2.87
29.20	20	48.7	47.8	46.8	45.7	44.5	43.1	41.6	39.9	38.0	35.7	32.8	1.93	2.29
	22	46.0	45.0	44.0	42.9	41.7	40.4	38.9	37.2	35.2	32.9	30.1	1.50	1.84
	24	43.7	42.8	41.8	40.7	39.5	38.1	36.6	35.0	33.0	30.7	27.9	1.19	1.53
	18	54.1	53.1	52.0	50.9	49.6	48.2	46.6	44.8	42.8	40.3	37.3	2.50	2.87
30.82	20	50.7	49.7	48.6	47.5	46.2	44.8	43.2	41.4	39.3	36.9	33.9	1.91	2.27
	22	47.9	46.9	45.8	44.6	43.4	41.9	40.4	38.6	36.5	34.1	31.1	1.48	1.83
	24	45.5	44.5	43.5	42.3	41.0	39.6	38.0	36.2	34.2	31.7	28.8	1.17	1.51
	18	56.2	55.2	54.0	52.8	51.5	50.0	48.3	46.4	44.3	41.7	38.5	2.50	2.87
32.44	20	52.6	51.6	50.5	49.2	47.9	46.4	44.8	42.9	40.7	38.1	35.0	1.90	2.26
	22	49.7	48.7	47.6	46.3	45.0	43.5	41.8	40.0	37.8	35.2	32.1	1.47	1.82
	24	47.3	46.2	45.1	43.9	42.5	41.0	39.4	37.5	35.3	32.8	29.6	1.15	1.50
	18	58.3	57.2	56.0	54.7	53.3	51.7	50.0	48.0	45.7	43.0	39.7	2.50	2.87
34.06	20	54.6	53.5	52.3	51.1	49.6	48.1	46.3	44.4	42.1	39.4	36.1	1.90	2.26
	22	51.6	50.5	49.3	48.0	46.6	45.0	43.3	41.3	49.0	36.3	33.0	1.45	1.81
	24	49.1	48.0	46.8	45.5	44.1	42.5	40.8	38.8	36.5	33.8	30.5	1.14	1.49

TABLE 227

Process Times (B) at Retort Temperature of 250°F for Conduction-Heating Foods in 300 x 206 Can

f_h	z	INITIAL FOOD TEMPERATURE (T_{ih})											Equivalent	
		100	110	120	130	140	150	160	170	180	190	200	F_c^{18}	F_s^{18}
	18	38.3	37.4	36.5	35.6	34.5	33.4	32.1	30.7	29.1	27.3	25.1	2.44	2.87
27.58	20	36.8	36.0	35.1	34.1	33.1	32.0	30.7	29.3	27.7	25.8	23.7	1.98	2.39
	22	35.6	34.7	33.8	32.9	31.8	30.7	29.4	28.0	26.4	24.6	22.4	1.62	2.02
	24	34.4	33.5	32.6	31.7	30.6	29.5	28.2	26.8	25.2	23.4	21.2	1.32	1.71
	18	40.1	39.2	38.3	37.3	36.1	34.9	33.6	32.1	30.4	28.5	26.1	2.44	2.87
29.20	20	38.6	37.7	36.8	35.7	34.6	33.4	32.1	30.6	28.9	26.9	24.6	1.98	2.40
	22	37.2	36.4	35.4	34.4	33.3	32.1	30.8	29.3	27.6	25.6	23.3	1.60	2.01
	24	36.0	35.1	34.1	33.1	32.0	30.8	29.5	28.0	26.3	24.3	22.0	1.30	1.70
	18	41.9	41.0	40.0	38.9	37.7	36.5	35.0	33.5	31.7	29.6	27.2	2.43	2.87
30.82	20	40.3	39.4	38.4	37.3	36.1	34.9	33.5	31.9	30.1	28.0	25.6	1.97	2.39
	22	38.9	38.0	37.0	35.9	34.8	33.5	32.1	30.5	28.7	26.6	24.2	1.59	2.00
	24	37.6	36.6	35.6	34.6	33.4	32.1	30.7	29.1	27.4	25.3	22.8	1.28	1.68
	18	43.7	42.7	41.7	40.5	39.3	38.0	36.5	34.8	32.9	30.8	28.2	2.43	2.87
32.44	20	42.0	41.0	40.0	38.9	37.6	36.3	34.8	33.2	31.3	29.1	26.5	1.95	2.38
	22	40.5	39.6	38.5	37.4	36.2	34.8	33.3	31.7	29.8	27.6	25.1	1.58	1.99
	24	39.1	38.1	37.1	36.0	34.8	33.4	31.9	30.3	28.4	26.2	23.6	1.26	1.66
	18	45.4	44.4	43.3	42.1	40.8	39.4	37.9	36.1	34.2	31.9	29.2	2.43	2.87
34.06	20	43.7	42.7	41.6	40.4	39.1	37.7	36.1	34.4	32.4	30.1	27.5	1.94	2.36
	22	42.2	41.2	40.1	38.9	37.6	36.2	34.6	32.9	30.9	28.6	25.9	1.56	1.98
	24	40.7	39.6	38.6	37.4	36.1	34.7	33.1	31.4	29.4	27.1	24.4	1.24	1.64

TABLE 228

Process Times (B) at Retort Temperature of 260°F for Conduction-Heating Foods in 300 x 206 Can

f_h	z	INITIAL FOOD TEMPERATURE (T_{ih})											Equivalent	
		100	110	120	130	140	150	160	170	180	190	200	F_c^{18}	F_s^{18}
	18	31.8	31.0	30.2	29.3	28.3	27.3	26.1	24.9	23.5	21.9	20.0	2.39	2.87
27.58	20	31.0	30.2	29.4	28.5	27.5	26.5	25.4	24.1	22.7	21.1	19.2	1.99	2.45
	22	30.2	29.4	28.6	27.7	26.7	25.7	24.6	23.3	21.9	20.3	18.4	1.64	2.09
	24	29.4	28.7	27.8	27.0	26.0	25.0	23.8	22.6	21.1	19.5	17.7	1.35	1.79
	18	33.4	32.6	31.7	30.7	29.7	28.6	27.4	26.1	24.6	22.9	20.9	2.39	2.87
29.20	20	32.5	31.7	30.8	29.9	28.9	27.8	26.6	25.2	23.7	22.0	20.1	1.98	2.44
	22	31.7	30.8	30.0	29.0	28.0	26.9	25.7	24.4	22.9	21.2	19.2	1.62	2.07
	24	30.9	30.1	29.2	28.3	27.2	26.1	24.9	23.6	22.1	20.4	18.5	1.33	1.77
	18	35.0	34.1	33.2	32.2	31.1	29.9	28.7	27.3	25.7	23.9	21.8	2.39	2.87
30.82	20	34.1	33.2	32.3	31.3	30.2	29.0	27.8	26.4	24.8	23.0	20.9	1.96	2.43
	22	33.1	32.3	31.3	30.4	29.3	28.1	26.8	25.4	23.9	22.1	20.0	1.60	2.05
	24	32.3	31.5	30.5	29.5	28.5	27.3	26.0	24.6	23.0	21.3	19.2	1.31	1.75
	18	36.5	35.6	34.7	33.6	32.5	31.3	29.9	28.4	26.8	24.9	22.7	2.39	2.87
32.44	20	35.6	34.7	33.7	32.6	31.5	30.3	29.0	27.5	25.8	23.9	21.8	1.95	2.42
	22	34.6	33.7	32.7	31.7	30.5	29.3	28.0	26.5	24.8	23.0	20.8	1.58	2.03
	24	33.7	32.8	31.8	30.8	29.7	28.4	27.1	25.6	24.0	22.1	19.9	1.29	1.73
	18	38.1	37.2	36.1	35.0	33.9	32.6	31.2	29.6	27.9	25.9	23.6	2.39	2.87
34.06	20	37.1	36.1	35.1	34.0	32.8	31.5	30.1	28.6	26.8	24.9	22.6	1.94	2.41
	22	36.0	35.1	34.1	33.0	31.8	30.5	29.1	27.5	25.8	23.8	21.5	1.56	2.01
	24	35.1	34.2	33.2	32.1	30.9	29.6	28.2	26.6	24.9	22.9	20.6	1.27	1.71

TABLE 229

Process Times (B) at Retort Temperature of 230°F for Conduction-Heating Foods in 300 x 308 Can

f_h	z	INITIAL FOOD TEMPERATURE (T_{ih})											Equivalent	
		100	110	120	130	140	150	160	170	180	190	200	F_c^{18}	F_s^{18}
	18	93.8	92.4	91.0	89.4	87.7	85.7	83.5	81.0	77.9	74.2	69.5	2.60	2.90
38.12	20	83.8	82.5	81.1	79.5	77.7	75.8	73.6	71.0	68.0	64.3	59.6	1.89	2.17
	22	75.6	74.3	72.8	71.3	69.5	67.6	65.3	62.8	59.8	56.1	51.3	1.43	1.70
	24	69.2	67.9	66.4	64.9	63.1	61.2	59.0	56.4	53.4	49.7	44.9	1.05	1.33
	18	97.3	95.9	94.4	92.7	90.9	88.8	86.5	83.8	80.6	76.7	71.6	2.60	2.91
40.37	20	86.9	85.5	84.0	82.3	80.4	78.4	76.0	73.3	70.1	66.2	61.2	1.89	2.17
	22	78.2	76.8	75.2	73.5	71.7	69.7	67.3	64.6	61.4	57.5	52.5	1.39	1.67
	24	72.0	70.5	69.0	67.4	65.5	63.4	61.1	58.4	55.2	51.3	46.2	1.05	1.32
	18	100.8	99.2	97.7	96.0	94.0	91.8	89.4	86.5	83.1	79.0	73.7	2.60	2.91
42.61	20	89.8	88.4	86.8	85.0	83.0	80.9	78.4	75.5	72.2	68.0	62.7	1.89	2.17
	22	80.8	79.3	77.7	75.9	74.0	71.8	69.3	66.5	63.1	59.0	53.6	1.36	1.65
	24	74.6	73.1	71.5	69.8	67.8	65.6	63.2	60.3	56.9	52.8	47.5	1.03	1.31
	18	104.2	102.7	101.0	99.1	97.1	94.8	92.2	89.2	85.6	81.3	75.7	2.59	2.90
44.85	20	92.7	91.1	89.4	87.6	85.5	83.2	80.6	77.6	74.1	69.7	64.1	1.89	2.17
	22	83.7	82.1	80.5	78.6	76.5	74.3	71.6	68.6	65.1	60.7	55.1	1.36	1.65
	24	77.2	75.7	74.0	72.1	70.1	67.8	65.2	62.2	58.6	54.3	48.7	1.01	1.29
	18	107.6	105.9	104.2	102.2	100.1	97.6	94.9	91.8	88.0	83.5	77.6	2.59	2.90
47.10	20	95.5	93.8	92.0	90.1	87.9	85.5	82.8	79.7	75.9	71.4	65.5	1.89	2.17
	22	86.6	84.9	83.2	81.2	79.0	76.6	73.9	70.8	67.0	62.5	56.6	1.35	1.65
	24	79.8	78.2	76.4	74.4	72.3	69.9	67.1	64.0	60.3	55.7	49.8	1.00	1.28

TABLE 230

Process Times (B) at Retort Temperature of 240°F for Conduction-Heating Foods in 300 x 308 Can

f_h	z	INITIAL FOOD TEMPERATURE (T_{ih})											Equivalent	
		100	110	120	130	140	150	160	170	180	190	200	F_c^{18}	F_s^{18}
	18	63.7	62.4	61.1	59.7	58.1	56.3	54.4	52.2	49.6	46.6	42.9	2.53	2.90
38.12	20	59.7	58.4	57.1	55.7	54.1	52.4	50.4	48.2	45.6	42.6	38.9	1.90	2.27
	22	56.3	55.1	53.8	52.3	50.8	49.0	47.1	44.9	42.3	39.3	35.6	1.45	1.81
	24	53.6	52.4	51.0	49.6	48.0	46.3	44.3	42.1	39.6	36.5	32.8	1.13	1.48
	18	66.5	65.2	63.8	62.3	60.6	58.7	56.7	54.3	51.6	48.4	44.5	2.52	2.90
40.37	20	62.3	61.0	59.6	58.1	56.4	54.6	52.5	50.1	47.4	44.2	40.3	1.89	2.26
	22	58.8	57.5	56.1	54.6	52.9	51.1	49.0	46.7	44.0	40.8	36.9	1.44	1.80
	24	56.0	54.7	53.2	51.7	50.1	48.2	46.1	43.8	41.1	37.9	34.0	1.12	1.47
	18	69.3	67.9	66.4	64.8	63.1	61.1	58.9	56.5	53.6	50.2	46.1	2.52	2.90
42.61	20	64.9	63.6	62.1	60.5	58.7	56.8	54.6	52.1	49.3	45.9	41.8	1.88	2.26
	22	61.3	59.9	58.4	56.8	55.1	53.1	50.9	48.5	45.6	42.2	38.1	1.42	1.79
	24	58.3	56.9	55.5	53.9	52.1	50.1	48.0	45.5	42.6	39.3	35.1	1.10	1.45
	18	72.0	70.6	69.0	67.3	65.5	63.4	61.1	58.5	55.5	52.0	47.6	2.52	2.90
44.85	20	67.6	66.1	64.5	62.9	61.0	58.9	56.7	54.1	51.0	47.5	43.1	1.87	2.25
	22	63.8	62.3	60.8	59.1	57.2	55.2	52.9	50.3	47.3	43.7	39.4	1.41	1.78
	24	60.6	59.2	57.6	55.9	54.1	52.0	49.7	47.1	44.1	40.6	36.2	1.08	1.44
	18	74.8	73.3	71.7	69.9	67.9	65.8	63.4	60.6	57.5	53.8	49.2	2.52	2.90
47.10	20	70.1	68.6	67.0	65.2	63.2	61.1	58.7	55.9	52.8	49.1	44.5	1.86	2.24
	22	66.2	64.7	63.1	61.3	59.3	57.2	54.8	52.0	48.9	45.2	40.6	1.40	1.77
	24	63.0	61.4	59.8	58.0	56.1	53.9	51.5	48.8	45.6	41.9	37.3	1.07	1.43

TABLE 231

Process Times (B) at Retort Temperature of 250°F for Conduction-Heating Foods in 300 x 308 Can

f_h	z	INITIAL FOOD TEMPERATURE (T_{ih})											Equivalent	
		100	110	120	130	140	150	160	170	180	190	200	F_c^{18}	F_s^{18}
	18	50.0	48.8	47.6	46.3	44.8	43.2	41.5	39.6	37.3	34.8	31.8	2.46	2.90
38.12	20	48.0	46.9	45.7	44.3	42.9	41.3	39.6	37.6	35.4	32.9	29.8	1.95	2.38
	22	46.3	45.2	44.0	42.6	41.2	39.6	37.9	35.9	33.7	31.2	28.1	1.56	1.97
	24	44.6	43.5	42.3	40.9	39.5	37.9	36.2	34.2	32.0	29.5	26.4	1.22	1.62
	18	52.4	51.2	49.9	48.5	47.0	45.3	43.4	41.4	39.0	36.3	33.1	2.46	2.90
40.37	20	50.4	49.2	47.9	46.4	44.9	43.3	41.4	39.3	37.0	34.3	31.1	1.94	2.37
	22	48.6	47.3	46.0	44.6	43.1	41.4	39.6	37.5	35.2	32.5	29.3	1.54	1.96
	24	46.8	45.6	44.3	42.9	41.3	39.7	37.8	35.7	33.4	30.7	27.5	1.20	1.61
	18	54.8	53.5	52.1	50.7	49.1	47.3	45.3	43.2	40.7	37.8	34.5	2.46	2.90
42.61	20	52.7	51.4	50.0	48.5	46.9	45.2	43.2	41.0	38.6	35.7	32.3	1.93	2.37
	22	50.8	49.5	48.1	46.6	45.0	43.3	41.3	39.1	36.7	33.8	30.4	1.53	1.95
	24	48.9	47.6	46.2	44.7	43.1	41.4	39.4	37.2	34.8	31.9	28.5	1.18	1.59
	18	57.2	55.8	54.4	52.8	51.1	49.3	47.2	44.9	42.3	39.3	35.8	2.46	2.90
44.85	20	54.9	53.6	52.1	50.6	48.9	47.0	45.0	42.7	40.1	37.1	33.5	1.92	2.36
	22	52.9	51.6	50.1	48.6	46.9	45.0	43.0	40.7	38.1	35.1	31.5	1.51	1.93
	24	50.9	49.6	48.1	46.6	44.9	43.0	41.0	38.7	36.1	33.1	29.5	1.16	1.57
	18	59.5	58.1	56.6	55.0	53.2	51.2	49.1	46.7	43.9	40.8	37.1	2.46	2.90
47.10	20	57.2	55.8	54.3	52.6	50.8	48.9	46.7	44.3	41.6	38.4	34.7	1.91	2.35
	22	55.1	53.7	52.2	50.5	48.7	46.8	44.6	42.2	39.5	36.3	32.6	1.50	1.92
	24	53.0	51.6	50.1	48.4	46.6	44.7	42.5	40.1	37.4	34.2	30.5	1.15	1.55

TABLE 232

Process Times (B) at Retort Temperature of 260°F for Conduction-Heating Foods in 300 x 308 Can

f_h	z	INITIAL FOOD TEMPERATURE (T_{ih})											Equivalent	
		100	110	120	130	140	150	160	170	180	190	200	F_c^{18}	F_s^{18}
38.12	18	42.1	41.0	39.9	38.7	37.3	35.9	34.3	32.6	30.6	28.4	25.9	2.42	2.90
	20	40.9	39.9	38.7	37.5	36.2	34.7	33.1	31.4	29.4	27.2	24.7	1.95	2.42
	22	39.7	38.7	37.5	36.3	35.0	33.5	32.0	30.2	28.3	26.1	23.5	1.55	2.00
	24	38.7	37.7	36.5	35.3	34.0	32.5	30.9	29.2	27.2	25.0	22.5	1.25	1.69
40.37	18	44.2	43.1	41.9	40.6	39.2	37.7	36.0	34.2	32.1	29.7	27.0	2.42	2.90
	20	43.0	41.9	40.6	39.3	37.9	36.4	34.7	32.9	30.8	28.5	25.8	1.94	2.41
	22	41.7	40.6	39.4	38.1	36.7	35.1	33.5	31.6	29.6	27.2	24.5	1.53	1.98
	24	40.6	39.5	38.3	37.0	35.6	34.1	32.4	30.5	28.5	26.1	23.4	1.22	1.67
42.61	18	46.4	45.2	43.9	42.5	41.0	39.4	37.7	35.7	33.5	31.1	28.2	2.42	2.90
	20	45.0	43.8	42.6	41.2	39.7	38.1	36.3	34.4	32.2	29.7	26.9	1.93	2.40
	22	43.7	42.5	41.2	39.8	38.3	36.7	35.0	33.0	30.8	28.4	25.5	1.51	1.96
	24	42.5	41.3	40.1	38.7	37.2	35.6	33.8	31.9	29.7	27.2	24.4	1.20	1.65
44.85	18	48.5	47.2	45.9	44.4	42.9	41.2	39.3	37.3	35.0	32.4	29.4	2.42	2.90
	20	47.1	45.8	44.5	43.0	41.4	39.8	37.9	35.8	33.6	31.0	27.9	1.91	2.39
	22	45.6	44.4	43.0	41.6	40.0	38.3	36.5	34.4	32.1	29.5	26.5	1.48	1.94
	24	44.4	43.2	41.8	40.4	38.8	37.1	35.3	33.2	30.9	28.3	25.3	1.19	1.63
47.10	18	50.6	49.3	47.8	46.3	44.7	42.9	41.0	38.8	36.4	33.7	30.5	2.42	2.90
	20	49.1	47.8	46.3	44.8	43.2	41.4	39.5	37.3	34.9	32.2	29.0	1.91	2.38
	22	47.6	46.2	44.8	43.3	41.7	39.9	37.9	35.8	33.4	30.6	27.5	1.47	1.93
	24	46.3	45.0	43.5	42.0	40.4	38.6	36.7	34.5	32.1	29.4	26.2	1.17	1.62

TABLE 233

Process Times (B) at Retort Temperature of 230°F for Conduction-Heating Foods in 300 x 400 Can

f_h	z	INITIAL FOOD TEMPERATURE (T_{ih}) 100	110	120	130	140	150	160	170	180	190	200	Equivalent F_c^{18}	F_s^{18}
40.91	18	98.3	96.9	95.4	93.7	91.8	89.7	87.3	84.6	81.4	77.4	72.3	2.61	2.92
	20	87.8	86.4	84.8	83.1	81.2	79.2	76.8	74.0	70.8	66.8	61.7	1.90	2.18
	22	78.9	77.5	76.0	74.3	72.4	70.3	67.9	65.2	62.0	58.0	52.9	1.39	1.67
	24	72.7	71.3	69.8	68.1	66.2	64.1	61.7	59.0	55.7	51.8	46.7	1.05	1.33
43.32	18	102.1	100.6	98.9	97.1	95.2	92.9	90.4	87.5	84.1	79.9	74.5	2.61	2.92
	20	90.9	89.4	87.8	86.0	84.0	81.8	79.3	76.4	73.0	68.8	63.3	1.90	2.18
	22	81.8	80.3	78.7	76.9	74.9	72.7	70.2	67.3	63.9	59.7	54.2	1.37	1.65
	24	75.6	74.1	72.4	70.6	68.7	66.4	63.9	61.0	57.6	53.4	48.0	1.03	1.31
45.73	18	105.7	104.1	102.4	100.5	98.4	96.1	93.4	90.4	86.8	82.3	76.6	2.61	2.92
	20	94.0	92.4	90.6	88.8	86.7	84.3	81.7	78.6	75.0	70.6	64.8	1.90	2.18
	22	85.0	83.4	81.6	79.8	77.7	75.3	72.7	69.6	66.0	61.6	55.8	1.36	1.66
	24	78.4	76.8	75.0	73.2	71.1	68.7	66.1	63.0	59.4	55.0	49.2	1.01	1.30
48.13	18	109.3	107.6	105.8	103.8	101.6	99.1	96.3	93.1	89.3	84.6	78.6	2.61	2.92
	20	96.9	95.2	93.4	91.4	89.2	86.8	84.0	80.7	76.9	72.3	66.3	1.90	2.18
	22	88.0	86.3	84.5	82.5	80.3	77.9	75.1	71.8	68.0	63.4	57.4	1.36	1.66
	24	81.1	79.4	77.6	75.6	73.4	71.0	68.2	64.9	61.1	56.5	50.5	1.00	1.28
50.54	18	112.7	111.0	109.1	107.0	104.7	102.1	99.2	95.8	91.8	86.9	80.6	2.61	2.92
	20	99.7	98.0	96.1	94.0	91.7	89.1	86.1	82.8	78.8	73.9	67.6	1.87	2.16
	22	91.0	89.2	87.3	85.2	82.9	80.3	77.4	74.0	70.0	65.1	58.8	1.35	1.65
	24	83.8	82.0	80.1	78.0	75.7	73.1	70.2	66.8	62.8	57.9	51.6	0.98	1.27

TABLE 234

Process Times (B) at Retort Temperature of 240°F for Conduction-Heating Foods in 300 x 400 Can

f_h	z	INITIAL FOOD TEMPERATURE (T_{ih})											Equivalent	
		100	110	120	130	140	150	160	170	180	190	200	F_c^{18}	F_s^{18}
	18	67.3	65.9	64.5	63.0	61.3	59.4	57.3	54.9	52.2	49.0	45.0	2.54	2.92
40.91	20	63.0	61.7	60.3	58.7	57.0	55.2	53.1	50.7	48.0	44.7	40.8	1.90	2.27
	22	59.5	58.2	56.8	55.2	53.5	51.7	49.6	47.2	44.5	41.2	37.3	1.44	1.81
	24	56.6	55.3	53.9	52.3	50.6	48.7	46.7	44.3	41.5	38.3	34.3	1.12	1.47
	18	70.3	68.9	67.3	65.7	63.9	61.9	59.7	57.2	54.3	50.9	46.7	2.53	2.92
43.32	20	65.9	64.5	63.0	61.3	59.5	57.5	55.3	52.8	49.9	46.5	42.3	1.89	2.26
	22	62.1	60.7	59.2	57.6	55.8	53.8	51.6	49.1	46.2	42.8	38.6	1.43	1.79
	24	59.1	57.7	56.2	54.6	52.8	50.8	48.6	46.1	43.2	39.8	35.6	1.10	1.46
	18	73.2	71.7	70.1	68.4	66.5	64.4	62.1	59.4	56.4	52.8	48.3	2.53	2.92
45.73	20	68.6	67.2	65.6	63.8	62.0	59.9	57.5	54.9	51.8	48.2	43.8	1.88	2.26
	22	64.8	63.3	61.7	60.0	58.1	56.0	53.7	51.0	48.0	44.4	39.9	1.42	1.78
	24	61.6	60.1	58.6	56.8	54.9	52.8	50.5	47.9	44.8	41.2	36.7	1.08	1.44
	18	76.2	74.6	73.0	71.1	69.2	67.0	64.5	61.7	58.5	54.7	50.0	2.53	2.92
48.13	20	71.4	69.8	68.2	66.3	64.3	62.1	59.7	56.9	53.7	49.9	45.2	1.87	2.25
	22	67.4	65.9	64.2	62.4	60.4	58.2	55.7	52.9	49.7	45.9	41.2	1.40	1.77
	24	64.1	62.6	60.9	59.1	57.1	54.9	52.4	49.6	46.4	42.6	37.9	1.07	1.43
	18	79.1	77.5	75.7	73.8	71.7	69.4	66.8	63.9	60.5	56.5	51.6	2.52	2.92
50.54	20	74.1	72.5	70.8	68.9	66.8	64.4	61.9	58.9	55.5	51.5	46.7	1.86	2.24
	22	70.0	68.4	66.6	64.7	62.6	60.3	57.7	54.8	51.4	47.4	42.5	1.39	1.76
	24	66.6	64.9	63.2	61.3	59.2	56.9	54.3	51.4	48.0	44.0	39.1	1.06	1.42

TABLE 235

Process Times (B) at Retort Temperature of 250°F for Conduction-Heating Foods in 300 x 400 Can

f_h	z	INITIAL FOOD TEMPERATURE (T_{ih})											Equivalent	
		100	110	120	130	140	150	160	170	180	190	200	F_c^{18}	F_s^{18}
40.91	18	53.0	51.8	50.5	49.1	47.5	45.8	43.9	41.9	39.5	36.7	33.5	2.47	2.92
	20	51.0	49.7	48.4	47.0	45.5	43.8	41.9	39.8	37.4	34.7	31.4	1.95	2.38
	22	49.1	47.9	46.6	45.2	43.6	41.9	40.1	38.0	35.6	32.9	29.6	1.55	1.97
	24	47.3	46.1	44.8	43.4	41.8	40.1	38.2	36.2	33.8	31.0	27.8	1.21	1.61
43.32	18	55.6	54.3	52.9	51.4	49.8	48.0	46.0	43.8	41.3	38.4	34.9	2.47	2.92
	20	53.4	52.1	50.7	49.2	47.6	45.8	43.8	41.6	39.1	36.2	32.8	1.94	2.37
	22	51.5	50.2	48.8	47.3	45.7	43.9	41.9	39.7	37.2	34.3	30.8	1.53	1.95
	24	49.6	48.3	46.9	45.4	43.7	41.9	40.0	37.7	35.2	32.3	28.9	1.19	1.59
45.73	18	58.1	56.8	55.3	53.7	52.0	50.1	48.0	45.7	43.0	40.0	36.3	2.47	2.92
	20	55.9	54.5	53.0	51.4	49.7	47.8	45.7	43.4	40.7	37.7	34.0	1.93	2.36
	22	53.8	52.4	51.0	49.4	47.7	45.8	43.7	41.3	38.7	35.6	32.0	1.52	1.94
	24	51.8	50.4	48.9	47.4	45.6	43.7	41.6	39.3	36.7	33.6	30.0	1.17	1.57
48.13	18	60.7	59.2	57.7	56.0	54.2	52.2	50.0	47.5	44.7	41.5	37.7	2.47	2.92
	20	58.3	56.8	55.3	53.6	51.8	49.8	47.6	45.1	42.3	39.1	35.3	1.92	2.35
	22	56.1	54.7	53.1	51.5	49.6	47.6	45.4	43.0	40.2	37.0	33.2	1.50	1.92
	24	54.0	52.5	51.0	49.3	47.5	45.5	43.3	40.8	38.1	34.8	31.0	1.14	1.55
50.54	18	63.2	61.7	60.0	58.3	56.4	54.3	52.0	49.4	46.5	43.1	39.1	2.47	2.92
	20	60.7	59.2	57.5	55.8	53.9	51.8	49.5	46.9	43.9	40.6	36.6	1.91	2.34
	22	58.4	56.9	55.3	53.5	51.6	49.5	47.2	44.6	41.7	38.3	34.3	1.48	1.90
	24	56.2	54.7	53.0	51.3	49.4	47.3	45.0	42.4	39.4	36.1	32.1	1.13	1.53

TABLE 236

Process Times (B) at Retort Temperature of 260°F for Conduction-Heating Foods in 300 x 400 Can

f_h	z	INITIAL FOOD TEMPERATURE (T_{ih})											Equivalent	
		100	110	120	130	140	150	160	170	180	190	200	F_c^{18}	F_s^{18}
40.91	18	44.8	43.6	42.4	41.1	39.7	38.1	36.4	34.6	32.5	30.1	27.4	2.43	2.92
	20	43.5	42.4	41.1	39.8	38.4	36.9	35.2	33.3	31.2	28.8	26.1	1.95	2.42
	22	42.2	41.1	39.9	38.5	37.1	35.6	33.9	32.0	29.9	27.5	24.8	1.53	1.99
	24	41.1	40.0	38.8	37.4	36.0	34.5	32.8	30.9	28.8	26.4	23.7	1.23	1.67
43.32	18	47.1	45.9	44.6	43.2	41.7	40.0	38.2	36.2	34.0	31.5	28.6	2.43	2.92
	20	45.7	44.5	43.2	41.8	40.3	38.7	36.9	34.9	32.7	30.2	27.3	1.93	2.41
	22	44.3	43.1	41.8	40.4	38.9	37.3	35.5	33.5	31.3	28.8	25.9	1.51	1.97
	24	43.2	41.9	40.6	39.3	37.7	36.1	34.3	32.3	30.1	27.6	24.7	1.21	1.65
45.73	18	49.3	48.1	46.7	45.2	43.6	41.9	40.0	37.9	35.6	32.9	29.9	2.43	2.92
	20	47.9	46.6	45.2	43.8	42.2	40.4	38.5	36.4	34.1	31.5	28.4	1.92	2.39
	22	46.4	45.1	43.8	42.3	40.7	39.0	37.1	35.0	32.6	30.0	26.9	1.49	1.95
	24	45.2	43.9	42.5	41.1	39.5	37.7	35.8	33.8	31.4	28.8	25.7	1.19	1.63
48.13	18	51.6	50.2	48.8	47.2	45.6	43.8	41.8	39.6	37.1	34.3	31.1	2.43	2.92
	20	50.0	48.7	47.2	45.7	44.0	42.2	40.2	38.0	35.5	32.8	29.5	1.91	2.39
	22	48.5	47.1	45.7	44.1	42.5	40.7	38.7	36.5	34.0	31.2	28.0	1.47	1.93
	24	47.2	45.8	44.4	42.8	41.2	39.3	37.4	35.2	32.7	29.9	26.7	1.17	1.62
50.54	18	53.8	52.4	50.9	49.3	47.5	45.6	43.5	41.2	38.6	35.7	32.3	2.43	2.92
	20	52.2	50.8	49.3	47.6	45.9	44.0	41.9	39.6	37.0	34.0	30.7	1.90	2.38
	22	50.5	49.1	47.6	46.0	44.2	42.3	40.2	37.9	35.3	32.4	29.0	1.45	1.91
	24	49.2	47.8	46.2	44.6	42.9	41.0	38.9	36.5	34.0	31.0	27.6	1.15	1.60

TABLE 237

Process Times (B) at Retort Temperature of 230°F for Conduction-Heating Foods in 300 x 407 Can

f_h	z	INITIAL FOOD TEMPERATURE (T_{ih})											Equivalent	
		100	110	120	130	140	150	160	170	180	190	200	F_c^{18}	F_s^{18}
42.76	18	101.3	99.9	98.2	96.5	94.5	92.3	89.9	87.0	83.6	79.5	74.1	2.62	2.93
	20	90.3	88.8	87.2	85.5	83.5	81.3	78.8	76.0	72.6	68.4	63.1	1.91	2.19
	22	81.2	79.7	78.1	76.3	74.3	72.2	69.7	66.8	63.4	59.3	53.9	1.38	1.66
	24	75.0	73.5	71.9	70.1	68.2	66.0	63.5	60.7	57.3	53.1	47.8	1.04	1.32
45.27	18	105.2	103.6	101.9	100.0	98.0	95.6	93.0	90.0	86.4	82.0	76.4	2.62	2.93
	20	93.5	92.0	90.3	88.4	86.3	84.0	81.4	78.3	74.8	70.4	64.7	1.91	2.19
	22	84.5	82.9	81.2	79.3	77.2	74.9	72.3	69.3	65.7	61.3	55.6	1.37	1.66
	24	77.9	76.4	74.7	72.8	70.7	68.4	65.8	62.7	59.2	54.8	49.1	1.02	1.30
47.79	18	108.9	107.3	105.5	103.5	101.3	98.8	96.1	92.9	89.1	84.5	78.5	2.62	2.93
	20	96.6	95.0	93.2	91.2	89.0	86.6	83.8	80.6	76.8	72.2	66.2	1.91	2.19
	22	87.7	86.0	84.2	82.2	80.0	77.6	74.8	71.6	67.8	63.2	57.2	1.36	1.66
	24	80.8	79.2	77.3	75.4	73.2	70.7	68.0	64.8	61.0	56.4	50.4	1.00	1.29
50.30	18	112.6	110.8	108.9	106.8	104.5	102.0	99.0	95.7	91.7	86.8	80.5	2.62	2.93
	20	99.6	97.9	96.0	93.9	91.6	89.0	86.1	82.7	78.7	73.9	67.6	1.88	2.17
	22	90.8	89.1	87.2	85.1	82.8	80.2	77.3	73.9	69.9	65.1	58.8	1.36	1.66
	24	83.6	81.9	80.0	77.9	75.6	73.0	70.1	66.8	62.8	57.9	51.6	0.99	1.28
52.82	18	116.1	114.3	112.3	110.1	107.7	105.0	101.9	98.4	94.2	89.1	82.5	2.62	2.93
	20	102.6	100.8	98.8	96.6	94.2	91.5	88.4	84.9	80.7	75.6	69.0	1.85	2.14
	22	93.9	92.0	90.0	87.8	85.4	82.7	79.7	76.1	71.9	66.8	60.2	1.35	1.65
	24	86.4	84.6	82.6	80.4	78.0	75.3	72.2	68.7	64.5	59.4	52.8	0.97	1.26

TABLE 238

Process Times (B) at Retort Temperature of 240°F for Conduction-Heating Foods in 300 x 407 Can

f_h	z	INITIAL FOOD TEMPERATURE (T_{ih}) 100	110	120	130	140	150	160	170	180	190	200	Equivalent F_c^{18}	F_s^{18}
42.76	18	69.6	68.2	66.8	65.1	63.4	61.4	59.2	56.7	53.9	50.5	46.4	2.54	2.93
	20	65.3	63.9	62.4	60.8	59.0	57.0	54.9	52.4	49.5	46.1	42.0	1.90	2.27
	22	61.6	60.2	58.7	57.1	55.3	53.4	51.2	48.7	45.9	42.5	38.3	1.44	1.80
	24	58.6	57.2	55.7	54.1	52.3	50.4	48.2	45.7	42.9	39.5	35.3	1.11	1.47
45.27	18	72.7	71.3	69.7	68.0	66.1	64.0	61.7	59.1	56.1	52.5	48.1	2.54	2.93
	20	68.2	66.7	65.1	63.4	61.6	59.5	57.2	54.5	51.5	47.9	43.5	1.89	2.27
	22	64.4	62.9	61.3	59.6	57.7	55.7	53.4	50.7	47.7	44.1	39.7	1.42	1.79
	24	61.2	59.7	58.2	56.5	54.6	52.5	50.2	47.6	44.5	41.0	36.6	1.09	1.45
47.79	18	75.8	74.3	72.6	70.8	68.8	66.7	64.2	61.4	58.2	54.5	49.8	2.54	2.93
	20	71.1	69.5	67.9	66.0	64.1	61.9	59.4	56.7	53.5	49.7	45.1	1.88	2.26
	22	67.1	65.6	63.9	62.1	60.1	57.9	55.5	52.7	49.5	45.7	41.1	1.41	1.78
	24	63.8	62.3	60.6	58.8	56.8	54.6	52.2	49.4	46.2	42.4	37.8	1.08	1.44
50.30	18	78.9	77.3	75.5	73.6	71.6	69.3	66.7	63.8	60.4	56.4	51.5	2.53	2.93
	20	73.9	72.3	70.6	68.7	66.6	64.3	61.7	58.8	55.4	51.4	46.6	1.87	2.25
	22	69.8	68.2	66.4	64.5	62.5	60.2	57.6	54.7	51.3	47.3	42.4	1.40	1.77
	24	66.4	64.8	63.0	61.1	59.0	56.7	54.2	51.2	47.9	43.9	39.0	1.06	1.43
52.82	18	81.9	80.2	78.4	76.4	74.2	71.8	69.1	66.0	62.5	58.3	53.2	2.53	2.93
	20	76.8	75.1	73.3	71.3	69.1	66.7	64.0	60.9	57.4	53.2	48.1	1.86	2.24
	22	72.5	70.8	69.0	67.0	64.8	62.4	59.7	56.6	53.1	48.9	43.8	1.39	1.76
	24	68.9	67.2	65.4	63.4	61.2	58.8	56.1	53.0	49.5	45.3	40.2	1.05	1.42

TABLE 239

Process Times ($\bar{B}$) at Retort Temperature of 250°F for Conduction-Heating Foods in 300 x 407 Can

f_h	z	INITIAL FOOD TEMPERATURE (T_{ih})											Equivalent	
		100	110	120	130	140	150	160	170	180	190	200	F_c^{18}	F_s^{18}
42.76	18	55.0	53.8	52.4	50.9	49.3	47.5	45.6	43.4	40.9	38.0	34.6	2.48	2.93
	20	52.9	51.6	50.2	48.8	47.1	45.4	43.4	41.2	38.7	35.9	32.5	1.95	2.38
	22	51.0	49.7	48.3	46.8	45.2	43.5	41.5	39.3	36.8	34.0	30.6	1.54	1.96
	24	49.1	47.8	46.4	44.9	43.3	41.6	39.6	37.4	34.9	32.1	28.7	1.20	1.60
45.27	18	57.7	56.4	54.9	53.3	51.6	49.7	47.7	45.3	42.7	39.7	36.1	2.48	2.93
	20	55.4	54.1	52.6	51.1	49.3	47.5	45.4	43.1	40.5	37.4	33.8	1.94	2.37
	22	53.4	52.1	50.6	49.0	47.3	45.4	43.4	41.1	38.4	35.4	31.8	1.53	1.95
	24	51.4	50.1	48.6	47.0	45.3	43.4	41.4	39.1	36.4	33.4	29.8	1.17	1.58
47.79	18	60.3	58.9	57.4	55.7	53.9	51.9	49.7	47.3	44.5	41.3	37.5	2.48	2.93
	20	58.0	56.5	55.0	53.3	51.5	49.6	47.4	44.9	42.2	39.0	35.2	1.93	2.36
	22	55.8	54.4	52.9	51.2	49.4	47.4	45.2	42.8	40.0	36.8	33.0	1.51	1.93
	24	53.7	52.3	50.7	49.1	47.3	45.3	43.1	40.7	37.9	34.7	30.9	1.15	1.56
50.30	18	63.0	61.5	59.8	58.1	56.2	54.1	51.8	49.2	46.3	43.0	39.0	2.48	2.93
	20	60.5	59.0	57.4	55.6	53.7	51.6	49.3	46.7	43.8	40.5	36.5	1.92	2.35
	22	58.2	56.7	55.1	53.3	51.4	49.4	47.1	44.5	41.6	38.2	34.2	1.49	1.91
	24	56.0	54.5	52.9	51.1	49.2	47.1	44.8	42.3	39.3	36.0	32.0	1.13	1.54
52.82	18	65.6	64.0	62.3	60.5	58.5	56.3	53.9	51.2	48.1	44.6	40.4	2.47	2.93
	20	63.0	61.4	59.7	57.9	55.9	53.7	51.3	48.6	45.5	42.0	37.8	1.91	2.35
	22	60.6	59.0	57.3	55.5	53.5	51.3	48.9	46.2	43.1	39.6	35.4	1.47	1.90
	24	58.3	56.7	55.0	53.2	51.2	49.0	46.6	43.9	40.8	37.3	33.1	1.12	1.53

TABLE 240

Process Times (B) at Retort Temperature of 260°F for Conduction-Heating Foods in 300 x 407 Can

f_h	z	INITIAL FOOD TEMPERATURE (T_{ih})											Equivalent	
		100	110	120	130	140	150	160	170	180	190	200	F_c^{18}	F_s^{18}
	18	46.6	45.4	44.1	42.7	41.2	39.6	37.8	35.9	33.7	31.2	28.4	2.44	2.93
42.76	20	45.2	44.0	42.7	41.4	39.9	38.3	36.5	34.5	32.3	29.9	27.0	1.95	2.42
	22	43.9	42.7	41.4	40.0	38.5	36.9	35.1	33.2	31.0	28.5	25.6	1.52	1.98
	24	42.7	41.5	40.2	38.9	37.4	35.8	34.0	32.0	29.8	27.4	24.5	1.22	1.66
	18	48.9	47.7	46.3	44.9	43.3	41.6	39.7	37.6	35.3	32.7	29.6	2.44	2.93
45.27	20	47.5	46.2	44.9	43.4	41.8	40.1	38.3	36.2	33.9	31.2	28.2	1.93	2.41
	22	46.0	44.8	43.4	42.0	40.4	38.7	36.8	34.7	32.4	29.8	26.8	1.50	1.96
	24	44.8	43.6	42.2	40.7	39.2	37.5	35.6	33.5	31.2	28.6	25.5	1.20	1.64
	18	51.3	49.9	48.5	47.0	45.3	43.5	41.5	39.3	36.9	34.1	30.9	2.44	2.93
47.79	20	49.8	48.4	47.0	45.4	43.8	42.0	40.0	37.8	35.4	32.6	29.4	1.92	2.40
	22	48.2	46.9	45.4	43.9	42.2	40.4	38.5	36.3	33.8	31.1	27.9	1.48	1.94
	24	46.9	45.6	44.2	42.6	41.0	39.1	37.2	35.0	32.5	29.8	26.6	1.18	1.63
	18	53.6	52.2	50.7	49.1	47.3	45.4	43.4	41.1	38.5	35.6	32.2	2.44	2.93
50.30	20	52.0	50.6	49.1	47.5	45.7	43.8	41.7	39.4	36.9	33.9	30.6	1.91	2.39
	22	50.4	49.0	47.5	45.8	44.1	42.2	40.1	37.8	35.2	32.3	28.9	1.46	1.92
	24	49.0	47.6	46.1	44.5	42.7	40.8	38.7	36.4	33.9	30.9	27.6	1.16	1.61
	18	56.0	54.5	52.9	51.2	49.4	47.4	45.2	42.8	40.1	37.0	33.5	2.44	2.93
52.82	20	54.2	52.8	51.2	49.5	47.6	45.6	43.5	41.0	38.3	35.3	31.7	1.90	2.38
	22	52.5	51.0	49.5	47.8	45.9	43.9	41.7	39.3	36.6	33.6	30.0	1.45	1.91
	24	51.1	49.6	48.0	46.3	44.5	42.5	40.3	37.9	35.2	32.1	28.6	1.14	1.59

TABLE 241

Process Times (B) at Retort Temperature of 230°F for Conduction-Heating Foods in 301 x 411 Can

f_h	z	INITIAL FOOD TEMPERATURE (T_{ih})											Equivalent	
		100	110	120	130	140	150	160	170	180	190	200	F_c^{18}	F_s^{18}
45.22	18	105.2	103.7	101.9	100.1	98.0	95.7	93.1	90.0	86.5	82.1	76.4	2.62	2.94
	20	93.6	92.0	90.3	88.4	86.4	84.1	81.4	78.4	74.8	70.4	64.8	1.91	2.20
	22	84.5	82.9	81.2	79.3	77.3	75.0	72.3	69.3	65.7	61.3	55.7	1.38	1.67
	24	78.0	76.4	74.7	72.8	70.7	68.4	65.8	62.8	59.2	54.8	49.2	1.03	1.31
47.88	18	109.2	107.5	105.7	103.7	101.5	99.1	96.3	93.1	89.3	84.7	78.7	2.62	2.94
	20	96.9	95.2	93.4	91.4	89.2	86.8	84.0	80.8	77.0	72.4	66.4	1.91	2.20
	22	87.9	86.2	84.4	82.4	80.2	77.8	75.0	71.8	68.0	63.4	57.4	1.37	1.67
	24	81.0	79.3	77.5	75.6	73.4	70.9	68.1	64.9	61.1	56.5	50.5	1.01	1.29
50.54	18	113.0	111.3	109.4	107.3	105.0	102.4	99.4	96.1	92.1	87.2	80.8	2.62	2.94
	20	100.0	98.3	96.4	94.3	92.0	89.4	86.4	83.1	79.1	74.2	67.8	1.89	2.18
	22	91.2	89.4	87.5	85.4	83.1	80.5	77.6	74.2	70.2	65.3	59.0	1.36	1.66
	24	84.0	82.2	80.3	78.2	75.9	73.3	70.4	67.0	63.0	58.1	51.8	0.99	1.28
53.20	18	116.8	114.9	112.9	110.7	108.3	105.5	102.5	98.9	94.7	89.5	82.9	2.62	2.94
	20	103.3	101.4	99.4	97.2	94.8	92.0	88.9	85.4	81.2	76.0	69.4	1.85	2.15
	22	94.4	92.6	90.6	88.4	85.9	83.2	80.1	76.6	72.3	67.2	60.5	1.36	1.66
	24	87.0	85.1	83.1	80.9	78.5	75.7	72.6	69.1	64.9	59.7	53.1	0.97	1.27
55.86	18	120.4	118.4	116.3	114.0	111.5	108.6	105.4	101.6	97.2	91.8	84.8	2.62	2.94
	20	106.9	104.9	102.8	100.5	97.9	95.1	91.8	88.1	83.7	78.3	71.3	1.85	2.15
	22	97.6	95.6	93.5	91.2	88.7	85.8	82.6	78.8	74.4	69.0	62.0	1.33	1.64
	24	90.1	88.1	86.0	83.7	81.1	78.3	75.0	71.3	66.9	61.5	54.5	0.96	1.26

TABLE 242

Process Times (B) at Retort Temperature of 240°F for Conduction-Heating Foods in 301 x 411 Can

f_h	z	INITIAL FOOD TEMPERATURE (T_{ih})											Equivalent	
		100	110	120	130	140	150	160	170	180	190	200	F_c^{18}	F_s^{18}
	18	72.7	71.3	69.7	68.0	66.1	64.0	61.7	59.1	56.1	52.5	48.1	2.55	2.94
45.22	20	68.2	66.7	65.1	63.4	61.6	59.5	57.2	54.6	51.5	48.0	43.6	1.89	2.27
	22	64.3	62.9	61.3	59.6	57.7	55.7	53.4	50.7	47.7	44.1	39.7	1.43	1.80
	24	61.2	59.7	58.2	56.5	54.6	52.5	50.2	47.6	44.6	41.0	36.6	1.10	1.45
	18	76.0	74.5	72.8	71.0	69.0	66.8	64.4	61.6	58.4	54.6	50.0	2.55	2.94
47.88	20	71.2	69.7	68.0	66.2	64.2	62.0	59.6	56.8	53.6	49.8	45.2	1.88	2.26
	22	67.3	65.7	64.1	62.2	60.3	58.1	55.6	52.8	49.6	45.8	41.2	1.42	1.79
	24	64.0	62.4	60.7	58.9	57.0	54.8	52.3	49.5	46.3	42.5	37.9	1.08	1.44
	18	79.3	77.6	75.9	74.0	71.9	69.6	67.0	64.0	60.7	56.7	51.8	2.54	2.94
50.54	20	74.3	72.6	70.9	69.0	66.9	64.6	62.0	59.1	55.7	51.7	46.8	1.87	2.26
	22	70.1	68.5	66.7	64.8	62.7	60.4	57.8	54.9	51.5	47.5	42.6	1.40	1.78
	24	66.7	65.1	63.3	61.4	59.3	57.0	54.4	51.5	48.1	44.1	39.2	1.07	1.43
	18	82.5	80.8	78.9	76.9	74.7	72.3	69.5	66.5	62.9	58.7	53.5	2.54	2.94
53.20	20	77.3	75.6	73.7	71.7	69.5	67.1	64.4	61.3	57.7	53.5	48.3	1.87	2.25
	22	73.0	71.3	69.4	67.4	65.2	62.8	60.1	57.0	53.4	49.2	44.0	1.39	1.76
	24	69.4	67.7	65.8	63.8	61.6	59.2	56.4	53.4	49.8	45.6	40.4	1.06	1.42
	18	85.7	83.9	81.9	79.8	77.5	74.9	72.1	68.8	65.1	60.7	55.3	2.54	2.94
55.86	20	80.3	78.5	76.5	74.4	72.1	69.6	66.7	63.5	59.7	55.3	49.9	1.85	2.24
	22	75.8	74.0	72.1	70.0	67.7	65.1	62.3	59.0	55.3	50.9	45.4	1.38	1.75
	24	72.1	70.3	68.3	66.2	63.9	61.3	58.5	55.2	51.5	47.1	41.7	1.05	1.41

TABLE 243

Process Times (B) at Retort Temperature of 250°F for Conduction-Heating Foods in 301 x 411 Can

f_h	z	INITIAL FOOD TEMPERATURE (T_{ih})											Equivalent	
		100	110	120	130	140	150	160	170	180	190	200	F_c^{18}	F_s^{18}
45.22	18	57.7	56.3	54.9	53.3	51.6	49.7	47.7	45.3	42.7	39.7	36.1	2.49	2.94
	20	55.4	54.1	52.6	51.0	49.3	47.5	45.4	43.1	40.5	37.4	33.9	1.95	2.38
	22	53.4	52.1	50.6	49.0	47.3	45.4	43.4	41.1	38.4	35.4	31.8	1.53	1.95
	24	51.4	50.0	48.6	47.0	45.3	43.4	41.4	39.1	36.4	33.4	29.8	1.18	1.59
47.88	18	60.5	59.0	57.5	55.8	54.0	52.1	49.9	47.4	44.6	41.4	37.6	2.49	2.94
	20	58.1	56.7	55.1	53.5	51.7	49.7	47.5	45.0	42.3	39.0	35.3	1.94	2.37
	22	56.0	54.5	53.0	51.3	49.5	47.5	45.3	42.9	40.1	36.9	33.1	1.51	1.93
	24	53.8	52.4	50.9	49.2	47.4	45.4	43.2	40.8	38.0	34.8	31.0	1.16	1.57
50.54	18	63.3	61.7	60.1	58.4	56.5	54.4	52.0	49.5	46.5	43.1	39.1	2.49	2.94
	20	60.8	59.2	57.6	55.9	53.9	51.9	49.5	47.0	44.0	40.6	36.6	1.92	2.36
	22	58.5	57.0	55.3	53.6	51.7	49.6	47.3	44.7	41.8	38.4	34.4	1.49	1.92
	24	56.2	54.7	53.1	51.3	49.4	47.3	45.0	42.4	39.5	36.1	32.1	1.14	1.55
53.20	18	66.0	64.5	62.7	60.9	58.9	56.7	54.2	51.5	48.4	44.9	40.7	2.48	2.94
	20	63.4	60.8	60.1	58.3	56.2	54.0	51.6	48.9	45.8	42.2	38.0	1.91	2.35
	22	61.0	59.4	57.7	55.9	53.8	51.6	49.2	46.5	43.4	39.8	35.6	1.48	1.90
	24	58.7	57.1	55.4	53.5	51.5	49.3	46.9	44.1	41.1	37.5	33.3	1.12	1.53
55.86	18	68.8	67.1	65.3	63.4	61.3	59.0	56.4	53.6	50.3	46.6	42.2	2.48	2.94
	20	66.0	64.4	62.6	60.6	58.5	56.2	53.7	50.8	47.6	43.8	39.4	1.91	2.35
	22	63.5	61.8	60.0	58.1	56.0	53.7	51.1	48.3	45.0	41.3	36.9	1.46	1.89
	24	61.1	59.4	57.6	55.7	53.5	51.2	48.7	45.8	42.6	38.8	34.4	1.11	1.52

TABLE 244

Process Times (B) at Retort Temperature of 260°F for Conduction-Heating Foods in 301 x 411 Can

f_h	z	INITIAL FOOD TEMPERATURE (T_{ih})											Equivalent	
		100	110	120	130	140	150	160	170	180	190	200	F_c^{18}	F_s^{18}
	18	48.9	47.6	46.3	44.8	43.3	41.6	39.7	37.6	35.3	32.7	29.6	2.45	2.94
45.22	20	47.5	46.2	44.8	43.4	41.8	40.1	38.2	36.2	33.9	31.2	28.2	1.94	2.41
	22	46.0	44.8	43.4	41.9	40.4	38.7	36.8	34.7	32.4	29.8	26.8	1.51	1.96
	24	44.8	43.5	42.2	40.7	39.2	37.4	35.6	33.5	31.2	28.6	25.5	1.20	1.65
	18	51.4	50.1	48.6	47.1	45.4	43.6	41.6	39.4	37.0	34.2	31.0	2.45	2.94
47.88	20	49.9	48.5	47.1	45.5	43.9	42.1	40.1	37.9	35.5	32.7	29.5	1.93	2.40
	22	48.3	47.0	45.5	44.0	42.3	40.5	38.5	36.4	33.9	31.1	27.9	1.48	1.94
	24	47.0	45.7	44.3	42.7	41.0	39.2	37.3	35.1	32.6	29.8	26.6	1.18	1.63
	18	53.9	52.5	50.9	49.3	47.6	45.7	43.6	41.2	38.7	35.7	32.3	2.45	2.94
50.54	20	52.2	50.8	49.3	47.7	45.9	44.0	41.9	39.6	37.0	34.1	30.7	1.92	2.39
	22	50.6	49.2	47.7	46.0	44.3	42.4	40.3	38.0	35.4	32.5	29.1	1.47	1.93
	24	49.2	47.8	46.3	44.7	42.9	41.0	38.9	36.6	34.0	31.1	27.7	1.16	1.61
	18	56.3	54.8	53.3	51.5	49.7	47.7	45.5	43.0	40.3	37.2	33.7	2.44	2.94
53.22	20	54.6	53.1	51.5	49.8	48.0	45.9	43.7	41.3	38.6	35.5	31.9	1.90	2.38
	22	52.9	51.4	49.8	48.1	46.2	44.2	42.0	39.6	36.9	33.8	30.2	1.45	1.92
	24	51.4	49.9	48.3	46.6	44.8	42.8	40.6	38.1	35.4	32.3	28.8	1.14	1.59
	18	58.8	57.2	55.5	53.7	51.8	49.7	47.4	44.8	42.0	38.7	35.0	2.44	2.94
55.86	20	57.0	55.4	53.7	51.9	50.0	47.9	45.6	43.0	40.1	36.9	33.2	1.89	2.37
	22	55.1	53.6	51.9	50.1	48.2	46.1	43.7	41.2	38.3	35.1	31.4	1.44	1.91
	24	53.6	52.0	50.4	48.6	46.6	44.5	42.2	39.6	36.8	33.5	29.8	1.13	1.58

TABLE 245

Process Times (B) at Retort Temperature of 230°F for Conduction-Heating Foods in 303 x 406 Can

f_h	z	INITIAL FOOD TEMPERATURE (T_{ih})											Equivalent	
		100	110	120	130	140	150	160	170	180	190	200	F_c^{18}	F_s^{18}
47.10	18	108.1	106.4	104.6	102.7	100.5	98.1	95.4	92.2	88.5	83.9	78.1	2.63	2.94
	20	95.9	94.3	92.5	90.6	88.4	86.0	83.3	80.1	76.4	71.8	65.9	1.91	2.20
	22	86.9	85.3	83.5	81.5	79.4	77.0	74.2	71.1	67.4	62.8	56.9	1.37	1.67
	24	80.1	78.5	76.7	74.8	72.6	70.2	67.5	64.3	60.6	56.0	50.1	1.01	1.30
49.87	18	112.1	110.4	108.5	106.4	104.1	101.6	98.7	95.3	91.4	86.6	80.3	2.62	2.94
	20	99.3	97.5	95.6	93.6	91.3	88.7	85.9	82.5	78.6	73.7	67.5	1.90	2.19
	22	90.4	88.6	86.8	84.7	82.4	79.9	77.0	73.6	69.7	64.8	58.6	1.37	1.66
	24	83.3	81.5	79.6	77.6	75.3	72.7	69.9	66.5	62.6	57.7	51.5	1.00	1.29
52.64	18	116.0	114.2	112.2	110.0	107.6	104.9	101.8	98.3	94.2	89.1	82.5	2.62	2.94
	20	102.5	100.7	98.7	96.5	94.1	91.4	88.3	84.8	80.6	75.5	69.0	1.85	2.15
	22	93.8	91.9	89.9	87.8	85.3	82.7	79.6	76.1	71.9	66.8	60.2	1.36	1.66
	24	86.3	84.5	82.5	80.3	77.9	75.2	72.2	68.6	64.5	59.4	52.8	0.98	1.27
55.42	18	119.8	117.9	115.8	113.5	110.9	108.1	104.9	101.2	96.8	91.4	84.5	2.62	2.94
	20	106.3	104.3	102.2	100.0	97.4	94.6	91.4	87.7	83.3	77.9	71.0	1.85	2.15
	22	97.1	95.1	93.0	90.7	88.2	85.4	82.2	78.4	74.1	68.7	61.8	1.34	1.64
	24	89.6	87.6	85.5	83.2	80.7	77.9	74.7	70.9	66.6	61.2	54.3	0.97	1.26
58.19	18	123.5	121.5	119.3	116.8	114.2	111.2	107.8	103.9	99.3	93.7	86.4	2.62	2.94
	20	110.0	107.9	105.7	103.3	100.7	97.7	94.3	90.4	85.8	80.2	72.9	1.84	2.15
	22	100.3	98.3	96.1	93.7	91.0	88.0	84.7	80.8	76.2	70.5	63.3	1.32	1.62
	24	92.7	90.7	88.5	86.1	83.5	80.5	77.1	73.2	68.6	63.0	55.7	0.96	1.26

TABLE 246

Process Times (B) at Retort Temperature of 240°F for Conduction-Heating Foods in 303 x 406 Can

f_h	z	INITIAL FOOD TEMPERATURE (T_{ih})											Equivalent	
		100	110	120	130	140	150	160	170	180	190	200	F_c^{18}	F_s^{18}
	18	75.0	73.5	71.9	70.1	68.2	66.0	63.6	60.9	57.7	54.0	49.4	2.55	2.94
47.10	20	70.3	68.8	67.2	65.4	63.5	61.3	58.9	56.2	53.0	49.3	44.7	1.89	2.27
	22	66.4	64.9	63.3	61.5	59.5	57.4	55.0	52.2	49.1	45.4	40.8	1.42	1.79
	24	63.1	61.6	60.0	58.2	56.3	54.1	51.7	49.0	45.8	42.1	37.5	1.08	1.44
	18	78.4	76.8	75.1	73.2	71.2	68.9	66.3	63.4	60.1	56.1	51.3	2.54	2.94
49.87	20	73.5	71.9	70.2	68.3	66.2	63.9	61.4	58.5	55.2	51.2	46.4	1.88	2.26
	22	69.4	67.8	66.1	64.2	62.1	59.8	57.3	54.4	51.1	47.1	42.3	1.41	1.78
	24	66.0	64.4	62.7	60.8	58.7	56.4	53.9	51.0	47.7	43.7	38.9	1.07	1.43
	18	81.8	80.1	78.3	76.3	74.1	71.7	69.0	66.0	62.4	58.3	53.2	2.54	2.94
52.64	20	76.7	75.0	73.1	71.1	69.0	66.6	63.9	60.8	57.3	53.1	48.0	1.87	2.25
	22	72.4	70.7	68.9	66.9	64.7	62.3	59.6	56.6	53.0	48.9	43.8	1.39	1.77
	24	68.8	67.1	65.3	63.3	61.1	58.7	56.0	53.0	49.4	45.3	40.2	1.06	1.42
	18	85.1	83.3	81.4	79.3	77.0	74.5	71.7	68.4	64.7	60.3	55.0	2.54	2.94
55.42	20	79.8	78.0	76.1	74.0	71.7	69.1	66.3	63.1	59.4	55.0	49.6	1.86	2.24
	22	75.4	73.6	71.7	69.6	67.3	64.7	61.9	58.7	55.0	50.6	45.2	1.38	1.76
	24	71.6	69.8	67.9	65.8	63.5	61.0	58.1	54.9	51.2	46.8	41.5	1.05	1.41
	18	88.4	86.6	84.6	82.4	79.9	77.3	74.3	70.9	67.0	62.4	56.8	2.54	2.94
58.19	20	82.9	81.0	79.0	76.8	74.4	71.7	68.8	65.4	61.5	56.9	51.2	1.85	2.24
	22	78.3	76.4	74.4	72.2	69.8	67.1	64.1	60.8	56.9	52.3	46.6	1.37	1.74
	24	74.4	72.5	70.5	68.3	65.9	63.2	60.2	56.9	53.0	48.4	42.7	1.04	1.40

TABLE 247

Process Times (B) at Retort Temperature of 250°F for Conduction-Heating Foods in 303 x 406 Can

f_h	z	INITIAL FOOD TEMPERATURE (T_{ih})											Equivalent	
		100	110	120	130	140	150	160	170	180	190	200	F_c^{18}	F_s^{18}
	18	59.7	58.3	56.7	55.1	53.3	51.4	49.2	46.8	44.1	40.9	37.2	2.49	2.94
47.10	20	57.3	55.9	54.4	52.8	51.0	49.0	46.9	44.5	41.7	38.6	34.8	1.94	2.38
	22	55.2	53.8	52.3	50.6	48.9	46.9	44.8	42.4	39.6	36.5	32.7	1.52	1.94
	24	53.1	51.7	50.2	48.6	46.8	44.8	42.7	40.3	37.5	34.4	30.7	1.17	1.57
	18	62.6	61.1	59.5	57.7	55.8	53.8	51.5	48.9	46.1	42.7	38.8	2.49	2.94
49.87	20	60.1	58.6	57.0	55.2	53.4	51.3	49.0	46.5	43.6	40.2	36.3	1.93	2.36
	22	57.8	56.4	54.7	53.0	51.1	49.1	46.8	44.2	41.3	38.0	34.1	1.50	1.92
	24	55.6	54.1	52.5	50.8	48.9	46.9	44.6	42.0	39.1	35.8	31.8	1.14	1.55
	18	65.5	63.9	62.2	60.4	58.4	56.2	53.8	51.1	48.0	44.5	40.4	2.48	2.94
52.64	20	62.9	61.3	59.6	57.8	55.8	53.6	51.2	48.5	45.4	41.9	37.7	1.92	2.35
	22	60.5	58.9	57.2	55.4	53.4	51.2	48.8	46.1	43.1	39.5	35.4	1.48	1.91
	24	58.2	56.6	54.9	53.1	51.1	48.9	46.5	43.8	40.7	37.2	33.0	1.13	1.53
	18	68.3	66.7	64.9	63.0	60.9	58.6	56.1	53.2	50.0	46.3	41.9	2.48	2.94
55.42	20	65.6	63.9	62.2	60.2	58.1	55.8	53.3	50.5	47.3	43.6	39.2	1.91	2.35
	22	63.1	61.4	59.7	57.7	55.6	53.3	50.8	48.0	44.8	41.0	36.7	1.47	1.89
	24	60.7	59.0	57.2	55.3	53.2	50.9	48.4	45.5	42.3	38.6	34.2	1.11	1.52
	18	71.2	69.5	67.6	65.6	63.4	61.0	58.3	55.3	51.9	48.0	43.4	2.48	2.94
58.19	20	68.3	66.6	64.7	62.7	60.5	58.1	55.4	52.4	49.1	45.2	40.6	1.90	2.34
	22	65.7	63.9	62.1	60.0	57.9	55.4	52.8	49.8	46.4	42.5	37.9	1.45	1.88
	24	63.1	61.4	59.5	57.5	55.3	52.9	50.2	47.3	43.9	40.0	35.4	1.09	1.50

TABLE 248

Process Times (B) at Retort Temperature of 260°F for Conduction-Heating Foods in 303 x 406 Can

f_h	z	INITIAL FOOD TEMPERATURE (T_{ih})											Equivalent	
		100	110	120	130	140	150	160	170	180	190	200	F_c^{18}	F_s^{18}
	18	50.7	49.4	47.9	46.4	44.8	43.0	41.1	38.9	36.5	33.8	30.6	2.45	2.94
47.10	20	49.2	47.8	46.4	44.9	43.3	41.5	39.5	37.4	35.0	32.3	29.1	1.93	2.41
	22	47.6	46.3	44.9	43.4	41.8	40.0	38.0	35.9	33.5	30.7	27.6	1.49	1.95
	24	46.4	45.1	43.6	42.1	40.5	38.7	36.8	34.6	32.2	29.5	26.3	1.19	1.64
	18	53.3	51.9	50.4	48.8	47.0	45.1	43.1	40.8	38.2	35.4	32.0	2.45	2.94
49.87	20	51.6	50.3	48.8	47.2	45.4	43.5	41.5	39.2	36.6	33.7	30.4	1.92	2.40
	22	50.0	48.6	47.1	45.5	43.8	41.9	39.9	37.6	35.0	32.1	28.8	1.47	1.93
	24	48.7	47.3	45.8	44.2	42.4	40.6	38.5	36.2	33.7	30.8	27.4	1.17	1.62
	18	55.8	54.3	52.8	51.1	49.2	47.3	45.1	42.7	40.0	36.9	33.4	2.45	2.94
52.64	20	54.1	52.6	51.1	49.4	47.5	45.5	43.4	41.0	38.3	35.2	31.7	1.91	2.38
	22	52.4	50.9	49.4	47.7	45.8	43.8	41.7	39.3	36.6	33.5	30.0	1.46	1.92
	24	51.0	49.5	47.9	46.2	44.4	42.4	40.2	37.8	35.1	32.1	28.5	1.15	1.60
	18	58.4	56.8	55.2	53.4	51.5	49.4	47.1	44.5	41.7	38.5	34.8	2.44	2.94
55.42	20	56.6	55.0	53.3	51.6	49.6	47.5	45.2	42.7	39.9	36.7	33.0	1.89	2.37
	22	54.8	53.2	51.6	49.8	47.8	45.8	43.5	40.9	38.1	34.9	31.2	1.44	1.91
	24	53.2	51.7	50.0	48.2	46.3	44.2	41.9	39.4	36.6	33.3	29.6	1.13	1.58
	18	60.9	59.3	57.5	55.7	53.6	51.4	49.0	46.4	43.4	40.0	36.1	2.44	2.94
58.19	20	59.0	57.4	55.6	53.8	51.7	49.5	47.1	44.5	41.5	38.1	34.2	1.88	2.36
	22	57.1	55.5	53.7	51.9	49.8	47.6	45.2	42.6	39.6	36.2	32.3	1.43	1.90
	24	55.5	53.9	52.1	50.3	48.2	46.0	43.6	41.0	38.0	34.6	30.7	1.11	1.56

TABLE 249

Process Times (B) at Retort Temperature of 230°F for Conduction-Heating Foods in 303 x 509 Can

f_h	z	INITIAL FOOD TEMPERATURE (T_{ih}) 100	110	120	130	140	150	160	170	180	190	200	Equivalent F_c^{18}	F_s^{18}
51.26	18	114.4	112.6	110.7	108.6	106.2	103.6	100.6	97.2	93.1	88.2	81.8	2.65	2.96
	20	101.2	99.4	97.5	95.4	93.0	90.4	87.4	84.0	80.0	75.0	68.6	1.90	2.19
	22	92.3	90.5	88.6	86.5	84.1	81.5	78.5	75.1	71.1	66.1	59.7	1.38	1.67
	24	85.0	83.3	81.3	79.2	76.9	74.2	71.3	67.8	63.8	58.8	52.4	1.00	1.29
54.28	18	118.6	116.7	114.7	112.4	109.9	107.2	104.0	100.4	96.1	90.8	84.1	2.65	2.96
	20	105.0	103.1	101.0	98.8	96.3	93.5	90.4	86.8	82.5	77.2	70.4	1.87	2.17
	22	96.0	94.1	92.0	89.8	87.3	84.5	81.4	77.7	73.4	68.2	61.4	1.36	1.66
	24	88.4	86.5	84.5	82.2	79.8	77.0	73.8	70.2	65.9	60.6	53.9	0.98	1.28
57.29	18	122.7	120.7	118.5	116.2	113.5	110.6	107.3	103.4	98.9	93.4	86.2	2.65	2.96
	20	109.1	107.1	104.9	102.5	99.9	97.0	93.7	89.8	85.3	79.7	72.6	1.86	2.17
	22	99.5	97.5	95.4	93.0	90.4	87.5	84.1	80.3	75.8	70.2	63.1	1.34	1.64
	24	91.9	90.0	87.8	85.4	82.8	79.9	76.5	72.7	68.2	62.6	55.5	0.97	1.27
60.31	18	126.6	124.5	122.3	119.8	117.0	113.9	110.4	106.4	101.6	95.8	88.2	2.65	2.96
	20	113.0	110.9	108.6	106.2	103.4	100.3	96.8	92.8	88.0	82.2	74.6	1.85	2.17
	22	103.1	101.0	98.7	96.2	93.4	90.3	86.8	82.8	78.0	72.2	64.7	1.32	1.63
	24	95.4	93.3	91.0	88.5	85.8	82.7	79.2	75.1	70.4	64.5	57.0	0.96	1.26
63.33	18	130.4	128.2	125.9	123.2	120.3	117.1	113.4	109.2	104.2	98.0	90.1	2.65	2.96
	20	116.9	114.7	112.3	109.7	106.8	103.6	99.9	95.6	90.6	84.5	76.6	1.85	2.17
	22	106.5	104.3	101.9	99.3	96.4	93.1	89.5	85.2	80.2	74.1	66.2	1.30	1.61
	24	98.8	96.6	94.2	91.5	88.6	85.4	81.7	77.5	72.5	66.3	58.4	0.95	1.25

TABLE 250

Process Times (B) at Retort Temperature of 240°F for Conduction-Heating Foods in 303 x 509 Can

f_h	z	INITIAL FOOD TEMPERATURE (T_{ih})											Equivalent	
		100	110	120	130	140	150	160	170	180	190	200	F_c^{18}	F_s^{18}
	18	80.3	78.6	76.9	74.9	72.8	70.5	67.8	64.9	61.4	57.4	52.4	2.57	2.96
51.26	20	75.2	73.6	71.8	69.9	67.7	65.4	62.8	59.8	56.4	52.3	47.3	1.89	2.27
	22	71.0	69.4	67.6	65.7	63.5	61.2	58.6	55.6	52.2	48.1	43.1	1.42	1.79
	24	67.5	65.9	64.1	62.2	60.1	57.7	55.1	52.1	48.7	44.6	39.7	1.08	1.44
	18	83.9	82.2	80.3	78.2	76.0	73.5	70.7	67.6	63.9	59.7	54.4	2.56	2.96
54.28	20	78.7	76.9	75.0	73.0	70.7	68.2	65.5	62.3	58.7	54.4	49.1	1.88	2.27
	22	74.3	72.5	70.7	68.6	66.4	63.9	61.1	58.0	54.3	50.0	44.8	1.40	1.78
	24	70.6	68.9	67.0	64.9	62.7	60.2	57.4	54.3	50.6	46.3	41.1	1.06	1.43
	18	87.5	85.7	83.7	81.5	79.2	76.5	73.6	70.3	66.5	61.9	56.4	2.56	2.96
57.29	20	82.0	80.2	78.2	76.0	73.7	71.0	68.1	64.8	61.0	56.4	50.9	1.87	2.26
	22	77.5	75.6	73.7	71.5	69.1	66.5	63.6	60.2	56.4	51.9	46.3	1.38	1.76
	24	73.6	71.8	69.8	67.6	65.3	62.6	59.7	56.4	52.6	48.0	42.5	1.05	1.42
	18	91.1	89.2	87.1	84.8	82.3	79.6	76.5	73.0	68.9	64.2	58.3	2.56	2.96
60.31	20	85.4	83.5	81.4	79.1	76.6	73.8	70.8	67.3	63.2	58.5	52.6	1.86	2.26
	22	80.7	78.7	76.6	74.4	71.9	69.1	66.0	62.5	58.5	53.7	47.9	1.37	1.75
	24	76.6	74.7	72.6	70.3	67.8	65.1	62.0	58.5	54.4	49.7	43.8	1.04	1.40
	18	94.7	92.6	90.4	88.0	85.4	82.5	79.3	75.6	71.4	66.4	60.2	2.55	2.96
63.33	20	88.8	86.7	84.5	82.1	79.5	76.6	73.4	69.7	65.5	60.4	54.3	1.85	2.25
	22	83.9	81.8	79.6	77.2	74.6	71.7	68.5	64.8	60.5	55.5	49.4	1.36	1.75
	24	79.6	77.6	75.4	73.0	70.4	67.5	64.2	60.6	56.3	51.3	45.2	1.02	1.39

TABLE 251

Process Times (B) at Retort Temperature of 250°F for Conduction-Heating Foods in 303 x 509 Can

f_h	z	Initial Food Temperature (T_{ih}): 100	110	120	130	140	150	160	170	180	190	200	Equivalent: F_c^{18}	F_s^{18}
51.26	18	64.1	62.6	60.9	59.1	57.2	55.1	52.7	50.1	47.1	43.7	39.7	2.51	2.96
	20	61.6	60.0	58.4	56.6	54.7	52.5	50.2	47.6	44.6	41.2	37.1	1.94	2.38
	22	59.3	57.7	56.1	54.3	52.4	50.2	47.9	45.3	42.3	38.9	34.8	1.51	1.93
	24	57.0	55.5	53.8	52.0	50.1	48.0	45.6	43.0	40.0	36.6	32.5	1.15	1.56
54.28	18	67.3	65.6	63.9	62.0	60.0	57.7	55.2	52.4	49.3	45.7	41.4	2.51	2.96
	20	64.6	62.9	61.2	59.3	57.3	55.0	52.5	49.8	46.6	43.0	38.7	1.93	2.37
	22	62.1	60.5	58.8	56.9	54.8	52.6	50.1	47.3	44.2	40.5	36.2	1.49	1.91
	24	59.7	58.1	56.4	54.5	52.4	50.2	47.7	44.9	41.8	38.1	33.8	1.13	1.54
57.29	18	70.4	68.7	66.8	64.8	62.7	60.3	57.7	54.7	51.4	47.6	43.0	2.50	2.96
	20	67.6	65.8	64.0	62.0	59.8	57.5	54.8	51.9	48.6	44.8	40.2	1.92	2.36
	22	65.0	63.2	61.4	59.4	57.2	54.9	52.2	49.3	46.0	42.2	37.6	1.47	1.90
	24	62.4	60.7	58.9	56.9	54.7	52.4	49.7	46.8	43.5	39.6	35.1	1.11	1.52
60.31	18	73.5	71.7	69.7	67.6	65.4	62.9	60.1	57.0	53.5	49.5	44.7	2.50	2.96
	20	70.5	68.7	66.8	64.7	62.4	59.9	57.1	54.0	50.5	46.5	41.7	1.91	2.35
	22	67.8	66.0	64.0	61.9	59.6	57.1	54.4	51.3	47.8	43.8	39.0	1.45	1.88
	24	65.1	63.3	61.4	59.3	57.0	54.5	51.7	48.7	45.2	41.1	36.4	1.09	1.50
63.33	18	76.6	74.7	72.6	70.4	68.0	65.4	62.5	59.3	55.6	51.4	46.3	2.50	2.96
	20	73.4	71.5	69.5	67.3	64.9	62.3	59.4	56.1	52.5	48.2	43.2	1.90	2.34
	22	70.5	68.6	66.6	64.4	62.0	59.4	56.5	53.2	49.6	45.3	40.3	1.43	1.86
	24	67.8	65.9	63.8	61.6	59.3	56.6	53.7	50.5	46.8	42.6	37.6	1.07	1.49

TABLE 252

Process Times (B) at Retort Temperature of 260°F for Conduction-Heating Foods in 303 x 509 Can

f_h	z	100	110	120	130	140	150	160	170	180	190	200	Equivalent F_c^{18}	Equivalent F_s^{18}
		INITIAL FOOD TEMPERATURE (T_{ih})												
51.26	18	54.6	53.2	51.6	50.0	48.2	46.3	44.1	41.8	39.2	36.2	32.8	2.47	2.96
	20	53.0	51.5	50.0	48.3	46.5	44.6	42.5	40.1	37.5	34.5	31.1	1.93	2.41
	22	51.3	49.9	48.3	46.7	44.9	42.9	40.8	38.5	35.9	32.9	29.5	1.48	1.94
	24	49.9	48.5	46.9	45.3	43.5	41.6	39.4	37.1	34.5	31.5	28.1	1.17	1.62
54.28	18	57.4	55.9	54.2	52.5	50.6	48.6	46.3	43.8	41.1	37.9	34.3	2.47	2.96
	20	55.6	54.1	52.5	50.7	48.8	46.8	44.5	42.1	39.3	36.1	32.5	1.92	2.40
	22	53.9	52.3	50.7	49.0	47.1	45.0	42.8	40.3	37.5	34.4	30.7	1.46	1.93
	24	52.4	50.9	49.2	47.5	45.6	43.5	41.3	38.8	36.0	32.9	29.3	1.15	1.60
57.29	18	60.2	58.6	56.8	55.0	53.0	50.8	48.5	45.8	42.9	39.6	35.8	2.47	2.96
	20	58.3	56.7	55.0	53.1	51.1	49.0	46.6	44.0	41.0	37.7	33.9	1.90	2.38
	22	56.4	54.8	53.1	51.3	49.3	47.1	44.7	42.1	39.2	35.9	32.0	1.45	1.92
	24	54.8	53.2	51.5	49.7	47.7	45.5	43.1	40.5	37.6	34.3	30.4	1.13	1.58
60.31	18	62.9	61.2	59.4	57.5	55.4	53.1	50.6	47.8	44.8	41.3	37.2	2.46	2.96
	20	60.9	59.2	57.4	55.5	53.4	51.1	48.6	45.9	42.8	39.3	35.2	1.89	2.37
	22	59.0	57.3	55.5	53.5	51.4	49.2	46.7	43.9	40.8	37.3	33.3	1.44	1.90
	24	57.3	55.6	53.8	51.9	49.8	47.5	45.0	42.2	39.1	35.6	31.6	1.11	1.57
63.33	18	65.7	63.9	62.0	59.9	57.7	55.4	52.7	49.8	46.6	42.9	38.7	2.46	2.96
	20	63.6	61.8	59.9	57.8	55.6	53.3	50.6	47.7	44.5	40.8	36.6	1.87	2.36
	22	61.5	59.7	57.8	55.8	53.6	51.2	48.6	45.7	42.4	38.8	34.5	1.42	1.89
	24	59.7	58.0	56.1	54.0	51.8	49.4	46.8	43.9	40.7	37.0	32.8	1.10	1.55

TABLE 253

Process Times (B) at Retort Temperature of 230°F for Conduction-Heating Foods in 307 x 113 Can

f_h	z	INITIAL FOOD TEMPERATURE (T_{ih})											Equivalent	
		100	110	120	130	140	150	160	170	180	190	200	F_c^{18}	F_s^{18}
	18	67.3	66.5	65.7	64.9	63.9	62.8	61.6	60.2	58.5	56.5	53.8	2.61	2.86
21.09	20	58.1	57.4	56.6	55.7	54.7	53.7	52.4	51.0	49.4	47.3	44.7	1.93	2.17
	22	51.9	51.1	50.3	49.5	48.5	47.4	46.2	44.8	43.1	41.1	38.4	1.44	1.69
	24	47.8	47.1	46.3	45.4	44.4	43.4	42.1	40.7	39.0	37.0	34.4	1.14	1.38
	18	69.2	68.4	67.6	66.6	65.6	64.5	63.2	61.7	59.9	57.7	55.0	2.61	2.86
22.33	20	59.9	59.1	58.3	57.4	56.4	55.2	53.9	52.4	50.6	48.5	45.7	1.93	2.17
	22	53.8	53.0	52.2	51.3	50.2	49.1	47.8	46.3	44.5	42.4	39.6	1.44	1.69
	24	49.6	48.8	47.9	47.0	46.0	44.9	43.6	42.1	40.3	38.1	35.3	1.14	1.37
	18	70.9	70.1	69.2	68.2	67.2	66.0	64.6	63.0	61.1	58.9	55.9	2.61	2.86
23.57	20	61.7	60.9	60.0	59.0	57.9	56.7	55.3	53.8	51.9	49.6	46.7	1.92	2.17
	22	55.7	54.9	54.0	53.0	51.9	50.7	49.4	47.8	45.9	43.6	40.7	1.43	1.69
	24	51.3	50.4	49.6	48.6	47.5	46.3	44.9	43.4	41.5	39.2	36.3	1.13	1.37
	18	72.9	72.0	71.1	70.0	68.9	67.6	66.2	64.5	62.6	60.2	57.1	2.60	2.86
24.81	20	63.5	62.6	61.7	60.6	59.5	58.2	56.8	55.1	53.2	50.8	47.7	1.91	2.17
	22	57.6	56.7	55.8	54.7	53.6	52.3	50.9	49.2	47.3	44.9	41.8	1.43	1.69
	24	52.9	52.1	51.1	50.1	49.0	47.7	46.3	44.6	42.6	40.2	37.1	1.13	1.37
	18	74.7	73.8	72.8	71.7	70.5	69.2	67.7	65.9	63.9	61.4	58.1	2.60	2.86
26.05	20	65.2	64.3	63.4	62.3	61.1	59.7	58.2	56.5	54.4	51.9	48.7	1.88	2.15
	22	59.4	58.5	57.5	56.4	55.2	53.9	52.4	50.6	48.6	46.0	42.8	1.43	1.68
	24	54.5	53.6	52.7	51.6	50.4	49.1	47.5	45.8	43.7	41.2	38.0	1.13	1.37

TABLE 254

Process Times (B) at Retort Temperature of 240°F for Conduction-Heating Foods in 307 x 113 Can

INITIAL FOOD TEMPERATURE (T_{ih})

f_h	z	100	110	120	130	140	150	160	170	180	190	200	Equivalent F_c^{18}	Equivalent F_s^{18}
21.09	18	41.1	40.5	39.7	38.9	38.1	37.1	36.0	34.8	33.4	31.7	29.7	2.53	2.86
	20	38.5	37.9	37.1	36.3	35.5	34.5	33.4	32.2	30.8	29.1	27.1	2.01	2.35
	22	36.3	35.7	34.9	34.1	33.3	32.3	31.2	30.0	28.6	26.9	24.9	1.59	1.92
	24	34.6	33.9	33.1	32.3	31.5	30.5	29.4	28.2	26.8	25.1	23.1	1.29	1.61
22.33	18	42.8	42.1	41.3	40.5	39.6	38.6	37.4	36.1	34.6	32.9	30.7	2.52	2.86
	20	40.1	39.4	38.6	37.8	36.8	35.8	34.7	33.4	31.9	30.1	28.0	1.99	2.33
	22	37.8	37.1	36.4	35.5	34.6	33.6	32.4	31.1	29.6	27.9	25.7	1.58	1.91
	24	36.0	35.3	34.5	33.7	32.7	31.7	30.6	29.3	27.8	26.0	23.9	1.27	1.60
23.57	18	44.5	43.7	42.9	42.0	41.1	40.0	38.8	37.4	35.8	34.0	31.7	2.52	2.86
	20	41.6	40.9	40.0	39.2	38.2	37.1	35.9	34.5	33.0	31.1	28.8	1.96	2.30
	22	39.4	38.6	37.8	36.9	35.9	34.8	33.6	32.3	30.7	28.8	26.5	1.57	1.90
	24	37.4	36.7	35.9	35.0	34.0	32.9	31.7	30.3	28.8	26.9	24.6	1.26	1.58
24.81	18	46.1	45.3	44.5	43.5	42.5	41.4	40.1	38.7	37.0	35.0	32.6	2.51	2.86
	20	43.2	42.4	41.6	40.6	39.6	38.5	37.2	35.7	34.1	32.1	29.7	1.96	2.30
	22	40.9	40.1	39.2	38.3	37.2	36.1	34.8	33.4	31.7	29.8	27.4	1.55	1.89
	24	38.8	38.0	37.2	36.2	35.2	34.1	32.8	31.4	29.7	27.7	25.3	1.24	1.57
26.05	18	47.8	46.9	46.0	45.0	43.9	42.8	41.4	39.9	38.2	36.1	33.6	2.51	2.86
	20	44.8	44.0	43.1	42.1	41.0	39.8	38.5	37.0	35.2	33.2	30.6	1.95	2.30
	22	42.3	41.5	40.6	39.6	38.5	37.3	36.0	34.5	32.7	30.7	28.1	1.53	1.88
	24	40.2	39.4	38.4	37.5	36.4	35.2	33.9	32.3	30.6	28.5	26.0	1.22	1.55

TABLE 255

Process Times (B) at Retort Temperature of 250°F for Conduction-Heating Foods in 307 x 113 Can

f_h	z	INITIAL FOOD TEMPERATURE (T_{ih}) 100	110	120	130	140	150	160	170	180	190	200	Equivalent F_c^{18}	F_s^{18}
21.09	18	30.8	30.1	29.5	28.7	27.9	27.1	26.1	25.0	23.8	22.4	20.7	2.45	2.86
	20	29.6	29.0	28.3	27.6	26.8	25.9	25.0	23.9	22.7	21.2	19.6	2.01	2.41
	22	28.6	28.0	27.3	26.6	25.8	24.9	24.0	22.9	21.7	20.3	18.6	1.66	2.06
	24	27.8	27.1	26.4	25.7	24.9	24.0	23.1	22.0	20.8	19.4	17.7	1.40	1.79
22.33	18	32.2	31.5	30.8	30.0	29.2	28.3	27.3	26.1	24.8	23.3	21.6	2.44	2.86
	20	31.0	30.4	29.6	28.9	28.0	27.1	26.1	24.9	23.6	22.1	20.4	1.99	2.40
	22	30.0	29.3	28.6	27.8	27.0	26.0	25.0	23.9	22.6	21.1	19.3	1.65	2.05
	24	29.0	28.4	27.6	26.9	26.0	25.1	24.1	22.9	21.6	20.1	18.4	1.37	1.77
23.57	18	33.6	32.9	32.2	31.4	30.5	29.5	28.4	27.2	25.8	24.3	22.4	2.44	2.86
	20	32.4	31.7	30.9	30.1	29.2	28.2	27.2	26.0	24.6	23.0	21.2	1.98	2.39
	22	31.3	30.6	29.8	29.0	28.1	27.2	26.1	24.9	23.5	21.9	20.1	1.64	2.04
	24	30.3	29.6	28.8	28.0	27.1	26.1	25.1	23.9	22.5	20.9	19.0	1.36	1.75
24.81	18	35.1	34.3	33.5	32.7	31.7	30.7	29.6	28.3	26.9	25.2	23.2	2.44	2.86
	20	33.8	33.0	32.2	31.4	30.4	29.4	28.3	27.0	25.6	23.9	21.9	1.97	2.39
	22	32.6	31.9	31.1	30.2	29.3	28.2	27.1	25.8	24.4	22.7	20.8	1.63	2.04
	24	31.5	30.8	30.0	29.1	28.2	27.2	26.0	24.8	23.3	21.7	19.7	1.34	1.73
26.05	18	36.5	35.7	34.9	34.0	33.0	31.9	30.7	29.4	27.9	26.1	24.1	2.44	2.86
	20	35.1	34.4	33.5	32.6	31.6	30.6	29.4	28.0	26.5	24.8	22.7	1.97	2.39
	22	33.9	33.2	32.3	31.4	30.4	29.4	28.2	26.8	25.3	23.6	21.5	1.62	2.03
	24	32.8	32.0	31.2	30.3	29.3	28.2	27.0	25.7	24.2	22.4	20.4	1.33	1.73

TABLE 256

Process Times (B) at Retort Temperature of 260°F for Conduction-Heating Foods in 307 x 113 Can

f_h	z	INITIAL FOOD TEMPERATURE (T_{ih})											Equivalent	
		100	110	120	130	140	150	160	170	180	190	200	F_c^{18}	F_s^{18}
21.09	18	25.2	24.7	24.0	23.3	22.6	21.8	20.9	20.0	18.9	17.7	16.3	2.40	2.86
	20	24.7	24.1	23.5	22.8	22.1	21.3	20.4	19.4	18.3	17.1	15.7	2.06	2.51
	22	24.1	23.6	22.9	22.2	21.5	20.7	19.8	18.9	17.8	16.6	15.2	1.75	2.19
	24	23.6	23.0	22.4	21.7	21.0	20.2	19.3	18.3	17.2	16.0	14.6	1.47	1.91
22.33	18	26.5	25.9	25.2	24.5	23.7	22.9	22.0	20.9	19.8	18.5	17.0	2.40	2.86
	20	25.9	25.3	24.6	23.9	23.1	22.3	21.4	20.3	19.2	17.9	16.4	2.04	2.50
	22	25.3	24.7	24.0	23.3	22.5	21.7	20.8	19.7	18.6	17.3	15.8	1.73	2.17
	24	24.7	24.1	23.4	22.7	21.9	21.1	20.2	19.1	18.0	16.7	15.2	1.44	1.88
23.57	18	27.8	27.1	26.4	25.6	24.8	23.9	23.0	21.9	20.7	19.3	17.7	2.40	2.86
	20	27.1	26.5	25.8	25.0	24.2	23.3	22.3	21.2	20.0	18.7	17.1	2.03	2.48
	22	26.5	25.8	25.1	24.4	23.5	22.6	21.7	20.6	19.4	18.0	16.4	1.71	2.15
	24	25.9	25.2	24.5	23.7	22.9	22.0	21.0	20.0	18.8	17.4	15.8	1.42	1.86
24.81	18	29.0	28.3	27.6	26.8	25.9	25.0	23.9	22.8	21.5	20.1	18.4	2.39	2.86
	20	28.3	27.6	26.9	26.1	25.2	24.3	23.3	22.1	20.9	19.4	17.8	2.02	2.47
	22	27.6	26.9	26.2	25.4	24.5	23.6	22.6	21.4	20.2	18.7	17.1	1.68	2.13
	24	27.0	26.3	25.5	24.7	23.9	22.9	21.9	20.8	19.5	18.1	16.4	1.40	1.84
26.05	18	30.2	29.5	28.7	27.9	27.0	26.0	24.9	23.7	22.4	20.9	19.2	2.39	2.86
	20	29.5	28.8	28.0	27.2	26.3	25.3	24.2	23.0	21.7	20.2	18.4	2.00	2.46
	22	28.8	28.1	27.3	26.4	25.5	24.5	23.5	22.3	20.9	19.4	17.7	1.66	2.11
	24	28.1	27.4	26.6	25.7	24.8	23.8	22.8	21.6	20.2	18.7	17.0	1.38	1.81

TABLE 257

Process Times (B) at Retort Temperature of 230°F for Conduction-Heating Foods in 307 x 203 Can

f_h	z	INITIAL FOOD TEMPERATURE (T_{ih}) 100	110	120	130	140	150	160	170	180	190	200	Equivalent F_c^{18}	Equivalent F_s^{18}
28.40	18	78.4	77.5	76.4	75.2	73.9	72.5	70.8	68.9	66.7	63.9	60.4	2.61	2.88
	20	69.2	68.2	67.1	66.0	64.7	63.2	61.6	59.7	57.4	54.7	51.1	1.89	2.16
	22	62.9	61.9	60.8	59.7	58.4	56.9	55.3	53.4	51.1	48.4	44.8	1.44	1.70
	24	57.6	56.7	55.6	54.4	53.1	51.7	50.0	48.1	45.9	43.1	39.6	1.14	1.38
30.07	18	80.9	79.8	78.7	77.5	76.1	74.5	72.8	70.8	68.4	65.5	61.7	2.61	2.88
	20	71.8	70.8	69.6	68.4	67.0	65.5	63.7	61.7	59.3	56.4	52.7	1.88	2.16
	22	65.2	64.2	63.0	61.8	60.4	58.9	57.1	55.1	52.7	49.8	46.1	1.44	1.70
	24	59.6	58.6	57.5	56.2	54.8	53.3	51.6	49.5	47.2	44.2	40.5	1.13	1.38
31.74	18	83.4	82.3	81.1	79.8	78.3	76.7	74.8	72.7	70.2	67.1	63.2	2.61	2.88
	20	74.3	73.2	72.0	70.7	69.3	67.7	65.8	63.7	61.2	58.1	54.1	1.88	2.16
	22	67.4	66.3	65.1	63.8	62.4	60.7	58.9	56.8	54.3	51.2	47.2	1.44	1.70
	24	61.6	60.5	59.3	57.9	56.5	54.9	53.0	50.9	48.4	45.3	41.3	1.10	1.36
33.41	18	85.8	84.6	83.3	81.9	80.4	78.7	76.8	74.5	71.9	68.6	64.5	2.60	2.88
	20	76.8	75.7	74.4	73.0	71.5	69.8	67.9	65.6	63.0	59.7	55.6	1.88	2.16
	22	69.6	68.4	67.2	65.8	64.3	62.5	60.6	58.4	55.7	52.5	48.3	1.44	1.70
	24	63.4	62.2	61.0	59.6	58.1	56.4	54.4	52.2	49.5	46.3	42.1	1.07	1.33
35.08	18	88.5	87.3	86.0	84.5	82.9	81.1	79.1	76.7	74.0	70.6	66.2	2.59	2.88
	20	79.3	78.1	76.7	75.3	73.7	71.9	69.8	67.5	64.7	61.3	56.9	1.87	2.16
	22	71.7	70.5	69.1	67.7	66.1	64.3	62.3	59.9	57.1	53.7	49.3	1.44	1.70
	24	65.2	64.0	62.6	61.2	59.6	57.8	55.7	53.4	50.6	47.2	42.8	1.05	1.31

TABLE 258

Process Times (B) at Retort Temperature of 240°F for Conduction-Heating Foods in 307 x 203 Can

f_h	z	INITIAL FOOD TEMPERATURE (T_{ih})											Equivalent	
		100	110	120	130	140	150	160	170	180	190	200	F_c^{18}	F_s^{18}
	18	51.0	50.0	49.1	48.0	46.8	45.5	44.1	42.4	40.5	38.3	35.5	2.53	2.88
28.40	20	47.8	46.9	45.9	44.9	43.7	42.4	40.9	39.3	37.4	35.1	32.4	1.96	2.31
	22	45.1	44.2	43.2	42.1	41.0	39.7	38.2	36.6	34.7	32.4	29.7	1.52	1.86
	24	42.9	42.0	41.0	40.0	38.8	37.5	36.0	34.4	32.5	30.2	27.5	1.20	1.54
	18	53.2	52.2	51.2	50.0	48.8	47.4	45.9	44.1	42.1	39.7	36.8	2.52	2.88
30.07	20	49.9	48.9	47.9	46.7	45.5	44.1	42.6	40.8	38.8	36.4	33.5	1.94	2.29
	22	47.1	46.1	45.1	43.9	42.7	41.3	39.8	38.0	36.0	33.6	30.7	1.50	1.85
	24	44.8	43.8	42.8	41.6	40.4	39.0	37.5	35.7	33.7	31.3	28.4	1.19	1.53
	18	55.4	54.4	53.3	52.1	50.7	49.3	47.7	45.8	43.7	41.2	38.1	2.52	2.88
31.74	20	51.9	50.8	49.7	48.5	47.2	45.8	44.2	42.3	40.2	37.7	34.6	1.92	2.28
	22	49.0	48.0	46.9	45.7	44.4	42.9	41.3	39.4	37.3	34.8	31.7	1.49	1.84
	24	46.6	45.6	44.5	43.3	42.0	40.5	38.9	37.0	34.9	32.4	29.3	1.17	1.51
	18	57.5	56.5	55.3	54.0	52.7	51.1	49.4	47.5	45.2	42.6	39.4	2.52	2.88
33.41	20	53.9	52.8	51.7	50.4	49.0	47.5	45.8	43.9	41.6	39.0	35.7	1.91	2.27
	22	50.9	49.8	48.7	47.4	46.0	44.5	42.8	40.9	38.6	36.0	32.7	1.47	1.83
	24	48.4	47.3	46.2	44.9	43.5	42.0	40.3	38.4	36.1	33.5	30.2	1.16	1.50
	18	59.7	58.5	57.3	56.0	54.5	52.9	51.1	49.1	46.7	44.0	40.6	2.51	2.88
35.08	20	55.9	54.8	53.6	52.3	50.8	49.2	47.4	45.4	43.0	40.2	36.8	1.90	2.27
	22	52.8	51.7	50.4	49.1	47.7	46.1	44.3	42.2	39.9	37.1	33.7	1.46	1.81
	24	50.2	49.1	47.9	46.6	45.1	43.5	41.7	39.7	37.3	34.5	31.1	1.14	1.49

TABLE 259

Process Times (B) at Retort Temperature of 250°F for Conduction-Heating Foods in 307 x 203 Can

f_h	z	INITIAL FOOD TEMPERATURE (T_{ih})											Equivalent	
		100	110	120	130	140	150	160	170	180	190	200	F_c^{18}	F_s^{18}
	18	39.2	38.4	37.5	36.5	35.4	34.2	32.9	31.5	29.8	27.9	25.7	2.45	2.88
28.40	20	37.8	36.9	36.0	35.0	33.9	32.8	31.5	30.0	28.4	26.5	24.2	1.99	2.41
	22	36.5	35.6	34.7	33.7	32.6	31.5	30.2	28.7	27.1	25.2	22.9	1.62	2.03
	24	35.2	34.4	33.5	32.5	31.4	30.2	28.9	27.5	25.8	23.9	21.7	1.32	1.71
	18	41.1	40.2	39.2	38.2	37.1	35.8	34.4	32.9	31.2	29.1	26.8	2.45	2.88
30.07	20	39.6	38.7	37.7	36.6	35.5	34.3	32.9	31.3	29.6	27.6	25.2	1.99	2.41
	22	38.2	37.3	36.3	35.3	34.1	32.9	31.5	30.0	28.2	26.2	23.8	1.61	2.02
	24	36.9	36.0	35.0	34.0	32.8	31.6	30.2	28.7	26.9	24.9	22.5	1.30	1.70
	18	43.0	42.0	41.0	39.9	38.7	37.4	35.9	34.3	32.5	30.3	27.8	2.45	2.88
31.74	20	41.3	40.4	39.4	38.3	37.1	35.7	34.3	32.7	30.8	28.7	26.2	1.97	2.39
	22	39.9	38.9	37.9	36.8	35.6	34.3	32.8	31.2	29.4	27.3	24.7	1.60	2.01
	24	38.5	37.5	36.5	35.4	34.2	32.9	31.5	29.8	28.0	25.9	23.4	1.28	1.68
	18	44.8	43.8	42.7	41.5	40.3	38.9	37.4	35.7	33.7	31.5	28.8	2.45	2.88
33.41	20	43.1	42.1	41.0	39.8	38.6	37.2	35.7	34.0	32.0	29.8	27.1	1.96	2.38
	22	41.6	40.6	39.5	38.3	37.1	35.7	34.2	32.5	30.5	28.3	25.6	1.58	2.00
	24	40.1	39.1	38.0	36.9	35.6	34.2	32.7	31.0	29.0	26.8	24.2	1.26	1.66
	18	46.6	45.5	44.4	43.2	41.9	40.4	38.8	37.0	35.0	32.6	29.9	2.44	2.88
35.08	20	44.8	43.8	42.6	41.4	40.1	38.6	37.0	35.2	33.2	30.9	28.1	1.95	2.37
	22	43.2	42.2	41.1	39.8	38.5	37.1	35.5	33.7	31.6	29.3	26.5	1.56	1.98
	24	41.7	40.6	39.5	38.3	37.0	35.5	33.9	32.1	30.1	27.7	25.0	1.24	1.64

TABLE 260

Process Times (B) at Retort Temperature of 260°F for Conduction-Heating Foods in 307 x 203 Can

f_h	z	INITIAL FOOD TEMPERATURE (T_{ih}) 100	110	120	130	140	150	160	170	180	190	200	Equivalent F_c^{18}	F_s^{18}
28.40	18	32.6	31.8	31.0	30.1	29.1	28.0	26.8	25.5	24.1	22.4	20.5	2.41	2.88
	20	31.8	31.0	30.2	29.2	28.2	27.2	26.0	24.7	23.2	21.6	19.7	2.00	2.46
	22	31.0	30.2	29.3	28.4	27.4	26.4	25.2	23.9	22.4	20.8	18.9	1.64	2.09
	24	30.2	29.4	28.6	27.7	26.7	25.6	24.4	23.1	21.7	20.0	18.1	1.35	1.79
30.07	18	34.3	33.4	32.5	31.5	30.5	29.4	28.1	26.7	25.2	23.5	21.4	2.41	2.88
	20	33.4	32.5	31.6	30.7	29.6	28.5	27.2	25.9	24.3	22.6	20.6	1.98	2.45
	22	32.5	31.7	30.7	29.8	28.7	27.6	26.4	25.0	23.4	21.7	19.7	1.62	2.07
	24	31.7	30.9	30.0	29.0	27.9	26.8	25.6	24.2	22.6	20.9	18.9	1.33	1.77
31.74	18	35.9	35.0	34.1	33.0	31.9	30.7	29.4	28.0	26.3	24.5	22.4	2.41	2.88
	20	35.0	34.1	33.1	32.1	31.0	29.8	28.5	27.0	25.4	23.6	21.4	1.97	2.44
	22	34.0	33.1	32.2	31.1	30.0	28.8	27.5	26.1	24.4	22.6	20.5	1.60	2.05
	24	33.2	32.3	31.3	30.3	29.2	28.0	26.7	25.2	23.6	21.8	19.6	1.31	1.75
33.41	18	37.5	36.6	35.6	34.5	33.3	32.1	30.7	29.2	27.5	25.5	23.3	2.41	2.88
	20	36.5	35.6	34.6	33.5	32.3	31.1	29.7	28.2	26.5	24.5	22.3	1.96	2.43
	22	35.5	34.6	33.6	32.5	31.3	30.1	28.7	27.2	25.4	23.5	21.3	1.58	2.03
	24	34.6	33.7	32.7	31.6	30.4	29.2	27.8	26.3	24.6	22.6	20.4	1.29	1.73
35.08	18	39.1	38.2	37.1	36.0	34.8	33.4	32.0	30.4	28.6	26.5	24.2	2.40	2.88
	20	38.1	37.1	36.0	34.9	33.7	32.4	30.9	29.3	27.5	25.5	23.1	1.95	2.41
	22	37.0	36.0	35.0	33.8	32.6	31.3	29.8	28.2	26.4	24.4	22.1	1.56	2.01
	24	36.1	35.1	34.0	32.9	31.7	30.3	28.9	27.3	25.5	23.5	21.1	1.27	1.71

TABLE 261

Process Times (B) at Retort Temperature of 230°F for Conduction-Heating Foods in 307 x 214 Can

f_h	z	INITIAL FOOD TEMPERATURE (T_{ih})											Equivalent	
		100	110	120	130	140	150	160	170	180	190	200	F_c^{18}	F_s^{18}
	18	95.8	94.5	93.0	91.3	89.5	87.5	85.2	82.6	79.5	75.7	70.7	2.61	2.91
39.38	20	85.6	84.3	82.8	81.1	79.3	77.3	75.0	72.4	69.3	65.5	60.5	1.89	2.18
	22	77.1	75.7	74.3	72.6	70.8	68.8	66.5	63.9	60.8	57.0	52.0	1.42	1.69
	24	70.8	69.4	67.9	66.3	64.5	62.5	60.2	57.6	54.5	50.6	45.7	1.05	1.33
	18	99.5	98.0	96.5	94.7	92.8	90.7	88.3	85.5	82.2	78.1	72.9	2.60	2.91
41.70	20	88.7	87.3	85.7	84.0	82.1	79.9	77.5	74.7	71.4	67.4	62.2	1.89	2.18
	22	79.7	78.2	76.7	74.9	73.0	70.9	68.5	65.7	62.4	58.3	53.1	1.37	1.65
	24	73.6	72.1	70.6	68.8	66.9	64.8	62.4	59.6	56.3	52.3	47.0	1.04	1.32
	18	103.0	101.5	99.8	98.0	96.0	93.8	91.2	88.3	84.8	80.5	75.0	2.60	2.91
44.01	20	91.7	90.2	88.5	86.7	84.7	82.4	79.9	76.9	73.4	69.2	63.7	1.89	2.18
	22	82.7	81.1	79.5	77.7	75.6	73.4	70.8	67.9	64.4	60.1	54.6	1.36	1.65
	24	76.3	74.8	73.1	71.3	69.3	67.0	64.5	61.5	58.1	53.8	48.3	1.02	1.30
	18	106.5	104.9	103.2	101.2	99.1	96.8	94.1	91.0	87.3	82.8	77.0	2.60	2.91
46.33	20	94.6	93.0	91.2	89.3	87.2	84.8	82.2	79.0	75.4	70.9	65.1	1.89	2.18
	22	85.7	84.0	82.3	80.4	78.3	75.9	73.2	70.1	66.4	61.9	56.2	1.36	1.65
	24	79.0	77.4	75.6	73.7	71.6	69.2	66.5	63.4	59.8	55.3	49.5	1.00	1.29
	18	109.9	108.2	106.4	104.4	102.1	99.7	96.8	93.6	89.7	85.0	78.9	2.60	2.91
48.65	20	97.4	95.7	93.9	91.9	89.6	87.1	84.3	81.1	77.2	72.5	66.4	1.89	2.18
	22	88.6	86.9	85.0	83.0	80.8	78.3	75.5	72.2	68.4	63.7	57.6	1.35	1.65
	24	81.6	79.9	78.1	76.1	73.8	71.4	68.5	65.3	61.4	56.7	50.6	0.99	1.28

TABLE 262

Process Times (B) at Retort Temperature of 240°F for Conduction-Heating Foods in 307 x 214 Can

f_h	z	INITIAL FOOD TEMPERATURE (T_{ih})											Equivalent	
		100	110	120	130	140	150	160	170	180	190	200	F_c^{18}	F_s^{18}
39.38	18	65.3	64.0	62.6	61.2	59.5	57.7	55.7	53.4	50.8	47.7	43.9	2.53	2.91
	20	61.2	59.9	58.5	57.0	55.4	53.6	51.6	49.3	46.7	43.6	39.7	1.90	2.27
	22	57.8	56.5	55.1	53.6	52.0	50.2	48.2	45.9	43.3	40.2	36.3	1.45	1.81
	24	54.9	53.7	52.3	50.8	49.2	47.4	45.4	43.1	40.4	37.3	33.5	1.12	1.48
41.70	18	68.2	66.8	65.4	63.8	62.1	60.2	58.1	55.6	52.8	49.5	45.5	2.53	2.91
	20	63.9	62.6	61.1	59.5	57.8	55.9	53.8	51.4	48.6	45.3	41.2	1.89	2.26
	22	60.3	59.0	57.5	56.0	54.2	52.3	50.2	47.8	45.0	41.7	37.6	1.43	1.80
	24	57.4	56.0	54.6	53.0	51.3	49.4	47.3	44.8	42.0	38.7	34.7	1.11	1.46
44.01	18	71.1	69.6	68.1	66.4	64.6	62.6	60.4	57.8	54.9	51.4	47.1	2.52	2.91
	20	66.6	65.2	63.7	62.0	60.2	58.2	55.9	53.4	50.4	46.9	42.7	1.88	2.26
	22	62.9	61.5	59.9	58.3	56.4	54.4	52.2	49.6	46.7	43.2	38.9	1.42	1.78
	24	59.8	58.4	56.9	55.2	53.4	51.4	49.1	46.6	43.6	40.1	35.9	1.09	1.45
46.33	18	73.9	72.4	70.8	69.1	67.1	65.0	62.7	60.0	56.9	53.2	48.7	2.52	2.91
	20	69.3	67.8	66.2	64.4	62.5	60.4	58.0	55.3	52.2	48.6	44.1	1.87	2.25
	22	65.4	63.9	62.3	60.6	58.6	56.5	54.2	51.5	48.4	44.7	40.2	1.41	1.78
	24	62.2	60.7	59.1	57.3	55.4	53.3	50.9	48.3	45.2	41.5	37.0	1.07	1.43
48.65	18	76.8	75.2	73.5	71.7	69.7	67.4	64.9	62.1	58.9	55.0	50.3	2.52	2.91
	20	71.9	70.4	68.7	66.8	64.8	62.6	60.1	57.3	54.0	50.2	45.5	1.86	2.24
	22	67.9	66.4	64.7	62.8	60.8	58.6	56.1	53.3	50.0	46.2	41.5	1.40	1.77
	24	64.6	63.0	61.3	59.5	57.5	55.3	52.8	49.9	46.7	42.8	38.1	1.06	1.42

TABLE 263

Process Times (B) at Retort Temperature of 250°F for Conduction-Heating Foods in 307 x 214 Can

f_h	z	INITIAL FOOD TEMPERATURE (T_{ih}) 100	110	120	130	140	150	160	170	180	190	200	Equivalent F_c^{18}	F_s^{18}
39.38	18	51.3	50.2	48.9	47.5	46.0	44.4	42.6	40.6	38.3	35.7	32.6	2.47	2.91
	20	49.4	48.2	46.9	45.5	44.1	42.4	40.6	38.6	36.3	33.7	30.6	1.95	2.38
	22	47.6	46.4	45.1	43.8	42.3	40.7	38.9	36.8	34.6	31.9	28.8	1.55	1.97
	24	45.8	44.7	43.4	42.0	40.5	38.9	37.1	35.1	32.8	30.2	27.1	1.21	1.62
41.70	18	53.8	52.6	51.2	49.8	48.2	46.5	44.6	42.5	40.0	37.2	33.9	2.47	2.91
	20	51.7	50.5	49.2	47.7	46.1	44.4	42.5	40.4	37.9	35.2	31.9	1.94	2.37
	22	49.9	48.6	47.3	45.8	44.3	42.5	40.6	38.5	36.1	33.3	30.0	1.54	1.95
	24	48.0	46.8	45.4	44.0	42.4	40.7	38.8	36.6	34.2	31.4	28.1	1.19	1.60
44.01	18	56.3	55.0	53.6	52.0	50.4	48.6	46.5	44.3	41.7	38.8	35.3	2.46	2.91
	20	54.1	52.8	51.4	49.8	48.2	46.4	44.3	42.1	39.5	36.6	33.1	1.93	2.36
	22	52.1	50.8	49.4	47.9	46.2	44.4	42.4	40.1	37.6	34.6	31.1	1.52	1.94
	24	50.2	48.9	47.4	45.9	44.3	42.4	40.4	38.2	35.6	32.7	29.2	1.17	1.58
46.33	18	58.8	57.4	55.9	54.3	52.5	50.6	48.5	46.1	43.4	40.3	36.6	2.46	2.91
	20	56.4	55.1	53.6	52.0	50.2	48.3	46.2	43.8	41.1	38.0	34.3	1.92	2.36
	22	54.4	53.0	51.5	49.9	48.1	46.2	44.1	41.7	39.0	35.9	32.3	1.51	1.93
	24	52.3	50.9	49.4	47.8	46.1	44.2	42.0	39.7	37.0	33.9	30.2	1.16	1.56
48.65	18	61.2	59.7	58.1	56.5	54.6	52.6	50.4	47.9	45.1	41.8	38.0	2.46	2.91
	20	58.8	57.3	55.7	54.0	52.2	50.2	48.0	45.5	42.7	39.4	35.5	1.91	2.34
	22	56.6	55.1	53.6	51.9	50.0	48.0	45.8	43.3	40.5	37.2	33.4	1.49	1.91
	24	54.4	53.0	51.4	49.7	47.9	45.9	43.6	41.1	38.3	35.1	31.2	1.14	1.54

TABLE 264

Process Times (B) at Retort Temperature of 260°F for Conduction-Heating Foods in 307 x 214 Can

f_h	z	INITIAL FOOD TEMPERATURE (T_{ih})											Equivalent	
		100	110	120	130	140	150	160	170	180	190	200	F_c^{18}	F_s^{18}
39.38	18	43.3	42.2	41.0	39.8	38.4	36.9	35.3	33.5	31.5	29.2	26.5	2.43	2.91
	20	42.1	41.0	39.8	38.5	37.2	35.7	34.1	32.3	30.2	28.0	25.3	1.95	2.42
	22	40.9	39.8	38.6	37.3	35.9	34.5	32.8	31.0	29.0	26.7	24.1	1.54	2.00
	24	39.8	38.7	37.5	36.3	34.9	33.4	31.8	30.0	28.0	25.7	23.0	1.24	1.68
41.70	18	45.5	44.3	43.1	41.8	40.3	38.7	37.0	35.1	33.0	30.5	27.8	2.43	2.91
	20	44.2	43.0	41.8	40.5	39.0	37.4	35.7	33.8	31.7	29.2	26.5	1.94	2.41
	22	42.9	41.7	40.5	39.1	37.7	36.1	34.4	32.5	30.3	27.9	25.1	1.52	1.98
	24	41.8	40.6	39.4	38.0	36.6	35.0	33.3	31.4	29.2	26.8	24.0	1.21	1.66
44.01	18	47.7	46.5	45.2	43.7	42.2	40.5	38.7	36.7	34.5	31.9	29.0	2.42	2.91
	20	46.3	45.1	43.8	42.3	40.8	39.2	37.3	35.3	33.1	30.5	27.6	1.92	2.40
	22	44.9	43.7	42.4	40.9	39.4	37.7	35.9	33.9	31.7	29.1	26.2	1.50	1.95
	24	43.7	42.5	41.2	39.8	38.2	36.6	34.7	32.7	30.5	27.9	25.0	1.20	1.64
46.33	18	49.9	48.6	47.2	45.7	44.1	42.3	40.4	38.3	35.9	33.2	30.1	2.42	2.91
	20	48.4	47.1	45.7	44.2	42.6	40.9	38.9	36.8	34.4	31.8	28.7	1.91	2.39
	22	46.9	45.6	44.2	42.7	41.1	39.4	37.5	35.3	33.0	30.3	27.2	1.48	1.94
	24	45.7	44.4	43.0	41.5	39.9	38.1	36.2	34.1	31.7	29.0	25.9	1.18	1.63
48.65	18	52.0	50.7	49.2	47.7	46.0	44.1	42.1	39.9	37.4	34.6	31.3	2.42	2.91
	20	50.5	49.1	47.7	46.1	44.4	42.6	40.5	38.3	35.8	33.0	29.8	1.90	2.38
	22	48.9	47.5	46.1	44.5	42.8	41.0	39.0	36.7	34.3	31.4	28.2	1.46	1.92
	24	47.6	46.2	44.8	43.2	41.5	39.7	37.7	35.4	32.9	30.1	26.9	1.16	1.61

TABLE 265

Process Times (B) at Retort Temperature of 230°F for Conduction-Heating Foods in 307 x 306 Can

f_h	z	INITIAL FOOD TEMPERATURE (T_{ih})											Equivalent	
		100	110	120	130	140	150	160	170	180	190	200	F_c^{18}	F_s^{18}
45.31	18	105.2	103.6	101.9	100.1	98.0	95.7	93.0	90.0	86.4	82.0	76.4	2.61	2.93
	20	93.6	92.0	90.3	88.4	86.3	84.0	81.4	78.3	74.8	70.4	64.7	1.90	2.19
	22	84.5	82.9	81.2	79.3	77.3	75.0	72.3	69.3	65.7	61.3	55.7	1.37	1.66
	24	78.0	76.4	74.7	72.8	70.7	68.4	65.8	62.8	59.2	54.8	49.1	1.02	1.30
47.98	18	109.2	107.5	105.7	103.7	101.5	99.1	96.3	93.1	89.3	84.6	78.6	2.61	2.93
	20	96.8	95.2	93.4	91.4	89.2	86.7	83.9	80.7	76.9	72.3	66.3	1.90	2.19
	22	87.9	86.2	84.4	82.4	80.2	77.8	75.0	71.8	68.0	63.3	57.3	1.36	1.66
	24	81.0	79.3	77.5	75.5	73.3	70.9	68.1	64.9	61.1	56.5	50.5	1.00	1.29
50.64	18	113.0	111.3	109.3	107.2	104.9	102.3	99.4	96.0	92.0	87.1	80.8	2.61	2.93
	20	100.0	98.2	96.3	94.2	91.9	89.3	86.4	83.0	79.0	74.1	67.7	1.88	2.17
	22	91.2	89.4	87.5	85.4	83.1	80.5	77.6	74.2	70.2	65.3	58.9	1.36	1.66
	24	84.0	82.2	80.3	78.2	75.9	73.3	70.4	67.0	63.0	58.1	51.8	0.99	1.28
53.31	18	116.7	114.9	112.9	110.7	108.2	105.5	102.4	98.8	94.6	89.5	82.8	2.61	2.93
	20	103.3	101.4	99.4	97.2	94.8	92.0	88.9	85.4	81.2	76.0	69.3	1.84	2.14
	22	94.4	92.6	90.6	88.4	85.9	83.2	80.1	76.5	72.3	67.1	60.5	1.35	1.65
	24	87.0	85.1	83.1	80.9	78.5	75.7	72.6	69.1	64.9	59.7	53.0	0.97	1.26
55.97	18	120.4	118.4	116.3	114.0	111.4	108.6	105.3	101.6	97.1	91.7	84.7	2.61	2.93
	20	106.9	104.9	102.8	100.5	97.9	95.1	97.9	95.1	91.8	78.2	71.2	1.84	2.14
	22	97.6	95.6	93.5	91.2	88.6	85.8	82.5	78.8	74.3	68.9	61.9	1.33	1.63
	24	90.1	88.1	86.0	83.7	81.2	78.3	75.0	71.3	66.9	61.4	54.4	0.96	1.26

TABLE 266

Process Times (B) at Retort Temperature of 240°F for Conduction-Heating Foods in 307 x 306 Can

f_h	z	INITIAL FOOD TEMPERATURE (T_{ih}) 100	110	120	130	140	150	160	170	180	190	200	Equivalent F_c^{18}	F_s^{18}
45.31	18	72.7	71.3	69.7	68.0	66.1	64.1	61.7	59.1	56.1	52.5	48.1	2.54	2.93
	20	68.2	66.8	65.2	63.5	61.6	59.5	57.2	54.6	51.5	47.9	43.6	1.89	2.26
	22	64.4	62.9	61.4	59.6	57.8	55.7	53.4	50.7	47.7	44.1	39.7	1.42	1.79
	24	61.2	59.8	58.2	56.5	54.6	52.5	50.2	47.6	44.6	41.0	36.6	1.09	1.45
47.98	18	76.1	74.5	72.8	71.0	69.0	66.8	64.4	61.6	58.4	54.6	49.9	2.54	2.93
	20	71.3	69.7	68.0	66.2	64.2	62.0	59.6	56.8	53.6	49.8	45.2	1.87	2.25
	22	67.3	65.8	64.1	62.3	60.3	58.1	55.6	52.9	49.6	45.8	41.2	1.41	1.78
	24	64.0	62.4	60.8	59.0	57.0	54.8	52.3	49.5	46.3	42.5	37.9	1.07	1.43
50.64	18	79.3	77.7	75.9	74.0	71.9	69.6	67.0	64.1	60.7	56.7	51.8	2.53	2.93
	20	74.3	72.7	70.9	69.0	66.9	64.6	62.0	59.1	55.7	51.7	46.8	1.86	2.25
	22	70.2	68.5	66.8	64.9	62.8	60.5	57.9	54.9	51.5	47.5	42.6	1.40	1.77
	24	66.7	65.1	63.3	61.4	59.3	57.0	54.4	51.5	48.1	44.1	39.2	1.06	1.42
53.31	18	82.5	80.8	79.0	76.9	74.7	72.3	69.6	66.5	62.9	58.7	53.5	2.53	2.93
	20	77.3	75.6	73.8	71.8	69.6	67.1	64.4	61.3	57.7	53.5	48.3	1.86	2.24
	22	73.0	71.3	69.5	67.5	65.3	62.8	60.1	57.0	53.4	49.2	44.0	1.38	1.76
	24	69.4	67.7	65.8	63.8	61.6	59.2	56.5	53.4	49.8	45.6	40.4	1.05	1.41
55.97	18	85.7	83.9	82.0	79.9	77.5	75.0	72.1	68.9	65.1	60.7	55.3	2.53	2.93
	20	80.3	78.5	76.6	74.5	72.1	69.6	66.7	63.5	59.7	55.3	49.9	1.85	2.23
	22	75.9	74.1	72.1	70.0	67.7	65.1	62.3	59.0	55.3	50.9	45.4	1.37	1.75
	24	72.1	70.3	68.4	66.2	63.9	61.4	58.5	55.3	51.5	41.7	41.7	1.04	1.41

TABLE 267

Process Times (B) at Retort Temperature of 250°F for Conduction-Heating Foods in 307 x 306 Can

f_h	z	INITIAL FOOD TEMPERATURE (T_{ih})											Equivalent	
		100	110	120	130	140	150	160	170	180	190	200	F_c^{18}	F_s^{18}
45.31	18	57.7	56.4	54.9	53.4	51.6	49.8	47.7	45.4	42.7	39.7	36.1	2.48	2.93
	20	55.5	54.1	52.7	51.1	49.4	47.5	45.4	43.1	40.5	37.4	33.9	1.94	2.37
	22	53.5	52.1	50.6	49.1	47.3	45.5	43.4	41.1	38.5	35.4	31.8	1.52	1.94
	24	51.4	50.1	48.6	47.0	45.3	43.5	41.4	39.1	36.4	33.4	29.8	1.17	1.58
47.98	18	60.5	59.1	57.6	55.9	54.1	52.1	49.9	47.4	44.7	41.4	37.6	2.48	2.93
	20	58.2	56.7	55.2	53.5	51.7	49.7	47.5	45.1	42.3	39.1	35.3	1.93	2.36
	22	56.0	54.6	53.0	51.4	49.5	47.6	45.4	42.9	40.1	36.9	33.1	1.50	1.92
	24	53.9	52.4	50.9	49.2	47.4	45.4	43.2	40.8	38.0	34.8	31.0	1.15	1.56
50.64	18	63.3	61.8	60.2	58.4	56.5	54.4	52.1	49.5	46.6	43.2	39.2	2.47	2.93
	20	60.8	59.3	57.7	55.9	54.0	51.9	49.6	47.0	44.1	40.7	36.6	1.91	2.35
	22	58.5	57.0	55.4	53.6	51.7	49.6	47.3	44.7	41.8	38.4	34.4	1.49	1.91
	24	56.3	54.8	53.1	51.4	49.5	47.4	45.1	42.5	39.5	36.1	32.1	1.13	1.54
53.31	18	66.1	64.5	62.8	60.9	58.9	56.7	54.3	51.6	48.5	44.9	40.7	2.47	2.93
	20	63.5	61.9	60.2	58.3	56.3	54.1	51.6	48.9	45.8	42.3	38.0	1.91	2.34
	22	61.1	59.5	57.8	55.9	53.9	51.7	49.2	46.5	43.4	39.9	35.6	1.47	1.89
	24	58.7	57.1	55.4	53.6	51.5	49.3	46.9	44.2	41.1	37.5	33.3	1.12	1.52
55.97	18	68.9	67.2	65.4	63.5	61.3	59.0	56.5	53.6	50.3	46.6	42.2	2.47	2.93
	20	66.1	64.4	62.6	60.7	58.6	56.3	53.7	50.8	47.6	43.8	39.4	1.90	2.34
	22	63.6	61.9	60.1	58.2	56.0	53.7	51.2	48.3	45.0	41.3	36.9	1.45	1.88
	24	61.1	59.4	57.6	55.7	53.6	51.3	48.7	45.8	42.6	38.8	34.4	1.10	1.51

TABLE 268

Process Times (B) at Retort Temperature of 260°F for Conduction-Heating Foods in 307 x 306 Can

f_h	z	INITIAL FOOD TEMPERATURE (T_{ih})											Equivalent	
		100	110	120	130	140	150	160	170	180	190	200	F_c^{18}	F_s^{18}
	18	49.0	47.7	46.3	44.9	43.3	41.6	39.7	37.6	35.3	32.7	29.7	2.44	2.93
45.31	20	47.5	46.3	44.9	43.4	41.9	40.2	38.3	36.2	33.9	31.3	28.2	1.93	2.40
	22	46.1	44.8	43.4	42.0	40.4	38.7	36.8	34.7	32.4	29.8	26.8	1.50	1.96
	24	44.9	43.6	42.2	40.8	39.2	37.5	35.6	33.5	31.2	28.6	25.6	1.20	1.64
	18	51.5	50.1	48.7	47.1	45.5	43.7	41.7	39.5	37.0	34.2	31.0	2.44	2.93
47.98	20	49.9	48.6	47.1	45.6	43.9	42.1	40.1	37.9	35.5	32.7	29.5	1.92	2.39
	22	48.4	47.0	45.6	44.0	42.4	40.6	38.6	36.4	33.9	31.1	27.9	1.48	1.94
	24	47.1	45.7	44.3	42.7	41.1	39.3	37.3	35.1	32.6	29.9	26.6	1.18	1.63
	18	53.9	52.5	51.0	49.4	47.6	45.7	43.6	41.3	38.7	35.8	32.4	2.44	2.93
50.64	20	52.3	50.9	49.4	47.7	46.0	44.1	42.0	39.6	37.1	34.1	30.7	1.91	2.38
	22	50.7	49.2	47.7	46.1	44.3	42.4	40.3	38.0	35.4	32.5	29.1	1.46	1.92
	24	49.3	47.9	46.3	44.7	43.0	41.0	38.9	36.6	34.0	31.1	27.7	1.16	1.61
	18	56.4	54.9	53.3	51.6	49.7	47.7	45.5	43.1	40.4	37.3	33.7	2.43	2.93
53.31	20	54.7	53.2	51.6	49.9	48.0	46.0	43.8	41.3	38.6	35.5	32.0	1.89	2.37
	22	52.9	51.4	49.9	48.1	46.3	44.3	42.1	39.6	36.9	33.8	30.2	1.45	1.91
	24	51.5	50.0	48.4	46.7	44.8	42.8	40.6	38.2	35.4	32.3	28.8	1.14	1.59
	18	58.9	57.3	55.6	53.8	51.9	49.7	47.4	44.9	42.0	38.8	35.0	2.43	2.93
55.97	20	57.0	55.5	53.8	52.0	50.0	47.9	45.6	43.0	40.2	36.9	33.2	1.88	2.36
	22	55.2	53.6	52.0	50.2	48.2	46.1	43.8	41.2	38.4	35.1	31.4	1.43	1.90
	24	53.7	52.1	50.4	48.6	46.7	44.5	42.2	39.7	36.8	33.6	29.8	1.12	1.57

TABLE 269

Process Times (B) at Retort Temperature of 230°F for Conduction-Heating Foods in 307 x 400 Can

f_h	z	INITIAL FOOD TEMPERATURE (T_{ih}) 100	110	120	130	140	150	160	170	180	190	200	Equivalent F_c^{18}	F_s^{18}
	18	113.5	111.7	109.8	107.7	105.4	102.8	99.8	96.4	92.4	87.5	81.1	2.63	2.94
50.79	20	100.4	98.6	96.7	94.6	92.3	89.7	86.8	83.4	79.3	74.4	68.1	1.89	2.18
	22	91.6	89.8	87.9	85.8	83.4	80.8	77.9	74.5	70.5	65.6	59.2	1.37	1.67
	24	84.3	82.6	80.7	78.6	76.2	73.6	70.7	67.3	63.3	58.3	52.0	0.99	1.28
	18	117.6	115.8	113.7	111.5	109.1	106.3	103.2	99.6	95.3	90.1	83.4	2.63	2.94
53.78	20	104.1	102.2	100.2	98.0	95.5	92.8	89.6	86.0	81.8	76.6	69.9	1.85	2.15
	22	95.2	93.3	91.3	89.0	86.6	83.8	80.7	77.1	72.9	67.6	60.9	1.35	1.65
	24	87.7	85.8	83.8	81.6	79.1	76.3	73.2	69.6	65.4	60.2	53.4	0.97	1.27
	18	121.7	119.7	117.6	115.2	112.6	109.7	106.4	102.6	98.1	92.6	85.5	2.63	2.94
56.77	20	108.1	106.2	104.0	101.7	99.1	96.2	92.9	89.1	84.6	79.1	72.0	1.85	2.16
	22	98.7	96.7	94.6	92.2	89.6	86.7	83.4	79.6	75.2	69.6	62.6	1.33	1.64
	24	91.2	89.2	87.0	84.7	82.1	79.2	75.9	72.1	67.6	62.1	55.0	0.96	1.26
	18	125.6	123.5	121.3	118.8	116.1	113.0	109.5	105.5	100.8	95.0	87.5	2.63	2.94
59.75	20	112.1	110.0	107.7	105.3	102.5	99.5	96.0	92.0	87.3	81.5	74.0	1.84	2.16
	22	102.2	100.1	97.9	95.4	92.7	89.6	86.1	82.1	77.4	71.6	64.1	1.31	1.62
	24	94.6	92.5	90.2	87.8	85.0	82.0	78.5	74.5	69.8	64.0	56.5	0.96	1.26
	18	129.4	127.2	124.8	122.2	119.4	116.2	112.5	108.3	103.4	97.3	89.4	2.63	2.94
62.74	20	115.9	113.7	111.4	108.8	105.9	102.7	99.1	94.9	89.9	83.8	76.0	1.84	2.16
	22	105.6	103.4	101.1	98.5	95.6	92.4	88.7	84.5	79.6	73.5	65.6	1.29	1.60
	24	97.9	95.7	93.4	90.8	87.9	84.7	81.1	76.9	71.9	65.8	58.0	0.94	1.25

TABLE 270

Process Times (B) at Retort Temperature of 240°F for Conduction-Heating Foods in 307 x 400 Can

f_h	z	100	110	120	130	140	150	160	170	180	190	200	Equivalent F_c^{18}	Equivalent F_s^{18}
		INITIAL FOOD TEMPERATURE (T_{ih})												
50.79	18	79.6	78.0	76.2	74.3	72.2	69.9	67.3	64.3	60.9	56.9	52.0	2.55	2.94
	20	74.6	73.0	71.2	69.3	67.2	64.8	62.2	59.3	55.9	51.9	47.0	1.88	2.26
	22	70.4	68.8	67.0	65.1	63.0	60.7	58.1	55.1	51.7	47.7	42.8	1.41	1.78
	24	67.0	65.3	63.6	61.6	59.5	57.2	54.6	51.7	48.3	44.3	39.3	1.07	1.43
53.78	18	83.2	81.5	79.6	77.6	75.3	72.9	70.1	67.0	63.4	59.2	53.9	2.55	2.94
	20	78.0	76.2	74.4	72.3	70.1	67.7	64.9	61.8	58.2	53.9	48.7	1.87	2.25
	22	73.6	71.9	70.0	68.0	65.8	63.3	60.6	57.5	53.9	49.6	44.4	1.39	1.77
	24	70.0	68.3	66.4	64.4	62.1	59.7	56.9	53.8	50.2	45.9	40.7	1.06	1.42
56.77	18	86.8	85.0	83.0	80.8	78.5	75.9	73.0	69.7	65.9	61.4	55.9	2.54	2.94
	20	81.3	79.5	77.5	75.4	73.0	70.4	67.5	64.2	60.4	55.9	50.4	1.86	2.25
	22	76.8	75.0	73.0	70.9	68.5	65.9	63.0	59.7	55.9	51.4	45.9	1.38	1.75
	24	73.0	71.2	69.2	67.1	64.7	62.1	59.2	55.9	52.1	47.6	42.1	1.05	1.41
59.75	18	90.3	88.4	86.3	84.1	81.6	78.9	75.8	72.4	68.4	63.6	57.8	2.54	2.94
	20	84.7	82.8	80.7	78.4	75.9	73.2	70.2	66.7	62.7	58.0	52.2	1.85	2.24
	22	80.0	78.1	76.0	73.7	71.3	68.5	65.5	62.0	58.0	53.3	47.5	1.36	1.74
	24	76.0	74.1	72.0	69.7	67.2	64.5	61.5	58.0	54.0	49.3	43.5	1.03	1.40
62.74	18	93.9	91.8	89.7	87.3	84.7	81.8	78.6	75.0	70.8	65.8	59.7	2.54	2.94
	20	88.0	86.0	83.8	81.4	78.8	75.9	72.7	69.1	64.9	59.9	53.8	1.84	2.24
	22	83.1	81.1	78.9	76.6	74.0	71.1	67.9	64.2	60.0	55.1	49.0	1.36	1.74
	24	78.9	76.9	74.7	72.4	69.8	66.9	63.7	60.1	55.9	50.9	44.8	1.02	1.39

TABLE 271

Process Times (B) at Retort Temperature of 250°F for Conduction-Heating Foods in 307 x 400 Can

f_h	z	INITIAL FOOD TEMPERATURE (T_{ih}) 100	110	120	130	140	150	160	170	180	190	200	Equivalent F_c^{18}	F_s^{18}
	18	63.5	62.0	60.4	58.6	56.7	54.6	52.3	49.7	46.7	43.3	39.3	2.49	2.94
50.79	20	61.0	59.5	57.9	56.1	54.2	52.1	49.8	47.2	44.2	40.8	36.8	1.93	2.36
	22	58.7	57.2	55.6	53.8	51.9	49.8	47.5	44.9	41.9	38.5	34.5	1.50	1.92
	24	56.5	55.0	53.3	51.6	49.7	47.6	45.2	42.6	39.7	36.3	32.3	1.14	1.55
	18	66.7	65.1	63.3	61.5	59.4	57.2	54.7	52.0	48.9	45.3	41.0	2.49	2.94
53.78	20	64.0	62.4	60.7	58.8	56.8	54.5	52.1	49.3	46.2	42.6	38.3	1.92	2.36
	22	61.6	60.0	58.2	56.4	54.3	52.1	49.7	46.9	43.8	40.2	35.9	1.48	1.90
	24	59.2	57.6	55.9	54.0	52.0	49.7	47.3	44.5	41.4	37.8	33.6	1.12	1.53
	18	69.8	68.1	66.2	64.3	62.1	59.8	57.2	54.3	51.0	47.2	42.7	2.49	2.94
56.77	20	67.0	65.3	63.4	61.5	59.3	57.0	54.4	51.5	48.2	44.4	39.9	1.91	2.35
	22	64.4	62.7	60.9	58.9	56.7	54.4	51.8	48.9	45.6	41.8	37.3	1.46	1.89
	24	61.9	60.2	58.4	56.4	54.3	51.9	49.3	46.4	43.1	39.3	34.8	1.10	1.51
	18	72.8	71.0	69.1	67.0	64.8	62.3	59.6	56.5	53.1	49.1	44.3	2.49	2.94
59.75	20	69.9	68.1	66.2	64.1	61.8	59.4	56.6	53.6	50.1	46.1	41.4	1.90	2.34
	22	67.2	65.4	63.5	61.4	59.1	56.6	53.9	50.9	47.4	43.4	38.7	1.44	1.87
	24	64.6	62.8	60.8	58.8	56.5	54.0	51.3	48.2	44.8	40.8	36.0	1.09	1.50
	18	75.9	74.0	72.0	69.8	67.4	64.8	62.0	58.7	55.1	50.9	45.9	2.48	2.94
62.74	20	72.8	70.9	68.9	66.7	64.3	61.7	58.9	55.6	52.0	47.8	42.8	1.88	2.33
	22	69.9	68.0	66.0	63.8	61.5	58.9	56.0	52.8	49.1	44.9	40.0	1.43	1.85
	24	67.2	65.3	63.3	61.1	58.7	56.1	53.3	50.1	46.4	42.2	37.3	1.07	1.48

TABLE 272

Process Times (B) at Retort Temperature of 260°F for Conduction-Heating Foods in 307 x 400 Can

f_h	z	INITIAL FOOD TEMPERATURE (T_{ih}) 100	110	120	130	140	150	160	170	180	190	200	Equivalent F_c^{18}	F_s^{18}
50.79	18	54.1	52.7	51.2	49.5	47.8	45.9	43.8	41.4	38.8	35.9	32.5	2.45	2.94
	20	52.5	51.1	49.5	47.9	46.1	44.2	42.1	39.8	37.2	34.2	30.8	1.92	2.40
	22	50.8	49.4	47.9	46.3	44.5	42.6	40.5	38.1	35.5	32.6	29.2	1.47	1.93
	24	49.5	48.0	46.5	44.9	43.1	41.2	39.1	36.8	34.2	31.2	27.8	1.17	1.62
53.78	18	56.9	55.4	53.8	52.0	50.2	48.1	45.9	43.4	40.7	37.6	34.0	2.45	2.94
	20	55.1	53.6	52.0	50.3	48.4	46.4	44.2	41.7	38.9	35.8	32.2	1.90	2.38
	22	53.4	51.9	50.3	48.5	46.7	44.6	42.4	40.0	37.2	34.1	30.5	1.45	1.92
	24	51.9	50.4	48.8	47.1	45.2	43.2	40.9	38.5	35.7	32.6	29.0	1.14	1.59
56.77	18	59.6	58.0	56.3	54.5	52.5	50.4	48.0	45.4	42.5	39.2	35.4	2.45	2.94
	20	57.8	56.2	54.5	52.6	50.7	48.5	46.2	43.6	40.7	37.4	33.6	1.89	2.37
	22	55.9	54.3	52.6	50.8	48.8	46.7	44.3	41.7	38.8	35.6	31.8	1.44	1.91
	24	54.4	52.8	51.1	49.2	47.3	45.1	42.8	40.2	37.3	34.0	30.2	1.12	1.58
59.75	18	62.4	60.7	58.9	57.0	54.9	52.6	50.2	47.4	44.4	40.9	36.9	2.45	2.94
	20	60.4	58.7	56.9	55.0	52.9	50.7	48.2	45.5	42.4	38.9	34.9	1.87	2.35
	22	58.4	56.8	55.0	53.1	51.0	48.7	46.3	43.5	40.5	37.0	33.0	1.43	1.89
	24	56.8	55.1	53.3	51.4	49.3	47.1	44.6	41.9	38.8	35.3	31.3	1.11	1.56
62.74	18	65.1	63.3	61.4	59.4	57.2	54.9	52.3	49.4	46.2	42.5	38.3	2.45	2.94
	20	63.0	61.2	59.4	57.3	55.2	52.8	50.2	47.3	44.1	40.5	36.3	1.86	2.34
	22	61.0	59.2	57.3	55.3	53.1	50.8	48.2	45.3	42.1	38.4	34.2	1.41	1.88
	24	59.2	57.4	55.6	53.5	51.4	49.0	46.4	43.5	40.3	36.7	32.5	1.09	1.54

TABLE 273

Process Times (B) at Retort Temperature of 230°F for Conduction-Heating Foods in 307 x 409 Can

f_h	z	INITIAL FOOD TEMPERATURE (T_{ih}) 100	110	120	130	140	150	160	170	180	190	200	Equivalent F_c^{18}	F_s^{18}
	18	118.7	116.8	114.7	112.5	110.0	107.2	104.0	100.4	96.1	90.8	84.0	2.64	2.95
54.37	20	105.1	103.2	101.1	98.9	96.4	93.6	90.4	86.8	82.5	77.2	70.4	1.86	2.16
	22	96.0	94.1	92.1	89.8	87.3	84.6	81.4	77.8	73.5	68.2	61.4	1.36	1.66
	24	88.5	86.6	84.5	82.3	79.8	77.0	73.9	70.2	65.9	60.7	53.9	0.98	1.27
	18	123.0	121.0	118.8	116.4	113.8	110.8	107.5	103.6	99.1	93.5	86.3	2.64	2.95
57.57	20	109.4	107.4	105.2	102.8	100.2	97.2	93.9	90.0	85.5	79.9	72.7	1.86	2.16
	22	99.8	97.8	95.6	93.2	90.6	87.7	84.3	80.5	75.9	70.3	63.1	1.33	1.64
	24	92.2	90.2	88.0	85.7	83.0	80.1	76.7	72.9	68.3	62.7	55.6	0.97	1.27
	18	127.1	125.0	122.7	120.2	117.4	114.3	110.8	106.7	101.9	96.0	88.4	2.64	2.95
60.77	20	113.6	111.4	109.1	106.6	103.9	100.7	97.2	93.2	88.3	82.5	74.9	1.85	2.16
	22	103.5	101.4	99.1	96.6	93.8	90.7	87.2	83.1	78.3	72.4	64.8	1.31	1.62
	24	95.9	93.7	91.4	88.9	86.1	83.0	79.5	75.4	70.6	64.7	57.2	0.96	1.26
	18	131.1	128.9	126.5	123.9	120.9	117.7	114.0	109.7	104.6	98.4	90.4	2.64	2.95
63.97	20	117.7	115.4	113.0	110.4	107.4	104.2	100.5	96.2	91.1	84.9	76.9	1.84	2.16
	22	107.2	105.0	102.6	99.9	97.0	93.7	90.0	85.7	80.7	74.5	66.5	1.30	1.61
	24	99.4	97.2	94.8	92.1	89.2	85.9	82.2	77.9	72.9	66.7	58.7	0.94	1.25
	18	135.0	132.7	130.1	127.3	124.3	120.8	116.9	112.4	107.1	100.6	92.2	2.64	2.95
67.12	20	121.7	119.3	116.8	114.0	110.9	107.5	103.6	99.1	93.8	87.3	78.9	1.84	2.16
	22	111.1	108.7	106.2	103.4	100.3	96.9	93.0	88.5	83.2	76.7	68.3	1.29	1.61
	24	102.9	100.6	98.0	95.2	92.2	88.7	84.8	80.3	75.0	68.5	60.1	0.93	1.24

TABLE 274

Process Times (B) at Retort Temperature of 240°F for Conduction-Heating Foods in 307 x 409 Can

f_h	z	INITIAL FOOD TEMPERATURE (T_{ih}) 100	110	120	130	140	150	160	170	180	190	200	Equivalent F_c^{18}	F_s^{18}
	18	84.0	82.2	80.4	78.3	76.1	73.6	70.8	67.6	64.0	59.7	54.4	2.56	2.95
54.37	20	78.7	77.0	75.1	73.0	70.8	68.3	65.5	62.4	58.7	54.4	49.1	1.88	2.26
	22	74.4	72.6	70.7	68.7	66.4	63.9	61.1	58.0	54.4	50.0	44.8	1.40	1.77
	24	70.7	68.9	67.0	65.0	62.7	60.2	57.5	54.3	50.7	46.4	41.1	1.06	1.42
	18	87.8	86.0	84.0	81.8	79.4	76.8	73.8	70.5	66.7	62.1	56.5	2.55	2.95
57.57	20	82.3	80.5	78.5	76.3	73.9	71.3	68.3	65.0	61.1	56.6	51.0	1.86	2.25
	22	77.8	75.9	73.9	71.7	69.3	66.7	63.8	60.4	56.6	52.0	46.4	1.38	1.76
	24	73.9	72.0	70.0	67.9	65.5	62.8	59.9	56.6	52.7	48.1	42.6	1.05	1.41
	18	91.6	89.7	87.6	85.3	82.8	80.0	76.9	73.3	69.3	64.5	58.6	2.55	2.95
60.77	20	85.9	83.9	81.8	79.5	77.0	74.2	71.1	67.6	63.5	58.7	52.8	1.86	2.25
	22	81.1	79.2	77.1	74.8	72.3	69.5	66.4	62.8	58.8	54.0	48.1	1.37	1.75
	24	77.1	75.1	73.0	70.7	68.2	65.4	62.3	58.8	54.7	49.9	44.0	1.03	1.40
	18	95.4	93.3	91.1	88.7	86.0	83.1	79.8	76.1	71.9	66.8	60.6	2.55	2.95
63.97	20	89.4	87.4	85.1	82.7	80.1	77.1	73.9	70.2	65.9	60.8	54.6	1.85	2.24
	22	84.5	82.4	80.2	77.8	75.1	72.2	68.9	65.2	60.9	55.9	49.7	1.36	1.74
	24	80.2	78.2	76.0	73.5	70.9	68.0	64.7	61.0	56.7	51.6	45.4	1.02	1.39
	18	99.2	97.0	94.7	92.1	89.3	86.3	82.8	78.9	74.4	69.1	62.6	2.55	2.95
67.17	20	92.9	90.8	88.4	85.9	83.1	80.1	76.6	72.7	68.2	62.9	56.4	1.84	2.24
	22	87.8	85.7	83.3	80.8	78.0	74.9	71.5	67.6	63.1	57.8	51.3	1.35	1.74
	24	83.4	81.2	78.9	76.3	73.6	70.5	67.1	63.2	58.7	53.3	46.8	1.01	1.38

TABLE 275

Process Times (B) at Retort Temperature of 250°F for Conduction-Heating Foods in 307 x 409 Can

f_h	z	INITIAL FOOD TEMPERATURE (T_{ih}) 100	110	120	130	140	150	160	170	180	190	200	Equivalent F_c^{18}	F_s^{18}
	18	67.3	65.7	64.0	62.1	60.0	57.8	55.3	52.5	49.3	45.7	41.4	2.50	2.95
54.37	20	64.6	63.0	61.3	59.4	57.3	55.1	52.6	49.8	46.6	43.0	38.7	1.93	2.36
	22	62.2	60.6	58.8	56.9	54.9	52.6	50.1	47.4	44.2	40.6	36.3	1.48	1.91
	24	59.8	58.2	56.4	54.5	52.5	50.2	47.7	45.0	41.8	38.2	33.9	1.13	1.54
	18	70.6	68.9	67.1	65.1	62.9	60.5	57.9	54.9	51.6	47.7	43.2	2.50	2.95
57.57	20	67.8	66.1	64.2	62.2	60.0	57.7	55.0	52.1	48.7	44.9	40.3	1.92	2.36
	22	65.2	63.5	61.6	59.6	57.4	55.1	52.4	49.5	46.1	42.3	37.7	1.47	1.89
	24	62.7	60.9	59.1	57.1	54.9	52.5	49.9	47.0	43.6	39.8	35.2	1.11	1.52
	18	73.9	72.1	70.1	68.0	65.7	63.2	60.4	57.3	53.8	49.7	44.9	2.50	2.95
60.77	20	70.9	69.1	67.1	65.0	62.7	60.2	57.4	54.3	50.8	46.7	41.9	1.90	2.34
	22	68.2	66.3	64.4	62.3	60.0	57.5	54.7	51.6	48.0	44.0	39.2	1.45	1.87
	24	65.5	63.7	61.7	59.6	57.3	54.8	52.0	48.9	45.4	41.3	36.5	1.09	1.50
	18	77.2	75.3	73.2	71.0	68.6	65.9	63.0	59.7	56.0	51.7	46.7	2.50	2.95
63.97	20	74.0	72.1	70.1	67.8	65.4	62.8	59.8	56.6	52.9	48.6	43.5	1.89	2.33
	22	71.1	69.2	67.1	64.9	62.5	59.8	56.9	53.6	49.9	45.7	40.6	1.43	1.86
	24	68.3	66.4	64.4	62.1	59.7	57.1	54.1	50.9	47.2	42.9	37.8	1.07	1.48
	18	80.4	78.4	76.3	73.9	71.4	68.6	65.5	62.1	58.2	53.7	48.4	2.49	2.95
67.17	20	77.1	75.1	72.9	70.6	68.1	65.3	62.2	58.8	54.9	50.4	45.1	1.88	2.33
	22	74.0	72.0	69.9	67.5	65.0	62.2	59.1	55.7	51.8	47.3	42.0	1.41	1.84
	24	71.1	69.1	67.0	64.6	62.1	59.3	56.2	52.8	48.9	44.4	39.1	1.05	1.47

TABLE 276

Process Times (B) at Retort Temperature of 260°F for Conduction-Heating Foods in 307 x 409 Can

f_h	z	INITIAL FOOD TEMPERATURE (T_{ih})											Equivalent	
		100	110	120	130	140	150	160	170	180	190	200	F_c^{18}	F_s^{18}
	18	57.5	55.9	54.3	52.6	50.7	48.6	46.4	43.9	41.1	37.9	34.3	2.46	2.95
54.37	20	55.7	54.2	52.5	50.8	48.9	46.8	44.6	42.1	39.3	36.2	32.5	1.91	2.39
	22	53.9	52.4	50.8	49.0	47.1	45.1	42.8	40.3	37.6	34.4	30.8	1.46	1.92
	24	52.4	50.9	49.3	47.5	45.6	43.6	41.3	38.9	36.1	32.9	29.3	1.15	1.60
	18	60.4	58.8	57.1	55.2	53.2	51.0	48.7	46.0	43.1	39.7	35.9	2.46	2.95
57.57	20	58.5	56.9	55.2	53.3	51.3	49.1	46.8	44.1	41.2	37.8	34.0	1.90	2.38
	22	56.7	55.0	53.3	51.5	49.5	47.3	44.9	42.3	39.3	36.0	32.1	1.45	1.91
	24	55.1	53.4	51.7	49.9	47.9	45.7	43.3	40.7	37.7	34.4	30.5	1.13	1.58
	18	63.3	61.6	59.8	57.8	55.7	53.4	50.9	48.1	45.0	41.5	37.4	2.46	2.95
60.77	20	61.3	59.6	57.8	55.8	53.7	51.4	48.9	46.1	43.0	39.5	35.4	1.88	2.36
	22	59.3	57.6	55.8	53.9	51.8	49.5	46.9	44.2	41.0	37.5	33.5	1.43	1.90
	24	57.7	55.9	54.1	52.2	50.1	47.8	45.2	42.5	39.4	35.8	31.8	1.11	1.56
	18	66.2	64.4	62.5	60.5	58.2	55.8	53.2	50.2	47.0	43.3	39.0	2.46	2.95
63.97	20	64.1	62.3	60.4	58.3	56.1	53.7	51.0	48.1	44.8	41.1	36.8	1.87	2.35
	22	62.0	60.2	58.3	56.3	54.0	51.6	49.0	46.1	42.8	39.1	34.8	1.42	1.88
	24	60.2	58.4	56.5	54.5	52.2	49.8	47.2	44.2	41.0	37.3	33.0	1.09	1.54
	18	69.1	67.2	65.2	63.1	60.7	58.2	55.4	52.3	48.9	45.0	40.5	2.46	2.95
67.17	20	66.9	65.0	63.0	60.8	58.5	55.9	53.2	50.1	46.6	42.8	38.3	1.86	2.34
	22	64.7	62.8	60.8	58.6	56.3	53.8	51.0	47.9	44.5	40.6	36.1	1.40	1.87
	24	62.8	60.9	58.9	56.7	54.4	51.9	49.1	46.0	42.6	38.7	34.2	1.07	1.53

TABLE 277

Process Times (B) at Retort Temperature of 230°F for Conduction-Heating Foods in 307 x 510 Can

f_h	z	INITIAL FOOD TEMPERATURE (T_{ih}) 100	110	120	130	140	150	160	170	180	190	200	Equivalent F_c^{18}	F_s^{18}
	18	125.0	123.0	120.8	118.3	115.6	112.6	109.2	105.3	100.6	94.9	87.5	2.66	2.97
58.89	20	111.3	109.3	107.1	104.6	101.9	98.9	95.5	91.6	86.9	81.2	73.8	1.87	2.18
	22	101.6	99.5	97.3	94.9	92.2	89.2	85.8	81.8	77.2	71.4	64.1	1.34	1.64
	24	93.9	91.9	89.6	87.2	84.5	81.5	78.1	74.1	69.5	63.8	56.4	0.97	1.27
	18	129.5	127.3	125.0	122.4	119.5	116.4	112.7	108.6	103.6	97.6	89.8	2.66	2.97
62.35	20	115.9	113.7	111.3	108.8	105.9	102.7	99.1	94.9	90.0	83.9	76.2	1.86	2.18
	22	105.6	103.4	101.1	98.5	95.6	92.4	88.8	84.6	79.7	73.7	65.9	1.32	1.63
	24	97.8	95.7	93.3	90.7	87.9	84.7	81.1	76.9	72.0	65.9	58.1	0.96	1.26
	18	133.8	131.5	129.0	126.3	123.3	119.9	116.1	111.7	106.5	100.1	91.9	2.66	2.97
65.82	20	120.3	118.0	115.5	112.8	109.8	106.4	102.6	98.2	92.9	86.6	78.3	1.85	2.18
	22	109.7	107.4	104.9	102.2	99.2	95.8	92.0	87.6	82.4	76.0	67.8	1.31	1.62
	24	101.7	99.4	96.9	94.2	91.1	87.8	84.0	79.6	74.3	68.0	59.7	0.94	1.25
	18	138.1	135.6	133.0	130.2	127.0	123.4	119.4	114.8	109.3	102.6	93.9	2.66	2.97
69.28	20	124.6	122.2	119.5	116.7	113.5	110.0	105.9	101.3	95.8	89.1	80.4	1.85	2.17
	22	113.8	111.4	108.8	105.9	102.8	99.2	95.2	90.6	85.1	78.4	69.7	1.30	1.61
	24	105.4	103.0	100.4	97.5	94.3	90.8	86.8	82.1	76.7	69.9	61.3	0.93	1.24
	18	143.0	140.4	137.7	134.7	131.4	127.6	123.4	118.5	112.8	105.7	96.6	2.65	2.97
72.75	20	128.8	126.3	123.5	120.5	117.2	113.5	109.2	104.4	98.6	91.6	82.5	1.84	2.16
	22	117.9	115.4	112.6	109.6	106.3	102.6	98.3	93.5	87.7	80.7	71.6	1.28	1.61
	24	109.2	106.6	103.9	100.9	97.5	93.8	89.6	84.7	79.0	71.9	62.8	0.92	1.23

TABLE 278

Process Times (B) at Retort Temperature of 240°F for Conduction-Heating Foods in 307 x 510 Can

f_h	z	INITIAL FOOD TEMPERATURE (T_{ih})											Equivalent	
		100	110	120	130	140	150	160	170	180	190	200	F_c^{18}	F_s^{18}
	18	89.6	87.7	85.6	83.4	81.0	78.3	75.2	71.8	67.9	63.2	57.5	2.57	2.97
58.89	20	83.9	82.0	80.0	77.8	75.3	72.6	69.6	66.2	62.3	57.6	51.9	1.88	2.27
	22	79.3	77.4	75.3	73.1	70.7	68.0	65.0	61.5	57.6	52.9	47.2	1.39	1.77
	24	75.3	73.4	71.4	69.2	66.7	64.0	61.0	57.6	53.7	49.0	43.3	1.05	1.42
	18	93.7	91.6	89.5	87.1	84.5	81.7	78.5	74.9	70.7	65.8	59.7	2.57	2.97
62.35	20	87.8	85.8	83.6	81.3	78.7	75.8	72.6	69.0	64.8	59.9	53.9	1.87	2.26
	22	82.9	80.9	78.8	76.4	73.8	71.0	67.8	64.2	60.0	55.0	49.0	1.37	1.76
	24	78.8	76.8	74.6	72.2	69.7	66.8	63.6	60.0	55.8	50.9	44.8	1.04	1.40
	18	97.7	95.6	93.3	90.8	88.1	85.1	81.7	77.9	73.5	68.3	61.9	2.57	2.97
65.82	20	91.6	89.5	87.2	84.7	82.0	79.0	75.6	71.8	67.4	62.2	55.8	1.86	2.25
	22	86.5	84.4	82.1	79.6	76.9	73.9	70.5	66.7	62.3	57.1	50.7	1.37	1.75
	24	82.2	80.1	77.8	75.3	72.6	69.6	66.2	62.4	58.0	52.7	46.4	1.02	1.39
	18	101.8	99.5	97.1	94.5	91.6	88.5	84.9	80.9	76.3	70.8	64.1	2.56	2.97
69.28	20	95.4	93.2	90.8	88.1	85.3	82.1	78.6	74.5	69.9	64.4	57.7	1.85	2.24
	22	90.1	87.9	85.5	82.9	80.0	76.9	73.3	69.3	64.7	59.2	52.5	1.36	1.75
	24	85.6	83.4	81.0	78.3	75.5	72.3	68.8	64.7	60.1	54.6	47.9	1.01	1.38
	18	105.8	103.4	100.9	98.2	95.1	91.8	88.1	83.9	79.0	73.2	66.2	2.56	2.97
72.75	20	99.2	96.8	94.3	91.5	88.5	85.2	81.5	77.3	72.4	66.6	59.6	1.83	2.23
	22	93.7	91.4	88.8	86.1	83.1	79.7	76.0	71.8	66.9	61.2	54.1	1.35	1.74
	24	89.0	86.7	84.1	81.4	78.4	75.0	71.3	67.1	62.2	56.5	49.4	1.00	1.38

TABLE 279

Process Times (B) at Retort Temperature of 250°F for Conduction-Heating Foods in 307 x 510 Can

f_h	z	INITIAL FOOD TEMPERATURE (T_{ih})											Equivalent	
		100	110	120	130	140	150	160	170	180	190	200	F_c^{18}	F_s^{18}
	18	72.1	70.3	68.4	66.4	64.2	61.7	59.0	56.0	52.6	48.7	44.0	2.52	2.97
58.89	20	69.2	67.4	65.5	63.5	61.2	58.8	56.1	53.1	49.7	45.7	41.1	1.93	2.37
	22	66.5	64.7	62.8	60.8	58.6	56.1	53.4	50.4	47.0	43.1	38.4	1.47	1.90
	24	63.9	62.2	60.3	58.2	56.0	53.6	50.9	47.9	44.4	40.5	35.8	1.11	1.52
	18	75.6	73.8	71.8	69.6	67.2	64.6	61.8	58.6	55.0	50.8	45.9	2.52	2.97
62.35	20	72.5	70.7	68.7	66.5	64.1	61.6	58.7	55.5	51.9	47.7	42.8	1.91	2.35
	22	69.7	67.8	65.8	63.7	61.3	58.7	55.9	52.7	49.1	44.9	40.0	1.45	1.88
	24	67.0	65.1	63.1	61.0	58.6	56.0	53.2	50.0	46.4	42.2	37.2	1.09	1.50
	18	79.2	77.2	75.1	72.8	70.3	67.6	64.6	61.2	57.4	53.0	47.8	2.51	2.97
65.82	20	75.9	73.9	71.8	69.5	67.0	64.3	61.3	57.9	54.1	49.7	44.5	1.90	2.35
	22	72.9	70.9	68.8	66.5	64.0	61.3	58.3	54.9	51.1	46.7	41.5	1.43	1.86
	24	70.0	68.1	66.0	63.7	61.2	58.5	55.4	52.1	48.3	43.9	38.6	1.07	1.48
	18	82.7	80.6	78.4	76.0	73.3	70.5	67.3	63.8	59.7	55.1	49.6	2.51	2.97
69.28	20	79.3	77.2	74.9	72.5	69.9	67.1	63.9	60.3	56.3	51.7	46.2	1.89	2.34
	22	76.1	74.0	71.8	69.4	66.7	63.9	60.7	57.2	53.1	48.5	43.0	1.42	1.85
	24	73.1	71.0	68.8	66.4	63.7	60.9	57.7	54.2	50.1	45.5	40.0	1.05	1.47
	18	86.2	84.0	81.6	79.1	76.4	73.3	70.0	66.3	62.1	57.2	51.4	2.51	2.97
72.75	20	82.6	80.4	78.0	75.5	72.8	69.8	66.4	62.7	58.5	53.6	47.9	1.88	2.33
	22	79.2	77.0	74.7	72.1	69.4	66.4	63.1	59.3	55.1	50.3	44.5	1.40	1.83
	24	76.1	73.9	71.6	69.0	66.3	63.3	59.9	56.2	52.0	47.1	41.4	1.04	1.45

TABLE 280

Process Times (B) at Retort Temperature of 260°F for Conduction-Heating Foods in 307 x 510 Can

f_h	z	INITIAL FOOD TEMPERATURE (T_{ih})											Equivalent	
		100	110	120	130	140	150	160	170	180	190	200	F_c^{18}	F_s^{18}
	18	61.7	60.0	58.3	56.4	54.3	52.1	49.6	47.0	43.9	40.5	36.6	2.48	2.97
58.89	20	59.7	58.1	56.3	54.4	52.4	50.1	47.7	45.0	42.0	38.6	34.6	1.91	2.39
	22	57.8	56.2	54.4	52.5	50.5	48.2	45.8	43.1	40.1	36.7	32.7	1.45	1.92
	24	56.2	54.5	52.8	50.9	48.8	46.6	44.2	41.5	38.5	35.0	31.1	1.13	1.58
	18	64.8	63.1	61.2	59.2	57.0	54.7	52.1	49.2	46.1	42.4	38.3	2.48	2.97
62.35	20	62.8	61.0	59.1	57.1	55.0	52.6	50.0	47.2	44.0	40.4	36.2	1.89	2.37
	22	60.7	59.0	57.1	55.1	53.0	50.6	48.0	45.2	42.0	38.4	34.2	1.44	1.90
	24	59.0	57.2	55.4	53.4	51.2	48.8	46.3	43.4	40.2	36.6	32.4	1.11	1.57
	18	68.0	66.1	64.1	62.0	59.7	57.3	54.5	51.5	48.2	44.3	39.9	2.48	2.97
65.82	20	65.8	63.9	62.0	59.8	57.5	55.1	52.3	49.3	46.0	42.1	37.7	1.88	2.36
	22	63.6	61.8	59.8	57.7	55.4	52.9	50.2	47.2	43.8	40.0	35.6	1.42	1.89
	24	61.8	59.9	58.0	55.8	53.6	51.1	48.3	45.3	42.0	38.1	33.7	1.09	1.54
	18	71.1	69.1	67.1	64.8	62.4	59.8	56.9	53.8	50.2	46.2	41.6	2.47	2.97
69.28	20	68.8	66.8	64.7	62.5	60.1	57.5	54.6	51.4	47.9	43.9	39.2	1.87	2.35
	22	66.5	64.6	62.5	60.3	57.9	55.3	52.4	49.2	45.7	41.7	37.0	1.41	1.88
	24	64.5	62.6	60.5	58.3	55.9	53.3	50.4	47.2	43.7	39.7	35.0	1.07	1.53
	18	74.2	72.2	70.0	67.7	65.1	62.4	59.4	56.0	52.3	48.1	43.2	2.47	2.97
72.75	20	71.7	69.7	67.5	65.2	62.6	59.9	56.9	53.6	49.8	45.6	40.7	1.86	2.35
	22	69.4	67.4	65.2	62.8	60.3	57.6	54.6	51.2	47.5	43.3	38.4	1.40	1.87
	24	67.3	65.2	63.1	60.7	58.2	55.5	52.4	49.1	45.4	41.2	36.3	1.06	1.51

TABLE 281

Process Times (B) at Retort Temperature of 230°F for Conduction-Heating Foods in 307 x 512 Can

f_h	z	INITIAL FOOD TEMPERATURE (T_{ih})											Equivalent	
		100	110	120	130	140	150	160	170	180	190	200	F_c^{18}	F_s^{18}
	18	125.6	123.5	121.3	118.8	116.1	113.1	109.7	105.7	101.0	95.3	87.8	2.66	2.98
59.29	20	111.9	109.8	107.6	105.1	102.4	99.4	96.0	92.0	87.3	81.5	74.1	1.87	2.18
	22	102.1	100.0	97.8	95.3	92.6	89.6	86.1	82.2	77.5	71.7	64.3	1.34	1.64
	24	94.4	92.3	90.1	87.6	84.9	81.9	78.5	74.5	69.8	64.0	56.6	0.97	1.27
	18	130.1	127.9	125.5	122.9	120.0	116.8	113.2	109.0	104.0	97.9	90.1	2.66	2.98
62.77	20	116.4	114.2	111.9	109.3	106.4	103.2	99.5	95.3	90.4	84.3	76.4	1.86	2.18
	22	106.1	103.9	101.5	98.9	96.1	92.9	89.2	85.0	80.0	74.0	66.1	1.32	1.63
	24	98.3	96.1	93.8	91.2	88.3	85.1	81.4	77.2	72.3	66.2	58.3	0.96	1.26
	18	134.4	132.1	129.6	126.8	123.8	120.4	116.6	112.1	106.9	100.5	92.2	2.66	2.98
66.26	20	120.8	118.5	116.0	113.3	110.3	106.9	103.0	98.6	93.3	86.9	78.6	1.85	2.18
	22	110.2	107.9	105.4	102.7	99.6	96.3	92.4	88.0	82.7	76.3	68.0	1.31	1.62
	24	102.2	99.9	97.4	94.6	91.6	88.2	84.3	79.9	74.7	68.2	60.0	0.94	1.25
	18	138.7	136.3	133.7	130.8	127.6	124.0	120.0	115.3	109.8	103.0	94.3	2.66	2.97
69.75	20	125.2	122.7	120.1	117.2	114.0	110.5	106.4	101.7	96.2	89.5	80.8	1.85	2.17
	22	114.4	112.0	109.3	106.5	103.3	99.7	95.7	91.0	85.5	78.7	70.0	1.30	1.61
	24	105.9	103.5	100.9	98.0	94.8	91.2	87.2	82.5	77.0	70.2	61.5	0.93	1.24
	18	143.7	141.1	138.4	135.3	132.0	128.2	124.0	119.1	113.3	106.2	97.0	2.65	2.98
73.23	20	129.4	126.9	124.1	121.1	117.7	114.0	109.7	104.8	99.0	91.9	82.8	1.83	2.16
	22	118.5	115.9	113.2	110.1	106.8	103.1	98.8	93.9	88.1	81.0	71.9	1.28	1.61
	24	109.7	107.2	104.4	101.4	98.0	94.3	90.0	85.1	79.3	72.2	63.1	0.92	1.23

TABLE 282

Process Times (B) at Retort Temperature of 240°F for Conduction-Heating Foods in 307 x 512 Can

f_h	z	INITIAL FOOD TEMPERATURE (T_{ih})											Equivalent	
		100	110	120	130	140	150	160	170	180	190	200	F_c^{18}	F_s^{18}
	18	90.0	88.1	86.1	83.8	81.4	78.7	75.6	72.2	68.2	63.5	57.8	2.57	2.98
59.29	20	84.4	82.5	80.4	78.2	75.7	73.0	70.0	66.5	62.6	57.9	52.1	1.88	2.27
	22	79.7	77.8	75.7	73.5	71.0	68.3	65.3	61.9	57.9	53.2	47.4	1.39	1.77
	24	75.7	73.8	71.8	69.5	67.1	64.4	61.3	57.9	53.9	49.2	43.5	1.05	1.42
	18	94.2	92.1	90.0	87.6	85.0	82.1	78.9	75.3	71.1	66.1	60.0	2.57	2.98
62.77	20	88.3	86.2	84.1	81.7	79.1	76.2	73.0	69.4	65.2	60.2	54.1	1.87	2.26
	22	83.4	81.4	79.2	76.8	74.2	71.3	68.1	64.5	60.3	55.3	49.2	1.37	1.76
	24	79.2	77.2	75.0	72.6	70.0	67.2	63.9	60.3	56.1	51.1	45.0	1.03	1.40
	18	98.3	96.1	93.8	91.3	88.6	85.5	82.2	78.3	73.9	68.6	62.2	2.57	2.98
66.26	20	92.1	90.0	87.7	85.2	82.4	79.4	76.0	72.2	67.7	62.5	56.1	1.86	2.26
	22	87.0	84.9	82.6	80.1	77.3	74.3	70.9	67.1	62.6	57.4	51.0	1.37	1.75
	24	82.6	80.5	78.2	75.7	72.9	69.9	66.5	62.7	58.2	53.0	46.6	1.02	1.39
	18	102.3	100.1	97.7	95.0	92.1	88.9	85.4	81.3	76.7	71.1	64.4	2.56	2.98
69.75	20	95.9	93.7	91.3	88.6	85.7	82.5	79.0	74.9	70.3	64.7	58.0	1.85	2.24
	22	90.6	88.4	86.0	83.3	80.5	77.3	73.7	69.6	65.0	59.5	52.7	1.36	1.75
	24	86.1	83.8	81.4	78.8	75.9	72.7	69.1	65.1	60.4	54.9	48.1	1.01	1.38
	18	106.3	104.0	101.4	98.7	95.6	92.3	88.5	84.3	79.4	73.6	66.5	2.56	2.98
73.23	20	99.7	97.3	94.8	92.0	89.0	85.6	81.9	77.7	72.7	67.0	59.9	1.83	2.23
	22	94.2	91.9	89.3	86.6	83.5	80.2	76.4	72.2	67.3	61.5	54.4	1.36	1.74
	24	89.5	87.1	84.6	81.8	78.8	75.4	71.7	67.5	62.5	56.8	49.7	1.00	1.38

TABLE 283

Process Times (B) at Retort Temperature of 250°F for Conduction-Heating Foods in 307 x 512 Can

f_h	z	Initial Food Temperature (T_{ih}) 100	110	120	130	140	150	160	170	180	190	200	Equivalent F_c^{18}	F_s^{18}
59.29	18	72.5	70.7	68.8	66.8	64.5	62.1	59.4	56.3	52.9	48.9	44.2	2.52	2.98
	20	69.6	67.8	65.9	63.8	61.6	59.1	56.4	53.4	50.0	46.0	41.3	1.93	2.37
	22	66.9	65.1	63.2	61.1	58.9	56.4	53.7	50.7	47.3	43.3	38.6	1.47	1.90
	24	64.3	62.5	60.6	58.5	56.3	53.9	51.1	48.1	44.7	40.7	36.0	1.11	1.52
62.77	18	76.1	74.2	72.2	70.0	67.6	65.0	62.1	58.9	55.3	51.1	46.1	2.52	2.98
	20	73.0	71.1	69.1	66.9	64.5	61.9	59.0	55.8	52.2	48.0	43.0	1.91	2.35
	22	70.1	68.2	66.2	64.0	61.6	59.0	56.2	53.0	49.3	45.1	40.2	1.45	1.88
	24	67.4	65.5	63.5	61.3	58.9	56.3	53.4	50.2	46.6	42.4	37.4	1.09	1.50
66.26	18	79.6	77.6	75.5	73.2	70.7	68.0	64.9	61.5	57.7	53.3	48.0	2.52	2.98
	20	76.4	74.4	72.2	69.9	67.4	64.7	61.7	58.3	54.4	50.0	44.7	1.90	2.35
	22	73.3	71.3	69.2	66.9	64.4	61.6	58.6	55.2	51.4	46.9	41.7	1.43	1.86
	24	70.4	68.5	66.3	64.0	61.5	58.8	55.7	52.4	48.5	44.1	38.8	1.07	1.48
69.75	18	83.2	81.1	78.8	76.4	73.8	70.9	67.7	64.1	60.1	55.4	49.9	2.51	2.98
	20	79.7	77.6	75.4	73.0	70.3	67.4	64.2	60.7	56.6	52.0	46.4	1.89	2.34
	22	76.5	74.4	72.2	69.7	67.1	64.2	61.0	57.5	53.4	48.7	43.2	1.42	1.85
	24	73.5	71.4	69.2	66.7	64.1	61.2	58.0	54.5	50.4	45.7	40.2	1.05	1.47
73.23	18	86.7	84.5	82.1	79.6	76.8	73.8	70.4	66.7	62.4	57.5	51.7	2.51	2.98
	20	83.0	80.8	78.5	75.9	73.2	70.1	66.8	63.0	58.8	53.9	48.1	1.88	2.33
	22	79.6	77.5	75.1	72.6	69.8	66.8	63.4	59.7	55.4	50.5	44.7	1.40	1.83
	24	76.5	74.3	72.0	69.4	66.6	63.6	60.3	56.5	52.3	47.4	41.6	1.04	1.45

TABLE 284

Process Times (B) at Retort Temperature of 260°F for Conduction-Heating Foods in 307 x 512 Can

f_h	z	INITIAL FOOD TEMPERATURE (T_{ih})											Equivalent	
		100	110	120	130	140	150	160	170	180	190	200	F_c^{18}	F_s^{18}
	18	62.0	60.4	58.6	56.7	54.6	52.4	49.9	47.2	44.2	40.8	36.8	2.48	2.98
59.29	20	60.1	58.4	56.6	54.7	52.7	50.4	48.0	45.3	42.2	38.8	34.8	1.91	2.39
	22	58.2	56.5	54.7	52.8	50.8	48.5	46.1	43.4	40.3	36.9	32.9	1.45	1.92
	24	56.5	54.9	53.1	51.2	49.1	46.9	44.4	41.7	38.7	35.2	31.3	1.13	1.58
	18	65.2	63.5	61.6	59.5	57.4	55.0	52.4	49.5	46.3	42.7	38.5	2.48	2.98
62.77	20	63.1	61.4	59.5	57.5	55.3	52.9	50.3	47.4	44.2	40.6	36.4	1.89	2.37
	22	61.1	59.3	57.5	55.4	53.3	50.9	48.3	45.4	42.2	38.6	34.4	1.44	1.90
	24	59.3	57.6	55.7	53.7	51.5	49.1	46.5	43.7	40.4	36.8	32.6	1.11	1.56
	18	68.4	66.5	64.5	62.4	60.1	57.6	54.8	51.8	48.4	44.6	40.1	2.48	2.98
66.26	20	66.2	64.3	62.3	60.2	57.9	55.4	52.6	49.6	46.2	42.4	37.9	1.88	2.36
	22	64.0	62.2	60.2	58.0	55.7	53.2	50.5	47.5	44.1	40.2	35.8	1.42	1.89
	24	62.1	60.3	58.3	56.2	53.9	51.4	48.6	45.6	42.2	38.3	33.9	1.09	1.54
	18	71.5	69.6	67.5	65.2	62.8	60.2	57.3	54.1	50.5	46.5	41.8	2.48	2.98
69.75	20	69.2	67.2	65.1	62.9	60.5	57.8	54.9	51.7	48.2	44.1	39.5	1.87	2.35
	22	66.9	65.0	62.9	60.6	58.2	55.6	52.7	49.5	45.9	41.9	37.2	1.41	1.88
	24	64.9	63.0	60.9	58.6	56.2	53.6	50.7	47.5	43.9	39.9	35.2	1.07	1.53
	18	74.7	72.6	70.4	68.1	65.5	62.7	59.7	56.4	52.6	48.4	43.5	2.47	2.98
73.23	20	72.2	70.1	67.9	65.6	63.0	60.2	57.2	53.9	50.1	45.9	41.0	1.86	2.35
	22	69.8	67.8	65.6	63.2	60.7	57.9	54.9	51.5	47.8	43.5	38.6	1.39	1.87
	24	67.7	65.6	63.4	61.1	58.5	55.8	52.7	49.4	45.6	41.4	36.5	1.05	1.51

TABLE 285

Process Times (B) at Retort Temperature of 230°F for Conduction-Heating Foods in 307 x 704 Can

f_h	z	100	110	120	130	140	150	160	170	180	190	200	Equivalent F_c^{18}	Equivalent F_s^{18}
		INITIAL FOOD TEMPERATURE (T_{ih})												
62.69	18	130.4	128.2	125.8	123.2	120.3	117.1	113.5	109.3	104.3	98.3	90.4	2.68	3.00
	20	116.6	114.4	112.0	109.4	106.6	103.4	99.7	95.5	90.6	84.5	76.7	1.88	2.20
	22	106.3	104.1	101.7	99.1	96.3	93.0	89.4	85.2	80.3	74.2	66.3	1.33	1.64
	24	98.4	96.3	93.9	91.3	88.4	85.2	81.6	77.4	72.4	66.4	58.5	0.97	1.27
66.37	18	134.9	132.6	130.1	127.4	124.3	120.9	117.1	112.6	107.4	101.0	92.7	2.68	3.00
	20	121.3	119.0	116.5	113.7	110.7	107.3	103.4	99.0	93.7	87.3	79.0	1.87	2.20
	22	110.6	108.3	105.8	103.0	100.0	96.6	92.8	88.3	83.1	76.6	68.3	1.32	1.63
	24	102.5	100.2	97.7	95.0	91.9	88.5	84.7	80.2	75.0	68.5	60.3	0.95	1.26
70.06	18	139.5	137.1	134.4	131.5	128.3	124.7	120.7	116.0	110.4	103.6	94.9	2.68	2.99
	20	125.9	123.4	120.8	117.9	114.7	111.1	107.0	102.3	96.8	90.0	81.2	1.86	2.19
	22	115.0	112.6	109.9	107.0	103.8	100.3	96.2	91.5	86.0	79.2	70.4	1.31	1.63
	24	106.5	104.1	101.4	98.5	95.3	91.7	87.7	83.0	77.4	70.6	61.9	0.94	1.25
73.75	18	144.7	142.2	139.4	136.3	132.9	129.2	124.9	120.0	114.1	107.0	97.8	2.67	3.00
	20	130.4	127.8	125.0	122.0	118.6	114.8	110.5	105.6	99.8	92.6	83.4	1.85	2.18
	22	119.4	116.8	114.0	110.9	107.6	103.8	99.5	94.6	88.7	81.6	72.4	1.29	1.62
	24	110.5	108.0	105.2	102.1	98.7	95.0	90.7	85.8	79.9	72.8	63.6	0.92	1.24
77.44	18	149.8	147.1	144.2	141.0	137.5	133.5	129.0	123.8	117.7	110.2	100.5	2.67	3.00
	20	134.8	132.1	129.2	126.0	122.4	118.5	114.0	108.8	102.7	95.2	85.5	1.83	2.16
	22	123.6	120.9	118.0	114.8	111.2	107.3	102.8	97.6	91.5	84.0	74.3	1.28	1.61
	24	114.6	111.9	108.9	105.7	102.2	98.2	93.7	88.6	82.4	74.9	65.2	0.91	1.23

TABLE 286

Process Times (B) at Retort Temperature of 240°F for Conduction-Heating Foods in 307 x 704 Can

f_h	z	INITIAL FOOD TEMPERATURE (T_{ih})											Equivalent	
		100	110	120	130	140	150	160	170	180	190	200	F_c^{18}	F_s^{18}
62.69	18	94.2	92.2	90.0	87.7	85.1	82.2	79.0	75.4	71.2	66.2	60.1	2.59	3.00
	20	88.3	86.3	84.1	81.8	79.2	76.3	73.1	69.5	65.3	60.3	54.2	1.89	2.28
	22	83.4	81.4	79.2	76.9	74.3	71.4	68.2	64.6	60.4	55.4	49.3	1.39	1.77
	24	79.2	77.2	75.1	72.7	70.1	67.2	64.0	60.4	56.2	51.2	45.1	1.05	1.41
66.37	18	98.6	96.4	94.1	91.6	88.9	85.8	82.4	78.6	74.1	68.9	62.4	2.59	3.00
	20	92.4	90.2	87.9	85.4	82.7	79.6	76.2	72.4	68.0	62.7	56.3	1.88	2.27
	22	87.3	85.1	82.8	80.3	77.6	74.5	71.1	67.3	62.9	57.6	51.2	1.38	1.76
	24	82.9	80.7	78.4	75.9	73.2	70.1	66.7	62.9	58.5	53.2	46.8	1.03	1.40
70.06	18	102.9	100.6	98.2	95.5	92.6	89.4	85.8	81.8	77.1	71.5	64.7	2.59	3.00
	20	96.4	94.2	91.7	89.1	86.2	83.0	79.4	75.3	70.6	65.1	58.3	1.86	2.26
	22	91.1	88.9	86.4	83.8	80.9	77.7	74.1	70.0	65.3	59.8	53.0	1.37	1.76
	24	86.5	84.3	81.8	79.2	76.3	73.1	69.5	65.4	60.7	55.2	48.4	1.02	1.39
73.75	18	107.1	104.7	102.2	99.4	96.3	93.0	89.2	84.9	80.0	74.1	67.0	2.58	3.00
	20	100.4	98.0	95.5	92.7	89.6	86.3	82.5	78.2	73.3	67.4	60.3	1.85	2.25
	22	94.9	92.5	90.0	87.2	84.1	80.8	77.0	72.7	67.8	61.9	54.8	1.37	1.75
	24	90.1	87.8	85.2	82.4	79.4	76.0	72.2	67.9	63.0	57.2	50.0	1.01	1.39
77.44	18	111.4	108.9	106.2	103.2	100.0	96.5	92.5	88.0	82.9	76.7	69.2	2.58	3.00
	20	104.4	101.9	99.2	96.3	93.1	89.5	85.6	81.1	75.9	69.8	62.3	1.84	2.24
	22	98.7	96.2	93.5	90.6	87.4	83.9	79.9	75.4	70.2	64.1	56.6	1.36	1.75
	24	93.7	91.2	88.5	85.6	82.4	78.9	74.9	70.4	65.2	59.1	51.6	1.00	1.37

TABLE 287

Process Times (B) at Retort Temperature of 250°F for Conduction-Heating Foods in 307 x 704 Can

f_h	z	INITIAL FOOD TEMPERATURE (T_{ih})											Equivalent	
		100	110	120	130	140	150	160	170	180	190	200	F_c^{18}	F_s^{18}
	18	76.1	74.2	72.2	70.0	67.6	65.0	62.2	59.0	55.3	51.1	46.2	2.54	3.00
62.69	20	73.0	71.1	69.1	66.9	64.5	61.9	59.1	55.9	52.2	48.0	43.1	1.93	2.37
	22	70.1	68.2	66.2	64.1	61.7	59.1	56.2	53.0	49.4	45.2	40.2	1.46	1.89
	24	67.4	65.5	63.5	61.3	59.0	56.4	53.5	50.3	46.6	42.5	37.5	1.10	1.51
	18	79.8	77.9	75.7	73.4	70.9	68.2	65.1	61.7	57.9	53.4	48.2	2.54	3.00
66.37	20	76.6	74.6	72.4	70.1	67.6	64.9	61.8	58.4	54.6	50.1	44.9	1.92	2.37
	22	73.5	71.5	69.4	67.1	64.6	61.8	58.8	55.4	51.6	47.1	41.9	1.45	1.88
	24	70.6	68.7	66.5	64.2	61.7	59.0	55.9	52.5	48.7	44.2	39.0	1.08	1.49
	18	83.6	81.5	79.2	76.8	74.1	71.2	68.0	64.5	60.4	55.7	50.1	2.54	3.00
70.06	20	80.1	78.0	75.8	73.3	70.7	67.8	64.6	61.0	56.9	52.2	46.7	1.91	2.36
	22	76.9	74.8	72.5	70.1	67.5	64.6	61.3	57.8	53.7	49.0	43.5	1.43	1.86
	24	73.9	71.8	69.5	67.1	64.4	61.5	58.3	54.7	50.7	46.0	40.4	1.06	1.48
	18	87.3	85.1	82.7	80.1	77.3	74.3	70.9	67.1	62.9	57.9	52.1	2.53	3.00
73.75	20	83.6	81.4	79.0	76.5	73.7	70.6	67.3	63.5	59.2	54.3	48.4	1.90	2.34
	22	80.2	78.0	75.6	73.1	70.3	67.2	63.9	60.1	55.8	50.9	45.0	1.41	1.84
	24	77.1	74.9	72.5	69.9	67.1	64.1	60.7	56.9	52.7	47.7	41.9	1.05	1.46
	18	91.0	88.6	86.1	83.5	80.5	77.3	73.8	69.8	65.3	60.1	54.0	2.53	3.00
77.44	20	87.1	84.8	82.3	79.6	76.7	73.5	69.9	66.0	61.5	56.3	50.2	1.88	2.33
	22	83.5	81.2	78.7	76.0	73.1	69.9	66.4	62.4	57.9	52.7	46.6	1.39	1.82
	24	80.2	77.9	75.4	72.7	69.8	66.6	63.1	59.1	54.6	49.4	43.3	1.03	1.44

TABLE 288

Process Times (B) at Retort Temperature of 260°F for Conduction-Heating Foods in 307 x 704 Can

f_h	z	INITIAL FOOD TEMPERATURE (T_{ih})											Equivalent	
		100	110	120	130	140	150	160	170	180	190	200	F_c^{18}	F_s^{18}
62.69	18	65.2	63.4	61.6	59.5	57.4	55.0	52.4	49.5	46.3	42.7	38.5	2.50	3.00
	20	63.1	61.4	59.5	57.5	55.3	52.9	50.3	47.5	44.3	40.6	36.4	1.91	2.39
	22	61.1	59.3	57.5	55.4	53.3	50.9	48.3	45.4	42.2	38.6	34.4	1.45	1.92
	24	59.3	57.6	55.7	53.7	51.5	49.1	46.5	43.7	40.5	36.8	32.6	1.12	1.58
66.37	18	68.5	66.7	64.7	62.6	60.3	57.7	55.0	52.0	48.6	44.7	40.3	2.50	3.00
	20	66.3	64.5	62.5	60.3	58.0	55.5	52.8	49.7	46.4	42.5	38.1	1.90	2.38
	22	64.2	62.3	60.3	58.2	55.9	53.4	50.6	47.6	44.2	40.4	35.9	1.43	1.90
	24	62.3	60.4	58.5	56.3	54.0	51.5	48.8	45.7	42.3	38.5	34.0	1.10	1.56
70.06	18	71.9	69.9	67.8	65.6	63.1	60.5	57.6	54.4	50.8	46.7	42.0	2.50	3.00
	20	69.5	67.6	65.5	63.2	60.8	58.1	55.2	52.0	48.4	44.4	39.7	1.88	2.37
	22	67.3	65.3	63.2	60.9	58.5	55.9	53.0	49.8	46.2	42.1	37.4	1.42	1.89
	24	65.2	63.3	61.2	58.9	56.5	53.8	50.9	47.7	44.2	40.1	35.4	1.08	1.54
73.75	18	75.2	73.1	70.9	68.5	66.0	63.2	60.1	56.8	53.0	48.7	43.8	2.49	3.00
	20	72.7	70.6	68.4	66.0	63.5	60.7	57.6	54.3	50.5	46.2	41.3	1.88	2.36
	22	70.3	68.3	66.0	63.7	61.1	58.3	55.3	51.9	48.1	43.8	38.9	1.41	1.88
	24	68.2	66.1	63.9	61.5	59.0	56.2	53.1	49.7	46.0	41.7	36.8	1.06	1.52
77.44	18	78.5	76.3	74.0	71.5	68.8	65.9	62.7	59.1	55.2	50.7	45.5	2.49	3.00
	20	75.8	73.7	71.3	68.8	66.2	63.2	60.0	56.5	52.5	48.0	42.8	1.87	2.36
	22	73.4	71.2	68.9	66.4	63.7	60.8	57.6	54.0	50.0	45.6	40.4	1.40	1.87
	24	71.1	68.9	66.6	64.1	61.4	58.5	55.3	51.7	47.8	43.3	38.1	1.05	1.50

TABLE 289

Process Times (B) at Retort Temperature of 230°F for Conduction-Heating Foods in 401 x 205 Can

f_h	z	INITIAL FOOD TEMPERATURE (T_{ih})											Equivalent	
		100	110	120	130	140	150	160	170	180	190	200	F_c^{18}	F_s^{18}
	18	89.2	87.9	86.6	85.2	83.5	81.7	79.7	77.3	74.6	71.1	66.7	2.63	2.92
35.23	20	79.9	78.7	77.3	75.9	74.3	72.4	70.4	68.0	65.3	61.8	57.4	1.90	2.18
	22	72.3	71.0	69.7	68.2	66.6	64.8	62.8	60.4	57.6	54.2	49.8	1.46	1.72
	24	65.7	64.5	63.1	61.7	60.1	58.3	56.2	53.9	51.1	47.7	43.3	1.06	1.33
	18	92.6	91.3	89.9	88.3	86.6	84.7	82.6	80.1	77.1	73.5	68.8	2.62	2.92
37.30	20	82.8	81.5	80.1	78.6	76.9	75.0	72.8	70.3	67.4	63.7	59.1	1.90	2.18
	22	74.8	73.5	72.1	70.5	68.8	66.9	64.7	62.2	59.3	55.7	51.0	1.46	1.72
	24	68.3	67.0	65.6	64.0	62.3	60.4	58.3	55.8	52.8	49.2	44.5	1.06	1.33
	18	95.9	94.5	93.1	91.4	89.6	87.6	85.3	82.7	79.6	75.8	70.8	2.61	2.92
39.38	20	85.7	84.3	82.9	81.2	79.4	77.4	75.1	72.5	69.4	65.6	60.6	1.90	2.18
	22	77.2	75.8	74.3	72.7	70.9	68.9	66.6	64.0	60.9	57.0	52.1	1.42	1.69
	24	70.9	69.5	68.0	66.4	64.6	62.6	60.3	57.6	54.5	50.7	45.8	1.05	1.33
	18	99.2	97.7	96.2	94.5	92.6	90.4	88.0	85.3	82.0	78.0	72.8	2.61	2.92
41.45	20	88.5	87.1	85.5	83.8	81.9	79.8	77.3	74.6	71.3	67.3	62.1	1.90	2.18
	22	79.5	78.1	76.5	74.8	72.9	70.8	68.4	65.6	62.3	58.3	53.1	1.38	1.66
	24	73.4	71.9	70.4	68.6	66.7	64.6	62.2	59.4	56.2	52.2	47.0	1.04	1.32
	18	102.4	100.9	99.2	97.4	95.4	93.2	90.7	87.8	84.3	80.1	74.7	2.61	2.92
43.52	20	91.2	89.7	88.0	86.2	84.2	82.0	79.5	76.6	73.1	68.9	63.5	1.90	2.18
	22	82.1	80.6	78.9	77.1	75.1	72.9	70.4	67.5	64.0	59.8	54.4	1.37	1.65
	24	75.8	74.3	72.7	70.9	68.9	66.6	64.1	61.2	57.8	53.5	48.1	1.03	1.31

TABLE 290

Process Times (B) at Retort Temperature of 240°F for Conduction-Heating Foods in 401 x 205 Can

f_h	z	INITIAL FOOD TEMPERATURE (T_{ih})											Equivalent	
		100	110	120	130	140	150	160	170	180	190	200	F_c^{18}	F_s^{18}
	18	60.1	58.9	57.7	56.4	54.9	53.3	51.5	49.4	47.1	44.3	40.9	2.55	2.92
35.23	20	56.3	55.2	53.9	52.6	51.2	49.5	47.7	45.7	43.3	40.5	37.1	1.93	2.30
	22	53.1	52.0	50.8	49.4	48.0	46.4	44.6	42.5	40.2	37.4	34.0	1.48	1.84
	24	50.6	49.4	48.2	46.9	45.4	43.8	42.0	40.0	37.6	34.8	31.4	1.16	1.51
	18	62.7	61.5	60.2	58.8	57.2	55.5	53.6	51.4	48.9	46.0	42.4	2.54	2.92
37.30	20	58.8	57.6	56.3	54.9	53.3	51.6	49.7	47.5	45.0	42.1	38.5	1.92	2.29
	22	55.5	54.3	53.0	51.6	50.0	48.3	46.4	44.2	41.7	38.8	35.2	1.47	1.82
	24	52.8	51.6	50.3	48.9	47.3	45.6	43.7	41.6	39.1	36.1	32.5	1.15	1.50
	18	65.3	64.1	62.7	61.2	59.6	57.8	55.8	53.5	50.8	47.7	43.9	2.54	2.92
39.38	20	61.2	59.9	58.6	57.1	55.5	53.7	51.6	49.4	46.7	43.6	39.8	1.90	2.27
	22	57.8	56.5	55.2	53.7	52.1	50.3	48.2	46.0	43.3	40.2	36.4	1.45	1.81
	24	55.0	53.7	52.3	50.8	49.2	47.4	45.4	43.1	40.5	37.4	33.5	1.13	1.48
	18	67.9	66.6	65.2	63.6	61.9	60.0	57.9	55.4	52.7	49.4	45.4	2.53	2.92
41.45	20	63.7	62.3	60.9	59.3	57.6	55.7	53.6	51.2	48.4	45.1	41.1	1.90	2.27
	22	60.1	58.8	57.3	55.8	54.0	52.1	50.0	47.6	44.8	41.6	37.5	1.44	1.80
	24	57.2	55.8	54.4	52.8	51.1	49.2	47.1	44.7	41.9	38.6	34.6	1.11	1.47
	18	70.5	69.1	67.6	65.9	64.1	62.1	59.9	57.4	54.5	51.0	46.8	2.53	2.92
43.52	20	66.1	64.7	63.2	61.5	59.7	57.7	55.5	53.0	50.1	46.6	42.4	1.89	2.26
	22	62.4	61.0	59.5	57.8	56.0	54.0	51.8	49.3	46.4	42.9	38.7	1.42	1.79
	24	59.3	57.9	56.4	54.8	53.0	51.0	48.8	46.2	43.3	39.9	35.7	1.10	1.45

TABLE 291

Process Times (B) at Retort Temperature of 250°F for Conduction-Heating Foods in 401 x 205 Can

f_h	z	INITIAL FOOD TEMPERATURE (T_{ih}) 100	110	120	130	140	150	160	170	180	190	200	Equivalent F_c^{18}	F_s^{18}
	18	46.9	45.8	44.7	43.5	42.1	40.7	39.1	37.3	35.2	32.9	30.1	2.48	2.92
35.23	20	45.1	44.0	42.9	41.7	40.3	38.9	37.3	35.5	33.4	31.1	28.3	1.98	2.40
	22	43.5	42.4	41.3	40.1	38.8	37.3	35.7	33.9	31.8	29.5	26.7	1.59	2.01
	24	41.9	40.9	39.8	38.5	37.2	35.7	34.1	32.3	30.3	27.9	25.1	1.26	1.66
	18	49.1	48.0	46.8	45.5	44.1	42.5	40.8	38.9	36.8	34.3	31.3	2.48	2.92
37.30	20	47.2	46.1	44.9	43.6	42.2	40.6	38.9	37.0	34.9	32.4	29.4	1.96	2.39
	22	45.5	44.4	43.2	41.9	40.5	39.0	37.3	35.4	33.2	30.7	27.8	1.57	1.99
	24	43.9	42.8	41.6	40.3	38.9	37.3	35.6	33.7	31.5	29.1	26.1	1.23	1.64
	18	51.4	50.2	48.9	47.6	46.1	44.4	42.6	40.6	38.3	35.7	32.6	2.48	2.92
39.38	20	49.4	48.2	46.9	45.6	44.1	42.4	40.6	38.6	36.3	33.7	30.6	1.96	2.39
	22	47.6	46.4	45.2	43.8	42.3	40.7	38.9	36.9	34.6	31.9	28.8	1.56	1.98
	24	45.9	44.7	43.4	42.1	40.6	38.9	37.1	35.1	32.8	30.2	27.1	1.22	1.62
	18	53.6	52.4	51.0	49.6	48.0	46.3	44.4	42.3	39.9	37.1	33.8	2.47	2.92
41.45	20	51.5	50.3	48.9	47.5	45.9	44.2	42.3	40.2	37.8	35.0	31.7	1.95	2.38
	22	49.7	48.4	47.1	45.6	44.1	42.4	40.5	38.3	35.9	33.2	29.9	1.54	1.96
	24	47.8	46.6	45.2	43.8	42.2	40.5	38.6	36.5	34.1	31.3	28.0	1.20	1.61
	18	55.8	54.5	53.1	51.6	50.0	48.2	46.2	43.9	41.4	38.5	35.1	2.47	2.92
43.52	20	53.6	52.3	50.9	49.4	47.8	46.0	44.0	41.8	39.2	36.3	32.9	1.94	2.37
	22	51.7	50.4	49.0	47.5	45.8	44.0	42.0	39.8	37.3	34.4	30.9	1.53	1.95
	24	49.8	48.5	47.1	45.5	43.9	42.1	40.1	37.9	35.4	32.4	29.0	1.18	1.59

TABLE 292

Process Times (B) at Retort Temperature of 260°F for Conduction-Heating Foods in 401 x 205 Can

f_h	z	INITIAL FOOD TEMPERATURE (T_{ih}) 100	110	120	130	140	150	160	170	180	190	200	Equivalent F_c^{18}	Equivalent F_s^{18}
35.23	18	39.4	38.4	37.3	36.2	35.0	33.6	32.2	30.5	28.7	26.7	24.3	2.44	2.92
	20	38.3	37.3	36.2	35.1	33.9	32.6	31.1	29.5	27.7	25.6	23.3	1.98	2.45
	22	37.2	36.2	35.2	34.0	32.8	31.5	30.0	28.4	26.6	24.6	22.2	1.59	2.04
	24	36.3	35.3	34.2	33.1	31.9	30.5	29.1	27.5	25.7	23.6	21.3	1.29	1.73
37.30	18	41.3	40.3	39.2	38.0	36.7	35.3	33.7	32.0	30.1	28.0	25.5	2.44	2.92
	20	40.2	39.2	38.0	36.8	35.5	34.1	32.6	30.9	29.0	26.8	24.3	1.97	2.43
	22	39.0	38.0	36.9	35.7	34.4	33.0	31.4	29.7	27.8	25.7	23.2	1.57	2.02
	24	38.0	37.0	35.9	34.7	33.4	32.0	30.4	28.7	26.8	24.7	22.2	1.26	1.71
39.38	18	43.3	42.2	41.0	39.8	38.4	36.9	35.3	33.5	31.5	29.2	26.6	2.43	2.92
	20	42.1	41.0	39.8	38.6	37.2	35.7	34.1	32.3	30.3	28.0	25.3	1.95	2.42
	22	40.9	39.8	38.6	37.3	36.0	34.5	32.8	31.0	29.0	26.7	24.1	1.55	2.00
	24	39.8	38.7	37.5	36.3	34.9	33.4	31.8	30.0	28.0	25.7	23.0	1.24	1.69
41.45	18	45.3	44.1	42.9	41.6	40.1	38.6	36.8	34.9	32.8	30.4	27.6	2.43	2.92
	20	44.0	42.8	41.6	40.3	38.8	37.3	35.5	33.6	31.5	29.1	26.3	1.94	2.41
	22	42.7	41.5	40.3	39.0	37.5	35.9	34.2	32.3	30.2	27.8	25.0	1.53	1.98
	24	41.6	40.4	39.2	37.8	36.4	34.8	33.1	31.2	29.1	26.7	23.9	1.22	1.67
43.52	18	47.3	46.0	44.7	43.3	41.8	40.2	38.4	36.4	34.2	31.6	28.7	2.43	2.92
	20	45.9	44.7	43.4	42.0	40.5	38.8	37.0	35.0	32.8	30.3	27.3	1.93	2.41
	22	44.5	43.3	42.0	40.6	39.1	37.4	35.6	33.6	31.4	28.9	26.0	1.51	1.96
	24	43.3	42.1	40.8	39.4	37.9	36.2	34.4	32.5	30.2	27.7	24.8	1.20	1.65

TABLE 293

Process Times (B) at Retort Temperature of 230°F for Conduction-Heating Foods in 401 x 211 Can

f_h	z	INITIAL FOOD TEMPERATURE (T_{ih})											Equivalent	
		100	110	120	130	140	150	160	170	180	190	200	F_c^{18}	F_s^{18}
	18	102.6	101.1	99.4	97.6	95.6	93.4	90.9	88.0	84.5	80.3	74.9	2.62	2.93
43.50	20	91.4	89.9	88.2	86.4	84.4	82.2	79.7	76.8	73.3	69.1	63.7	1.91	2.20
	22	82.2	80.7	79.1	77.3	75.3	73.0	70.5	67.6	64.2	59.9	54.5	1.38	1.66
	24	75.9	74.4	72.8	71.0	69.0	66.8	64.2	61.3	57.9	53.7	48.2	1.04	1.32
	18	106.4	104.8	103.1	101.2	99.1	96.7	94.1	91.0	87.3	82.9	77.1	2.62	2.93
46.06	20	94.6	93.0	91.3	89.4	87.2	84.9	82.2	79.1	75.5	71.0	65.3	1.91	2.20
	22	85.5	83.9	82.2	80.3	78.2	75.8	73.2	70.1	66.4	62.0	56.2	1.37	1.66
	24	78.9	77.3	75.6	73.7	71.5	69.2	66.5	63.4	59.8	55.3	49.6	1.02	1.30
	18	110.2	108.5	106.7	104.7	102.5	100.0	97.2	93.9	90.0	85.3	79.3	2.62	2.93
48.62	20	97.7	96.0	94.2	92.2	90.0	87.5	84.6	81.4	77.5	72.8	66.8	1.91	2.20
	22	88.8	87.1	85.3	83.2	81.0	78.5	75.7	72.5	68.6	63.9	57.8	1.37	1.66
	24	81.8	80.1	78.3	76.3	74.1	71.6	68.7	65.5	61.6	56.9	50.9	1.00	1.29
	18	113.9	112.1	110.2	108.1	105.7	103.1	100.1	96.7	92.6	87.7	81.3	2.62	2.93
51.18	20	100.7	98.9	97.0	94.9	92.5	89.9	86.9	83.5	79.5	74.5	68.1	1.87	2.17
	22	91.9	90.2	88.2	86.1	83.8	81.1	78.2	74.8	70.7	65.7	59.3	1.36	1.66
	24	84.7	82.9	81.0	78.8	76.5	73.9	70.9	67.5	63.4	58.5	52.1	0.99	1.28
	18	117.5	115.6	113.6	111.3	108.9	106.1	103.0	99.4	95.1	89.9	83.2	2.62	2.93
53.74	20	103.9	102.1	100.0	97.8	95.4	92.6	89.5	85.9	81.6	76.4	69.7	1.85	2.15
	22	95.0	93.2	91.1	88.9	86.4	83.7	80.6	77.0	72.7	67.5	60.8	1.35	1.65
	24	87.6	85.7	83.7	81.4	79.0	76.2	73.1	69.5	65.3	60.0	53.3	0.97	1.27

TABLE 294

Process Times (B) at Retort Temperature of 240°F for Conduction-Heating Foods in 401 x 211 Can

f_h	z	INITIAL FOOD TEMPERATURE (T_{ih})											Equivalent	
		100	110	120	130	140	150	160	170	180	190	200	F_c^{18}	F_s^{18}
43.50	18	70.6	69.2	67.7	66.0	64.2	62.2	60.0	57.5	54.6	51.1	46.9	2.55	2.93
	20	66.2	64.8	63.2	61.6	59.8	57.8	55.6	53.1	50.1	46.7	42.5	1.90	2.28
	22	62.4	61.0	59.5	57.9	56.1	54.1	51.9	49.3	46.4	43.0	38.8	1.43	1.80
	24	59.4	58.0	56.5	54.8	53.0	51.1	48.8	46.3	43.4	39.9	35.7	1.11	1.46
46.06	18	73.7	72.2	70.6	68.9	67.0	64.9	62.5	59.9	56.8	53.1	48.7	2.54	2.93
	20	69.1	67.6	66.0	64.3	62.4	60.3	57.9	55.3	52.2	48.5	44.1	1.89	2.27
	22	65.3	63.8	62.2	60.4	58.5	56.4	54.1	51.4	48.3	44.7	40.2	1.42	1.79
	24	62.1	60.6	59.0	57.2	55.3	53.2	50.9	48.2	45.1	41.5	37.0	1.09	1.45
48.62	18	76.9	75.3	73.6	71.8	69.8	67.6	65.1	62.3	59.0	55.1	50.4	2.54	2.93
	20	72.0	70.5	68.8	66.9	64.9	62.7	60.2	57.4	54.2	50.3	45.6	1.88	2.26
	22	68.0	66.5	64.8	62.9	60.9	58.7	56.2	53.4	50.1	46.3	41.6	1.41	1.78
	24	64.7	63.1	61.4	59.6	57.6	55.4	52.9	50.1	46.8	43.0	38.2	1.07	1.44
51.18	18	80.0	78.4	76.6	74.7	72.5	70.2	67.6	64.6	61.2	57.1	52.2	2.54	2.93
	20	75.0	73.3	71.6	69.6	67.5	65.2	62.5	59.6	56.1	52.1	47.1	1.87	2.25
	22	70.8	69.1	67.4	65.4	63.3	61.0	58.4	55.4	52.0	47.9	42.9	1.40	1.77
	24	67.3	65.7	63.9	61.9	59.8	57.5	54.9	51.9	48.5	44.4	39.5	1.06	1.42
53.74	18	83.1	81.4	79.5	77.5	75.2	72.8	70.0	66.9	63.3	59.1	53.9	2.54	2.93
	20	77.9	76.1	74.3	72.2	70.0	67.6	64.8	61.7	58.1	53.8	48.6	1.86	2.25
	22	73.6	71.8	70.0	67.9	65.7	63.2	60.5	57.4	53.8	49.5	44.3	1.38	1.76
	24	69.9	68.2	66.3	64.3	62.0	59.6	56.8	53.7	50.1	45.9	40.7	1.05	1.42

TABLE 295

Process Times (B) at Retort Temperature of 250°F for Conduction-Heating Foods in 401 x 211 Can

f_h	z	INITIAL FOOD TEMPERATURE (T_{ih})											Equivalent	
		100	110	120	130	140	150	160	170	180	190	200	F_c^{18}	F_s^{18}
43.50	18	55.9	54.6	53.2	51.6	50.0	48.2	46.2	44.0	41.5	38.5	35.1	2.49	2.93
	20	53.7	52.4	51.0	49.5	47.8	46.0	44.0	41.8	39.3	36.4	32.9	1.95	2.39
	22	51.7	50.4	49.0	47.5	45.9	44.1	42.1	39.9	37.3	34.4	31.0	1.54	1.96
	24	49.8	48.5	47.1	45.6	43.9	42.1	40.1	37.9	35.4	32.5	29.0	1.19	1.60
46.06	18	58.6	57.2	55.7	54.1	52.4	50.5	48.3	46.0	43.3	40.2	36.6	2.49	2.93
	20	56.3	54.9	53.4	51.8	50.1	48.2	46.0	43.7	41.0	37.9	34.3	1.94	2.38
	22	54.2	52.8	51.3	49.7	48.0	46.1	44.0	41.6	39.0	35.9	32.2	1.52	1.94
	24	52.2	50.8	49.3	47.7	46.0	44.0	41.9	39.6	36.9	33.8	30.2	1.17	1.58
48.62	18	61.2	59.8	58.2	56.5	54.7	52.7	50.5	48.0	45.1	41.9	38.0	2.48	2.93
	20	58.8	57.4	55.8	54.1	52.3	50.3	48.0	45.6	42.7	39.5	35.6	1.93	2.37
	22	56.6	55.2	53.6	51.9	50.1	48.1	45.9	43.4	40.6	37.3	33.4	1.50	1.93
	24	54.5	53.0	51.5	49.8	47.9	45.9	43.7	41.2	38.4	35.1	31.3	1.15	1.56
51.18	18	63.9	62.4	60.7	59.0	57.0	54.9	52.6	49.9	47.0	43.6	39.5	2.48	2.93
	20	61.4	59.8	58.2	56.4	54.5	52.4	50.0	47.4	44.4	41.0	37.0	1.92	2.35
	22	59.1	57.5	55.9	54.1	52.2	50.1	47.7	45.1	42.1	38.7	34.7	1.49	1.91
	24	56.8	55.3	53.6	51.9	49.9	47.8	45.5	42.8	39.9	36.4	32.4	1.13	1.54
53.74	18	66.6	65.0	63.3	61.4	59.4	57.1	54.7	51.9	48.8	45.2	41.0	2.48	2.93
	20	63.9	62.3	60.6	58.7	56.7	54.5	52.0	49.3	46.1	42.5	38.3	1.91	2.35
	22	61.5	59.9	58.2	56.3	54.3	52.0	49.6	46.8	43.7	40.1	35.9	1.47	1.90
	24	59.1	57.5	55.8	53.9	51.9	49.7	47.2	44.5	41.4	37.8	33.5	1.12	1.53

TABLE 296

Process Times (B) at Retort Temperature of 260°F for Conduction-Heating Foods in 401 x 211 Can

f_h	z	INITIAL FOOD TEMPERATURE (T_{ih})											Equivalent	
		100	110	120	130	140	150	160	170	180	190	200	F_c^{18}	F_s^{18}
	18	47.3	46.1	44.8	43.4	41.8	40.2	38.4	36.4	34.2	31.7	28.8	2.45	2.93
43.50	20	45.9	44.7	43.4	42.0	40.5	38.8	37.0	35.0	32.8	30.3	27.4	1.95	2.42
	22	44.5	43.3	42.0	40.6	39.1	37.4	35.6	33.7	31.4	28.9	26.0	1.52	1.98
	24	43.4	42.1	40.8	39.4	37.9	36.3	34.5	32.5	30.3	27.7	24.8	1.21	1.66
	18	49.7	48.4	47.0	45.5	43.9	42.2	40.3	38.2	35.8	33.2	30.1	2.45	2.93
46.06	20	48.2	46.9	45.5	44.1	42.5	40.7	38.8	36.7	34.4	31.7	28.6	1.93	2.41
	22	46.7	45.4	44.1	42.6	41.0	39.2	37.3	35.2	32.9	30.2	27.1	1.50	1.96
	24	45.5	44.2	42.8	41.3	39.7	38.0	36.1	34.0	31.6	29.0	25.9	1.19	1.64
	18	52.1	50.7	49.3	47.7	46.0	44.2	42.2	39.9	37.4	34.6	31.4	2.44	2.93
48.62	20	50.5	49.2	47.7	46.1	44.4	42.6	40.6	38.4	35.9	33.1	29.8	1.92	2.40
	22	48.9	47.6	46.1	44.6	42.9	41.0	39.0	36.8	34.3	31.5	28.2	1.48	1.94
	24	47.6	46.3	44.8	43.2	41.6	39.7	37.7	35.5	33.0	30.2	26.9	1.18	1.63
	18	54.5	53.0	51.5	49.8	48.1	46.1	44.0	41.7	39.1	36.1	32.7	2.44	2.93
51.18	20	52.8	51.4	49.8	48.2	46.4	44.5	42.4	40.0	37.4	34.4	31.0	1.91	2.39
	22	51.1	49.7	48.2	46.5	44.7	42.8	40.7	38.4	35.7	32.8	29.3	1.46	1.92
	24	49.7	48.3	46.8	45.1	43.4	41.4	39.3	37.0	34.3	31.4	27.9	1.16	1.61
	18	56.8	55.3	53.7	52.0	50.1	48.1	45.9	43.4	40.6	37.5	33.9	2.44	2.93
53.74	20	55.1	53.6	52.0	50.2	48.4	46.3	44.1	41.6	38.9	35.8	32.2	1.90	2.37
	22	53.3	51.8	50.2	48.5	46.6	44.6	42.4	39.9	37.2	34.0	30.4	1.45	1.91
	24	51.9	50.3	48.7	47.0	45.1	43.1	40.9	38.4	35.7	32.6	29.0	1.14	1.59

TABLE 297

Process Times (B) at Retort Temperature of 230°F for Conduction-Heating Foods in 401 x 411 Can

f_h	z	INITIAL FOOD TEMPERATURE (T_{ih})											Equivalent	
		100	110	120	130	140	150	160	170	180	190	200	F_c^{18}	F_s^{18}
71.80	18	141.8	139.3	136.6	133.6	130.4	126.7	122.5	117.7	112.0	105.1	96.1	2.66	2.99
	20	127.8	125.3	122.6	119.7	116.4	112.7	108.5	103.7	98.0	91.1	82.1	1.85	2.18
	22	116.9	114.5	111.7	108.8	105.5	101.8	97.6	92.8	87.2	80.2	71.2	1.30	1.62
	24	108.2	105.7	103.0	100.1	96.8	93.1	88.9	84.1	78.5	71.5	62.5	0.93	1.24
76.02	18	147.7	145.1	142.2	139.1	135.6	131.7	127.3	122.2	116.2	108.8	99.3	2.66	2.99
	20	133.0	130.3	127.4	124.3	120.8	116.9	112.5	107.4	101.4	94.0	84.5	1.83	2.16
	22	121.8	119.2	116.3	113.2	109.7	105.8	101.4	96.3	90.3	82.9	73.4	1.28	1.60
	24	112.9	110.3	107.4	104.2	100.8	96.9	92.5	87.4	81.3	74.0	64.5	0.91	1.23
80.24	18	153.5	150.7	147.7	144.3	140.7	136.6	131.9	126.5	120.2	112.4	102.4	2.65	2.99
	20	138.1	135.3	132.3	128.9	125.3	121.2	116.5	111.1	104.8	97.0	87.0	1.81	2.14
	22	126.6	123.8	120.8	117.5	113.8	109.7	105.1	99.7	93.3	85.6	75.5	1.27	1.59
	24	117.5	114.7	111.6	108.3	104.7	100.5	95.9	90.5	84.2	76.4	66.4	0.90	1.22
84.47	18	159.1	156.2	153.0	149.5	145.6	141.3	136.4	130.8	124.1	115.9	105.3	2.64	2.99
	20	143.4	140.5	137.3	133.8	129.9	125.6	120.7	115.0	108.3	100.2	89.6	1.80	2.14
	22	131.3	128.4	125.2	121.7	117.8	113.5	108.6	103.0	96.3	88.1	77.5	1.25	1.58
	24	122.0	119.0	115.8	112.3	108.5	104.2	99.3	93.6	86.9	78.7	68.2	0.89	1.21
88.69	18	164.6	161.6	158.2	154.5	150.5	145.9	140.8	134.9	127.8	119.2	108.2	2.64	2.99
	20	148.6	145.5	142.2	138.5	134.4	129.9	124.8	118.8	111.8	103.2	92.1	1.80	2.14
	22	136.1	133.0	129.7	126.0	122.0	117.4	112.3	106.3	99.3	90.7	79.6	1.24	1.57
	24	126.4	123.3	119.9	116.3	112.2	107.7	102.5	96.6	89.6	81.0	69.9	0.88	1.20

TABLE 298

Process Times (B) at Retort Temperature of 240°F for Conduction-Heating Foods in 401 x 411 Can

f_h	z	INITIAL TOOD TEMPERATURE (T_{ih})											Equivalent	
		100	110	120	130	140	150	160	170	180	190	200	F_c^{18}	F_s^{18}
71.80	18	104.8	102.5	100.0	97.3	94.3	91.0	87.3	83.2	78.4	72.7	65.7	2.57	2.99
	20	98.2	95.9	93.4	90.7	87.7	84.5	80.8	76.6	71.8	66.1	59.2	1.85	2.25
	22	92.8	90.5	88.0	85.3	82.3	79.1	75.4	71.2	66.4	60.7	53.8	1.36	1.75
	24	88.2	85.9	83.4	80.6	77.7	74.4	70.7	66.5	61.7	56.1	49.1	1.01	1.38
76.02	18	109.6	107.2	104.6	101.7	98.5	95.1	91.2	86.8	81.7	75.7	68.3	2.57	2.99
	20	102.8	100.4	97.7	94.8	91.7	88.2	84.3	79.9	74.8	68.8	61.4	1.83	2.24
	22	97.2	94.8	92.1	89.2	86.1	82.6	78.7	74.3	69.2	63.2	55.8	1.36	1.74
	24	92.3	89.8	87.2	84.3	81.2	77.7	73.8	69.4	64.3	58.3	50.9	1.00	1.37
80.24	18	114.5	111.9	109.1	106.1	102.7	99.1	95.0	90.3	84.9	78.6	70.8	2.57	2.99
	20	107.3	104.7	102.0	98.9	95.6	91.9	87.8	83.2	77.8	71.4	63.7	1.82	2.23
	22	101.5	99.0	96.2	93.1	89.8	86.1	82.0	77.4	72.0	65.7	57.9	1.35	1.74
	24	96.3	93.8	91.0	87.9	84.6	80.9	76.8	72.2	66.8	60.5	52.7	0.99	1.36
84.47	18	119.2	116.5	113.6	110.4	106.9	103.0	98.7	93.8	88.2	81.5	73.3	2.57	2.99
	20	111.9	109.2	106.2	103.0	99.5	95.7	91.4	86.5	80.8	74.1	65.9	1.82	2.23
	22	105.8	103.1	100.2	97.0	93.5	89.6	85.3	80.4	74.8	68.1	59.9	1.34	1.73
	24	100.3	97.6	94.7	91.5	88.0	84.1	79.8	74.9	69.3	62.6	54.4	0.97	1.35
88.69	18	124.0	121.1	118.1	114.7	111.0	107.0	102.4	97.3	91.4	84.3	75.7	2.56	2.99
	20	116.4	113.5	110.5	107.1	103.4	99.4	94.8	89.7	83.8	76.7	68.1	1.82	2.23
	22	110.1	107.2	104.1	100.8	97.1	93.1	88.5	83.4	77.4	70.4	61.8	1.33	1.72
	24	104.3	101.5	98.4	95.0	91.3	87.3	82.8	77.6	71.7	64.6	56.1	0.96	1.33

TABLE 299

Process Times (B) at Retort Temperature of 250°F for Conduction-Heating Foods in 401 x 411 Can

f_h	z	INITIAL FOOD TEMPERATURE (T_{ih})											Equivalent	
		100	110	120	130	140	150	160	170	180	190	200	F_c^{18}	F_s^{18}
71.80	18	85.3	83.1	80.8	78.3	75.6	72.6	69.3	65.7	61.5	56.7	51.0	2.52	2.99
	20	81.7	79.6	77.3	74.8	72.1	69.1	65.8	62.1	58.0	53.2	47.5	1.89	2.34
	22	78.4	76.3	73.9	71.5	68.7	65.8	62.5	58.8	54.6	49.8	44.2	1.41	1.84
	24	75.3	73.2	70.9	68.4	65.7	62.7	59.4	55.7	51.6	46.8	41.1	1.05	1.46
76.02	18	89.5	87.2	84.8	82.1	79.2	76.1	72.6	68.7	64.3	59.2	53.2	2.52	2.99
	20	85.7	83.5	81.0	78.4	75.5	72.3	68.9	65.0	60.6	55.5	49.5	1.88	2.33
	22	82.2	79.9	77.5	74.8	72.0	68.8	65.3	61.5	57.0	52.0	45.9	1.39	1.82
	24	79.0	76.7	74.2	71.6	68.7	65.6	62.1	58.2	53.8	48.7	42.7	1.03	1.44
80.24	18	93.7	91.3	88.7	85.9	82.9	79.6	75.9	71.8	67.1	61.8	55.4	2.52	2.99
	20	89.7	87.3	84.7	82.0	78.9	75.6	71.9	67.8	63.2	57.8	51.4	1.87	2.32
	22	86.0	83.6	81.0	78.2	75.2	71.9	68.2	64.1	59.4	54.1	47.7	1.37	1.81
	24	82.6	80.2	77.6	74.8	71.8	68.5	64.8	60.7	56.0	50.7	44.3	1.01	1.43
84.47	18	97.9	95.3	92.6	89.7	86.5	83.0	79.1	74.8	69.9	64.3	57.6	2.52	2.99
	20	93.7	91.2	88.4	85.5	82.3	78.8	74.9	70.6	65.7	60.1	53.4	1.86	2.31
	22	89.7	87.2	84.5	81.5	78.4	74.9	71.0	66.7	61.8	56.1	49.4	1.36	1.79
	24	86.2	83.6	80.9	78.0	74.8	71.3	67.4	63.1	58.2	52.6	45.9	1.00	1.41
88.69	18	102.0	99.4	96.5	93.4	90.1	86.4	82.3	77.8	72.7	66.7	59.7	2.52	2.99
	20	97.6	95.0	92.1	89.0	85.7	82.0	77.9	73.4	68.3	62.3	55.3	1.85	2.30
	22	93.4	90.8	87.9	84.8	81.5	77.8	73.8	69.2	64.1	58.1	51.1	1.34	1.77
	24	89.7	87.1	84.2	81.1	77.8	74.1	70.1	65.5	60.4	54.4	47.4	0.98	1.40

TABLE 300

Process Times (B) at Retort Temperature of 260°F for Conduction-Heating Foods in 401 x 411 Can

f_h	z	INITIAL FOOD TEMPERATURE (T_{ih})											Equivalent	
		100	110	120	130	140	150	160	170	180	190	200	F_c^{18}	F_s^{18}
	18	73.4	71.4	69.2	66.9	64.4	61.7	58.7	55.5	51.8	47.6	42.8	2.49	2.99
71.80	20	71.0	69.0	66.8	64.5	62.0	59.3	56.3	53.0	49.4	45.2	40.4	1.87	2.36
	22	68.7	66.7	64.5	62.2	59.7	57.0	54.0	50.7	47.1	42.9	38.1	1.41	1.88
	24	66.6	64.6	62.4	60.1	57.6	54.9	51.9	48.6	45.0	40.8	36.0	1.07	1.52
	18	77.2	75.1	72.8	70.3	67.7	64.8	61.7	58.2	54.3	49.9	44.8	2.48	2.99
76.02	20	74.6	72.5	70.2	67.7	65.1	62.2	59.1	55.6	51.7	47.3	42.2	1.86	2.35
	22	72.2	70.0	67.7	65.3	62.7	59.8	56.6	53.2	49.3	44.9	39.8	1.39	1.87
	24	69.9	67.8	65.5	63.1	60.4	57.5	54.4	50.9	47.0	42.6	37.5	1.05	1.51
	18	81.0	78.7	76.3	73.7	70.9	67.9	64.6	60.9	56.8	52.1	46.8	2.48	2.99
80.24	20	78.2	75.9	73.5	70.9	68.2	65.1	61.8	58.1	54.0	49.4	44.0	1.85	2.34
	22	75.6	73.4	71.0	68.4	65.6	62.6	59.2	55.6	51.5	46.8	41.4	1.38	1.85
	24	73.2	71.0	68.6	66.0	63.2	60.2	56.8	53.2	49.1	44.4	39.0	1.03	1.49
	18	84.7	82.3	79.8	77.1	74.1	70.9	67.4	63.6	59.3	54.4	48.7	2.48	2.99
84.47	20	81.8	79.4	76.9	74.2	71.2	68.0	64.5	60.7	56.3	51.4	45.8	1.84	2.33
	22	79.1	76.7	74.2	71.4	68.5	65.3	61.8	58.0	53.6	48.7	43.1	1.36	1.84
	24	76.5	74.1	71.6	68.9	66.0	62.8	59.3	55.4	51.1	46.2	40.5	1.01	1.47
	18	88.4	85.9	83.3	80.4	77.3	74.0	70.3	66.2	61.7	56.6	50.6	2.48	2.99
88.69	20	85.3	82.9	80.2	77.3	74.3	70.9	67.2	63.2	58.6	53.5	47.6	1.83	2.33
	22	82.5	80.0	77.3	74.5	71.4	68.1	64.4	60.3	55.8	50.7	44.7	1.35	1.83
	24	79.8	77.3	74.6	71.8	68.7	65.4	61.7	57.6	53.1	47.9	42.0	0.99	1.46

TABLE 301

Process Times (B) at Retort Temperature of 230°F for Conduction-Heating Foods in 401 x 602 Can

f_h	z	INITIAL FOOD TEMPERATURE (T_{ih}) 100	110	120	130	140	150	160	170	180	190	200	Equivalent F_c^{18}	F_s^{18}
81.11	18	155.1	152.2	149.2	145.8	142.1	138.0	133.3	127.8	121.4	113.5	103.4	2.67	3.01
	20	139.5	136.7	133.6	130.3	126.6	122.4	117.7	112.3	105.9	98.0	87.9	1.82	2.16
	22	127.9	125.1	122.1	118.7	115.0	110.8	106.1	100.7	94.3	86.4	76.3	1.28	1.61
	24	118.7	115.9	112.8	109.4	105.7	101.6	96.9	91.5	85.0	77.2	67.0	0.91	1.23
85.88	18	161.4	158.4	155.2	151.6	147.7	143.3	138.3	132.6	125.8	117.5	106.7	2.67	3.01
	20	145.5	142.5	139.3	135.7	131.8	127.4	122.4	116.7	109.9	101.6	90.8	1.82	2.16
	22	133.2	130.2	127.0	123.4	119.5	115.1	110.1	104.4	97.6	89.3	78.5	1.26	1.59
	24	123.8	120.8	117.5	114.0	110.0	105.7	100.7	94.9	88.1	79.8	69.1	0.90	1.22
90.65	18	167.6	164.5	161.1	157.3	153.2	148.5	143.3	137.2	130.0	121.2	109.9	2.66	3.01
	20	151.4	148.2	144.8	141.1	136.9	132.3	127.0	120.9	113.8	105.0	93.7	1.81	2.15
	22	138.7	135.5	132.1	128.4	124.2	119.6	114.3	108.2	101.1	92.3	81.0	1.25	1.58
	24	128.8	125.6	122.2	118.4	114.3	109.7	104.4	98.3	91.1	82.4	71.0	0.88	1.21
95.43	18	173.8	170.5	166.9	162.9	158.5	153.7	148.1	141.7	134.2	124.9	113.0	2.66	3.01
	20	157.1	153.8	150.2	146.3	141.9	137.0	131.5	125.1	117.5	108.3	96.4	1.80	2.15
	22	144.1	140.7	137.1	133.2	128.8	123.9	118.4	112.0	104.5	95.2	83.3	1.24	1.57
	24	133.8	130.5	126.9	123.0	118.6	113.7	108.2	101.8	94.2	85.0	73.1	0.87	1.20
100.20	18	179.8	176.3	172.5	168.4	163.8	158.7	152.9	146.2	138.2	128.5	116.0	2.66	3.01
	20	162.8	159.3	155.5	151.4	146.8	141.7	135.9	129.1	121.2	111.5	99.0	1.79	2.14
	22	149.3	145.9	142.1	137.9	133.3	128.2	122.4	115.7	107.8	98.1	85.5	1.22	1.56
	24	138.8	135.3	131.5	127.4	122.8	117.7	111.9	105.1	97.2	87.5	75.0	0.86	1.19

TABLE 302

Process Times (B) at Retort Temperature of 240°F for Conduction-Heating Foods in 401 x 602 Can

f_h	z	INITIAL FOOD TEMPERATURE (T_{ih}) 100	110	120	130	140	150	160	170	180	190	200	Equivalent F_c^{18}	F_s^{18}
	18	115.7	113.1	110.2	107.2	103.8	100.1	96.0	91.3	85.8	79.4	71.5	2.59	3.01
81.11	20	108.5	105.8	103.0	100.0	96.6	92.9	88.7	84.0	78.6	72.2	64.3	1.84	2.25
	22	102.6	100.0	97.2	94.1	90.8	87.0	82.9	78.2	72.8	66.3	58.5	1.36	1.75
	24	97.4	94.7	91.9	88.9	85.5	81.8	77.6	72.9	67.5	61.1	53.2	1.00	1.37
	18	121.1	118.3	115.3	112.1	108.5	104.6	100.2	95.2	89.5	82.7	74.3	2.59	3.01
85.88	20	113.6	110.8	107.9	104.6	101.1	97.1	92.7	87.7	82.0	75.2	66.9	1.84	2.25
	22	107.5	104.7	101.7	98.5	94.9	91.0	86.6	81.6	75.9	69.1	60.7	1.35	1.74
	24	101.9	99.1	96.1	92.9	89.3	85.4	81.0	76.0	70.3	63.5	55.2	0.98	1.36
	18	126.4	123.5	120.4	116.9	113.2	109.0	104.4	99.1	93.1	85.9	77.1	2.59	3.01
90.65	20	118.7	115.8	112.6	109.2	105.5	101.3	96.7	91.4	85.3	78.2	69.4	1.84	2.25
	22	112.2	109.3	106.2	102.7	99.0	94.8	90.2	85.0	78.9	71.7	62.9	1.34	1.74
	24	106.3	103.4	100.3	96.8	93.1	88.9	84.3	79.0	73.0	65.8	57.0	0.96	1.34
	18	131.8	128.7	125.4	121.8	117.8	113.5	108.6	103.1	96.7	89.1	79.9	2.59	3.01
95.43	20	123.7	120.7	117.4	113.7	109.8	105.4	100.5	95.0	88.6	81.1	71.8	1.84	2.25
	22	117.0	113.9	110.6	107.0	103.0	98.7	93.8	88.2	81.8	74.3	65.0	1.33	1.73
	24	110.7	107.7	104.3	100.7	96.8	92.4	87.5	82.0	75.6	68.1	58.8	0.95	1.32
	18	137.1	133.9	130.4	126.6	122.5	117.9	112.8	107.0	100.3	92.3	82.6	2.58	3.01
100.20	20	128.7	125.5	122.0	118.2	114.1	109.5	104.4	98.6	91.9	83.9	74.2	1.84	2.25
	22	121.6	118.4	114.9	111.1	107.0	102.4	97.3	91.5	84.8	76.8	67.1	1.32	1.71
	24	115.1	111.9	108.4	104.6	100.4	95.9	90.7	84.9	78.2	70.3	60.6	0.93	1.31

TABLE 303

Process Times (B) at Retort Temperature of 250°F for Conduction-Heating Foods in 401 x 602 Can

f_h	z	INITIAL FOOD TEMPERATURE (T_{ih})											Equivalent	
		100	110	120	130	140	150	160	170	180	190	200	F_c^{18}	F_s^{18}
81.11	18	94.7	92.3	89.7	86.8	83.8	80.4	76.7	72.6	67.9	62.4	56.0	2.55	3.01
	20	90.7	88.3	85.6	82.8	79.8	76.4	72.7	68.5	63.8	58.4	52.0	1.89	2.34
	22	86.9	84.5	81.9	79.0	76.0	72.6	68.9	64.8	60.1	54.6	48.2	1.39	1.82
	24	83.5	81.0	78.4	75.6	72.5	69.2	65.5	61.3	56.6	51.2	44.8	1.02	1.44
85.88	18	99.4	96.8	94.1	91.1	87.8	84.3	80.4	76.0	71.0	65.2	58.4	2.54	3.01
	20	95.1	92.6	89.8	86.8	83.6	80.0	76.1	71.7	66.7	61.0	54.2	1.87	2.33
	22	91.1	88.6	85.8	82.8	79.6	76.0	72.1	67.7	62.7	56.9	50.1	1.37	1.80
	24	87.5	84.9	82.2	79.2	76.0	72.4	68.5	64.1	59.1	53.3	46.5	1.00	1.42
90.65	18	104.1	101.4	98.5	95.3	91.9	88.1	84.0	79.3	74.1	68.0	60.8	2.54	3.01
	20	99.6	96.9	94.0	90.8	87.4	83.6	79.5	74.8	69.6	63.5	56.3	1.86	2.31
	22	95.3	92.6	89.7	86.5	83.1	79.4	75.2	70.6	65.3	59.2	52.1	1.35	1.78
	24	91.5	88.8	85.9	82.8	79.3	75.6	71.4	66.8	61.5	55.5	48.3	0.99	1.41
95.43	18	108.8	105.9	102.8	99.5	95.9	91.9	87.6	82.7	77.2	70.8	63.2	2.54	3.01
	20	104.0	101.1	98.1	94.8	91.1	87.2	82.8	78.0	72.4	66.0	58.5	1.85	2.30
	22	99.5	96.6	93.6	90.3	86.6	82.7	78.3	73.4	67.9	61.5	54.0	1.33	1.77
	24	95.5	92.7	89.6	86.3	82.7	78.7	74.4	69.5	64.0	57.6	50.0	0.97	1.39
100.20	18	113.4	110.4	107.2	103.7	99.9	95.7	91.1	86.0	80.2	73.5	65.6	2.54	3.01
	20	108.4	105.4	102.2	98.7	94.9	90.7	86.2	81.0	75.2	68.5	60.6	1.84	2.29
	22	103.6	100.6	97.4	93.9	90.1	86.0	81.4	76.3	70.5	63.8	55.8	1.31	1.75
	24	99.5	96.5	93.3	89.8	86.0	81.9	77.3	72.2	66.4	59.6	51.7	0.96	1.37

TABLE 304

Process Times (B) at Retort Temperature of 260°F for Conduction-Heating Foods in 401 x 602 Can

f_h	z	INITIAL FOOD TEMPERATURE (T_{ih})											Equivalent	
		100	110	120	130	140	150	160	170	180	190	200	F_c^{18}	F_s^{18}
	18	81.8	79.5	77.1	74.5	71.7	68.6	65.3	61.6	57.4	52.7	47.3	2.51	3.01
81.11	20	79.0	76.7	74.3	71.7	68.9	65.8	62.5	58.7	54.6	49.9	44.5	1.87	2.36
	22	76.4	74.2	71.7	69.1	66.3	63.2	59.9	56.2	52.0	47.3	41.9	1.39	1.87
	24	74.0	71.7	69.3	66.7	63.9	60.8	57.5	53.7	49.6	44.9	39.5	1.04	1.50
	18	86.0	83.6	81.1	78.3	75.3	72.1	68.5	64.6	60.2	55.2	49.5	2.50	3.01
85.88	20	83.1	80.7	78.1	75.3	72.3	69.1	65.5	61.6	57.2	52.2	46.5	1.86	2.35
	22	80.3	77.9	75.3	72.6	60.6	66.3	62.8	58.9	54.5	49.5	43.7	1.38	1.85
	24	77.7	75.3	72.7	70.0	67.0	63.7	60.2	56.3	51.9	46.9	41.1	1.02	1.48
	18	90.2	87.7	85.0	82.1	78.9	75.5	71.7	67.6	62.9	57.7	51.6	2.50	3.01
90.65	20	87.1	84.6	81.8	78.9	75.8	72.3	68.6	64.4	59.8	54.6	48.5	1.85	2.34
	22	84.2	81.6	78.9	76.0	72.9	69.4	65.7	61.5	56.9	51.6	45.6	1.36	1.84
	24	81.4	78.9	76.2	73.2	70.1	66.7	62.9	58.8	54.1	48.9	42.8	1.00	1.46
	18	94.4	91.7	88.8	85.8	82.5	78.9	74.9	70.5	65.7	60.1	53.7	2.50	3.01
95.43	20	91.1	88.4	85.6	82.5	79.2	75.6	71.6	67.2	62.4	56.8	50.4	1.84	2.33
	22	88.1	85.4	82.5	79.4	76.1	72.5	68.6	64.2	59.3	53.8	47.4	1.35	1.83
	24	85.1	82.4	79.5	76.5	73.2	69.5	65.6	61.2	56.4	50.8	44.4	0.98	1.45
	18	98.5	95.7	92.7	89.5	86.0	82.2	78.1	73.5	68.3	62.5	55.8	2.50	3.01
100.20	20	95.1	92.3	89.2	86.0	82.5	78.8	74.6	70.0	64.9	59.1	52.4	1.83	2.33
	22	91.9	89.1	86.1	82.8	79.4	75.6	71.4	66.8	61.7	55.9	49.2	1.34	1.82
	24	88.7	85.9	82.9	79.7	76.2	72.4	68.3	63.7	58.6	52.8	46.1	0.97	1.44

TABLE 305

Process Times (B) at Retort Temperature of 230°F for Conduction-Heating Foods in 404 x 200 Can

f_h	z	INITIAL FOOD TEMPERATURE (T_{ih})											Equivalent	
		100	110	120	130	140	150	160	170	180	190	200	F_c^{18}	F_s^{18}
	18	79.0	78.0	76.9	75.7	74.4	72.9	71.3	69.4	67.1	64.4	60.8	2.64	2.91
28.49	20	69.6	68.6	67.5	66.4	65.1	63.6	61.9	60.0	57.8	55.0	51.5	1.91	2.18
	22	63.3	62.3	61.2	60.0	58.7	57.3	55.6	53.7	51.4	48.7	45.1	1.45	1.71
	24	58.0	57.0	55.9	54.7	53.4	52.0	50.3	48.4	46.2	43.4	39.9	1.16	1.40
	18	81.4	80.4	79.2	78.0	76.6	75.1	73.3	71.3	68.9	66.0	62.2	2.64	2.91
30.16	20	72.2	71.2	70.0	68.8	67.4	65.9	64.1	62.1	59.7	56.8	53.0	1.90	2.19
	22	65.6	64.5	63.4	62.1	60.8	59.2	57.5	55.5	53.1	50.1	46.4	1.45	1.71
	24	60.0	59.0	57.8	56.6	55.2	53.6	51.9	49.9	47.5	44.6	40.8	1.15	1.39
	18	83.9	82.8	81.6	80.3	78.8	77.2	75.3	73.2	70.7	67.6	63.6	2.63	2.91
31.84	20	74.8	73.7	72.5	71.1	69.7	68.1	66.2	64.1	61.6	58.5	54.5	1.90	2.18
	22	67.8	66.7	65.5	64.2	62.8	61.1	59.3	57.1	54.6	51.5	47.6	1.45	1.71
	24	61.9	60.8	59.6	58.3	56.9	55.2	53.4	51.3	48.7	45.6	41.7	1.12	1.37
	18	86.3	85.1	83.9	82.5	81.0	79.2	77.3	75.1	72.4	69.2	65.0	2.63	2.91
33.51	20	77.3	76.1	74.9	73.5	71.9	70.2	68.3	66.0	63.4	60.1	55.9	1.90	2.18
	22	70.0	68.8	67.6	66.2	64.7	62.9	61.0	58.8	56.1	52.9	48.7	1.45	1.71
	24	63.8	62.6	61.4	60.0	58.5	56.7	54.8	52.6	49.9	46.7	42.5	1.09	1.35
	18	89.0	87.8	86.5	85.0	83.4	81.6	79.6	77.2	74.4	71.0	66.6	2.62	2.91
35.19	20	79.7	78.5	77.2	75.7	74.1	72.3	70.3	67.9	65.1	61.7	57.3	1.89	2.18
	22	72.1	70.9	69.6	68.1	66.5	64.7	62.7	60.3	57.5	54.1	49.7	1.45	1.71
	24	65.6	64.3	63.0	61.6	69.9	58.1	56.1	53.8	51.0	47.6	43.2	1.06	1.33

TABLE 306

Process Times (B) at Retort Temperature of 240°F for Conduction-Heating Foods in 404 x 200 Can

f_h	z	INITIAL FOOD TEMPERATURE (T_{ih})											Equivalent	
		100	110	120	130	140	150	160	170	180	190	200	F_c^{18}	F_s^{18}
	18	51.2	50.3	49.3	48.2	47.0	45.7	44.3	42.6	40.7	38.5	35.7	2.55	2.91
28.49	20	48.1	47.2	46.2	45.1	43.9	42.6	41.2	39.5	37.6	35.3	32.6	1.98	2.33
	22	45.4	44.4	43.4	42.4	41.2	39.9	38.4	36.8	34.9	32.6	29.9	1.54	1.88
	24	43.1	42.2	41.2	40.2	39.0	37.7	36.2	34.6	32.7	30.4	27.6	1.22	1.56
	18	53.5	52.5	51.4	50.3	49.0	47.7	46.1	44.4	42.4	40.0	37.0	2.55	2.91
30.16	20	50.1	49.2	48.1	47.0	45.7	44.3	42.8	41.0	39.0	36.6	33.7	1.96	2.32
	22	47.3	46.3	45.3	44.1	42.9	41.5	40.0	38.2	36.2	33.8	30.9	1.52	1.87
	24	45.0	44.0	43.0	41.9	40.6	39.2	37.7	35.9	33.9	31.5	28.6	1.21	1.55
	18	55.7	54.6	53.5	52.3	51.0	49.6	47.9	46.1	43.9	41.4	38.3	2.55	2.91
31.84	20	52.1	51.1	50.0	48.8	47.5	46.0	44.4	42.6	40.4	37.9	34.8	1.94	2.30
	22	49.2	48.2	47.1	45.9	44.6	43.1	41.5	39.7	37.5	35.0	31.9	1.51	1.86
	24	46.8	45.8	44.7	43.5	42.2	40.7	39.1	37.3	35.1	32.6	29.5	1.19	1.53
	18	57.8	56.7	55.6	54.3	52.9	51.4	49.7	47.7	45.5	42.8	39.6	2.54	2.91
33.51	20	54.2	53.1	51.9	50.7	49.3	47.7	46.0	44.1	41.8	39.2	35.9	1.93	2.30
	22	51.2	50.1	48.9	47.7	46.3	44.7	43.0	41.1	38.8	36.2	32.9	1.49	1.85
	24	48.7	47.6	46.4	45.1	43.8	42.2	40.5	38.6	36.3	33.7	30.4	1.17	1.52
	18	60.0	58.8	57.6	56.3	54.8	53.2	51.4	49.4	47.0	44.2	40.8	2.54	2.91
35.19	20	56.2	55.1	53.9	52.5	51.1	49.5	47.7	45.6	43.3	40.5	37.1	1.93	2.29
	22	53.1	51.9	50.7	49.4	47.9	46.3	44.5	42.5	40.1	37.3	33.9	1.48	1.83
	24	50.5	49.3	48.1	46.8	45.3	43.7	41.9	39.9	37.5	34.7	31.3	1.16	1.51

TABLE 307

Process Times (B) at Retort Temperature of 250°F for Conduction-Heating Foods in 404 x 200 Can

f_h	z	INITIAL FOOD TEMPERATURE (T_{ih})											Equivalent	
		100	110	120	130	140	150	160	170	180	190	200	F_c^{18}	F_s^{18}
28.49	18	39.4	38.6	37.6	36.6	35.6	34.4	33.1	31.6	30.0	28.1	25.8	2.48	2.91
	20	37.9	37.1	36.2	35.2	34.1	32.9	31.6	30.1	28.5	26.6	24.3	2.01	2.43
	22	36.6	35.8	34.9	33.9	32.8	31.6	30.3	28.8	27.2	25.3	23.0	1.64	2.05
	24	35.4	34.5	33.6	32.6	31.5	30.4	29.1	27.6	26.0	24.0	21.8	1.33	1.73
30.16	18	41.3	40.4	39.4	38.4	37.2	36.0	34.6	33.1	31.3	29.3	26.9	2.48	2.91
	20	39.7	38.8	37.9	36.8	35.7	34.4	33.0	31.5	29.7	27.7	25.3	2.01	2.43
	22	38.4	37.5	36.5	35.4	34.3	33.0	31.7	30.1	28.4	26.4	24.0	1.63	2.04
	24	37.0	36.1	35.2	34.1	33.0	31.7	30.3	28.8	27.1	25.0	22.6	1.32	1.71
31.84	18	43.2	42.2	41.2	40.1	38.9	37.5	36.1	34.5	32.6	30.5	28.0	2.48	2.91
	20	41.5	40.6	39.5	38.4	37.2	35.9	34.5	32.8	31.0	28.8	26.3	2.00	2.42
	22	40.1	39.1	38.1	37.0	35.8	34.5	33.0	31.4	29.5	27.4	24.9	1.62	2.03
	24	38.7	37.7	36.7	35.6	34.4	33.1	31.6	30.0	28.1	26.0	23.5	1.30	1.70
33.51	18	45.0	44.0	42.9	41.7	40.5	39.1	37.6	35.8	33.9	31.7	29.0	2.47	2.91
	20	43.3	42.3	41.2	40.0	38.8	37.4	35.8	34.1	32.2	29.9	27.3	1.98	2.41
	22	41.8	40.8	39.7	38.5	37.2	35.9	34.3	32.6	30.7	28.4	25.8	1.60	2.02
	24	40.3	39.3	38.2	37.0	35.8	34.4	32.9	31.1	29.2	27.0	24.3	1.28	1.68
35.19	18	46.8	45.8	44.6	43.4	42.1	40.6	39.0	37.2	35.2	32.8	30.0	2.47	2.91
	20	45.0	44.0	42.8	41.6	40.3	38.8	37.2	35.4	33.4	31.0	28.2	1.97	2.40
	22	43.4	42.4	41.3	40.0	38.7	37.2	35.6	33.8	31.8	29.4	26.6	1.58	2.00
	24	41.9	40.8	39.7	38.5	37.1	35.7	34.1	32.3	30.2	27.9	25.1	1.26	1.66

TABLE 308

Process Times (B) at Retort Temperature of 260°F for Conduction-Heating Foods in 404 x 200 Can

f_h	z	INITIAL FOOD TEMPERATURE (T_{ih})											Equivalent	
		100	110	120	130	140	150	160	170	180	190	200	F_c^{18}	F_s^{18}
28.49	18	32.8	32.0	31.1	30.2	29.2	28.1	26.9	25.6	24.2	22.5	20.6	2.44	2.91
	20	31.9	31.1	30.3	29.4	28.4	27.3	26.1	24.8	23.4	21.7	19.8	2.03	2.49
	22	31.1	30.3	29.5	28.5	27.6	26.5	25.3	24.0	22.5	20.9	19.0	1.66	2.12
	24	30.3	29.5	28.7	27.8	26.8	25.7	24.5	23.2	21.8	20.1	18.2	1.37	1.81
30.16	18	34.4	33.6	32.7	31.7	30.6	29.5	28.2	26.9	25.3	23.6	21.6	2.44	2.91
	20	33.5	32.7	31.8	30.8	29.8	28.6	27.4	26.0	24.4	22.7	20.7	2.01	2.47
	22	32.6	31.8	30.9	29.9	28.9	27.7	26.5	25.1	23.6	21.8	19.8	1.64	2.09
	24	31.8	31.0	30.1	29.1	28.1	26.9	25.7	24.3	22.8	21.0	19.0	1.35	1.79
31.84	18	36.0	35.2	34.2	33.2	32.1	30.9	29.5	28.1	26.5	24.6	22.5	2.43	2.91
	20	35.1	34.2	33.3	32.2	31.1	29.9	28.6	27.1	25.5	23.7	21.5	2.00	2.46
	22	34.2	33.3	32.3	31.3	30.2	29.0	27.7	26.2	24.6	22.7	20.6	1.62	2.07
	24	33.3	32.4	31.5	30.4	29.3	28.1	26.8	25.3	23.7	21.9	19.7	1.33	1.77
33.51	18	37.7	36.7	35.7	34.6	33.5	32.2	30.8	29.3	27.6	25.6	23.4	2.43	2.91
	20	36.7	35.7	34.7	33.6	32.5	31.5	29.8	28.3	26.6	24.6	22.4	1.99	2.45
	22	35.7	34.7	33.7	32.6	31.5	30.2	28.8	27.3	25.6	23.6	21.4	1.60	2.05
	24	34.8	33.8	32.8	31.7	30.6	29.3	27.9	26.4	24.7	22.7	20.5	1.31	1.75
35.19	18	39.3	38.3	37.3	36.1	34.9	33.6	32.1	30.5	28.7	26.7	24.3	2.43	2.91
	20	38.2	37.2	36.2	35.1	33.8	32.5	31.0	29.4	27.6	25.6	23.2	1.97	2.44
	22	37.2	36.2	35.1	34.0	32.8	31.4	30.0	28.4	26.6	24.5	22.2	1.58	2.04
	24	36.2	35.2	34.2	33.0	31.8	30.5	29.0	27.4	25.6	23.6	21.2	1.29	1.73

TABLE 309

Process Times (B) at Retort Temperature of 230°F for Conduction-Heating Foods in 404 x 211 Can

f_h	z	INITIAL FOOD TEMPERATURE (T_{ih})											Equivalent	
		100	110	120	130	140	150	160	170	180	190	200	F_c^{18}	F_s^{18}
	18	105.4	103.8	102.1	100.3	98.2	95.9	93.2	90.2	86.6	82.2	76.6	2.63	2.94
45.30	20	93.8	92.2	90.5	88.6	86.5	84.2	81.6	78.6	75.0	70.6	64.9	1.92	2.20
	22	84.6	83.1	81.4	79.5	77.4	75.1	72.5	69.4	65.8	61.5	55.8	1.38	1.67
	24	78.1	76.5	74.8	72.9	70.9	68.6	65.9	62.9	59.3	54.9	49.3	1.03	1.31
	18	109.4	107.7	105.9	103.9	101.7	99.3	96.5	93.3	89.5	84.8	78.8	2.63	2.94
47.97	20	97.0	95.4	93.6	91.6	89.4	86.9	84.2	80.9	77.1	72.5	66.5	1.92	2.20
	22	88.0	86.4	84.6	82.6	80.4	77.9	75.1	71.9	68.1	63.5	57.5	1.37	1.67
	24	81.2	79.5	77.7	75.7	73.5	71.0	68.3	65.0	61.2	56.6	50.6	1.01	1.30
	18	113.2	111.5	109.6	107.5	105.1	102.6	99.6	96.2	92.2	87.3	81.0	2.63	2.94
50.63	20	100.2	98.5	96.5	94.4	92.1	89.5	86.6	83.2	79.2	74.3	68.0	1.89	2.18
	22	91.4	89.6	87.7	85.6	83.3	80.7	77.7	74.4	70.3	65.4	59.1	1.37	1.67
	24	84.2	82.4	80.5	78.4	76.1	73.5	70.5	67.2	63.1	58.2	51.9	0.99	1.28
	18	117.0	115.1	113.1	110.9	108.5	105.7	102.6	99.1	94.9	89.7	83.0	2.63	2.94
53.30	20	103.4	101.6	99.6	97.4	94.9	92.2	89.1	85.5	81.3	76.2	69.5	1.85	2.15
	22	94.6	92.7	90.7	88.5	86.1	83.4	80.3	76.7	72.5	67.3	60.6	1.36	1.66
	24	87.1	85.3	83.2	81.0	78.6	75.9	72.8	69.2	65.0	59.8	53.2	0.98	1.27
	18	120.6	118.7	116.5	114.2	111.7	108.8	105.6	101.8	97.4	92.0	85.0	2.63	2.94
55.96	20	107.1	105.1	103.0	100.7	98.1	95.3	92.0	88.3	83.8	78.4	71.4	1.85	2.15
	22	97.7	95.8	93.7	91.4	88.8	85.9	82.7	79.0	74.5	69.1	62.1	1.34	1.64
	24	90.2	88.3	86.2	83.9	81.3	78.4	75.2	71.4	67.0	61.6	54.6	0.97	1.26

TABLE 310

Process Times (B) at Retort Temperature of 240°F for Conduction-Heating Foods in 404 x 211 Can

f_h	z	INITIAL FOOD TEMPERATURE (T_{ih})											Equivalent	
		100	110	120	130	140	150	160	170	180	190	200	F_c^{18}	F_s^{18}
	18	72.8	71.4	69.8	68.1	66.2	64.1	61.8	59.2	56.2	52.6	48.2	2.55	2.94
45.30	20	68.3	66.8	65.3	63.5	61.7	59.6	57.3	54.7	51.6	48.0	43.6	1.90	2.28
	22	64.5	63.0	61.4	59.7	57.8	55.8	53.5	50.8	47.8	44.2	39.8	1.43	1.80
	24	61.3	59.9	58.3	56.6	54.7	52.6	50.3	47.7	44.6	41.1	36.7	1.10	1.46
	18	76.1	74.6	72.9	71.1	69.1	66.9	64.5	61.7	58.5	54.7	50.0	2.55	2.94
47.97	20	71.3	69.8	68.1	66.3	64.3	62.1	59.7	56.9	53.7	49.9	45.2	1.89	2.27
	22	67.4	65.8	64.2	62.4	60.4	58.2	55.7	52.9	49.7	45.9	41.3	1.42	1.79
	24	64.1	62.5	60.9	59.0	57.1	54.9	52.4	49.6	46.4	42.6	38.0	1.08	1.44
	18	79.4	77.8	76.0	74.1	72.0	69.7	67.1	64.2	60.8	56.8	51.9	2.55	2.94
50.63	20	74.4	72.8	71.0	69.1	67.0	64.7	62.1	59.2	55.8	51.8	46.9	1.88	2.26
	22	70.2	68.6	66.9	64.9	62.8	60.5	57.9	55.0	51.6	47.6	42.7	1.41	1.78
	24	66.8	65.2	63.4	61.5	59.4	57.1	54.5	51.6	48.2	44.2	39.3	1.07	1.43
	18	82.6	80.9	79.0	77.0	74.8	72.4	69.7	66.6	63.0	58.8	53.6	2.54	2.94
53.30	20	77.4	75.7	73.9	71.8	69.6	67.2	64.5	61.4	57.8	53.6	48.4	1.87	2.25
	22	73.1	71.4	69.6	67.5	65.3	62.9	60.2	57.1	53.5	49.3	44.1	1.39	1.77
	23	69.5	67.8	65.9	63.9	61.7	59.3	56.5	53.5	49.9	45.7	40.5	1.06	1.42
	18	85.8	84.0	82.1	80.0	77.6	75.1	72.2	69.0	65.2	60.8	55.4	2.54	2.94
55.96	20	80.4	78.6	76.7	74.6	72.2	69.7	66.8	63.6	59.8	55.4	50.0	1.86	2.25
	22	76.0	74.2	72.2	70.1	67.8	65.2	62.4	59.1	55.4	50.9	45.5	1.38	1.76
	24	72.2	70.4	68.4	66.3	64.0	61.5	58.6	55.3	51.6	47.2	41.7	1.05	1.41

TABLE 311

Process Times (B) at Retort Temperature of 250°F for Conduction-Heating Foods in 404 x 211 Can

f_h	z	INITIAL FOOD TEMPERATURE (T_{ih})											Equivalent	
		100	110	120	130	140	150	160	170	180	190	200	F_c^{18}	F_s^{18}
	18	57.8	56.4	55.0	53.4	51.7	49.8	47.7	45.4	42.8	39.8	36.2	2.49	2.94
45.30	20	55.5	54.2	52.7	51.1	49.4	47.6	45.5	43.2	40.5	37.5	33.9	1.95	2.39
	22	53.5	52.1	50.7	49.1	47.4	45.5	43.5	41.1	38.5	35.5	31.9	1.54	1.96
	24	51.5	50.1	48.7	47.1	45.4	43.5	41.4	39.1	36.5	33.5	29.9	1.18	1.59
	18	60.6	59.2	57.6	55.9	54.1	52.1	49.9	47.5	44.7	41.5	37.7	2.49	2.94
47.97	20	58.2	56.8	55.2	53.6	51.7	49.8	47.6	45.1	42.3	39.1	35.3	1.94	2.38
	22	56.1	54.6	53.1	51.4	49.6	47.6	45.4	43.0	40.2	37.0	33.2	1.51	1.94
	24	53.9	52.5	50.9	49.3	47.5	45.5	43.3	40.8	38.1	34.8	31.0	1.16	1.57
	18	63.4	61.9	60.2	58.5	56.6	54.5	52.1	49.6	46.6	43.2	39.2	2.49	2.94
50.63	20	60.9	59.3	57.7	56.0	54.0	51.9	49.6	47.0	44.1	40.7	36.7	1.93	2.36
	22	58.6	57.1	55.4	53.7	51.8	49.7	47.4	44.8	41.8	38.4	34.4	1.50	1.92
	24	56.3	54.8	53.2	51.4	49.5	47.4	45.1	42.5	39.6	36.2	32.2	1.14	1.55
	18	66.2	64.6	62.9	61.0	59.0	56.8	54.3	51.6	48.5	45.0	40.7	2.49	2.94
53.30	20	63.5	61.9	60.2	58.4	56.3	54.1	51.7	49.0	45.9	42.3	38.1	1.92	2.36
	22	61.1	59.5	57.8	56.0	53.9	51.7	49.3	46.6	43.5	39.9	35.7	1.48	1.91
	24	58.8	57.2	55.5	53.6	51.6	49.4	46.9	44.2	41.1	37.6	33.3	1.12	1.53
	18	68.9	67.3	65.5	63.5	61.4	59.1	56.5	53.7	50.4	46.7	42.2	2.49	2.94
55.96	20	66.2	64.5	62.7	60.7	58.6	56.3	53.7	50.9	47.6	43.9	39.5	1.91	2.35
	22	63.6	62.0	60.2	58.2	56.1	53.8	51.2	48.4	45.1	41.4	36.9	1.47	1.89
	24	61.2	59.5	57.7	55.8	53.6	51.3	48.8	45.9	42.7	38.9	34.5	1.11	1.52

ABLE 312

Process Times (B) at Retort Temperature of 260°F for Conduction-Heating Foods in 404 x 211 Can

f_h	z	INITIAL FOOD TEMPERATURE (T_{ih})											Equivalent	
		100	110	120	130	140	150	160	170	180	190	200	F_c^{18}	F_s^{18}
	18	49.0	47.7	46.4	44.9	43.3	41.6	39.8	37.7	35.4	32.7	29.7	2.45	2.94
45.30	20	47.6	46.3	44.9	43.5	41.9	40.2	38.3	36.2	33.9	31.3	28.3	1.94	2.42
	22	46.1	44.8	43.5	42.0	40.4	38.7	36.9	34.8	32.5	29.8	26.8	1.51	1.97
	24	44.9	43.6	42.3	40.8	39.2	37.5	35.6	33.6	31.3	28.6	25.6	1.20	1.65
	18	51.5	50.1	48.7	47.2	45.5	43.7	41.7	39.5	37.1	34.3	31.1	2.45	2.94
47.97	20	50.0	48.6	47.2	45.6	44.0	42.1	40.2	38.0	35.5	32.7	29.5	1.93	2.41
	22	48.4	47.1	45.6	44.1	42.4	40.6	38.6	36.4	34.0	31.2	28.0	1.49	1.95
	24	47.1	45.8	44.3	42.8	41.1	39.3	37.3	35.1	32.7	29.9	26.7	1.19	1.63
	18	54.0	52.6	51.0	49.4	47.6	45.7	43.6	41.3	38.7	35.8	32.4	2.45	2.94
50.63	20	52.3	50.9	49.4	47.8	46.0	44.1	42.0	39.7	37.1	34.2	30.8	1.92	2.40
	22	50.7	49.3	47.8	46.1	44.4	42.5	40.4	38.0	35.5	32.5	29.1	1.47	1.93
	24	49.3	47.9	46.4	44.8	43.0	41.1	39.0	36.7	34.1	31.1	27.8	1.17	1.62
	18	56.4	54.9	53.3	51.6	49.8	47.8	45.6	43.1	40.4	37.3	33.7	2.45	2.94
53.30	20	54.7	53.2	51.6	49.9	48.0	46.0	43.8	41.4	38.7	35.6	32.0	1.91	2.38
	22	53.0	51.5	49.9	48.2	46.3	44.3	42.1	39.7	36.9	33.8	30.3	1.46	1.92
	24	51.5	50.0	48.4	46.7	44.9	42.8	40.6	38.2	35.5	32.4	28.8	1.15	1.60
	18	58.9	57.3	55.6	53.8	51.9	49.8	47.5	44.9	42.0	38.8	35.1	2.45	2.94
55.96	20	57.1	55.5	53.8	52.0	50.1	47.9	45.6	43.1	40.2	37.0	33.2	1.89	2.37
	22	55.2	53.7	52.0	50.2	48.3	46.1	43.8	41.3	38.4	35.2	31.4	1.44	1.91
	24	53.7	52.1	50.5	48.7	46.7	44.6	42.3	39.7	36.9	33.6	29.9	1.13	1.58

TABLE 313

Process Times (B) at Retort Temperature of 230°F for Conduction-Heating Foods in 404 x 307 Can

f_h	z	INITIAL FOOD TEMPERATURE (T_{ih}) 100	110	120	130	140	150	160	170	180	190	200	Equivalent F_c^{18}	F_s^{18}
60.21	18	126.6	124.5	122.2	119.7	117.0	113.9	110.4	106.4	101.6	95.8	88.3	2.65	2.97
	20	113.0	110.9	108.6	106.1	103.4	100.3	96.8	92.8	88.0	82,1	74.6	1.86	2.17
	22	103.0	100.9	98.6	96.2	93.4	90.3	86.8	82.8	78.0	72.2	64.7	1.32	1.63
	24	95.3	93.2	91.0	88.5	85.7	82.6	79.1	75.1	70.3	64.5	57.0	0.96	1.27
63.75	18	131.1	128.9	126.5	123.8	120.9	117.6	113.9	109.7	104.6	98.5	90.5	2.65	2.97
	20	117.5	115.3	112.9	110.3	107.3	104.1	100.4	96.1	91.1	84.9	76.9	1.85	2.17
	22	107.1	104.8	102.4	99.8	96.9	93.6	89.9	85.7	80.6	74.4	66.5	1.30	1.61
	24	99.3	97.1	94.7	92.0	89.1	85.8	82.2	77.9	72.8	66.7	58.7	0.95	1.25
67.29	18	135.4	133.0	130.5	127.7	124.6	121.2	117.3	112.8	107.5	100.9	92.5	2.65	2.96
	20	122.0	119.6	117.1	114.3	111.2	107.8	103.9	99.4	94.1	87.5	79.1	1.84	2.17
	22	111.4	109.0	106.5	103.7	100.6	97.2	93.3	88.8	83.4	76.9	68.5	1.30	1.61
	24	103.2	100.8	98.3	95.5	92.4	89.0	85.1	80.6	75.2	68.7	60.3	0.93	1.24
70.83	18	140.1	137.7	135.0	132.1	128.8	125.2	121.1	116.4	110.7	103.9	95.0	2.64	2.96
	20	126.3	123.9	121.2	118.3	115.0	111.4	107.3	102.5	96.9	90.1	81.2	1.84	2.16
	22	115.6	113.1	110.4	107.5	104.2	100.6	96.5	91.8	86.2	79.3	70.4	1.29	1.61
	24	106.9	104.5	101.8	98.9	95.6	92.0	87.9	83.2	77.6	70.7	61.8	0.92	1.23
74.37	18	145.1	142.5	139.7	136.6	133.2	129.4	125.1	120.1	114.3	107.0	97.8	2.64	2.97
	20	130.7	128.1	125.3	122.2	118.8	115.0	110.7	105.7	99.8	92.6	83.3	1.82	2.15
	22	119.7	117.1	114.3	111.2	107.8	104.0	99.7	94.7	88.8	81.6	72.3	1.27	1.60
	24	110.9	108.3	105.5	102.4	99.0	95.2	90.9	85.9	80.0	72.8	63.5	0.91	1.22

TABLE 314

Process Times (B) at Retort Temperature of 240°F for Conduction-Heating Foods in 404 x 307 Can

f_h	z	INITIAL FOOD TEMPERATURE (T_{ih})											Equivalent	
		100	110	120	130	140	150	160	170	180	190	200	F_c^{18}	F_s^{18}
	18	91.1	89.1	87.0	84.8	82.3	79.5	76.4	72.9	68.9	64.1	58.3	2.56	2.97
60.21	20	85.3	83.4	81.3	79.0	76.5	73.8	70.7	67.2	63.2	58.4	52.6	1.87	2.26
	22	80.6	78.7	76.6	74.3	71.8	69.1	66.0	62.5	58.5	53.7	47.9	1.38	1.76
	24	76.6	74.6	72.5	70.3	67.8	65.0	61.9	58.5	54.4	49.7	43.8	1.04	1.41
	18	95.2	93.2	91.0	88.5	85.9	83.0	79.7	76.0	71.8	66.7	60.5	2.56	2.97
63.75	20	89.3	87.2	85.0	82.6	79.9	77.0	73.8	70.1	65.8	60.8	54.6	1.86	2.25
	22	84.3	82.3	80.1	77.7	75.0	72.1	68.8	65.1	60.9	55.8	49.6	1.37	1.75
	24	80.1	78.0	75.8	73.4	70.8	67.9	64.6	60.9	56.6	51.6	45.4	1.03	1.39
	18	99.4	97.2	94.9	92.3	89.5	86.5	83.0	79.1	74.6	69.3	62.8	2.56	2.97
67.29	20	93.2	91.0	88.7	86.1	83.3	80.2	76.8	72.9	68.4	63.1	56.5	1.85	2.24
	22	88.0	85.9	83.5	81.0	78.2	75.1	71.7	67.8	63.3	57.9	51.4	1.36	1.74
	24	83.6	81.4	79.1	76.5	73.7	70.7	67.2	63.3	58.8	53.5	47.0	1.01	1.38
	18	103.5	101.2	98.8	96.1	93.1	89.9	86.3	82.2	77.4	71.8	65.0	2.55	2.97
70.83	20	97.0	94.7	92.3	89.6	86.7	83.4	79.8	75.7	71.0	65.3	58.5	1.83	2.23
	22	91.7	89.4	86.9	84.3	81.3	78.1	74.5	70.4	65.6	60.0	53.1	1.35	1.74
	24	87.1	84.8	82.3	79.7	76.7	73.5	69.9	65.7	61.0	55.4	48.5	1.01	1.38
	18	107.6	105.2	102.6	99.8	96.7	93.3	89.5	85.2	80.2	74.3	67.1	2.55	2.97
74.37	20	100.9	98.5	95.9	93.1	90.0	86.6	82.8	78.5	73.5	67.6	60.4	1.82	2.22
	22	95.3	92.9	90.4	87.6	84.5	81.1	77.3	73.0	68.0	62.1	54.9	1.35	1.73
	24	90.5	88.1	85.6	82.7	79.7	76.3	72.5	68.1	63.2	57.3	50.1	0.99	1.37

TABLE 315

Process Times (B) at Retort Temperature of 250°F for Conduction-Heating Foods in 404 x 307 Can

f_h	z	INITIAL FOOD TEMPERATURE (T_{ih})											Equivalent	
		100	110	120	130	140	150	160	170	180	190	200	F_c^{18}	F_s^{18}
60.21	18	73.4	71.6	69.7	67.6	65.3	62.8	60.0	57.0	53.5	49.4	44.7	2.51	2.97
	20	70.4	68.6	66.7	64.6	62.3	59.8	57.1	54.0	50.5	46.5	41.7	1.91	2.36
	22	67.7	65.9	63.9	61.9	59.6	57.1	54.3	51.3	47.8	43.7	39.0	1.46	1.88
	24	65.1	63.3	61.3	59.2	57.0	54.5	51.7	48.6	45.1	41.1	36.3	1.10	1.51
63.75	18	77.0	75.1	73.1	70.8	68.4	65.8	62.9	59.6	55.9	51.6	46.6	2.51	2.97
	20	73.9	72.0	69.9	67.7	65.3	62.6	59.7	56.5	52.8	48.5	43.4	1.90	2.34
	22	71.0	69.0	67.0	64.8	62.4	59.7	56.8	53.6	49.9	45.6	40.5	1.44	1.87
	24	68.2	66.3	64.2	62.0	59.6	57.0	54.0	50.8	47.1	42.8	37.8	1.08	1.49
67.29	18	80.6	78.6	76.4	74.1	71.6	68.8	65.7	62.3	58.3	53.8	48.5	2.51	2.97
	20	77.3	75.3	73.1	70.8	68.2	65.4	62.4	58.9	55.0	50.5	45.2	1.89	2.34
	22	74.2	72.2	70.0	67.7	65.1	62.4	59.3	55.8	51.9	47.4	42.1	1.42	1.85
	24	71.3	69.3	67.1	64.8	62.2	59.5	56.4	52.9	49.0	44.5	39.2	1.06	1.47
70.83	18	84.2	82.1	79.8	77.3	74.7	71.7	68.5	64.9	60.7	56.0	50.4	2.50	2.97
	20	80.7	78.6	76.3	73.8	71.2	68.2	65.0	61.4	57.2	52.5	46.9	1.88	2.33
	22	77.4	75.3	73.0	70.6	67.9	65.0	61.7	58.1	54.0	49.2	43.6	1.40	1.83
	24	74.4	72.3	70.0	67.5	64.8	61.9	58.7	55.0	50.9	46.2	40.6	1.04	1.46
74.37	18	87.7	85.5	83.1	80.5	77.7	74.6	71.2	67.4	63.1	58.1	52.2	2.50	2.97
	20	84.1	81.8	79.4	76.9	74.0	71.0	67.6	63.8	59.4	54.5	48.6	1.87	2.32
	22	80.6	78.4	76.0	73.4	70.6	67.5	64.1	60.3	56.0	51.0	45.1	1.38	1.81
	24	77.4	75.2	72.8	70.2	67.4	64.3	60.9	57.1	52.8	47.8	41.9	1.03	1.44

TABLE 316

Process Times (B) at Retort Temperature of 260°F for Conduction-Heating Foods in 404 x 307 Can

f_h	z	INITIAL FOOD TEMPERATURE (T_{ih})											Equivalent	
		100	110	120	130	140	150	160	170	180	190	200	F_c^{18}	F_s^{18}
	18	62.8	61.2	59.4	57.4	55.3	53.0	50.6	47.8	44.7	41.2	37.2	2.47	2.97
60.21	20	60.9	59.2	57.4	55.4	53.3	51.1	48.6	45.8	42.7	39.2	35.2	1.89	2.37
	22	58.9	57.2	55.4	53.5	51.4	49.1	46.6	43.9	40.8	37.3	33.3	1.44	1.91
	24	57.2	55.5	53.7	51.8	49.7	47.4	44.9	42.2	39.1	35.6	31.6	1.12	1.57
	18	66.1	64.3	62.4	60.3	58.1	55.7	53.1	50.1	46.9	43.2	38.9	2.47	2.97
63.75	20	63.9	62.2	60.2	58.2	56.0	53.6	50.9	48.0	44.8	41.1	36.8	1.88	2.36
	22	61.9	60.1	58.2	56.1	53.9	51.5	48.9	46.0	42.7	39.0	34.7	1.43	1.89
	24	60.1	58.3	56.4	54.3	52.1	49.7	47.1	44.2	40.9	37.2	32.9	1.10	1.55
	18	69.3	67.4	65.4	63.2	60.9	58.3	55.5	52.5	49.0	45.1	40.6	2.47	2.97
67.29	20	67.0	65.1	63.1	60.9	58.6	56.1	53.3	50.2	46.8	42.9	38.4	1.87	2.35
	22	64.8	63.0	60.9	58.8	56.4	53.9	51.1	48.0	44.6	40.7	36.2	1.41	1.88
	24	62.9	61.0	59.0	56.9	54.5	52.0	49.2	46.1	42.7	38.8	34.3	1.08	1.53
	18	72.5	70.5	68.4	66.1	63.6	60.9	58.0	54.8	51.1	47.0	42.3	2.46	2.97
70.83	20	70.1	68.1	66.0	63.7	61.2	58.5	55.6	52.4	48.7	44.6	39.9	1.86	2.34
	22	67.8	65.8	63.7	61.4	58.9	56.3	53.3	50.1	46.5	42.4	37.6	1.40	1.87
	24	65.7	63.8	61.6	59.4	56.9	54.2	51.3	48.0	44.4	40.3	35.6	1.06	1.52
	18	75.6	73.6	71.3	68.9	66.4	63.5	60.5	57.1	53.3	48.9	44.0	2.46	2.97
74.37	20	73.1	71.0	68.8	66.4	63.8	61.0	57.9	54.5	50.7	46.4	41.4	1.85	2.34
	22	70.7	68.6	66.4	64.0	61.4	58.6	55.5	52.1	48.3	44.0	39.0	1.38	1.86
	24	68.5	66.5	64.2	61.8	59.2	56.4	53.4	50.0	46.1	41.8	36.9	1.04	1.50

TABLE 317

Process Times (B) at Retort Temperature of 230°F for Conduction-Heating Foods in 404 x 309 Can

f_h	z	INITIAL FOOD TEMPERATURE (T_{ih})											Equivalent	
		100	110	120	130	140	150	160	170	180	190	200	F_C^{18}	F_S^{18}
	18	129.3	127.2	124.8	122.2	119.4	116.2	112.6	108.4	103.5	97.4	89.7	2.66	2.97
62.30	20	115.7	113.6	111.2	108.6	105.8	102.6	99.0	94.8	89.9	83.8	76.0	1.86	2.18
	22	105.5	103.3	100.9	98.4	95.5	92.3	88.7	84.5	79.6	73.6	65.8	1.31	1.62
	24	97.7	95.6	93.2	90.6	87.8	84.6	81.0	76.8	71.9	65.8	58.0	0.96	1.26
	18	133.9	131.6	129.1	126.4	123.3	120.0	116.1	111.7	106.5	100.1	91.9	2.65	2.97
65.96	20	120.4	118.1	115.6	112.9	109.8	106.5	102.6	98.2	93.0	86.6	78.4	1.85	2.17
	22	109.8	107.5	105.0	102.3	99.3	95.9	92.1	87.6	82.4	76.0	67.8	1.30	1.62
	24	101.8	99.5	97.0	94.2	91.2	87.8	84.0	79.6	74.4	68.0	59.8	0.94	1.25
	18	138.5	136.1	133.4	130.5	127.4	123.8	119.8	115.1	109.6	102.8	94.1	2.65	2.97
73.29	20	129.4	122.5	119.9	117.0	113.8	110.2	106.2	101.5	96.0	89.3	80.6	1.84	2.17
	22	114.2	111.8	109.1	106.2	103.1	99.5	95.5	90.8	85.3	78.5	69.8	1.29	1.61
	24	105.7	103.3	100.7	97.8	94.6	91.0	87.0	82.3	76.8	70.1	61.4	0.93	1.23
	18	143.7	141.1	138.3	135.3	132.0	128.2	124.0	119.0	113.2	106.1	97.0	2.64	2.97
73.29	20	129.4	126.8	124.1	121.0	117.7	113.9	109.7	104.8	99.0	91.9	82.7	1.83	2.15
	22	118.5	115.9	113.2	110.1	106.8	103.0	98.8	93.9	88.1	81.0	71.8	1.28	1.60
	24	109.7	107.2	104.4	101.4	98.0	94.3	90.0	85.1	79.3	72.2	63.0	0.91	1.22
	18	148.7	146.0	143.1	140.0	136.4	132.5	128.0	122.9	116.8	109.3	99.7	2.64	2.97
76.96	20	133.8	131.1	128.2	125.0	121.5	117.6	113.1	108.0	101.9	94.4	84.8	1.80	2.13
	22	122.7	120.0	117.1	113.9	110.4	106.5	102.0	96.8	90.7	83.3	73.7	1.27	1.59
	24	113.7	111.0	108.1	104.9	101.4	97.5	93.0	87.9	81.8	74.3	64.7	0.90	1.22

TABLE 318

Process Times (B) at Retort Temperature of 240° for Conduction-Heating Foods in 404 x 309 Can

f_h	z	INITIAL FOOD TEMPERATURE (T_{ih})											Equivalent	
		100	110	120	130	140	150	160	170	180	190	200	F_c^{18}	F_s^{18}
	18	93.5	91.5	89.4	87.0	84.4	81.6	78.4	74.8	70.6	65.7	59.7	2.56	2.97
62.30	20	87.7	85.7	83.5	81.2	78.6	75.7	72.5	68.9	64.8	59.8	53.8	1.86	2.26
	22	82.8	80.8	78.7	76.3	73.7	70.9	67.7	64.1	59.9	55.5	48.9	1.37	1.75
	24	78.7	76.7	74.5	72.2	69.6	66.7	63.5	59.9	55.8	50.8	44.8	1.03	1.40
	18	97.9	95.7	93.4	90.9	88.2	85.2	81.8	78.0	73.6	68.4	62.0	2.56	2.97
65.96	20	91.7	89.6	87.3	84.8	82.1	79.1	75.7	71.9	67.5	62.2	55.8	1.85	2.25
	22	86.7	84.5	82.2	79.8	77.0	74.0	70.6	66.8	62.4	57.2	50.8	1.36	1.75
	24	82.3	80.2	77.9	75.4	72.6	69.6	66.3	62.4	58.0	52.8	46.4	1.02	1.39
	18	102.1	99.9	97.5	94.8	92.0	88.8	85.2	81.2	76.5	71.0	64.2	2.56	2.97
69.63	20	95.7	93.5	91.9	88.4	85.6	82.4	78.8	74.8	70.1	64.6	57.9	1.84	2.24
	22	90.5	88.2	85.8	83.2	80.3	77.1	73.5	69.5	64.8	59.3	52.6	1.36	1.74
	24	85.9	83.7	81.2	78.6	75.7	72.5	69.0	64.9	60.3	54.8	48.0	1.01	1.38
	18	106.4	104.0	101.4	98.7	95.6	92.3	88.5	84.3	79.4	73.6	66.5	2.56	2.97
73.29	20	99.7	97.3	94.8	92.0	89.0	85.6	81.9	77.6	72.7	66.9	59.8	1.83	2.23
	22	94.2	91.9	89.3	86.6	83.5	80.2	76.4	72.2	67.3	61.5	54.4	1.35	1.74
	24	89.5	87.1	84.6	81.8	78.8	75.4	71.7	67.4	62.5	56.7	49.6	1.00	1.37
	18	110.6	108.1	105.4	102.5	99.3	95.8	91.9	87.4	82.2	76.2	68.7	2.55	2.97
76.96	20	103.7	101.2	98,5	95.6	92.4	88.9	85.0	80.5	75.3	69.3	61.8	1.82	2.22
	22	98.0	95.6	92.9	90.0	86.8	83.3	79.3	74.9	69.7	63.6	56.2	1.34	1.73
	24	93.1	90.6	87.9	85.0	81.8	78.3	74.4	69.9	64.7	58.6	51.2	0.99	1.36

TABLE 319

Process Times (B) at Retort Temperature of 250°F for Conduction-Heating Foods in 404 x 309 Can

f_h	z	INITIAL FOOD TEMPERATURE (T_{ih})											Equivalent	
		100	110	120	130	140	150	160	170	180	190	200	F_c^{18}	F_s^{18}
	18	75.5	73.7	71.7	69.5	67.2	64.6	61.7	58.5	54.9	50.8	45.8	2.51	2.97
62.30	20	72.5	70.6	68.6	66.4	64.1	61.5	58.7	55.5	51.9	47.7	42.7	1.91	2.35
	22	69.6	67.8	65.8	63.6	61.2	58.7	55.8	52.6	49.0	44.8	39.9	1.45	1.87
	24	66.9	65.1	63.0	60.9	58.5	56.0	53.1	49.9	46.3	42.1	37.2	1.09	1.50
	18	79.3	77.3	75.2	72.9	70.4	67.7	64.7	61.3	57.5	53.0	47/8	2.51	2.97
65.96	20	76.0	74.1	71.9	69.6	67.1	64.4	61.4	58.0	54.2	49.8	44.6	1.90	2.34
	22	73.0	71.0	68.9	66.6	64.1	61.4	58.4	55.0	51.2	46.8	41.5	1.43	1.86
	24	70.2	68.2	66.1	63.8	61.3	58.5	55.5	52.1	48.3	43.9	38.7	1.07	1.48
	18	83.0	80.9	78.7	76.3	73.6	70.7	67.6	64.0	60.0	55.3	49.8	2.51	2.97
69.63	20	79.6	77.5	75.2	72.8	70.2	67.3	64.1	60.6	56.5	51.9	46.3	1.89	2.33
	22	76.4	74.3	72.0	69.6	67.0	64.1	60.9	57.3	53.3	48.6	43.1	1.41	1.84
	24	73.4	71.3	69.0	66.6	64.0	61.1	57.9	54.3	50.3	45.6	40.1	1.05	1.46
	18	86.7	84.5	82.1	79.6	76.8	73.8	70.4	66.7	62.4	57.5	51.7	2.51	2.97
73.29	20	83.1	80.9	78.5	75.9	73.2	70.1	66.8	63.0	58.8	53.9	48.1	1.87	2.32
	22	79.7	77.5	75.1	72.6	69.8	66.8	63.4	59.7	55.4	50.5	44.7	1.39	1.82
	24	76.5	74.3	72.0	69.4	66.6	63.6	60.3	56.5	52.3	47.4	41.6	1.03	1.45
	18	90.3	88.0	85.5	82.9	80.0	76.8	73.3	69.3	64.9	59.7	53.6	2.50	2.97
76.96	20	86.5	84.2	81.7	79.1	76.2	73.0	69.5	65.5	61.1	55.9	49.8	1.86	2.31
	22	83.0	80.6	78.2	75.5	72.6	69.4	65.9	61.9	57.5	52.3	46.2	1.37	1.81
	24	79.7	77.4	74.9	72.2	69.3	66.1	62.6	58.7	54.2	49.0	43.0	1.02	1.43

TABLE 320

Process Times (B) at Retort Temperature of 260°F for Conduction-Heating Foods in 404 x 309 Can

f_h	z	INITIAL FOOD TEMPERATURE (T_{ih})											Equivalent	
		100	110	120	130	140	150	160	170	180	190	200	F_c^{18}	F_s^{18}
62.30	18	64.8	63.0	61.1	59.1	57.0	54.6	52.0	49.2	46.0	42.4	38.2	2.47	2.97
	20	62.7	60.9	59.1	57.1	54.9	52.6	50.0	47.1	43.9	40.3	36.2	1.89	2.37
	22	60.7	58.9	57.1	55.1	52.9	50.5	48.0	45.1	41.9	38.3	34.1	1.43	1.90
	24	58.9	57.2	55.3	53.3	51.1	48.8	46.2	43.4	40.2	36.6	32.4	1.11	1.56
65.96	18	68.1	66.2	64.3	62.1	59.8	57.3	54.6	51.6	48.2	44.4	40.0	2.47	2.97
	20	65.9	64.0	62.1	59.9	57.6	55.1	52.4	49.4	46.0	42.2	37.8	1.87	2.36
	22	63.8	61.9	59.9	57.8	55.5	53.0	50.3	47.3	43.9	40.1	35.7	1.42	1.89
	24	61.9	60.0	58.0	55.9	53.6	51.1	48.4	45.4	42.0	38.2	33.8	1.09	1.54
69.63	18	71.4	69.4	67.3	65.1	62.7	60.1	57.2	54.0	50.4	46.4	41.7	2.47	2.97
	20	69.0	67.1	65.0	62.8	60.3	57.7	54.8	51.6	48.1	44.0	39.4	1.86	2.35
	22	66.8	64.8	62.8	60.5	58.1	55.5	52.6	49.4	45.8	41.8	37.1	1.40	1.87
	24	64.8	62.8	60.8	58.5	56.1	53.5	50.6	47.4	43.8	39.8	35.1	1.07	1.52
73.29	18	74.7	72.6	70.4	68.1	65.5	62.8	59.7	56.4	52.6	48.4	43.5	2.47	2.97
	20	72.2	70.1	67.9	65.6	63.0	60.3	57.2	53.9	50.1	45.9	41.0	1.85	2.34
	22	69.8	67.8	65.6	63.2	60.7	57.9	54.9	51.5	47.8	43.5	38.6	1.39	1.86
	24	67.7	65.6	63.4	61.1	58.5	55.8	52.7	49.4	45.6	41.4	36.5	1.05	1.51
76.96	18	78.0	75.8	73.5	71.0	68.3	65.4	62.3	58.7	54.8	50.3	45.2	2.46	2.97
	20	75.3	73.2	70.8	68.4	65.7	62.8	59.6	56.1	52.1	47.7	42.5	1.85	2.34
	22	72.9	70.7	68.4	65.9	63.2	60.3	57.1	53.6	49.7	45.2	40.1	1.38	1.85
	24	70.6	68.4	66.1	63.6	61.0	58.1	54.9	51.4	47.4	43.0	37.8	1.03	1.49

TABLE 321

Process Times (B) at Retort Temperature of 230°F for Conduction-Heating Foods in 404 x 700 Can

f_h	z	INITIAL FOOD TEMPERATURE (T_{ih}) 100	110	120	130	140	150	160	170	180	190	200	Equivalent F^{18}	F^{18}
91.67	18	169.3	166.1	162.7	158.9	154.7	150.0	144.7	138.5	131.3	122.4	111.0	2.68	3.03
	20	152.9	149.7	146.3	142.5	138.3	133.6	128.3	122.1	114.9	106.0	94.5	1.83	2.17
	22	140.1	136.9	133.5	129.7	125.5	120.8	115.5	109.3	102.1	93.2	81.7	1.26	1.59
	24	130.1	126.9	123.4	119.6	115.5	110.8	105.4	9913	92.1	83.2	71.7	0.89	1.21
97.06	18	176.2	172.9	169.2	165.2	160.7	155.8	150.2	143.7	136.0	126.6	114.4	2.68	3.03
	20	159.4	156.0	152.4	148.4	143.9	139.0	133.3	126.8	119.1	109.7	97.6	1.82	2.16
	22	146.2	142.8	139.1	135.1	130.7	125.7	120.1	113.6	105.9	96.5	84.3	1.24	1.58
	24	135.8	132.4	128.8	124.7	120.3	115.3	109.7	103.2	95.5	86.1	74.0	0.88	1.20
102.45	18	183.0	179.5	175.6	171.4	166.7	161.4	155.5	148.6	140.5	130.6	117.8	2.67	3.03
	20	165.8	162.2	158.3	154.1	149.4	144.2	138.2	131.4	123.3	113.3	100.5	1.80	2.15
	22	152.1	148.6	144.7	140.4	135.7	130.5	124.6	117.7	109.6	99.7	86.9	1.23	1.57
	24	141.4	137.8	134.0	129.7	125.0	119.8	113.8	107.0	98.9	88.9	76.1	0.87	1.19
107.85	18	190.1	186.3	182.3	177.8	172.9	167.3	161.1	153.9	145.3	134.9	121.4	2.67	3.03
	20	172.1	168.3	164.3	159.8	154.9	149.3	143.1	135.9	127.3	116.9	103.4	1.78	2.14
	22	158.0	154.2	150.1	145.7	140.7	135.2	129.0	121.7	113.2	102.8	89.3	1.22	1.56
	24	146.9	143.1	139.1	134.6	129.7	124.1	117.9	110.7	102.1	91.7	78.2	0.85	1.18
113.24	18	197.1	193.2	188.9	184.2	179.0	173.3	166.7	159.1	150.1	139.2	125.0	2.67	3.03
	20	178.5	174.6	170.3	165.6	160.4	154.6	148.1	140.5	131.5	120.5	106.4	1.78	2.14
	22	163.9	160.0	155.7	151.0	145.8	140.0	133.5	125.9	116.9	106.0	91.8	1.21	1.55
	24	152.4	148.5	144.2	139.5	134.3	128.6	122.0	114.4	105.4	94.5	80.3	0.84	1.17

TABLE 322

Process Times (B) at Retort Temperature of 240°F for Conduction-Heating Foods in 404 x 700 Can

f_h	z	INITIAL FOOD TEMPERATURE (T_{ih})											Equivalent	
		100	110	120	130	140	150	160	170	180	190	200	F_c^{18}	F_s^{18}
91.67	18	127.8	124.8	121.6	118.2	114.4	110.2	105.5	100.2	94.0	86.8	77.9	2.61	3.03
	20	119.9	117.0	113.8	110.3	106.6	102.4	97.7	92.4	86.2	79.0	70.1	1.85	2.26
	22	113.4	110.5	107.3	103.8	100.0	95.8	91.1	85.8	79.7	72.4	63.5	1.35	1.75
	24	107.4	104.5	101.3	97.8	94.1	89.9	85.2	79.9	73.7	66.5	57.6	0.97	1.35
97.06	18	133.8	130.7	127.3	123.6	119.6	115.2	110.2	104.6	98.1	90.4	81.0	2.60	3.03
	20	125.6	122.5	119.1	115.5	111.5	107.0	102.0	96.4	89.9	82.2	72.8	1.85	2.27
	22	118.7	115.6	112.3	108.6	104.6	100.1	95.2	89.5	83.0	75.3	65.9	1.34	1.74
	24	112.4	109.3	105.9	102.2	98.2	93.8	88.8	83.2	76.7	69.0	59.6	0.95	1.33
102.45	18	139.8	136.6	133.0	129.1	124.9	120.2	114.9	109.0	102.1	94.0	84.1	2.60	3.03
	20	131.3	128.0	124.4	120.5	116.3	111.6	106.4	100.4	93.6	85.4	75.5	1.85	2.26
	22	124.0	120.7	117.1	113.3	109.0	104.3	99.1	93.2	86.3	78.2	68.3	1.32	1.72
	24	117.3	114.0	110.5	106.6	102.4	97.7	92.4	86.5	79.6	71.5	61.6	0.93	1.31
107.85	18	145.8	142.3	138.6	134.5	130.0	125.1	119.6	113.3	106.1	97.6	87.1	2.60	3.03
	20	136.8	133.3	129.6	125.5	121.0	116.1	110.6	104.3	97.1	88.6	78.1	1.84	2.25
	22	129.2	125.7	122.0	117.9	113.4	108.5	103.0	96.7	89.5	81.0	70.5	1.31	1.71
	24	122.3	118.8	115.1	111.0	106.5	101.6	96.1	89.8	82.6	74.1	63.6	0.92	1.30
113.24	18	151.7	148.1	144.1	139.8	135.2	130.0	124.2	117.6	110.0	101.1	90.1	2.60	3.03
	20	142.3	138.6	134.7	130.4	125.7	120.6	114.8	108.2	100.6	91.6	80.7	1.82	2.24
	22	134.4	130.7	126.8	122.5	117.8	112.7	106.9	100.3	92.7	83.7	72.8	1.30	1.70
	24	127.2	123.6	119.6	115.4	110.7	105.5	99.7	93.1	85.6	76.6	65.6	0.91	1.29

TABLE 323

Process Times (B) at Retort Temperature of 250°F for Conduction-Heating Foods in 404 x 700 Can

f_h	z	INITIAL FOOD TEMPERATURE (T_{ih})											Equivalent	
		100	110	120	130	140	150	160	170	180	190	200	F_c^{18}	F_s^{18}
91.67	18	105.2	102.5	99.5	96.3	92.9	89.1	84.9	80.2	74.9	68.7	61.5	2.56	3.03
	20	100.6	97.9	95.0	91.8	88.3	84.5	80.3	75.6	70.3	64.2	56.9	1.87	2.33
	22	96.3	93.6	90.6	87.4	84.0	80.2	76.0	71.3	66.0	59.9	52.6	1.36	1.79
	24	92.5	89.8	86.8	83.6	80.2	76.4	72.2	67.5	62.2	56.0	48.8	0.99	1.41
97.06	18	110.5	107.6	104.4	101.1	97.4	93.4	88.9	84.0	78.3	71.8	64.2	2.56	3.03
	20	105.6	102.7	99.6	96.2	92.6	88.5	84.1	79.1	73.5	67.0	59.3	1.86	2.32
	22	101.1	98.1	95.0	91.6	88.0	84.0	79.5	74.6	68.9	62.4	54.7	1.34	1.77
	24	97.0	94.1	91.0	87.6	84.0	79.9	75.5	70.5	64.9	58.4	50.7	0.98	1.40
102.45	18	115.7	112.6	109.3	105.8	101.9	97.6	93.0	87.7	81.8	74.9	66.8	2.56	3.03
	20	110.6	107.5	104.2	100.7	96.8	92.5	87.9	82.6	76.7	69.8	61.7	1.85	2.31
	22	105.7	102.7	99.4	95.8	91.9	87.7	83.0	77.8	71.8	65.0	56.8	1.32	1.76
	24	101.5	98.4	95.1	91.6	87.7	83.5	78.8	73.5	67.6	60.7	52.6	0.96	1.38
107.85	18	120.9	117.7	114.2	110.4	106.4	101.9	97.0	91.4	85.2	78.0	69.4	2.56	3.03
	20	115.5	112.3	108.8	105.1	101.0	96.5	91.6	86.1	79.8	72.6	64.1	1.84	2.30
	22	110.4	107.2	103.7	99.9	95,9	91.4	86.5	80.9	74.7	67.5	58.9	1.31	1.74
	24	106.0	102.7	99.3	95.5	91.5	87.0	82.1	76.5	70.3	63.1	54.5	0.94	1.36
113.24	18	126.1	122.7	119.0	115.1	110.8	106.1	100.9	95.1	88.6	81.0	72.0	2.55	3.03
	20	120.4	117.0	113.3	109.4	105.1	100.4	95.3	89.5	82.9	75.3	66.4	1.83	2.29
	22	115.0	111.6	108.0	104.0	99.8	95.1	89.9	84.1	77.5	69.9	61.0	1.29	1.73
	24	110.4	107.0	103.4	99.4	95.1	90.5	85.3	79.5	72.9	65.3	56.4	0.93	1.35

TABLE 324

Process Times (B) at Retort Temperature of 260°F for Conduction-Heating Foods in 404 x 700 Can

f_h	z	INITIAL FOOD TEMPERATURE (T_{ih})											Equivalent	
		100	110	120	130	140	150	160	170	180	190	200	F_c^{18}	F_s^{18}
	18	91.2	88.6	85.9	82.9	79.7	76.3	72.5	68.3	63.6	58.3	52.2	2.52	3.03
91.67	20	88.0	85.5	82.7	79.8	76.6	73.1	69.3	65.1	60.4	55.1	49.0	1.86	2.36
	22	85.1	82.5	79.8	76.8	73.6	70.2	66.4	62.2	57.5	52.2	46.0	1.37	1.85
	24	82.3	79.7	77.0	74.0	70.8	67.4	63.6	59.4	54.7	49.4	43.2	1.01	1.47
	18	95.9	93.2	90.3	87.1	83.8	80.1	76.1	71.6	66.7	61.0	54.5	2.52	3.03
97.06	20	92.5	89.8	86.9	83.8	80.4	76.8	72.7	68.3	63.3	57.7	51.2	1.85	2.35
	22	89.5	86.7	83.8	80.7	77.3	73.7	69.6	65.2	60.2	54.6	48.1	1.36	1.84
	24	86.4	83.7	80.8	77.7	74.3	70.6	66.6	62.2	57.2	51.6	45.1	0.99	1.45
	18	100.5	97.7	94.6	91.3	87.7	83.9	79.6	74.9	69.7	63.8	56.9	2.52	3.03
102.45	20	97.0	94.2	91.1	87.8	84.2	80.4	76.1	71.4	66.2	60.2	53.4	1.84	2.34
	22	93.8	90.9	87.8	84.5	81.0	77.1	72.9	68.2	62.9	57.0	50.1	1.35	1.83
	24	90.6	87.7	84.6	81.3	77.8	73.9	69.7	65.0	59.7	53.8	46.9	0.97	1.44
	18	105.2	102.2	98.9	95.5	91.7	87.7	83.2	78.3	72.7	66.5	59.3	2.52	3.03
107.85	20	101.5	98.4	95.2	91.7	88.0	83.9	79.5	74.5	69.0	62.7	55.5	1.83	2.32
	22	98.1	95.1	91.8	88.3	84.6	80.5	76.1	71.1	65.6	59.4	52.1	1.34	1.82
	24	94.7	91.7	88.4	85.0	81.2	77.1	72.7	67.7	62.2	56.0	48.7	0.96	1.43
	18	109.9	106.7	103.3	99.6	95.7	91.4	86.7	81.6	75.8	69.2	61.6	2.51	3.03
113.24	20	105.9	102.7	99.3	95.7	91.7	87.5	82.8	77.6	71.8	65.2	57.6	1.81	2.31
	22	102.3	99.2	95.8	92.1	88.2	83.9	79.2	74.0	68.2	61.7	54.1	1.33	1.81
	24	98.8	95.6	92.2	88.6	84.6	80.3	75.7	70.5	64.7	58.1	50.5	0.95	1.42

TABLE 325

Process Times (B) at Retort Temperature of 230°F for Conduction-Heating Foods in 603 x 700 Can

f_h	z	INITIAL FOOD TEMPERATURE (T_{ih})											Equivalent	
		100	110	120	130	140	150	160	170	180	190	200	F_c^{18}	F_s^{18}
170.00	18	268.8	262.9	256.5	249.5	241.7	233.0	223.1	211.8	198.3	181.8	160.6	2.71	3.10
	20	244.3	238.3	231.9	224.9	217.1	208.4	198.6	187.2	173.7	157.2	136.0	1.75	2.13
	22	225.0	219.1	212.7	205.6	197.8	189.2	179.3	167.9	154.5	138.0	116.7	1.16	1.52
	24	209.4	203.5	197.1	190.0	182.3	173.6	163.7	152.3	138.9	122.4	101.1	0.79	1.13
180.00	18	280.9	274.6	267.8	260.4	252.1	242.9	232.5	220.4	206.2	188.7	166.2	2.70	3.10
	20	255.3	249.0	242.2	234.8	226.5	217.3	206.9	193.8	180.6	163.1	140.7	1.74	2.12
	22	235.3	229.0	222.2	214.7	206.5	197.3	186.9	174.8	160.6	143.1	120.6	1.15	1.51
	24	218.9	212.7	205.9	198.4	190.2	181.0	170.5	158.5	144.2	126.8	104.3	0.78	1.12
190.00	18	292.9	286.3	279.1	271.2	262.5	252.8	241.8	229.1	214.0	195.6	171.9	2.70	3.10
	20	266.2	259.6	252.4	244.5	235.8	226.1	215.1	202.4	187.3	168.9	145.2	1.73	2.11
	22	245.4	238.8	231.7	223.8	215.1	205.4	194.4	181.6	166.6	148.2	124.4	1.14	1.50
	24	228.5	221.9	214.7	206.8	198.1	188.4	177.4	164.7	149.6	131.2	107.5	0.77	1.12
200.00	18	304.7	297.7	290.1	281.9	272.7	262.5	250.9	237.5	221.7	202.3	177.3	2.70	3.10
	20	277.1	270.1	262.6	254.3	245.1	234.9	223.3	209.9	194.1	174.7	149.7	1.73	2.11
	22	255.5	248.6	241.0	232.8	223.6	213.4	201.8	188.4	172.6	153.2	128.2	1.13	1.50
	24	238.0	231.0	223.5	215.2	206.1	195.8	184.2	170.8	155.0	135.6	110.6	0.76	1.11
210.00	18	316.3	309.0	301.1	292.4	282.8	272.0	259.9	245.8	229.2	208.8	182.6	2.70	3.10
	20	287.8	280.5	272.6	263.9	254.3	243.5	231.4	217.3	200.7	180.3	154.1	1.72	2.11
	22	265.6	258.3	250.4	241.7	232.1	221.3	209.1	195.1	178.4	158.1	131.9	1.13	1.50
	24	247.4	240.1	232.1	223.4	213.8	203.1	190.9	176.9	160.2	139.9	113.6	0.75	1.10

TABLE 326

Process Times (B) at Retort Temperature of 240°F for Conduction-Heating Foods in 603 x 700 Can

f_h	z	INITIAL FOOD TEMPERATURE (T_{ih})											Equivalent	
		100	110	120	130	140	150	160	170	180	190	200	F_c^{18}	F_s^{18}
	18	212.4	206.9	201.0	194.6	187.5	179.8	171.1	161.2	149.8	136.4	119.9	2.65	3.10
170.00	20	199.2	193.8	187.9	181.4	174.4	166.6	157.9	148.1	136.7	123.2	106.7	1.80	2.23
	22	188.0	182.6	176.7	170.2	163.2	155.4	146.7	136.9	125.5	112.0	95.5	1.23	1.64
	24	177.7	172.2	166.3	159.9	152.8	145.0	136.4	126.5	115.1	101.7	85.2	0.83	1.22
	18	222.6	216.8	210.6	203.8	196.3	188.1	178.9	168.4	156.4	142.1	124.7	2.65	3.10
180.00	20	208.9	203.1	196.9	190.1	182.6	174.4	165.2	154.7	142.7	128.4	111.0	1.79	2.22
	22	197.0	191.2	185.0	178.2	170.7	162.5	153.3	142.9	130.8	116.6	99.1	1.21	1.63
	24	186.2	180.4	174.1	167.3	159.9	151.6	142.4	132.0	120.0	105.7	88.3	0.82	1.20
	18	232.7	226.6	220.0	212.8	205.0	196.3	186.6	175.5	162.8	147.8	129.4	2.64	3.10
190.00	20	218.5	212.4	205.8	198.6	190.7	182.1	172.3	161.3	148.6	133.6	115.1	1.78	2.22
	22	206.0	199.8	193.2	186.1	178.2	169.5	159.8	148.8	136.0	121.0	102.6	1.20	1.61
	24	194.6	188.5	181.9	174.7	166.9	158.2	148.5	137.4	124.7	109.7	91.3	0.80	1.19
	18	243.0	236.5	229.6	222.0	213.7	204.6	194.3	182.8	169.4	153.5	134.1	2.64	3.10
200.00	20	228.0	221.6	214.6	207.0	198.8	189.6	179.4	167.8	154.4	138.6	119.2	1.77	2.21
	22	214.9	208.4	201.5	193.9	185.6	176.5	166.3	154.7	141.3	125.4	106.0	1.19	1.60
	24	203.0	196.5	189.6	182.0	173.8	164.6	154.4	142.8	129.4	113.6	94.2	0.79	1.18
	18	253.1	246.3	239.0	231.1	222.4	212.8	202.0	189.9	175.8	159.2	138.8	2.64	3.10
210.00	20	237.4	230.6	223.3	215.4	206.7	197.1	186.4	174.2	160.1	143.5	123.1	1.76	2.20
	22	223.7	216.9	209.6	201.7	193.0	183.4	172.4	160.4	146.4	129.8	109.4	1.17	1.59
	24	211.3	204.5	197.2	189.3	180.6	171.0	160.2	148.1	134.0	117.4	97.0	0.78	1.17

TABLE 327

Process Times (B) at Retort Temperature of 250°F for Conduction-Heating Foods in 603 x 700 Can

f_h	z	INITIAL FOOD TEMPERATURE (T_{ih}) 100	110	120	130	140	150	160	170	180	190	200	Equivalent F_c^{18}	F_s^{18}
170.00	18	179.5	174.4	169.0	163.0	156.6	149.6	141.8	133.1	123.3	111.9	98.4	2.61	3.10
	20	171.0	165.9	160.4	154.5	148.1	141.0	133.3	124.6	114.7	103.3	89.9	1.79	2.27
	22	163.0	157.9	152.4	146.5	140.1	133.0	125.3	116.6	106.7	95.3	81.9	1.21	1.66
	24	156.2	151.1	145.6	139.7	133.3	126.2	118.5	109.8	99.9	88.5	75.1	0.85	1.28
180.00	18	188.6	183.2	177.4	171.2	164.4	156.9	148.7	139.5	129.0	117.0	102.7	2.61	3.10
	20	179.6	174.2	168.4	162.1	155.3	147.9	139.6	130.4	120.0	107.9	93.7	1.78	2.25
	22	171.1	165.7	159.9	153.7	146.9	139.4	131.2	122.0	111.5	99.5	85.2	1.20	1.65
	24	163.9	158.5	152.7	146.5	139.7	132.2	124.0	114.8	104.3	92.3	78.0	0.83	1.26
190.00	18	197.7	192.0	185.9	179.3	172.1	164.2	155.5	145.8	134.8	122.1	107.0	2.60	3.10
	20	188.1	182.4	176.3	169.7	162.5	154.7	146.0	136.2	125.2	112.5	97.5	1.77	2.24
	22	179.3	173.6	167.5	160.9	153.7	145.8	137.1	127.4	116.4	103.7	88.6	1.19	1.64
	24	171.6	165.9	159.8	153.2	146.0	138.2	129.5	119.8	108.7	96.0	81.0	0.82	1.25
200.00	18	206.7	200.7	194.2	187.3	179.7	171.4	162.3	152.1	140.5	127.1	111.2	2.60	3.10
	20	196.6	190.6	184.2	177.2	169.7	161.4	152.2	142.0	130.4	117.0	101.2	1.75	2.23
	22	187.4	181.4	174.9	168.0	160.4	152.1	143.0	132.9	121.2	107.8	91.9	1.18	1.63
	24	179.3	173.3	166.8	159.9	152.3	144.1	134.9	124.7	113.1	99.7	83.8	0.80	1.24
210.00	18	215.6	109.3	202.5	195.2	187.3	178.6	169.0	158.3	146.1	132.0	115.4	2.60	3.10
	20	205.0	198.7	192.0	184.7	176.8	168.1	158.5	147.7	135.5	121.5	104.8	1.74	2.22
	22	195.4	189.1	182.3	175.0	167.1	158.4	148.8	138.1	125.9	111.8	95.2	1.17	1.62
	24	186.9	180.6	173.8	166.5	158.6	149.9	140.3	129.5	117.3	103.3	86.7	0.79	1.22

TABLE 328

Process Times (B) at Retort Temperature of 260°F for Conduction-Heating Foods in 603 x 700 Can

f_h	z	INITIAL FOOD TEMPERATURE (T_{ih})											Equivalent	
		100	110	120	130	140	150	160	170	180	190	200	F_c^{18}	F_s^{18}
	18	157.9	153.2	148.1	142.6	136.7	130.3	123.2	115.5	106.8	96.9	85.5	2.57	3.10
170.00	20	151.8	147.0	141.0	136.4	130.5	124.1	117.1	109.3	100.6	90.7	79.3	1.77	2.29
	22	146.3	141.5	136.4	130.9	125.0	118.6	111.6	103.8	95.1	85.2	73.9	1.25	1.75
	24	140.9	136.1	131.0	125.6	119.7	113.2	106.2	98.4	89.7	79.9	68.5	0.87	1.35
	18	166.2	161.1	155.7	149.9	143.7	136.9	129.4	121.2	112.0	101.5	89.5	2.56	3.10
180.00	20	159.6	154.6	149.2	143.4	137.1	130.3	122.9	114.6	105.4	95.0	82.9	1.76	2.28
	22	153.7	148.7	143.3	137.5	131.2	124.4	117.0	108.7	99.5	89.1	77.1	1.23	1.73
	24	148.1	143.0	137.6	131.8	125.6	118.8	111.3	103.1	93.9	83.5	71.4	0.85	1.33
	18	174.4	169.0	163.3	157.2	150.6	143.4	135.6	126.9	117.2	106.1	93.4	2.56	3.10
190.00	20	167.4	162.1	156.4	150.3	143.7	136.5	128.6	119.9	110.2	99.2	86.5	1.75	2.27
	22	161.2	155.8	150.1	144.0	137.4	130.2	122.4	113.7	104.0	92.9	80.2	1.22	1.72
	24	155.2	149.9	144.2	138.1	131.5	124.3	116.4	107.7	98.0	87.0	74.3	0.84	1.32
	18	182.5	176.9	170.9	164.5	157.5	150.0	141.7	143.5	122.3	110.7	97.3	2.56	3.10
200.00	20	175.2	169.6	163.6	157.1	150.2	142.6	134.4	125.2	115.0	103.4	90.0	1.74	2.26
	22	168.5	162.9	156.9	150.5	143.5	136.0	127.7	118.6	108.3	96.7	83.3	1.20	1.70
	24	162.3	156.7	150.7	144.2	137.3	129.7	121.5	112.3	102.1	90.5	77.1	0.82	1.30
	18	190.6	184.7	178.4	171.7	164.4	156.4	147.7	138.1	127.4	115.2	101.1	2.56	3.10
210.00	20	182.9	177.0	170.7	164.0	156.7	148.7	140.0	130.4	119.7	107.5	93.4	1.74	2.26
	22	175.9	170.0	163.7	156.9	149.6	141.7	133.0	123.4	112.6	100.5	86.4	1.19	1.69
	24	169.4	163.5	157.2	150.4	143.1	135.2	126.5	116.9	106.1	94.0	79.9	0.81	1.29

SECTION III: COMMERCIAL STERILITY WITH z VALUES FROM 16 TO 22; TABLES 329 TO 492

Hypothetical Processing Criteria to Achieve Commercial Sterility in Conduction-Heating Products

Thermobacteriological considerations

Organism of concern	: *C. sporogenes*
Initial population	: One per gram of food
Extent of reduction	: 4 log cycles
D_{250} Value	: 1.5 min
z Values	: 16, 18, 20, and 22F°

Processing conditions

Initial food temperature (T_{ih})	: 100 to 200°F
Retort temperatures (T_r)	: 230 to 260°F
Heating rate function (f_h)	: Based on 5 values for No. 10 can
Heating lag factor (j_{ch})	: 2.00
Cooling lag factor (j_{cc})	: 2.00

TABLE 329

Process Times (B) at Retort Temperature of 230°F for Conduction-Heating Foods in 202 x 204 Can

f_h	z	INITIAL FOOD TEMPERATURE (T_{ih})											Equivalent	
		100	110	120	130	140	150	160	170	180	190	200	F^{18}_c	F^{18}_s
16.91	16	150.1	149.5	148.8	148.1	147.4	146.5	145.5	144.4	143.1	141.4	139.3	11.48	12.29
	18	127.8	127.2	126.6	125.9	125.1	124.3	123.3	122.1	120.8	119.2	117.1	8.31	8.98
	20	109.0	108.5	107.8	107.1	106.4	105.5	104.5	103.4	102.0	100.4	98.3	6.33	6.87
	22	94.2	93.6	92.9	92.2	91.5	90.6	89.6	88.5	87.1	85.5	83.4	5.10	5.53
17.90	16	154.7	154.1	153.4	152.7	151.9	151.0	149.9	148.7	147.3	145.6	143.3	11.48	12.30
	18	131.1	130.5	129.8	129.0	128.2	127.3	126.3	125.1	123.6	121.9	119.7	8.30	8.98
	20	111.3	110.6	110.0	109.2	108.4	107.5	106.5	105.3	103.8	102.1	99.9	6.33	6.87
	22	95.5	94.9	94.2	93.5	92.7	91.7	90.7	89.5	88.1	86.4	84.1	5.10	5.54
18.89	16	159.1	158.5	157.8	157.0	156.2	155.2	154.1	152.9	151.4	149.5	147.2	11.49	12.32
	18	134.1	133.4	132.7	131.9	131.1	130.1	129.0	127.8	126.3	124.4	122.1	8.29	8.98
	20	113.3	112.6	111.9	111.1	110.3	109.3	108.2	107.0	105.5	103.6	101.3	6.33	6.89
	22	96.6	96.0	95.3	94.5	93.6	92.7	91.6	90.3	88.8	87.0	84.6	5.10	5.55
19.89	16	163.4	162.7	162.0	161.2	160.3	159.2	158.1	156.8	155.2	153.3	150.8	11.49	12.33
	18	136.9	136.2	135.5	134.6	133.7	132.7	131.6	130.2	128.7	126.7	124.2	8.29	8.98
	20	115.1	114.4	113.6	112.8	111.9	110.9	109.7	108.4	106.8	104.9	102.4	6.33	6.89
	22	97.6	96.9	96.2	95.3	94.4	93.4	92.2	90.9	89.3	87.4	84.9	5.09	5.58
20.88	16	167.5	166.8	166.0	165.1	164.1	163.1	161.9	160.5	158.8	156.8	154.2	11.49	12.35
	18	139.5	138.8	138.0	137.1	136.2	135.1	133.9	132.5	130.9	128.8	126.2	8.28	8.98
	20	116.7	115.9	115.1	114.3	113.3	112.3	111.0	109.6	108.0	106.0	103.4	6.33	6.90
	22	97.6	96.9	96.1	95.3	94.3	93.2	92.0	90.6	89.0	87.0	84.3	4.94	5.61

TABLE 330

Process Times (B) at Retort Temperature of 240°F for Conduction-Heating Foods in 202 x 204 Can

f_h	z	INITIAL FOOD TEMPERATURE (T_{ih})											Equivalent	
		100	110	120	130	140	150	160	170	180	190	200	F_c^{18}	F_s^{18}
16.91	16	61.5	60.9	60.3	59.7	59.0	58.2	57.4	56.4	55.3	53.9	52.3	9.46	10.68
	18	55.2	54.6	54.1	53.4	52.7	51.9	51.1	50.1	49.0	47.6	46.0	7.74	8.95
	20	50.6	50.1	49.5	48.9	48.2	47.4	46.5	45.5	44.4	43.1	41.4	6.50	7.70
	22	47.1	46.5	45.9	45.3	44.6	43.8	43.0	42.0	40.9	39.5	37.9	5.55	6.73
17.90	16	63.0	62.4	61.8	61.1	60.4	59.6	58.7	57.6	56.4	55.0	53.3	9.42	10.71
	18	56.8	56.2	55.6	54.9	54.2	53.4	52.4	51.4	50.2	48.8	47.1	7.73	9.00
	20	52.1	51.5	50.9	50.2	49.5	48.6	47.7	46.7	45.5	44.1	42.3	6.47	7.71
	22	48.4	47.8	47.2	46.5	45.8	45.0	44.1	43.0	41.8	40.4	38.7	5.50	6.72
18.89	16	64.3	63.7	63.0	62.3	61.6	60.7	59.7	58.6	57.4	55.9	54.0	9.34	10.67
	18	58.2	57.6	56.9	56.2	55.4	54.5	53.6	52.5	51.2	49.7	47.9	7.69	8.98
	20	53.5	52.9	52.2	51.5	50.7	49.9	48.9	47.8	46.5	45.0	43.2	6.44	7.70
	22	49.7	49.1	48.4	47.7	46.9	46.1	45.1	44.0	42.8	41.3	39.4	5.44	6.68
19.89	16	65.8	65.2	64.5	63.7	62.9	62.0	61.0	59.8	58.5	56.9	55.0	9.34	10.67
	18	59.6	58.9	58.3	57.5	56.7	55.8	54.8	53.6	52.3	50.7	48.8	7.65	8.96
	20	54.8	54.2	53.5	52.8	51.9	51.0	50.0	48.9	47.5	46.0	44.0	6.39	7.68
	22	51.1	50.4	49.7	49.0	48.2	47.3	46.2	45.1	43.8	42.2	40.3	5.36	6.66
20.88	16	67.4	66.8	66.0	65.2	64.4	63.4	62.4	61.1	59.8	58.1	56.1	9.35	10.71
	18	61.1	60.5	59.7	58.9	58.1	57.1	56.1	54.8	53.4	51.8	49.8	7.64	8.99
	20	56.2	55.5	54.8	54.0	53.1	52.2	51.1	49.9	48.5	46.9	44.8	6.34	7.66
	22	52.4	51.7	51.0	50.2	49.4	48.4	47.3	46.1	44.7	43.1	41.0	5.24	6.61

TABLE 331

Process Times (B) at Retort Temperature of 250°F for Conduction-Heating Foods in 202 x 204 Can

f_h	z	INITIAL FOOD TEMPERATURE (T_{ih})											Equivalent	
		100	110	120	130	140	150	160	170	180	190	200	F_c^{18}	F_s^{18}
16.91	16	34.2	33.7	33.2	32.6	31.9	31.2	30.5	29.6	28.6	27.5	26.1	7.90	9.73
	18	33.3	32.8	32.2	31.6	31.0	30.3	29.5	28.7	27.7	26.6	25.2	7.13	9.00
	20	32.4	31.9	31.4	30.8	30.1	29.4	28.7	27.8	26.8	25.7	24.3	6.48	8.37
	22	31.6	31.1	30.6	30.0	29.4	28.7	27.9	27.0	26.1	24.9	23.6	5.96	7.84
17.90	16	35.6	35.1	34.5	33.9	33.2	32.5	31.7	30.7	29.7	28.5	27.1	7.85	9.75
	18	34.6	34.1	33.5	32.9	32.2	31.5	30.7	29.8	28.7	27.5	26.1	7.09	9.02
	20	33.7	33.2	32.6	32.0	31.3	30.6	29.8	28.8	27.8	26.6	25.2	6.45	8.38
	22	32.9	32.4	31.8	31.2	30.5	29.8	28.9	28.0	27.0	25.8	24.4	5.91	7.81
18.89	16	37.0	36.4	35.8	35.2	34.4	33.7	32.8	31.8	30.7	29.5	28.0	7.81	9.76
	18	36.0	35.4	34.8	34.1	33.4	32.6	31.8	30.8	29.7	28.4	26.9	7.05	9.02
	20	35.0	34.4	33.8	33.2	32.4	31.7	30.8	29.8	28.7	27.5	26.0	6.41	8.34
	22	34.1	33.6	33.0	32.3	31.6	30.8	29.9	29.0	27.9	26.6	25.1	5.79	7.71
19.89	16	38.3	37.7	37.1	36.4	35.7	34.8	33.9	32.9	31.7	30.4	28.8	7.77	9.76
	18	37.2	36.6	36.0	35.3	34.6	33.7	32.8	31.8	30.7	29.3	27.8	7.01	9.01
	20	36.2	35.6	35.0	34.3	33.5	32.7	31.8	30.8	29.6	28.3	26.7	6.31	8.27
	22	35.3	34.7	34.1	33.4	32.6	31.8	30.9	29.9	28.7	27.4	25.8	5.68	7.62
20.88	16	39.7	39.0	38.4	37.6	36.8	36.0	35.0	34.0	32.7	31.4	29.7	7.74	9.78
	18	38.5	37.9	37.2	36.5	35.7	34.8	33.9	32.8	31.6	30.2	28.5	6.98	8.98
	20	37.4	36.8	36.1	35.4	34.6	33.7	32.8	31.7	30.5	29.1	27.5	6.20	8.18
	22	36.5	35.8	35.2	34.4	33.7	32.8	31.8	30.8	29.6	28.2	26.5	5.58	7.54

TABLE 332

Process Times (B) at Retort Temperature of 260°F for Conduction-Heating Foods in 202 x 204 Can

f_h	z	INITIAL FOOD TEMPERATURE (T_{ih})											Equivalent	
		100	110	120	130	140	150	160	170	180	190	200	F_c^{18}	F_s^{18}
	16	25.0	24.5	24.0	23.4	22.9	22.2	21.5	20.7	19.9	18.9	17.8	6.80	9.27
16.91	18	24.8	24.3	23.8	23.2	22.7	22.0	21.3	20.5	19.7	18.7	17.6	6.52	8.98
	20	24.5	24.1	23.5	23.0	22.4	21.8	21.1	20.3	19.4	18.5	17.3	6.19	8.63
	22	24.3	23.8	23.3	22.8	22.2	21.5	20.8	20.1	19.2	18.2	17.1	5.86	8.28
	16	26.2	25.7	25.1	24.6	23.9	23.3	22.5	21.7	20.8	19.7	18.5	6.83	9.33
17.90	18	25.9	25.4	24.9	24.3	23.7	23.0	22.3	21.5	20.5	19.5	18.3	6.50	8.98
	20	25.7	25.2	24.6	24.1	23.4	22.8	22.0	21.2	20.3	19.2	18.0	6.14	8.60
	22	25.4	24.9	24.4	23.8	23.2	22.5	21.7	20.9	20.0	19.0	17.8	5.77	8.22
	16	27.4	26.8	26.3	25.7	25.0	24.3	23.5	22.7	21.7	20.6	19.3	6.87	9.38
18.89	18	27.1	26.6	26.0	25.4	24.7	24.0	23.2	22.4	21.4	20.3	19.0	6.48	8.98
	20	26.8	26.3	25.7	25.1	24.4	23.7	22.9	22.1	21.1	20.0	18.7	6.08	8.56
	22	26.5	26.0	25.4	24.8	24.1	23.4	22.6	21.8	20.8	19.7	18.4	5.70	8.16
	16	28.6	28.0	27.4	26.8	26.1	25.3	24.5	23.6	22.6	21.4	20.1	6.87	9.40
19.89	18	28.3	27.7	27.1	26.5	25.8	25.0	24.2	23.3	22.3	21.1	19.8	6.46	8.98
	20	27.9	27.4	26.8	26.1	25.4	24.7	23.9	22.9	21.9	20.8	19.4	6.03	8.53
	22	27.6	27.0	26.4	25.8	25.1	24.4	23.5	22.6	21.6	20.5	19.1	5.65	8.12
	16	29.7	29.1	28.5	27.8	27.1	26.3	25.5	24.5	23.4	22.2	20.8	6.87	9.42
20.88	18	29.4	28.8	28.2	27.5	26.8	26.0	25.1	24.2	23.1	21.9	20.5	6.45	8.98
	20	29.0	28.4	27.8	27.1	26.4	25.6	24.8	23.8	22.7	21.5	20.1	5.99	8.50
	22	28.7	28.1	27.5	26.8	26.1	25.3	24.4	23.5	22.4	21.2	19.8	5.60	8.09

TABLE 333

Process Times (B) at Retort Temperature of 230°F for Conduction-Heating Foods in 202 x 214 Can

f_h	z	INITIAL FOOD TEMPERATURE (T_{ih}) 100	110	120	130	140	150	160	170	180	190	200	Equivalent F_c^{18}	F_s^{18}
19.73	16	164.4	163.8	163.0	162.2	161.3	160.3	159.1	157.8	156.3	154.3	151.9	11.73	12.58
	18	138.2	137.5	136.7	135.9	135.0	134.0	132.9	131.6	130.0	128.1	125.6	8.47	9.16
	20	116.5	115.8	115.0	114.2	113.3	112.3	111.2	109.9	108.3	106.4	103.9	6.47	7.03
	22	99.1	98.4	97.7	96.8	95.9	94.9	93.8	92.5	90.9	89.0	86.5	5.21	5.67
20.89	16	169.3	168.5	167.8	166.9	165.9	164.9	163.7	162.3	160.6	158.6	156.0	11.73	12.60
	18	141.3	140.6	139.8	139.0	138.0	136.9	135.7	134.3	132.7	130.6	128.0	8.46	9.16
	20	118.4	117.7	116.9	116.1	115.1	114.0	112.8	111.4	109.8	107.7	105.1	6.46	7.04
	22	99.6	98.9	98.1	97.2	96.2	95.2	94.0	92.6	90.9	88.9	86.3	5.10	5.75
22.05	16	173.8	173.1	172.2	171.3	170.3	169.2	167.9	166.4	164.7	162.6	159.8	11.74	12.61
	18	144.2	143.5	142.6	141.7	140.7	139.6	138.3	136.8	135.1	132.9	130.2	8.45	9.16
	20	120.1	119.4	118.5	117.6	116.6	115.5	114.2	112.7	111.0	108.8	106.1	6.46	7.05
	22	100.5	99.8	98.9	98.0	97.0	95.9	94.6	93.1	91.4	89.3	86.5	5.01	5.68
23.21	16	178.2	177.4	176.5	175.5	174.5	173.3	171.9	170.4	168.5	166.3	163.4	11.74	12.62
	18	146.9	146.1	145.2	144.2	143.2	142.0	140.6	139.1	137.2	135.0	132.1	8.44	9.16
	20	121.6	120.8	119.9	118.9	117.9	116.7	115.3	113.8	111.9	109.7	106.8	6.46	7.06
	22	102.3	101.5	100.6	99.7	98.6	97.4	96.1	94.5	92.7	90.4	87.5	5.00	5.67
24.37	16	182.2	181.4	180.5	179.5	178.4	177.1	175.7	174.1	172.1	169.8	166.7	11.75	12.64
	18	149.3	148.4	147.5	146.5	145.4	144.1	142.7	141.1	139.2	136.8	133.8	8.43	9.17
	20	122.8	121.9	121.0	120.0	118.9	117.6	116.2	114.6	112.6	110.3	107.2	6.46	7.06
	22	103.9	103.0	102.1	101.1	100.0	98.8	97.3	95.7	93.8	91.4	88.4	5.00	5.66

TABLE 334

Process Times (B) at Retort Temperature of 240°F for Conduction-Heating Foods in 202 x 214 Can

f_h	z	INITIAL FOOD TEMPERATURE (T_{ih})											Equivalent	
		100	110	120	130	140	150	160	170	180	190	200	F_c^{18}	F_s^{18}
19.73	16	66.3	65.7	65.0	64.2	63.4	62.5	61.5	60.4	59.0	57.5	55.6	9.53	10.87
	18	60.0	59.4	58.7	57.9	57.1	56.2	55.2	54.1	52.8	51.2	49.3	7.85	9.15
	20	55.2	54.6	53.9	53.2	52.4	51.5	50.4	49.3	48.0	46.4	44.5	6.56	7.85
	22	51.4	50.8	50.1	49.3	48.5	47.6	46.6	45.5	44.1	42.6	40.7	5.55	6.82
20.89	16	68.2	67.5	66.8	66.0	65.2	64.2	63.1	61.9	60.5	58.9	56.8	9.56	10.92
	18	61.8	61.1	60.4	59.6	58.7	57.8	56.7	55.5	54.1	52.5	50.4	7.82	9.16
	20	56.9	56.2	55.5	54.7	53.8	52.8	51.8	50.6	49.2	47.5	45.5	6.52	7.83
	22	53.0	52.3	51.6	50.8	49.9	49.0	47.9	46.7	45.3	43.6	41.6	5.42	6.78
22.05	16	70.0	69.2	68.5	67.6	66.7	65.7	64.6	63.3	61.8	60.1	58.0	9.52	10.93
	18	63.5	62.8	62.0	61.2	60.3	59.3	58.1	56.9	55.4	53.6	51.5	7.80	9.17
	20	58.4	57.7	57.0	56.1	55.2	54.2	53.1	51.8	50.3	48.6	46.4	6.46	7.81
	22	54.7	54.0	53.2	52.4	51.4	50.4	49.3	48.0	46.6	44.8	42.7	5.33	6.75
23.21	16	71.6	70.9	70.1	69.2	68.2	67.2	66.0	64.6	63.1	61.2	59.0	9.49	10.92
	18	65.1	64.4	63.6	62.7	61.7	60.7	59.5	58.2	56.6	54.8	52.5	7.75	9.15
	20	60.1	59.3	58.5	57.6	56.7	55.6	54.4	53.1	51.5	49.7	47.4	6.42	7.79
	22	56.5	55.8	55.0	54.1	53.1	52.1	50.9	49.5	48.0	46.1	43.9	5.32	6.79
24.37	16	73.4	72.6	71.8	70.9	69.9	68.7	67.5	66.1	64.4	62.5	60.2	9.49	10.93
	18	66.8	66.0	65.2	64.2	63.2	62.1	60.9	59.5	57.8	55.9	53.5	7.72	9.14
	20	61.7	61.0	60.1	59.2	58.2	57.1	55.8	54.4	52.8	50.8	48.5	6.30	7.76
	22	58.3	57.5	56.7	55.8	54.8	53.7	52.4	51.0	49.4	47.4	45.1	5.30	6.79

TABLE 335

Process Times (B) at Retort Temperature of 250°F for Conduction-Heating Foods in 202 x 214 Can

f_h	z	INITIAL FOOD TEMPERATURE (T_{ih}) 100	110	120	130	140	150	160	170	180	190	200	Equivalent F_c^{18}	F_s^{18}
	16	38.4	37.8	37.2	36.5	35.7	34.9	34.0	33.0	31.9	30.5	29.0	7.98	9.97
19.73	18	37.3	36.7	36.1	35.4	34.7	33.8	32.9	31.9	30.8	29.5	27.9	7.21	9.21
	20	36.3	35.7	35.1	34.4	33.6	32.8	31.9	30.9	29.8	28.5	26.9	6.54	8.50
	22	35.4	34.8	34.2	33.5	32.7	31.9	31.0	30.0	28.9	27.6	26.0	5.89	7.83
	16	40.0	39.3	38.7	37.9	37.1	36.3	35.3	34.2	33.0	31.6	30.0	7.94	9.97
20.89	18	38.8	38.2	37.5	36.8	36.0	35.1	34.2	33.1	31.9	30.5	28.8	7.17	9.18
	20	37.7	37.1	36.4	35.7	34.9	34.1	33.1	32.0	30.8	29.4	27.8	6.41	8.39
	22	36.8	36.1	35.5	34.7	34.0	33.1	32.1	31.1	29.9	28.5	26.8	5.76	7.73
	16	41.6	40.9	40.2	39.4	38.6	37.7	36.7	35.5	34.3	32.8	31.0	7.95	10.03
22.05	18	40.3	39.7	39.0	38.2	37.4	36.5	35.4	34.3	33.0	31.6	29.8	7.13	9.16
	20	39.2	38.5	37.8	37.1	36.2	35.3	34.3	33.2	31.9	30.4	28.7	6.33	8.34
	22	38.2	37.5	36.8	36.0	35.2	34.3	33.3	32.1	30.9	29.4	27.6	5.69	7.68
	16	43.2	42.5	41.7	40.9	40.0	39.1	38.0	36.8	35.5	33.9	32.1	8.00	10.08
23.21	18	41.9	41.2	40.5	39.7	38.8	37.8	36.8	35.6	34.2	32.7	30.8	7.10	9.15
	20	40.7	40.0	39.2	38.4	37.6	36.6	35.5	34.3	33.0	31.5	29.6	6.30	8.33
	22	39.6	38.9	38.2	37.4	36.5	35.5	34.5	33.3	31.9	30.4	28.5	5.64	7.65
	16	44.8	44.0	43.3	42.4	41.5	40.5	39.4	38.1	36.7	35.1	33.1	8.03	10.12
24.37	18	43.5	42.7	41.9	41.1	40.2	39.2	38.1	36.8	35.4	33.8	31.8	7.09	9.16
	20	42.2	41.4	40.7	39.8	38.9	37.9	36.8	35.5	34.1	32.5	30.6	6.28	8.33
	22	41.0	40.3	39.5	38.7	37.8	36.8	35.6	34.4	33.0	31.3	29.4	5.58	7.63

TABLE 336

Process Times (B) at Retort Temperature of 260°F for Conduction-Heating Foods in 202 x 214 Can

f_h	z	INITIAL FOOD TEMPERATURE (T_{ih})											Equivalent	
		100	110	120	130	140	150	160	170	180	190	200	F_c^{18}	F_s^{18}
19.73	16	28.5	27.9	27.3	26.7	26.0	25.3	24.5	23.6	22.6	21.4	20.1	7.05	9.59
	18	28.2	27.6	27.1	26.4	25.7	25.0	24.2	23.3	22.3	21.1	19.8	6.65	9.17
	20	27.9	27.3	26.7	26.1	25.4	24.7	23.9	22.9	21.9	20.8	19.5	6.22	8.72
	22	27.6	27.0	26.4	25.8	25.1	24.4	23.5	22.6	21.6	20.5	19.2	5.83	8.31
20.89	16	29.9	29.3	28.7	28.0	27.3	26.5	25.6	24.7	23.6	22.4	21.0	7.05	9.61
	18	29.6	29.0	28.3	27.7	26.9	26.2	25.3	24.3	23.3	22.1	20.7	6.63	9.17
	20	29.2	28.6	28.0	27.3	26.6	25.8	24.9	24.0	22.9	21.7	20.3	6.17	8.69
	22	28.8	28.3	27.6	27.0	26.2	25.4	24.6	23.6	22.5	21.3	19.9	5.77	8.27
22.05	16	31.2	30.6	30.0	29.2	28.5	27.6	26.7	25.7	24.6	23.3	21.8	7.05	9.62
	18	30.9	30.3	29.6	28.9	28.1	27.3	26.4	25.4	24.2	23.0	21.5	6.61	9.17
	20	30.5	29.9	29.2	28.5	27.7	26.9	26.0	25.0	23.8	22.6	21.1	6.15	8.68
	22	30.1	29.6	28.8	28.1	27.3	26.5	25.6	24.6	23.5	22.2	20.7	5.73	8.24
23.21	16	32.6	31.9	31.2	30.5	29.7	28.8	27.8	26.8	25.6	24.2	22.7	7.04	9.64
	18	32.2	31.6	30.9	30.1	29.3	28.4	27.5	26.4	25.2	23.9	22.3	6.60	9.17
	20	31.8	31.1	30.4	29.7	28.9	28.0	27.0	26.0	24.8	23.5	21.9	6.14	8.68
	22	31.4	30.7	30.0	29.3	28.5	27.6	26.6	25.6	24.4	23.0	21.5	5.69	8.21
24.37	16	33.9	33.3	32.5	31.7	30.9	30.0	29.0	27.8	26.6	25.2	23.6	7.07	9.68
	18	33.5	32.8	32.1	31.3	30.5	29.5	28.5	27.4	26.2	24.8	23.1	6.58	9.17
	20	33.1	32.4	31.7	30.9	30.0	29.1	28.1	27.0	25.7	24.3	22.7	6.13	8.69
	22	32.6	31.9	31.2	30.4	29.6	28.6	27.6	26.5	25.3	23.9	22.2	5.65	8.18

TABLE 337

Process Times (B) at Retort Temperature of 230°F for Conduction-Heating Foods in 202 x 308 Can

f_h	z	Initial Food Temperature (T_{ih}) 100	110	120	130	140	150	160	170	180	190	200	Equivalent F_c^{18}	F_s^{18}
21.36	16	172.6	171.9	171.1	170.2	169.2	168.1	166.9	165.4	163.8	161.7	159.0	11.92	12.80
	18	144.0	143.3	142.5	141.6	140.6	139.5	138.3	136.8	135.1	133.1	130.4	8.59	9.31
	20	120.6	119.8	119.0	118.1	117.1	116.1	114.8	113.4	111.7	109.6	106.9	6.57	7.16
	22	101.3	100.5	99.7	99.9	97.9	96.8	95.5	94.1	92.4	90.3	87.7	5.16	5.86
22.64	16	177.5	176.7	175.9	174.9	173.9	172.8	171.4	169.9	168.1	165.9	163.1	11.93	12.81
	18	147.1	146.3	145.5	144.5	143.5	142.3	141.0	139.5	137.7	135.5	132.7	8.58	9.31
	20	122.3	121.6	120.7	119.8	118.7	117.6	116.3	114.7	112.9	110.8	107.9	6.56	7.16
	22	102.5	101.8	100.9	100.0	98.9	97.8	96.5	94.9	93.1	91.0	88.1	5.09	5.77
23.89	16	182.1	181.3	180.4	179.4	178.3	177.1	175.7	174.1	172.2	169.9	166.9	11.93	12.83
	18	149.9	149.1	148.2	147.2	146.1	144.9	143.5	141.9	140.0	137.7	134.7	8.57	9.31
	20	123.8	123.0	122.1	121.1	120.0	118.8	117.4	115.8	113.9	111.6	108.6	6.56	7.17
	22	104.4	103.6	102.7	101.7	100.6	99.4	98.0	96.4	94.5	92.2	89.2	5.08	5.76
25.15	16	186.5	185.6	184.7	183.6	182.5	181.2	179.7	178.1	176.1	173.6	170.5	11.94	12.84
	18	152.4	151.6	150.6	149.6	148.4	147.1	145.7	144.0	142.0	139.6	136.4	8.56	9.31
	20	125.1	124.2	123.2	122.2	121.0	119.8	118.3	116.6	114.6	112.2	109.0	6.56	7.18
	22	106.1	105.2	104.2	103.2	102.1	100.8	99.3	97.6	95.6	93.2	90.1	5.08	5.75
26.41	16	190.6	189.7	188.7	187.6	186.4	185.0	183.5	181.7	179.6	177.1	173.8	11.94	12.85
	18	154.7	153.8	152.8	151.7	150.5	149.1	147.6	145.8	143.7	141.2	137.9	8.56	9.31
	20	125.7	124.8	123.8	122.7	121.5	120.2	118.6	116.9	114.8	112.2	108.9	6.43	7.24
	22	107.5	106.6	105.6	104.5	103.3	101.9	100.4	98.6	96.6	94.0	90.7	5.06	5.75

TABLE 338

Process Times (B) at Retort Temperature of 240°F for Conduction-Heating Foods in 202 x 308 Can

f_h	z	INITIAL FOOD TEMPERATURE (T_{ih})											Equivalent	
		100	110	120	130	140	150	160	170	180	190	200	F_c^{18}	F_s^{18}
	16	69.6	68.9	68.2	67.4	66.5	65.5	64.4	63.2	61.7	60.0	58.0	9.73	11.10
21.38	18	63.1	62.4	61.6	60.8	59.9	59.0	57.9	56.6	55.2	53.5	51.4	7.96	9.31
	20	58.0	57.3	56.6	55.8	54.9	53.9	52.8	51.6	50.2	48.5	46.4	6.63	7.96
	22	54.1	53.4	52.7	51.8	51.0	50.0	48.9	47.7	46.2	44.5	42.5	5.50	6.88
	16	71.5	70.7	69.9	69.1	68.1	67.1	66.0	64.6	63.1	61.3	59.1	9.68	11.10
22.64	18	64.9	64.1	63.4	62.5	61.6	60.5	59.4	58.1	56.5	54.7	52.6	7.93	9.32
	20	59.8	59.0	58.2	57.4	56.4	55.4	54.2	52.9	51.4	49.6	47.4	6.57	7.93
	22	55.9	55.2	54.4	53.6	52.6	51.6	50.4	49.1	47.6	45.8	43.6	5.42	6.86
	16	73.3	72.5	71.7	70.8	69.8	68.7	67.5	66.1	64.5	62.6	60.3	9.66	11.10
23.89	18	66.7	65.9	65.1	64.2	63.2	62.1	60.9	59.5	57.9	56.0	53.7	7.88	9.29
	20	61.5	60.7	59.9	59.0	58.0	56.9	55.7	54.3	52.7	50.8	48.5	6.50	7.91
	22	58.0	57.2	56.4	55.5	54.5	53.4	52.2	50.8	49.2	47.3	45.0	5.41	6.90
	16	75.3	74.4	73.6	72.6	71.6	70.4	69.1	67.7	66.0	64.0	61.6	9.65	11.11
25.15	18	68.5	67.6	66.8	65.8	64.8	63.6	62.3	60.9	59.2	57.2	54.8	7.85	9.28
	20	63.4	62.6	61.7	60.8	59.7	58.6	57.3	55.8	54.2	52.2	49.7	6.40	7.89
	22	59.9	59.1	58.2	57.3	56.2	55.1	53.8	52.3	50.6	48.6	46.2	5.39	6.88
	16	77.1	76.3	75.4	74.4	73.3	72.1	70.7	69.2	67.4	65.3	62.8	9.62	11.11
26.41	18	70.3	69.4	68.5	67.5	66.4	65.2	63.9	62.3	60.6	58.5	55.9	7.81	9.28
	20	65.5	64.6	63.7	62.7	61.6	60.4	59.1	57.5	55.8	53.7	51.1	6.39	7.93
	22	61.7	60.9	60.0	59.0	57.9	56.7	55.3	53.8	52.0	49.9	47.4	5.37	6.86

TABLE 339

Process Times (B) at Retort Temperature of 250°F for Conduction-Heating Foods in 202 x 308 Can

f_h	z	INITIAL FOOD TEMPERATURE (T_{ih})											Equivalent	
		100	110	120	130	140	150	160	170	180	190	200	F_c^{18}	F_s^{18}
21.38	16	40.8	40.2	39.5	38.8	38.0	37.1	36.1	35.0	33.8	32.3	30.6	8.08	10.13
	18	39.7	39.0	38.3	37.6	36.8	35.9	34.9	33.8	32.6	31.2	29.5	7.30	9.32
	20	38.6	37.9	37.2	36.5	35.7	34.8	33.8	32.7	31.5	30.0	28.4	6.51	8.51
	22	37.6	36.9	36.2	35.5	34.7	33.8	32.8	31.7	30.5	29.1	27.4	5.86	7.84
22.64	16	42.6	41.9	41.2	40.4	39.5	38.6	37.6	36.4	35.1	33.6	31.8	8.11	10.20
	18	41.3	40.7	39.9	39.1	38.3	37.3	36.3	35.1	33.8	32.3	30.5	7.26	9.30
	20	40.2	39.5	38.7	38.0	37.1	36.2	35.1	34.0	32.7	31.1	29.4	6.44	8.46
	22	39.1	38.4	37.7	36.9	36.1	35.1	34.1	32.9	31.6	30.1	28.3	5.79	7.79
23.89	16	44.3	43.6	42.8	42.0	41.1	40.1	39.0	37.8	36.4	34.8	32.9	8.16	10.25
	18	43.0	42.3	41.5	40.7	39.8	38.8	37.7	36.5	35.1	33.5	31.6	7.23	9.30
	20	41.8	41.1	40.3	39.5	38.6	37.6	36.5	35.2	33.9	32.3	30.4	6.41	8.46
	22	40.7	39.9	39.2	38.3	37.4	36.5	35.4	34.1	32.8	31.2	29.3	5.73	7.77
25.15	16	46.1	45.3	44.5	43.6	42.7	41.6	40.5	39.2	37.7	36.1	34.1	8.17	10.28
	18	44.7	44.0	43.1	42.3	41.3	40.3	39.1	37.8	36.4	34.7	32.7	7.22	9.31
	20	43.4	42.6	41.8	40.9	40.0	39.0	37.8	36.5	35.1	33.4	31.4	6.39	8.47
	22	42.2	41.5	40.6	39.8	38.8	37.8	36.6	35.3	33.9	32.2	30.2	5.67	7.74
26.41	16	47.8	47.0	46.1	45.2	44.2	43.1	41.9	40.5	39.0	37.2	35.2	8.14	10.27
	18	46.3	45.6	44.7	43.8	42.8	41.7	40.5	39.1	37.6	35.8	33.7	7.19	9.31
	20	44.9	44.2	43.3	42.4	41.4	40.3	39.1	37.7	36.2	34.4	32.3	6.34	8.44
	22	43.7	42.9	42.1	41.2	40.2	39.1	37.9	36.5	35.0	33.2	31.1	5.60	7.69

TABLE 340

Process Times (B) at Retort Temperature of 260°F for Conduction-Heating Foods in 202 x 308 Can

f_h	z	INITIAL FOOD TEMPERATURE (T_{ih})											Equivalent	
		100	110	120	130	140	150	160	170	180	190	200	F_c^{18}	F_s^{18}
	16	30.6	30.0	29.3	28.6	27.9	27.1	26.2	25.2	24.1	22.9	21.4	7.19	9.76
21.38	18	30.2	29.6	29.0	28.3	27.6	26.7	25.9	24.9	23.8	22.6	21.1	6.76	9.31
	20	29.8	29.2	28.6	27.9	27.2	26.4	25.5	24.5	23.4	22.2	20.7	6.29	8.82
	22	29.5	28.9	28.3	27.6	26.8	26.0	25.1	24.1	23.1	21.8	20.4	5.88	8.39
	16	32.0	31.4	30.7	30.0	29.2	28.3	27.4	26.4	25.2	23.9	22.4	7.19	9.78
22.64	18	31.7	31.0	30.4	29.6	28.8	28.0	27.0	26.0	24.9	23.5	22.0	6.74	9.32
	20	31.3	30.6	29.9	29.2	28.4	27.6	26.6	25.6	24.4	23.1	21.6	6.27	8.81
	22	30.9	30.2	29.5	28.8	28.0	27.2	26.2	25.2	24.0	22.7	21.2	5.84	8.36
	16	33.5	32.8	32.1	31.3	30.5	29.6	28.6	27.5	26.3	24.9	23.3	7.18	9.79
23.89	18	33.1	32.4	31.7	30.9	30.1	29.2	28.2	27.1	25.9	24.5	22.9	6.73	9.32
	20	32.7	32.0	31.3	30.5	29.7	28.8	27.8	26.7	25.5	24.1	22.5	6.26	8.82
	22	32.2	31.5	30.8	30.1	29.2	28.3	27.3	26.2	25.0	23.6	22.0	5.80	8.33
	16	35.0	34.3	33.5	32.7	31.8	30.9	29.8	28.7	27.4	25.9	24.2	7.22	9.85
25.15	18	34.5	33.8	33.0	32.2	31.4	30.4	29.4	28.2	26.9	25.5	23.8	6.71	9.32
	20	34.1	33.4	32.6	31.8	30.9	30.0	28.9	27.8	26.5	25.0	23.3	6.25	8.83
	22	33.6	32.9	32.1	31.3	30.4	29.5	28.4	27.3	26.0	24.5	22.9	5.75	8.30
	16	36.4	35.7	34.9	34.0	33.1	32.1	31.0	29.8	28.5	26.9	25.2	7.26	9.91
26.41	18	35.9	35.2	34.4	33.5	32.6	31.6	30.5	29.3	27.9	26.4	24.7	6.70	9.32
	20	35.4	34.7	33.9	33.1	32.1	31.1	30.0	28.8	27.5	26.0	24.2	6.23	8.82
	22	34.9	34.2	33.4	32.6	31.6	30.6	29.5	28.3	27.0	25.5	23.7	5.71	8.27

TABLE 341

Process Times (B) at Retort Temperature of 230°F for Conduction-Heating Foods in 202 x 314 Can

f_h	z	INITIAL FOOD TEMPERATURE (T_{ih})											Equivalent	
		100	110	120	130	140	150	160	170	180	190	200	F_c^{18}	F_s^{18}
	16	176.0	175.2	174.4	173.5	172.5	171.3	170.0	168.6	166.8	164.7	161.9	12.02	12.91
22.04	18	146.4	145.6	144.8	143.9	142.9	141.8	140.5	139.0	137.3	135.1	132.4	8.65	9.38
	20	122.3	121.5	120.7	119.7	118.7	117.6	116.3	114.9	113.1	111.0	108.2	6.62	7.22
	22	102.3	101.6	100.7	99.8	98.8	97.7	96.4	94.9	93.2	91.0	88.3	5.15	5.85
	16	180.9	180.1	179.2	178.3	177.2	176.0	174.6	173.1	171.2	169.0	166.0	12.03	12.92
23.34	18	149.5	148.7	147.8	146.8	145.7	144.6	143.2	141.6	139.8	137.5	134.6	8.65	9.38
	20	124.0	123.2	122.3	121.3	120.2	119.1	117.7	116.1	114.3	112.0	109.1	6.61	7.22
	22	104.2	103.4	102.5	101.5	100.4	99.2	97.9	96.3	94.5	92.2	89.3	5.13	5.82
	16	185.6	184.7	183.8	182.7	181.6	180.4	178.9	177.3	175.3	172.9	169.9	12.03	12.93
24.64	18	152.2	151.4	150.5	149.4	148.3	147.0	145.6	144.0	142.0	139.6	136.6	8.64	9.38
	20	125.4	124.5	123.6	122.6	121.5	120.2	118.8	117.1	115.2	112.8	109.7	6.61	7.23
	22	106.0	105.1	104.2	103.2	102.1	100.8	99.4	97.7	95.8	93.4	90.3	5.12	5.80
	16	189.9	189.0	188.0	187.0	185.8	184.5	183.0	181.2	179.2	176.7	173.4	12.03	12.95
25.93	18	154.7	153.8	152.8	151.8	150.6	149.3	147.7	146.0	144.0	141.4	138.2	8.63	9.38
	20	126.5	125.6	124.6	123.5	122.3	121.0	119.5	117.8	115.7	113.2	110.0	6.57	7.26
	22	107.6	106.7	105.8	104.7	103.5	102.2	100.7	98.9	96.9	94.4	91.1	5.12	5.79
	16	194.0	193.1	192.1	190.9	189.7	188.3	186.7	184.9	182.7	180.1	176.7	12.04	12.96
27.23	18	156.9	156.0	155.0	153.8	152.6	151.2	149.6	147.8	145.6	143.0	139.6	8.62	9.38
	20	127.1	126.2	125.2	124.0	122.8	121.4	119.8	118.0	115.8	113.2	109.8	6.42	7.26
	22	109.0	108.1	107.0	105.9	104.7	103.3	101.7	99.9	97.7	95.1	91.7	5.06	5.81

TABLE 342

Process Times (B) at Retort Temperature of 240°F for Conduction-Heating Foods in 202 x 314 Can

f_h	z	INITIAL FOOD TEMPERATURE (T_{ih})											Equivalent	
		100	110	120	130	140	150	160	170	180	190	200	F_c^{18}	F_s^{18}
	16	70.9	70.2	69.5	68.6	67.7	66.7	65.6	64.3	62.8	61.1	58.9	9.80	11.19
22.04	18	64.3	63.6	62.8	62.0	61.1	60.1	59.0	57.7	56.2	54.5	52.3	8.02	9.39
	20	59.2	58.5	57.7	56.9	56.0	54.9	53.8	52.5	51.1	49.3	47.2	6.66	8.01
	22	55.2	54.5	53.7	52.9	52.0	51.0	49.8	48.6	47.1	45.3	43.2	5.50	6.91
	16	72.8	72.0	71.2	70.3	69.4	68.3	67.1	65.8	64.2	62.3	60.1	9.74	11.19
23.34	18	66.2	65.4	64.6	63.7	62.8	61.7	60.5	59.1	57.6	55.7	53.5	7.98	9.38
	20	61.0	60.2	59.4	58.5	57.6	56.5	55.3	54.0	52.4	50.6	48.3	6.61	7.99
	22	57.2	56.5	55.7	54.8	53.8	52.8	51.6	50.2	48.7	46.8	44.5	5.46	6.93
	16	74.8	74.0	73.1	72.2	71.2	70.0	68.8	67.3	65.7	63.7	61.4	9.75	11.19
24.64	18	68.0	67.2	66.4	65.4	64.4	63.3	62.0	60.6	59.0	57.0	54.6	7.93	9.36
	20	62.8	62.0	61.1	60.2	59.2	58.0	56.8	55.4	53.7	51.8	49.4	6.48	7.94
	22	59.3	58.5	57.7	56.7	55.7	54.6	53.3	51.9	50.2	48.3	45.9	5.45	6.95
	16	76.8	75.9	75.0	74.0	73.0	71.8	70.5	69.0	67.2	65.2	62.6	9.72	11.20
25.93	18	69.9	69.0	68.1	67.2	66.1	64.9	63.6	62.1	60.3	58.3	55.8	7.90	9.36
	20	64.9	64.1	63.2	62.2	61.1	59.9	58.6	57.1	55.4	53.3	50.8	6.45	7.97
	22	61.3	60.4	59.5	58.5	57.5	56.3	54.9	53.4	51.7	49.7	47.1	5.43	6.93
	16	78.7	77.8	76.9	75.9	74.7	73.5	72.1	70.5	68.7	66.5	63.9	9.71	11.22
27.23	18	71.7	70.9	69.9	68.9	67.8	66.5	65.1	63.5	61.7	59.6	56.9	7.86	9.35
	20	67.0	66.1	65.2	64.2	63.0	61.8	60.4	58.8	57.0	54.8	52.2	6.44	8.01
	22	63.1	62.3	61.3	60.3	59.2	57.9	56.5	55.0	53.1	51.0	48.3	5.41	6.90

TABLE 343

Process Times (B) at Retort Temperature of 250°F for Conduction-Heating Foods in 202 x 314 Can

f_h	z	INITIAL FOOD TEMPERATURE (T_{ih})											Equivalent	
		100	110	120	130	140	150	160	170	180	190	200	F_c^{18}	F_s^{18}
22.04	16	41.8	41.2	40.5	39.7	38.9	38.0	37.0	35.8	34.5	33.1	31.3	8.15	10.23
	18	40.6	40.0	39.3	38.5	37.7	36.7	35.7	34.6	33.3	31.8	30.1	7.35	9.38
	20	39.5	38.8	38.1	37.3	36.5	35.6	34.6	33.5	32.2	30.7	29.0	6.52	8.54
	22	38.5	37.8	37.1	36.3	35.5	34.6	33.6	32.4	31.2	29.7	27.9	5.87	7.86
23.34	16	43.7	43.0	42.2	41.4	40.5	39.6	38.5	37.3	35.9	34.4	32.5	8.21	10.30
	18	42.4	41.7	40.9	40.1	39.2	38.3	37.2	36.0	34.7	33.1	31.2	7.32	9.37
	20	41.2	40.5	39.7	38.9	38.0	37.1	36.0	34.8	33.4	31.9	30.0	6.49	8.53
	22	40.1	39.4	38.6	37.8	36.9	36.0	34.9	33.7	32.4	30.8	28.9	5.83	7.85
24.64	16	45.5	44.7	43.9	43.1	42.1	41.1	40.0	38.7	37.3	35.7	33.7	8.26	10.36
	18	44.1	43.4	42.6	41.7	40.8	39.8	38.7	37.4	36.0	34.3	32.4	7.29	9.38
	20	42.8	42.1	41.3	40.4	39.5	38.5	37.4	36.1	34.7	33.0	31.1	6.46	8.53
	22	41.7	41.0	40.2	39.3	38.4	37.4	36.2	35.0	33.5	31.9	29.9	5.76	7.81
25.93	16	47.2	46.5	45.6	44.7	43.7	42.7	41.5	40.2	38.7	36.9	34.9	8.24	10.37
	18	45.8	45.1	44.2	43.3	42.4	41.3	40.1	38.8	37.3	35.5	33.5	7.28	9.39
	20	44.5	43.7	42.9	42.0	41.0	39.9	38.7	37.4	35.9	34.2	32.1	6.44	8.53
	22	43.3	42.5	41.7	40.8	39.8	38.7	37.5	36.2	34.7	32.9	30.9	5.70	7.78
27.23	16	49.0	48.2	47.3	46.3	45.3	44.2	42.9	41.5	40.0	38.1	36.0	8.20	10.35
	18	47.5	46.7	45.8	44.9	43.8	42.7	41.5	40.1	38.5	36.7	34.5	7.25	9.38
	20	46.1	45.3	44.4	43.4	42.4	41.3	40.0	38.6	37.1	35.2	33.1	6.36	8.48
	22	44.8	44.0	43.1	42.2	41.1	40.0	38.8	37.4	35.8	34.0	31.8	5.62	7.72

TABLE 344

Process Times (B) at Retort Temperature of 260°F for Conduction-Heating Foods in 202 x 314 Can

f_h	z	INITIAL FOOD TEMPERATURE (T_{ih})											Equivalent	
		100	110	120	130	140	150	160	170	180	190	200	F_c^{18}	F_s^{18}
22.04	16	31.4	30.8	30.1	29.4	28.6	27.8	26.9	25.9	24.8	23.5	22.0	7.26	9.85
	18	31.0	30.4	29.8	29.1	28.3	27.5	26.5	25.5	24.4	23.1	21.7	6.82	9.39
	20	30.6	30.0	29.4	28.7	27.9	27.1	26.1	25.1	24.0	22.7	21.3	6.33	8.88
	22	30.3	29.7	29.0	28.3	27.5	26.7	25.8	24.8	23.6	22.4	20.9	5.92	8.44
23.34	16	32.9	32.2	31.5	30.8	30.0	29.1	28.1	27.1	25.9	24.5	23.0	7.26	9.86
	18	32.5	31.9	31.2	30.4	29.6	28.7	27.8	26.7	25.5	24.2	22.6	6.80	9.39
	20	32.1	31.5	30.8	30.0	29.2	28.3	27.3	26.3	25.1	23.7	22.2	6.32	8.88
	22	31.7	31.0	30.3	29.6	28.8	27.9	26.9	25.9	24.7	23.3	21.7	5.88	8.41
24.64	16	34.4	33.7	33.0	32.2	31.3	30.4	29.4	28.3	27.0	25.6	23.9	7.27	9.89
	18	34.0	33.3	32.6	31.8	30.9	30.0	29.0	27.8	26.6	25.1	23.5	6.79	9.39
	20	33.6	32.9	32.1	31.3	30.5	29.5	28.5	27.4	26.1	24.7	23.1	6.32	8.89
	22	33.1	32.4	31.7	30.9	30.0	29.1	28.1	26.9	25.7	24.2	22.6	5.84	8.38
25.93	16	35.9	35.2	34.4	33.6	32.7	31.7	30.6	29.4	28.1	26.6	24.9	7.31	9.95
	18	35.4	34.7	33.9	33.1	32.2	31.2	30.1	29.0	27.6	26.1	24.4	6.77	9.39
	20	35.0	34.3	33.5	32.6	31.7	30.8	29.7	28.5	27.2	25.7	23.9	6.31	8.90
	22	34.5	33.8	33.0	32.2	31.2	30.3	29.2	28.0	26.7	25.2	23.4	5.79	8.35
27.23	16	37.4	36.7	35.9	35.0	34.0	33.0	31.9	30.6	29.2	27.7	25.8	7.35	10.01
	18	36.9	36.1	35.3	34.4	33.5	32.4	31.3	30.1	28.7	27.1	25.3	6.76	9.39
	20	36.4	35.6	34.8	33.9	33.0	32.0	30.8	29.6	28.2	26.6	24.8	6.27	8.87
	22	35.9	35.1	34.3	33.4	32.5	31.5	30.3	29.1	27.7	26.1	24.3	5.75	8.32

TABLE 345

Process Times (B) at Retort Temperature of 230°F for Conduction-Heating Foods in 211 x 200 Can

f_h	z	INITIAL FOOD TEMPERATURE (T_{ih})											Equivalent	
		100	110	120	130	140	150	160	170	180	190	200	F_c^{18}	F_s^{18}
20.00	16	166.0	165.3	164.5	163.7	162.8	161.8	160.6	159.3	157.7	155.7	153.2	11.79	12.64
	18	139.3	138.6	137.9	137.1	136.1	135.1	134.0	132.6	131.0	129.1	126.6	8.50	9.21
	20	117.3	116.6	115.9	115.1	114.1	113.1	112.0	110.6	109.0	107.1	104.6	6.49	7.07
	22	99.7	99.0	98.3	97.4	96.5	95.5	94.3	93.0	91.4	89.5	87.0	5.23	5.70
21.18	16	170.8	170.1	169.3	168.4	167.5	166.4	165.1	163.7	162.0	160.0	157.4	11.79	12.66
	18	142.5	141.8	141.0	140.1	139.1	138.0	136.8	135.4	133.7	131.7	129.0	8.49	9.21
	20	119.3	118.5	117.7	116.9	115.9	114.8	113.6	112.2	110.5	108.4	105.8	6.49	7.08
	22	100.1	99.4	98.6	97.7	96.7	95.7	94.4	93.0	91.3	89.3	86.6	5.10	5.79
22.35	16	175.4	174.6	173.8	172.9	171.9	170.7	169.4	167.9	166.1	164.0	161.2	11.79	12.67
	18	145.4	144.6	143.8	142.8	141.8	140.7	139.4	137.9	136.1	133.9	131.1	8.48	9.21
	20	120.9	120.2	119.3	118.4	117.4	116.2	114.9	113.4	111.7	109.5	106.7	6.49	7.08
	22	101.3	100.6	99.7	98.8	97.8	96.6	95.3	93.8	92.1	89.9	87.1	5.03	5.71
23.53	16	179.8	178.9	178.1	177.1	176.0	174.8	173.4	171.9	170.0	167.7	164.8	11.80	12.68
	18	148.0	147.2	146.3	145.3	144.3	143.1	141.7	140.1	138.3	136.0	133.0	8.48	9.21
	20	122.4	121.5	120.7	119.7	118.6	117.4	116.0	114.5	112.6	110.3	107.4	6.49	7.09
	22	103.1	102.3	101.4	100.4	99.3	98.1	96.8	95.2	93.3	91.0	88.1	5.03	5.70
24.71	16	183.9	183.0	182.1	181.0	179.9	178.7	177.2	175.6	173.6	171.2	168.1	11.80	12.70
	18	150.4	149.6	148.6	147.6	146.5	145.2	143.8	142.1	140.2	137.8	134.7	8.47	9.21
	20	123.5	122.7	121.7	120.7	119.6	118.3	116.9	115.2	113.3	110.9	107.8	6.49	7.09
	22	104.7	103.8	102.9	101.9	100.7	99.5	98.0	96.4	94.4	92.0	88.9	5.02	5.69

TABLE 346

Process Times (B) at Retort Temperature of 240°F for Conduction-Heating Foods in 211 x 200 Can

f_h	z	INITIAL FOOD TEMPERATURE (T_{ih}) 100	110	120	130	140	150	160	170	180	190	200	Equivalent F_c^{18}	F_s^{18}
20.00	16	66.9	66.2	65.5	64.8	64.0	63.0	62.0	60.9	59.5	57.9	56.0	9.57	10.92
	18	60.6	59.9	59.2	58.5	57.7	56.7	55.7	54.6	53.2	51.6	49.7	7.88	9.19
	20	55.8	55.1	54.4	53.7	52.8	51.9	50.9	49.7	48.4	46.8	44.9	6.58	7.88
	22	51.9	51.3	50.6	49.8	49.0	48.1	47.0	45.9	44.5	43.0	41.0	5.57	6.85
21.18	16	68.8	68.2	67.4	66.6	65.8	64.8	63.7	62.5	61.1	59.4	57.3	9.61	10.97
	18	62.4	61.7	61.0	60.2	59.3	58.3	57.3	56.0	54.6	52.9	50.9	7.86	9.21
	20	57.4	56.7	56.0	55.2	54.3	53.3	52.2	51.0	49.6	47.9	45.9	6.54	7.87
	22	53.5	52.8	52.1	51.3	50.4	49.4	48.4	47.1	45.7	44.0	42.0	5.43	6.80
22.35	16	70.6	69.9	69.1	68.2	67.3	66.3	65.2	63.9	62.4	60.6	58.4	9.56	10.98
	18	64.1	63.4	62.6	61.7	60.8	59.8	58.6	57.3	55.8	54.1	51.9	7.83	9.21
	20	59.0	58.3	57.5	56.7	55.7	54.7	53.6	52.3	50.8	49.0	46.9	6.49	7.84
	22	55.2	54.5	53.8	52.9	52.0	51.0	49.8	48.5	47.0	45.3	43.1	5.36	6.79
23.53	16	72.3	71.5	70.7	69.8	68.9	67.8	66.6	65.2	63.6	61.8	59.5	9.54	10.98
	18	65.8	65.0	64.2	63.3	62.3	61.2	60.0	58.7	57.1	55.2	53.0	7.79	9.19
	20	60.7	59.9	59.1	58.2	57.2	56.1	54.9	53.6	52.0	50.1	47.9	6.42	7.82
	22	57.1	56.4	55.6	54.7	53.7	52.6	51.4	50.1	48.5	46.6	44.3	5.34	6.83
24.71	16	74.1	73.3	72.5	71.5	70.5	69.4	68.1	66.7	65.0	63.1	60.7	9.53	10.99
	18	67.4	66.6	65.8	64.8	63.8	62.7	61.4	60.0	58.3	56.4	54.0	7.75	9.18
	20	62.4	61.6	60.8	59.8	58.8	57.7	56.4	55.0	53.3	51.4	49.0	6.33	7.80
	22	59.0	58.2	57.3	56.4	55.3	54.2	52.9	51.5	49.9	47.9	45.5	5.33	6.81

TABLE 347

Process Times (B) at Retort Temperature of 250°F for Conduction-Heating Foods in 211 x 200 Can

f_h	z	INITIAL FOOD TEMPERATURE (T_{ih})											Equivalent	
		100	110	120	130	140	150	160	170	180	190	200	F_c^{18}	F_s^{18}
20.00	16	38.8	38.2	37.6	36.9	36.1	35.3	34.4	33.4	32.2	30.9	29.3	8.02	10.01
	18	37.7	37.1	36.5	35.8	35.0	34.2	33.3	32.3	31.1	29.8	28.2	7.24	9.25
	20	36.7	36.1	35.5	34.8	34.0	33.2	32.3	31.2	30.1	28.7	27.2	6.56	8.52
	22	35.8	35.2	34.5	33.9	33.1	32.3	31.4	30.3	29.2	27.8	26.3	5.90	7.85
21.18	16	40.4	39.8	39.1	38.3	37.5	36.7	35.7	34.6	33.4	32.0	30.3	7.97	10.02
	18	39.2	38.6	37.9	37.2	36.4	35.5	34.5	33.5	32.2	30.8	29.1	7.20	9.22
	20	38.1	37.5	36.8	36.1	35.3	34.4	33.4	32.4	31.1	29.7	28.0	6.42	8.41
	22	37.2	36.5	35.9	35.1	34.3	33.4	32.5	31.4	30.2	28.8	27.1	5.78	7.75
22.35	16	42.0	41.4	40.7	39.9	39.0	38.1	37.1	35.9	34.6	33.1	31.4	8.00	10.08
	18	40.8	40.1	39.4	38.6	37.8	36.9	35.8	34.7	33.4	31.9	30.1	7.17	9.20
	20	39.6	39.0	38.3	37.5	36.6	35.7	34.7	33.5	32.2	30.7	29.0	6.36	8.37
	22	38.6	37.9	37.2	36.4	35.6	34.7	33.6	32.5	31.2	29.7	27.9	5.71	7.71
23.53	16	43.7	43.0	42.2	41.4	40.5	39.5	38.5	37.3	35.9	34.3	32.5	8.05	10.14
	18	42.4	41.7	40.9	40.1	39.2	38.2	37.2	36.0	34.6	33.0	31.2	7.14	9.20
	20	41.2	40.5	39.7	38.9	38.0	37.0	35.9	34.7	33.4	31.8	29.9	6.33	8.37
	22	40.1	39.4	38.6	37.8	36.9	35.9	34.8	33.6	32.3	30.7	28.8	5.66	7.68
24.71	16	45.3	44.6	43.8	42.9	42.0	40.9	39.8	38.6	37.1	35.5	33.5	8.07	10.17
	18	44.0	43.2	42.4	41.6	40.6	39.6	38.5	37.2	35.8	34.1	32.2	7.12	9.21
	20	42.7	41.9	41.1	40.3	39.3	38.3	37.2	35.9	34.5	32.8	30.9	6.31	8.37
	22	41.5	40.8	40.0	39.1	38.2	37.2	36.0	34.8	33.3	31.7	29.7	5.60	7.66

TABLE 348

Process Times (B) at Retort Temperature of 260°F for Conduction-Heating Foods in 211 x 200 Can

f_h	z	INITIAL FOOD TEMPERATURE (T_{ih}) 100	110	120	130	140	150	160	170	180	190	200	Equivalent F_c^{18}	F_s^{18}
20.00	16	28.8	28.3	27.7	27.0	26.3	25.6	24.8	23.9	22.8	21.7	20.3	7.09	9.63
	18	28.6	28.0	27.4	26.7	26.1	25.3	24.5	23.6	22.5	21.4	20.0	6.68	9.21
	20	28.2	27.7	27.1	26.4	25.7	25.0	24.1	23.2	22.2	21.0	19.7	6.25	8.76
	22	27.9	27.3	26.7	26.1	25.4	24.6	23.8	22.9	21.9	20.7	19.4	5.85	8.34
21.18	16	30.2	29.6	29.0	28.3	27.6	26.8	25.9	25.0	23.9	22.6	21.2	7.09	9.65
	18	29.9	29.3	28.7	28.0	27.3	26.5	25.6	24.6	23.5	22.3	20.9	6.66	9.21
	20	29.5	28.9	28.3	27.6	26.9	26.1	25.2	24.2	23.2	21.9	20.5	6.20	8.72
	22	29.2	28.6	28.0	27.3	26.5	25.7	24.9	23.9	22.8	21.6	20.2	5.80	8.30
22.35	16	31.6	31.0	30.3	29.6	28.8	28.0	27.1	26.0	24.9	23.6	22.1	7.09	9.67
	18	31.3	30.6	30.0	29.3	28.5	27.6	26.7	25.7	24.5	23.2	21.7	6.65	9.21
	20	30.9	30.2	29.6	28.8	28.1	27.2	26.3	25.3	24.1	22.8	21.3	6.18	8.72
	22	30.5	29.8	29.2	28.5	27.7	26.8	25.9	24.9	23.7	22.4	20.9	5.75	8.27
23.53	16	33.0	32.3	31.6	30.9	30.0	29.2	28.2	27.1	25.9	24.5	23.0	7.08	9.68
	18	32.6	31.9	31.2	30.5	29.7	28.8	27.8	26.7	25.5	24.2	22.6	6.63	9.21
	20	32.2	31.5	30.8	30.1	29.2	28.4	27.4	26.3	25.1	23.7	22.2	6.17	8.73
	22	31.7	31.1	30.4	29.6	28.8	27.9	26.9	25.9	24.7	23.3	21.7	5.72	8.24
24.71	16	34.4	33.7	32.9	32.1	31.3	30.3	29.3	28.2	26.9	25.5	23.8	7.12	9.74
	18	33.9	33.2	32.5	31.7	30.8	29.9	28.9	27.7	26.5	25.0	23.4	6.62	9.21
	20	33.5	32.8	32.0	31.3	30.4	29.5	28.4	27.3	26.0	24.6	23.0	6.16	8.73
	22	33.0	32.3	31.6	30.8	29.9	29.0	28.0	26.8	25.6	24.1	22.5	5.68	8.21

TABLE 349

Process Times (B) at Retort Temperature of 230°F for Conduction-Heating Foods in 211 x 210 Can

f_h	z	INITIAL FOOD TEMPERATURE (T_{ih})											Equivalent	
		100	110	120	130	140	150	160	170	180	190	200	F_c^{18}	F_s^{18}
26.54	16	192.3	191.4	190.4	189.3	188.0	186.7	185.1	183.4	181.3	178.7	175.4	12.08	13.00
	18	156.2	155.3	154.3	153.2	152.0	150.6	149.1	147.3	145.2	142.6	139.3	8.66	9.42
	20	127.2	126.2	125.2	124.1	122.9	121.6	120.0	118.3	116.2	113.6	110.3	6.53	7.32
	22	108.6	107.7	106.7	105.6	104.4	103.0	101.5	99.7	97.6	95.0	91.7	5.13	5.81
28.10	16	197.1	196.1	195.0	193.9	192.6	191.1	189.5	187.6	185.4	182.7	179.2	12.09	13.02
	18	158.7	157.7	156.7	155.5	154.2	152.8	151.1	149.3	147.0	144.3	140.8	8.65	9.42
	20	128.6	127.6	126.6	125.4	124.1	122.7	121.1	119.2	117.0	114.2	110.7	6.42	7.26
	22	110.6	109.6	108.6	107.4	106.1	104.7	103.0	101.2	98.9	96.2	92.7	5.07	5.88
29.66	16	201.5	200.5	199.4	198.1	196.8	195.3	193.5	191.6	189.2	186.3	182.6	12.09	13.03
	18	160.8	159.8	158.7	157.5	156.1	154.6	152.9	150.9	148.5	145.7	142.0	8.64	9.42
	20	131.1	130.1	129.0	127.7	126.4	124.9	123.1	121.1	118.8	115.9	112.2	6.42	7.25
	22	112.2	111.1	110.0	108.8	107.4	105.9	104.2	102.2	99.8	97.0	93.3	4.99	5.81
31.22	16	205.6	204.5	203.4	202.1	200.6	199.0	197.2	195.1	192.7	189.6	185.7	12.09	13.04
	18	162.7	161.6	160.4	159.1	157.7	156.1	154.3	152.2	149.7	146.7	142.8	8.63	9.42
	20	133.3	132.3	131.1	129.8	128.4	126.8	125.0	122.9	120.4	117.4	113.5	6.42	7.25
	22	114.0	112.9	111.8	110.5	109.0	107.4	105.6	103.5	101.1	98.0	94.1	4.97	5.77
32.78	16	209.4	208.3	207.0	205.7	204.2	202.5	200.6	198.4	195.8	192.6	188.6	12.10	13.05
	18	164.1	163.0	161.8	160.4	158.9	157.2	155.3	153.1	150.5	147.4	143.3	8.62	9.42
	20	135.3	134.2	132.9	131.6	130.1	128.4	126.5	124.3	121.7	118.5	114.5	6.42	7.24
	22	116.0	114.8	113.6	112.2	110.7	109.1	107.2	105.0	102.4	99.2	95.1	4.93	5.77

TABLE 350

Process Times (B) at Retort Temperature of 240°F for Conduction-Heating Foods in 211 x 210 Can

f_h	z	INITIAL FOOD TEMPERATURE (T_{ih})											Equivalent	
		100	110	120	130	140	150	160	170	180	190	200	F_c^{18}	F_s^{18}
	16	77.8	76.9	76.0	75.0	73.9	72.7	71.4	69.8	68.0	65.9	63.4	9.75	11.24
26.54	18	70.9	70.0	69.1	68.1	67.0	65.8	64.4	62.9	61.1	59.0	56.4	7.92	9.39
	20	66.0	65.1	64.2	63.2	62.1	60.9	59.5	58.0	56.2	54.1	51.5	6.48	8.02
	22	62.2	61.4	60.5	59.5	58.4	57.1	55.8	54.2	52.5	50.4	47.8	5.44	6.94
	16	80.2	79.3	78.3	77.2	76.1	74.8	73.4	71.7	69.8	67.6	64.9	9.75	11.28
28.10	18	73.1	72.2	71.2	70.2	69.0	67.7	66.3	64.6	62.8	60.5	57.8	7.88	9.37
	20	68.5	67.6	66.6	65.5	64.4	63.1	61.6	60.0	58.1	55.9	53.2	6.45	8.05
	22	64.5	63.6	62.6	61.6	60.4	59.1	57.7	56.0	54.2	51.9	49.2	5.42	6.92
	16	82.4	81.5	80.5	79.3	78.1	76.7	75.2	73.5	71.5	69.2	66.3	9.69	11.25
29.66	18	75.7	74.8	73.7	72.6	71.4	70.0	68.5	66.8	64.8	62.5	59.6	7.85	9.43
	20	70.8	69.9	68.9	67.7	66.5	65.1	63.6	61.9	59.9	57.6	54.7	6.41	8.02
	22	66.7	65.8	64.7	63.6	62.4	61.0	59.5	57.8	55.8	53.5	50.6	5.41	6.90
	16	84.8	83.8	82.7	81.6	80.3	78.8	77.2	75.4	73.3	70.9	67.8	9.70	11.28
31.22	18	78.4	77.3	76.3	75.1	73.8	72.4	70.8	69.0	66.9	64.4	61.4	7.84	9.47
	20	73.2	72.2	71.1	69.9	68.6	67.2	65.6	63.8	61.7	59.2	56.2	6.39	8.00
	22	68.9	67.9	66.8	65.6	64.3	62.9	61.3	59.5	57.4	54.9	51.9	5.39	6.89
	16	87.2	86.1	85.0	83.7	82.4	80.9	79.2	77.3	75.1	72.5	69.3	9.68	11.29
32.78	18	80.8	79.8	78.6	77.4	76.0	74.5	72.8	70.9	68.7	66.2	63.0	7.79	9.48
	20	75.4	74.4	73.2	72.0	70.7	69.2	67.5	65.6	63.4	60.8	57.6	6.37	7.97
	22	71.0	70.0	68.8	67.6	66.2	64.7	63.1	61.2	59.0	56.4	53.2	5.39	6.90

TABLE 351

Process Times (B) at Retort Temperature of 250°F for Conduction-Heating Foods in 211 x 210 Can

f_h	z	INITIAL FOOD TEMPERATURE (T_{ih})											Equivalent	
		100	110	120	130	140	150	160	170	180	190	200	F_c^{18}	F_s^{18}
	16	48.1	47.3	46.5	45.5	44.5	43.4	42.2	40.9	39.3	37.5	35.4	8.26	10.40
26.54	18	46.7	45.9	45.0	44.1	43.1	42.0	40.8	39.4	37.9	36.1	34.0	7.30	9.42
	20	45.3	44.5	43.6	42.7	41.7	40.6	39.4	38.0	36.5	34.7	32.6	6.44	8.54
	22	44.0	43.2	42.4	41.5	40.5	39.4	38.2	36.8	35.3	33.5	31.4	5.69	7.79
	16	50.2	49.3	48.4	47.4	46.4	45.2	43.9	42.5	40.9	39.0	36.8	8.21	10.38
28.10	18	48.7	47.8	46.9	46.0	44.9	43.7	42.4	41.0	39.4	37.5	35.3	7.27	9.41
	20	47.2	46.3	45.4	44.5	43.4	42.2	40.9	39.5	37.9	36.0	33.8	6.35	8.49
	22	45.9	45.0	44.1	43.1	42.1	40.9	39.6	38.2	36.6	34.7	32.5	5.61	7.72
	16	52.2	51.4	50.4	49.4	48.2	47.0	45.7	44.1	42.4	40.4	38.1	8.20	10.40
29.66	18	50.7	49.8	48.8	47.8	46.7	45.4	44.1	42.6	40.9	38.9	36.5	7.23	9.41
	20	49.1	48.2	47.2	46.2	45.1	43.9	42.5	41.0	39.3	37.3	34.9	6.29	8.45
	22	47.7	46.8	45.8	44.8	43.7	42.5	41.1	39.6	37.9	35.9	33.5	5.52	7.65
	16	54.3	53.4	52.4	51.3	50.1	48.9	47.4	45.8	44.0	41.9	39.5	8.23	10.45
31.22	18	52.7	51.8	50.8	49.7	48.5	47.2	45.8	44.2	42.4	40.3	37.8	7.22	9.43
	20	51.0	50.1	49.1	48.0	46.8	45.5	44.1	42.5	40.7	38.6	36.1	6.27	8.45
	22	49.6	48.6	47.6	46.5	45.3	44.1	42.6	41.0	39.2	37.1	34.7	5.47	7.62
	16	56.4	55.4	54.4	53.2	52.0	50.6	49.1	47.5	45.6	43.4	40.8	8.26	10.50
32.78	18	54.7	53.7	52.7	51.5	50.3	48.9	47.4	45.7	43.8	41.6	39.0	7.20	9.44
	20	52.9	52.0	50.9	49.8	48.5	47.2	45.7	44.0	42.1	39.9	37.3	6.22	8.42
	22	51.4	50.4	49.3	48.2	47.0	45.6	44.1	42.4	40.5	38.3	35.7	5.42	7.59

TABLE 352

Process Times (B) at Retort Temperature of 260°F for Conduction-Heating Foods in 211 x 210 Can

f_h	z	INITIAL FOOD TEMPERATURE (T_{ih})											Equivalent	
		100	110	120	130	140	150	160	170	180	190	200	F_c^{18}	F_s^{18}
26.54	16	36.7	35.9	35.1	34.3	33.3	32.3	31.2	30.0	28.7	27.1	25.4	7.36	10.01
	18	36.1	35.4	34.6	33.7	32.8	31.8	30.7	29.5	28.2	26.6	24.8	6.80	9.43
	20	35.7	34.9	34.1	33.3	32.4	31.4	30.3	29.0	27.7	26.1	24.4	6.33	8.93
	22	35.2	34.4	33.6	32.8	31.9	30.9	29.8	28.5	27.2	25.6	23.9	5.80	8.36
28.10	16	38.5	37.7	36.8	35.9	35.0	33.9	32.7	31.4	30.0	28.4	26.5	7.41	10.08
	18	37.9	37.1	36.2	35.3	34.3	33.3	32.1	30.8	29.4	27.8	25.9	6.78	9.42
	20	37.4	36.6	35.7	34.8	33.9	32.8	31.6	30.3	28.9	27.3	25.4	6.27	8.88
	22	36.8	36.0	35.2	34.3	33.3	32.3	31.1	29.8	28.4	26.7	24.9	5.75	8.33
29.66	16	40.3	39.4	38.5	37.6	36.5	35.4	34.2	32.8	31.3	29.6	27.6	7.46	10.15
	18	39.6	38.8	37.9	36.9	35.9	34.8	33.5	32.2	30.7	28.9	26.9	6.77	9.42
	20	39.0	38.2	37.3	36.4	35.3	34.2	33.0	31.6	30.1	28.4	26.4	6.22	8.84
	22	38.5	37.7	36.8	35.8	34.8	33.7	32.4	31.1	29.6	27.8	25.8	5.70	8.29
31.22	16	42.0	41.1	40.2	39.2	38.1	36.9	35.6	34.2	32.6	30.8	28.7	7.50	10.21
	18	41.3	40.4	39.5	38.5	37.4	36.2	34.9	33.5	31.9	30.1	28.0	6.75	9.42
	20	40.7	39.8	38.9	37.9	36.8	35.6	34.3	32.9	31.3	29.5	27.4	6.16	8.80
	22	40.1	39.2	38.3	37.3	36.2	35.0	33.7	32.3	30.7	28.9	26.8	5.66	8.25
32.78	16	43.8	42.9	41.9	40.8	39.7	38.5	37.1	35.6	33.9	32.0	29.8	7.52	10.24
	18	43.0	42.1	41.1	40.1	38.9	37.7	36.3	34.8	33.1	31.2	29.0	6.74	9.42
	20	42.3	41.4	40.4	39.4	38.2	37.0	35.6	34.1	32.5	30.6	28.4	6.12	8.76
	22	41.7	40.8	39.8	38.8	37.6	36.4	35.0	33.5	31.8	29.9	27.8	5.59	8.19

TABLE 353

Process Times (B) at Retort Temperature of 230°F for Conduction-Heating Foods in 211 x 212 Can

f_h	z	INITIAL FOOD TEMPERATURE (T_{ih})											Equivalent	
		100	110	120	130	140	150	160	170	180	190	200	F_c^{18}	F_s^{18}
	16	195.8	194.9	193.8	192.7	191.4	190.0	188.4	186.6	184.4	181.7	178.3	12.13	13.06
27.54	18	158.3	157.3	156.3	155.1	153.9	152.5	150.9	149.0	146.9	144.2	140.7	8.68	9.45
	20	128.2	127.3	126.2	125.1	123.8	122.4	120.8	119.0	116.8	114.1	110.7	6.47	7.31
	22	110.0	109.0	108.0	106.8	105.6	104.1	102.6	100.7	98.5	95.9	92.4	5.09	5.86
	16	200.6	199.6	198.5	197.3	195.9	194.4	192.8	190.8	188.5	185.7	182.0	12.13	13.07
29.16	18	160.7	159.6	158.5	157.3	156.0	154.5	152.8	150.9	148.6	145.7	142.1	8.67	9.45
	20	130.7	129.7	128.6	127.3	126.0	124.5	122.8	120.9	118.6	115.7	112.1	6.45	7.28
	22	112.0	111.0	109.9	108.7	107.3	105.8	104.1	102.2	99.9	97.0	93.4	5.04	5.87
	16	205.0	203.9	202.8	201.5	200.1	198.5	196.7	194.6	192.2	189.2	185.4	12.14	13.09
30.78	18	162.7	161.6	160.4	159.2	157.8	156.2	154.4	152.3	149.9	146.9	143.1	8.67	9.45
	20	133.1	132.0	130.9	129.6	128.2	126.6	124.8	122.7	120.3	117.3	113.5	6.45	7.28
	22	113.7	112.6	111.5	110.2	108.8	107.2	105.4	103.4	100.9	97.9	94.1	4.99	5.80
	16	209.0	207.9	206.7	205.3	203.9	202.2	200.3	198.2	195.6	192.4	188.4	12.14	13.10
32.40	18	164.3	163.2	162.0	160.6	159.1	157.5	155.6	153.4	150.9	147.7	143.7	8.66	9.45
	20	135.3	134.1	132.9	131.6	130.1	128.4	126.5	124.4	121.8	118.7	114.6	6.44	7.27
	22	115.8	114.7	113.5	112.1	110.7	109.0	107.1	104.9	102.4	99.2	95.2	4.97	5.79
	16	212.8	211.6	210.3	208.9	207.3	205.6	203.6	201.3	198.6	195.3	191.1	12.15	13.11
34.02	18	165.8	164.7	163.4	162.0	160.4	158.7	156.7	154.4	151.7	148.4	144.2	8.62	9.49
	20	137.2	136.0	134.7	133.3	131.7	130.0	128.0	125.8	123.1	119.8	115.5	6.40	7.28
	22	117.9	116.7	115.4	114.0	112.5	110.7	108.7	106.5	103.8	100.5	96.2	4.92	5.81

TABLE 354

Process Times (B) at Retort Temperature of 240°F for Conduction-Heating Foods in 211 x 212 Can

f_h	z	INITIAL FOOD TEMPERATURE (T_{ih})											Equivalent	
		100	110	120	130	140	150	160	170	180	190	200	F_c^{18}	F_s^{18}
27.54	16	79.5	78.6	77.7	76.6	75.5	74.2	72.8	71.2	69.4	67.2	64.5	9.79	11.31
	18	72.5	71.6	70.6	69.6	68.4	67.2	65.8	64.2	62.3	60.1	57.5	7.93	9.42
	20	67.7	66.8	65.9	64.8	63.7	62.4	61.0	59.4	57.6	55.4	52.7	6.49	8.07
	22	63.8	62.9	62.0	60.9	59.8	58.5	57.1	55.5	53.7	51.5	48.8	5.45	6.95
29.16	16	81.9	81.0	80.0	78.9	77.6	76.3	74.8	73.1	71.2	68.9	66.0	9.76	11.30
	18	75.0	74.0	73.0	71.9	70.7	69.4	67.9	66.2	64.2	61.9	59.1	7.89	9.44
	20	70.2	69.3	68.2	67.1	65.9	64.6	63.1	61.4	59.5	57.2	54.3	6.45	8.06
	22	66.1	65.2	64.2	63.1	61.9	60.5	59.0	57.3	55.4	53.1	50.3	5.43	6.94
30.78	16	84.3	83.3	82.3	81.1	79.8	78.4	76.8	75.1	73.0	70.6	67.6	9.74	11.31
	18	77.7	76.7	75.7	74.5	73.2	71.8	70.2	68.5	66.4	64.0	61.0	7.88	9.49
	20	72.6	71.6	70.6	69.4	68.1	66.7	65.2	63.4	61.3	58.9	55.9	6.43	8.03
	22	68.4	67.4	66.3	65.2	63.9	62.5	60.9	59.1	57.1	54.6	51.6	5.42	6.92
32.40	16	86.8	85.7	84.6	83.4	82.0	80.5	78.9	77.0	74.8	72.3	69.1	9.72	11.33
	18	80.3	79.3	78.2	76.9	75.6	74.1	72.5	70.6	68.4	65.9	62.7	7.84	9.51
	20	75.0	74.0	72.8	71.6	70.3	68.8	67.1	65.3	63.1	60.5	57.4	6.40	8.01
	22	70.6	69.6	68.4	67.2	65.9	64.4	62.7	60.9	58.7	56.1	53.0	5.42	6.92
34.02	16	89.5	88.4	87.2	85.9	84.5	82.9	81.2	79.2	76.9	74.3	71.0	9.78	11.41
	18	82.9	81.8	80.6	79.3	77.9	76.3	74.6	72.6	70.4	67.7	64.4	7.80	9.52
	20	77.3	76.2	75.1	73.8	72.4	70.8	69.1	67.1	64.8	62.1	58.8	6.38	7.99
	22	72.8	71.7	70.5	69.2	67.8	66.3	64.5	62.6	60.3	57.6	54.3	5.42	6.92

TABLE 355

Process Times (B) at Retort Temperature of 250°F for Conduction-Heating Foods in 211 x 212 Can

f_h	z	INITIAL FOOD TEMPERATURE (T_{ih})											Equivalent	
		100	110	120	130	140	150	160	170	180	190	200	F_{c}^{18}	F_{s}^{18}
27.54	16	49.5	48.7	47.8	46.8	45.8	44.6	43.4	42.0	40.4	38.5	36.4	8.27	10.43
	18	48.0	47.2	46.3	45.4	44.3	43.2	41.9	40.5	38.9	37.1	34.9	7.31	9.45
	20	46.6	45.7	44.9	43.9	42.9	41.7	40.5	39.0	37.8	35.6	33.4	6.41	8.54
	22	45.3	44.5	43.6	42.6	41.6	40.4	39.2	37.8	36.2	34.3	32.1	5.67	7.78
29.16	16	51.6	50.8	49.8	48.8	47.7	46.5	45.2	43.7	42.0	40.0	37.7	8.23	10.42
	18	50.1	49.2	48.3	47.2	46.1	44.9	43.6	42.1	40.4	38.5	36.2	7.28	9.44
	20	48.5	47.6	46.7	45.7	44.6	43.4	42.0	40.6	38.9	36.9	34.6	6.32	8.49
	22	47.2	46.3	45.3	44.3	43.2	42.0	40.7	39.2	37.5	35.5	33.2	5.57	7.69
30.78	16	53.8	52.9	51.9	50.8	49.7	48.4	47.0	45.4	43.6	41.6	39.1	8.26	10.47
	18	52.2	51.3	50.3	49.2	48.0	46.8	45.4	43.8	42.0	39.9	37.5	7.25	9.46
	20	50.5	49.6	48.6	47.6	46.4	45.1	43.7	42.1	40.4	38.3	35.9	6.31	8.48
	22	49.1	48.2	47.2	46.1	44.9	43.7	42.3	40.7	38.9	36.8	34.4	5.51	7.66
32.40	16	56.0	55.0	54.0	52.8	51.6	50.3	48.8	47.1	45.3	43.1	40.5	8.29	10.53
	18	54.3	53.3	52.3	51.1	49.9	48.6	47.1	45.4	43.5	41.4	38.8	7.24	9.47
	20	52.5	51.6	50.5	49.4	48.2	46.8	45.4	43.7	41.8	39.6	37.1	6.27	8.47
	22	51.0	50.0	49.0	47.9	46.6	45.3	43.8	42.2	40.3	38.1	35.5	5.46	7.63
34.02	16	58.1	57.1	56.0	54.8	53.5	52.1	50.6	48.8	46.8	44.6	41.9	8.29	10.55
	18	56.3	55.3	54.2	53.0	51.7	50.3	48.8	47.0	45.1	42.8	40.1	7.21	9.47
	20	54.5	53.5	52.4	51.2	49.9	48.5	46.9	45.2	43.2	41.0	38.3	6.22	8.43
	22	52.9	51.9	50.8	49.6	48.3	46.9	45.3	43.6	41.6	39.3	36.6	5.40	7.58

TABLE 356

Process Times (B) at Retort Temperature of 260°F for Conduction-Heating Foods in 211 x 212 Can

f_h	z	INITIAL FOOD TEMPERATURE (T_{ih})											Equivalent	
		100	110	120	130	140	150	160	170	180	190	200	F_c^{18}	F_s^{18}
27.54	16	37.9	37.1	36.3	35.4	34.4	33.4	32.2	31.0	29.6	28.0	26.1	7.42	10.09
	18	37.3	36.5	35.7	34.8	33.8	32.8	31.7	30.4	29.0	27.4	25.5	6.83	9.46
	20	36.8	36.0	35.2	34.3	33.4	32.3	31.2	29.9	28.5	26.9	25.1	6.33	8.93
	22	36.3	35.5	34.7	33.8	32.8	31.8	30.7	29.4	28.0	26.4	24.5	5.80	8.37
29.16	16	39.7	38.9	38.0	37.1	36.1	35.0	33.8	32.4	30.9	29.2	27.3	7.47	10.16
	18	39.1	38.2	37.4	36.4	35.4	34.3	33.1	31.8	30.3	28.6	26.6	6.81	9.45
	20	38.5	37.7	36.9	35.9	34.9	33.8	32.6	31.3	29.8	28.1	26.1	6.27	8.89
	22	38.0	37.2	36.3	35.4	34.4	33.2	32.0	30.7	29.2	27.5	25.6	5.75	8.33
30.78	16	41.6	40.7	39.8	38.8	37.7	36.6	35.3	33.9	32.3	30.5	28.4	7.52	10.22
	18	40.9	40.0	39.1	38.1	37.0	35.8	34.6	33.2	31.6	29.8	27.7	6.79	9.46
	20	40.3	39.4	38.5	37.5	36.4	35.3	34.0	32.6	31.0	29.2	27.2	6.21	8.85
	22	39.7	38.8	37.9	36.9	35.8	34.7	33.4	32.0	30.4	28.6	26.6	5.70	8.30
32.40	16	43.4	42.5	41.5	40.5	39.3	38.1	36.8	35.3	33.6	31.8	29.6	7.55	10.26
	18	42.6	41.7	40.8	39.7	38.6	37.4	36.0	34.5	32.9	31.0	28.8	6.78	9.46
	20	42.0	41.0	40.1	39.0	37.9	36.7	35.3	33.9	32.2	30.3	28.2	6.16	8.80
	22	41.4	40.5	39.5	38.4	37.3	36.1	34.8	33.3	31.6	29.7	27.6	5.64	8.24
34.02	16	45.2	44.3	43.3	42.2	41.0	39.7	38.3	36.7	35.0	33.0	30.7	7.57	10.30
	18	44.4	43.4	42.4	41.3	40.1	38.9	37.5	35.9	34.2	32.2	29.9	6.77	9.46
	20	43.7	42.7	41.7	40.6	39.4	38.2	36.7	35.2	33.4	31.5	29.2	6.15	8.80
	22	43.0	42.1	41.1	40.0	38.8	37.5	36.1	34.5	32.8	30.8	28.5	5.57	8.18

TABLE 357

Process Times (B) at Retort Temperature of 230°F For Conduction-Heating Foods in 211 x 214 Can

f_h	z	INITIAL FOOD TEMPERATURE (T_{ih})											Equivalent	
		100	110	120	130	140	150	160	170	180	190	200	F_c^{18}	F_s^{18}
	16	199.0	198.0	196.9	195.8	194.5	193.0	191.3	189.4	187.2	184.4	180.9	12.17	13.11
28.46	18	160.1	159.1	158.0	156.9	155.6	154.1	152.4	150.5	148.3	145.5	142.0	8.71	9.49
	20	129.8	128.9	127.8	126.6	125.3	123.8	122.2	120.3	118.0	115.3	111.7	6.47	7.31
	22	111.6	110.6	109.5	108.4	107.1	105.6	103.9	102.0	99.8	97.0	93.5	5.10	5.93
	16	203.7	202.7	201.5	200.3	198.9	197.4	195.6	193.6	191.2	188.3	184.5	12.18	13.13
30.14	18	162.4	161.3	160.2	158.9	157.5	156.0	154.3	152.2	149.9	146.9	143.2	8.70	9.48
	20	132.5	131.4	130.3	129.0	127.7	126.1	124.4	122.4	120.0	117.0	113.3	6.47	7.31
	22	113.3	112.2	111.1	109.8	108.4	106.9	105.2	103.1	100.8	97.8	94.1	5.02	5.84
	16	208.1	207.0	205.8	204.4	203.0	201.4	199.5	197.4	194.9	191.8	187.8	12.18	13.14
31.81	18	164.2	163.1	161.9	160.6	159.1	157.5	155.7	153.5	151.0	147.9	144.0	8.69	9.48
	20	134.8	133.7	132.5	131.2	129.7	128.1	126.3	124.1	121.6	118.5	114.6	6.47	7.30
	22	115.4	114.5	113.1	111.7	110.3	108.7	106.8	104.7	102.2	99.1	95.1	5.00	5.81
	16	212.0	210.9	209.6	208.2	206.7	205.0	203.0	200.8	198.1	194.9	190.7	12.19	13.15
33.49	18	165.7	164.6	163.3	161.9	160.4	158.7	156.7	154.5	151.8	148.6	144.4	8.68	9.48
	20	136.9	135.7	134.4	133.1	131.5	129.8	127.9	125.6	123.0	119.7	115.6	6.46	7.29
	22	117.4	116.2	115.0	113.6	112.1	110.4	108.4	106.2	103.5	100.3	96.1	4.95	5.81
	16	215.7	214.5	213.1	211.7	210.1	208.3	206.2	203.9	201.1	197.7	193.3	12.19	13.16
35.16	18	167.2	165.9	164.6	163.2	161.6	159.8	157.7	155.4	152.6	149.2	144.8	8.54	9.55
	20	139.2	138.1	136.7	135.3	133.7	131.9	129.8	127.5	124.7	121.3	116.9	6.41	7.36
	22	119.9	118.7	117.3	115.9	114.3	112.5	110.4	108.1	105.3	101.9	97.5	4.94	5.86

TABLE 358

Process Times (B) at Retort Temperature of 240°F for Conduction-Heating Foods in 211 x 214 Can

f_h	z	INITIAL FOOD TEMPERATURE (T_{ih}) 100	110	120	130	140	150	160	170	180	190	200	Equivalent F_c^{18}	F_s^{18}
28.46	16	81.0	80.1	79.1	78.1	76.9	75.6	74.1	72.5	70.6	68.3	65.6	9.83	11.36
	18	73.9	73.0	72.0	70.9	79.7	68.4	67.0	65.3	63.4	61.1	58.4	7.94	9.44
	20	69.2	68.3	67.3	66.3	65.1	63.8	62.3	60.7	58.8	56.5	53.8	6.50	8.11
	22	65.2	64.3	63.3	62.2	61.1	59.8	58.3	56.7	54.8	52.5	49.7	5.46	6.97
30.14	16	83.5	82.5	81.5	80.3	79.1	77.7	76.1	74.4	72.4	70.0	67.1	9.77	11.33
	18	76.7	75.8	74.7	73.6	72.3	71.0	69.4	67.7	65.6	63.3	60.3	7.91	9.50
	20	71.8	70.8	69.8	68.6	67.4	66.0	64.4	62.7	60.7	58.3	55.4	6.46	8.07
	22	67.6	66.6	65.6	64.4	63.2	61.8	60.3	58.5	56.5	54.1	51.2	5.45	6.95
31.81	16	86.0	85.0	83.9	82.7	81.4	79.9	78.3	76.5	74.3	71.8	68.7	9.78	11.37
	18	79.5	78.5	77.4	76.2	74.9	73.4	71.8	69.9	67.8	65.3	62.2	7.89	9.54
	20	74.3	73.2	72.1	70.9	69.6	68.2	66.5	64.7	62.6	60.0	57.0	6.44	8.05
	22	69.9	68.9	67.8	66.6	65.3	63.8	62.2	60.3	58.2	55.7	52.6	5.44	6.94
33.49	16	88.7	87.6	86.4	85.2	83.8	82.2	80.5	78.6	76.3	73.7	70.4	9.78	11.40
	18	82.2	81.1	79.9	78.6	77.3	75.7	74.0	72.1	69.8	67.2	63.9	7.84	9.55
	20	76.7	75.6	74.4	73.2	71.8	70.3	68.6	66.6	64.4	61.7	58.5	6.42	8.03
	22	72.2	71.1	70.0	68.7	67.3	65.8	64.1	62.1	59.9	57.2	54.0	5.44	6.95
35.16	16	91.5	90.4	89.2	87.9	86.4	84.8	83.0	81.0	78.6	75.8	72.4	9.87	11.52
	18	84.8	83.6	82.4	81.1	79.6	78.0	76.2	74.2	71.8	69.0	65.6	7.81	9.55
	20	79.1	77.9	76.7	75.4	73.9	72.3	70.5	68.5	66.1	63.4	60.0	6.41	8.02
	22	74.4	73.3	72.1	70.7	69.3	67.7	65.9	63.8	61.5	58.7	55.3	5.44	6.95

TABLE 359

Process Times (B) at Retort Temperature of 250°F for Conduction-Heating Foods in 211 x 214 Can

f_h	z	INITIAL FOOD TEMPERATURE (T_{ih})											Equivalent	
		100	110	120	130	140	150	160	170	180	190	200	F_c^{18}	F_s^{18}
	16	50.8	49.9	49.0	48.0	46.9	45.8	44.5	43.0	41.3	39.4	37.2	8.28	10.46
28.46	18	49.3	48.4	47.5	46.5	45.4	44.2	42.9	41.5	39.8	37.9	35.7	7.33	9.48
	20	47.7	46.9	46.0	45.0	43.9	42.7	41.4	40.0	38.3	36.4	34.2	6.40	8.54
	22	46.4	45.5	44.6	43.6	42.6	41.4	40.1	38.6	37.0	35.1	32.8	5.65	7.76
	16	53.0	52.1	51.1	50.1	48.9	47.7	46.3	44.8	43.0	41.0	38.6	8.28	10.48
30.14	18	51.4	50.5	49.5	48.5	47.3	46.1	44.7	43.2	41.4	39.4	37.0	7.29	9.48
	20	49.8	48.9	47.9	46.9	45.7	44.5	43.1	41.6	39.8	37.8	35.4	6.34	8.51
	22	48.4	47.5	46.5	45.4	44.3	43.1	41.7	40.1	38.4	36.4	34.0	5.56	7.70
	16	55.3	54.3	53.3	52.2	51.0	49.6	48.2	46.6	44.7	42.6	40.1	8.31	10.54
31.81	18	53.6	52.6	51.6	50.5	49.3	48.0	46.5	44.9	43.0	40.9	38.4	7.27	9.50
	20	51.9	50.9	49.9	48.8	47.6	46.3	44.8	43.2	41.3	39.2	36.7	6.32	8.51
	22	50.4	49.4	48.4	47.3	46.1	44.8	43.3	41.7	39.8	37.7	35.2	5.51	7.67
	16	57.5	56.5	55.4	54.2	53.0	51.6	50.0	48.3	46.4	44.1	41.5	8.34	10.59
33.49	18	55.7	54.7	53.6	52.5	51.2	49.8	48.3	46.6	44.6	42.4	39.7	7.25	9.51
	20	53.9	52.9	51.8	50.7	49.4	48.0	46.5	44.8	42.8	40.6	37.9	6.26	8.47
	22	52.3	51.3	50.2	49.1	47.8	46.4	44.9	43.2	41.2	39.0	36.3	5.45	7.63
	16	59.6	58.6	57.5	56.2	54.9	53.4	51.8	50.0	48.0	45.6	42.9	8.31	10.59
35.16	18	57.8	56.7	55.6	54.4	53.1	51.6	50.0	48.2	46.2	43.8	41.0	7.23	9.50
	20	55.9	54.9	53.7	52.5	51.2	49.7	48.1	46.3	44.3	41.9	39.1	6.21	8.44
	22	54.2	53.2	52.1	50.8	49.5	48.0	46.4	44.6	42.6	40.2	37.5	5.38	7.58

TABLE 360

Process Times (B) at Retort Temperature of 260°F for Conduction-Heating Foods in 211 x 214 Can

f_h	z	INITIAL FOOD TEMPERATURE (T_{ih})											Equivalent	
		100	110	120	130	140	150	160	170	180	190	200	F_c^{18}	F_s^{18}
28.46	16	38.9	38.1	37.3	36.4	35.4	34.3	33.1	31.8	30.4	28.7	26.8	7.48	10.16
	18	38.3	37.5	36.7	35.7	34.8	33.7	32.5	31.2	29.7	28.1	26.2	6.85	9.49
	20	37.8	37.0	36.2	35.3	34.3	33.2	32.0	30.7	29.3	27.6	25.7	6.33	8.94
	22	37.3	36.5	35.6	24.7	33.7	32.7	31.5	30.2	28.7	27.1	25.2	5.80	8.38
30.14	16	40.9	40.0	39.1	38.1	37.1	36.0	34.7	33.3	31.8	30.0	28.0	7.53	10.23
	18	40.2	39.3	38.4	37.5	36.4	35.3	34.0	32.6	31.1	29.4	27.3	6.83	9.49
	20	39.6	38.8	37.9	36.9	35.9	34.7	33.5	32.1	30.5	28.8	26.8	6.27	8.90
	22	39.1	38.2	37.3	36.3	35.3	34.1	32.9	31.5	30.0	28.2	26.2	5.75	8.34
31.81	16	42.8	41.9	40.9	39.9	38.8	37.6	36.3	34.8	33.2	31.3	29.2	7.58	10.29
	18	42.0	41.1	40.2	39.2	38.0	36.8	35.5	34.1	32.4	30.6	28.5	6.81	9.49
	20	41.4	40.5	39.5	38.5	37.4	36.2	34.9	33.4	31.8	30.0	27.8	6.21	8.85
	22	40.8	39.9	38.9	37.9	36.8	35.6	34.3	32.8	31.2	29.4	27.2	5.70	8.30
33.49	16	44.6	43.7	42.7	41.6	40.5	39.2	37.8	36.3	34.6	32.6	30.4	7.59	10.32
	18	43.8	42.9	41.9	40.8	39.7	38.4	37.0	35.5	33.8	31.8	29.6	6.80	9.49
	20	43.2	42.2	41.2	40.1	39.0	37.7	36.3	34.8	33.1	31.1	28.9	6.18	8.83
	22	42.5	41.6	40.6	39.5	38.3	37.1	35.7	34.1	32.4	30.5	28.2	5.62	8.24
35.16	16	46.5	45.6	44.5	43.4	42.1	40.8	39.4	37.8	36.0	33.9	31.6	7.62	10.37
	18	45.7	44.7	43.6	42.5	41.3	39.9	38.5	36.9	35.1	33.0	30.7	6.79	9.49
	20	44.9	43.9	42.9	41.8	40.5	39.2	37.8	36.1	34.3	32.3	30.0	6.15	8.82
	22	44.2	43.2	42.2	41.0	39.8	38.5	37.0	35.4	33.6	31.6	29.2	5.55	8.17

TABLE 361

Process Times (B) at Retort Temperature of 230°F for Conduction-Heating Foods in 211 x 300 Can

f_h	z	INITIAL FOOD TEMPERATURE (T_{ih}) 100	110	120	130	140	150	160	170	180	190	200	Equivalent F_c^{18}	F_s^{18}
	16	201.8	200.8	199.7	198.5	197.1	195.6	193.9	192.0	189.7	186.8	183.2	122.2	13.16
29.31	18	161.7	160.7	159.6	158.4	157.0	155.5	153.8	151.9	149.5	146.7	143.0	8.74	9.52
	20	131.5	130.5	129.4	128.2	126.8	125.3	123.6	121.7	119.3	116.5	112.8	6.49	7.33
	22	112.7	111.7	110.6	109.4	108.0	106.5	104.8	102.9	100.6	97.7	94.0	5.08	5.91
	16	206.5	205.4	204.3	203.0	201.5	200.0	198.2	196.1	193.6	190.6	186.7	12.22	13.18
31.03	18	163.3	162.8	161.6	160.3	158.9	157.3	155.5	153.4	151.0	148.0	144.1	8.73	9.52
	20	134.1	133.0	131.8	130.5	129.1	127.5	125.7	123.7	121.2	118.2	114.3	6.49	7.33
	22	114.6	113.5	112.3	111.0	109.6	108.0	106.2	104.1	101.7	98.7	94.8	5.02	5.84
	16	210.8	209.7	208.4	207.1	205.6	203.9	202.0	199.8	197.2	194.0	189.9	12.23	13.19
32.76	18	165.6	164.4	163.2	161.8	160.4	158.7	156.8	154.6	152.0	148.8	144.7	8.72	9.52
	20	136.4	135.2	134.0	132.6	131.1	129.5	127.6	125.4	122.8	119.6	115.5	6.49	7.32
	22	116.8	115.7	114.4	113.1	111.6	109.9	108.0	105.8	103.2	100.0	96.0	5.00	5.83
	16	214.7	213.5	212.2	210.8	209.2	207.4	205.4	203.1	200.4	197.1	192.8	12.23	13.20
34.48	18	167.2	166.0	164.7	163.2	161.7	159.9	157.9	155.6	152.9	149.5	145.2	8.65	9.56
	20	138.5	137.3	136.0	134.6	133.0	131.3	129.3	126.9	124.2	120.9	116.6	6.45	7.35
	22	119.1	117.9	116.6	115.1	113.6	118.8	109.8	107.5	104.8	101.4	97.1	4.96	5.85
	16	218.3	217.0	215.7	214.2	212.5	210.7	208.6	206.1	203.3	199.8	195.2	12.23	13.21
36.20	18	168.5	167.2	165.8	164.4	162.7	160.8	158.7	156.3	153.5	149.9	145.4	8.49	9.52
	20	140.8	139.5	138.1	136.6	135.0	133.1	131.0	128.6	125.7	122.2	117.7	6.39	7.38
	22	121.5	120.2	118.9	117.4	115.7	113.9	111.8	109.3	106.5	103.0	98.4	4.94	5.86

TABLE 362

Process Times (B) at Retort Temperature of 240°F for Conduction-Heating Foods in 211 x 300 Can

f_h	z	INITIAL FOOD TEMPERATURE (T_{ih})											Equivalent	
		100	110	120	130	140	150	160	170	180	190	200	F_c^{18}	F_s^{18}
29.31	16	82.4	81.5	80.5	79.4	78.1	76.8	75.3	73.6	71.6	69.3	66.5	9.84	11.39
	18	75.4	74.5	73.4	72.3	71.1	69.8	68.3	66.6	64.6	62.3	59.5	7.95	9.50
	20	70.6	69.7	68.7	67.6	66.3	65.0	63.5	61.8	59.8	57.5	54.7	6.51	8.12
	22	66.5	65.4	64.6	63.5	62.2	60.9	59.4	57.7	55.7	53.4	50.6	5.48	6.98
31.03	16	85.0	84.0	82.9	81.7	80.5	79.0	77.4	75.6	73.6	71.1	68.1	9.81	11.39
	18	78.3	77.3	76.3	75.1	73.8	72.4	70.8	69.0	66.9	64.5	61.5	7.94	9.56
	20	73.2	72.2	71.1	70.0	68.7	67.3	65.7	63.9	61.8	59.3	56.3	6.47	8.09
	22	68.9	67.9	66.8	65.7	64.4	63.0	61.4	59.6	57.5	55.0	52.0	5.46	6.97
32.76	16	87.6	86.5	85.4	84.1	82.8	81.3	79.6	77.7	75.5	72.9	69.8	9.79	11.41
	18	81.1	80.1	78.9	77.7	76.3	74.8	73.2	71.3	69.1	66.5	63.3	7.89	9.58
	20	75.7	74.7	73.6	72.3	71.0	69.5	67.8	65.9	63.7	61.1	57.9	6.45	8.06
	22	71.3	70.2	69.1	67.9	66.5	65.0	63.3	61.4	59.2	56.7	53.5	5.46	6.97
34.48	16	90.5	89.4	88.2	86.9	85.5	83.9	82.1	80.1	77.8	75.1	71.7	9.87	11.50
	18	83.8	82.7	81.5	80.2	78.8	77.2	75.4	73.4	71.1	68.4	65.1	7.86	9.59
	20	78.2	77.1	75.9	74.6	73.2	71.6	69.8	67.8	65.5	62.8	59.4	6.43	8.04
	22	73.6	72.5	71.3	70.0	68.6	67.0	65.3	63.3	60.9	58.2	54.9	5.46	6.97
36.20	16	93.5	92.3	91.0	89.7	88.2	86.5	84.7	82.6	80.1	77.3	73.8	9.93	11.60
	18	86.5	85.3	84.0	82.7	81.2	79.5	77.7	75.6	73.1	70.3	66.8	7.83	9.56
	20	80.7	79.5	78.3	76.9	75.4	73.7	71.9	69.9	67.4	64.5	61.0	6.43	8.04
	22	75.9	74.7	73.5	72.1	70.6	68.9	67.1	65.0	62.6	59.7	56.2	5.46	6.98

TABLE 363

Process Times (B) at Retort Temperature of 250°F for Conduction-Heating Foods in 211 x 300 Can

f_h	z	INITIAL FOOD TEMPERATURE (T_{ih}) 100	110	120	130	140	150	160	170	180	190	200	Equivalent F_c^{18}	F_s^{18}
	16	51.9	51.0	50.1	49.1	48.0	46.8	45.4	43.9	42.2	40.3	37.9	8.30	10.49
29.31	18	50.4	49.5	48.5	47.5	46.4	45.2	43.9	42.4	40.7	38.7	36.4	7.34	9.51
	20	48.8	47.9	47.0	46.0	44.9	43.6	42.3	40.8	39.1	37.1	34.8	6.38	8.55
	22	47.4	46.6	45.6	44.6	43.5	42.3	40.9	39.4	37.7	35.8	33.4	5.62	7.75
	16	54.3	53.3	52.3	51.2	50.1	48.8	47.4	45.8	44.0	41.9	39.4	8.33	10.55
31.03	18	52.6	51.7	50.7	49.6	48.4	47.1	45.7	44.1	42.3	40.3	37.8	7.31	9.52
	20	51.0	50.0	49.0	47.9	46.8	45.5	44.1	42.5	40.7	38.6	36.1	6.36	8.54
	22	49.5	48.6	47.6	46.5	45.3	44.0	42.6	41.0	39.2	37.1	34.7	5.56	7.71
	16	56.6	55.6	54.5	53.4	52.1	50.8	49.3	47.6	45.7	43.5	40.9	8.36	10.61
32.76	18	54.8	53.8	52.8	51.7	50.4	49.1	47.6	45.9	44.0	41.8	39.2	7.29	9.53
	20	53.1	52.1	51.0	49.9	48.7	47.3	45.8	44.1	42.2	40.0	37.5	6.32	8.52
	22	51.5	50.5	49.5	48.4	47.1	45.8	44.3	42.6	40.7	38.5	35.9	5.51	7.68
	16	58.8	57.8	56.7	55.5	54.2	52.7	51.2	49.4	47.4	45.1	42.4	8.35	10.63
34.48	18	57.0	56.0	54.9	53.7	52.4	50.9	49.4	47.6	45.6	43.3	40.5	7.27	9.53
	20	55.2	54.1	53.0	51.8	50.5	49.1	47.5	45.7	43.7	41.4	38.7	6.26	8.48
	22	53.5	52.5	51.4	50.2	48.9	47.4	45.9	44.1	42.1	39.8	37.1	5.44	7.63
	16	61.0	59.9	58.8	57.5	56.2	54.7	53.0	51.1	49.0	46.6	43.8	8.32	10.63
36.20	18	59.1	58.1	56.9	55.6	54.3	52.8	51.1	49.3	47.2	44.7	41.9	7.25	9.53
	20	57.2	56.1	54.9	53.7	52.3	50.8	49.2	47.3	45.2	42.8	39.9	6.21	8.45
	22	55.5	54.4	53.2	52.0	50.6	49.1	47.4	45.6	43.5	41.1	38.2	5.36	7.58

TABLE 364

Process Times (B) at Retort Temperature of 260°F for Conduction-Heating Foods in 211 x 300 Can

f_h	z	INITIAL FOOD TEMPERATURE (T_{ih})											Equivalent	
		100	110	120	130	140	150	160	170	180	190	200	F_c^{18}	F_s^{18}
	16	39.9	39.1	38.2	37.3	36.3	35.2	34.0	32.6	31.1	29.4	27.5	7.54	10.23
29.31	18	39.3	38.5	37.6	36.6	35.6	34.5	33.3	32.0	30.5	28.8	26.8	6.87	9.52
	20	38.8	37.9	37.1	36.1	35.1	34.0	32.8	31.4	29.9	28.2	26.3	6.33	8.95
	22	38.2	37.4	36.5	35.6	34.5	33.4	32.2	30.9	29.4	27.7	25.7	5.80	8.39
	16	41.9	41.0	40.1	39.1	38.0	36.9	35.6	34.1	32.6	30.8	28.7	7.59	10.29
31.03	18	41.2	40.3	39.4	38.4	37.3	36.1	34.9	33.4	31.9	30.1	28.0	6.85	9.52
	20	40.6	39.7	38.8	37.8	36.7	35.5	34.3	32.8	31.3	29.5	27.4	6.27	8.91
	22	40.0	39.1	38.2	37.2	36.1	35.0	33.7	32.3	30.7	28.9	26.8	5.75	8.35
	16	43.8	42.9	41.9	40.9	39.8	38.5	37.2	35.7	34.0	32.1	29.9	7.61	10.33
32.76	18	43.1	42.2	41.2	40.1	39.0	37.8	36.4	34.9	33.2	31.3	29.1	6.84	9.52
	20	42.4	41.5	40.5	39.4	38.3	37.1	35.7	34.2	32.5	30.6	28.4	6.21	8.86
	22	41.8	40.9	39.9	38.8	37.7	36.5	35.1	33.6	31.9	30.0	27.8	5.68	8.30
	16	45.8	44.8	43.8	42.7	41.5	40.2	38.8	37.2	35.4	33.4	31.1	7.64	10.38
34.48	18	45.0	44.0	43.0	41.8	40.6	39.3	37.9	36.3	34.6	32.6	30.3	6.82	9.52
	20	44.2	43.3	42.2	41.1	39.9	38.6	37.2	35.6	33.9	31.9	29.6	6.20	8.86
	22	43.6	42.6	41.6	40.5	39.3	37.9	36.5	34.9	33.2	31.2	28.9	5.61	8.23
	16	47.7	46.7	45.6	44.5	43.2	41.8	40.3	38.7	36.8	34.7	32.3	7.67	10.43
36.20	18	46.8	45.8	44.7	43.5	42.3	40.9	39.4	37.8	35.9	33.8	31.4	6.81	9.52
	20	46.1	45.0	44.0	42.8	41.5	40.2	38.7	37.0	35.2	33.1	30.6	6.16	8.83
	22	45.3	44.3	43.2	42.0	40.8	39.4	37.9	36.2	34.4	32.3	29.9	5.53	8.16

TABLE 365

Process Times (B) at Retort Temperature of 230°F for Conduction-Heating Foods in 211 x 304 Can

f_h	z	INITIAL FOOD TEMPERATURE (T_{ih})											Equivalent	
		100	110	120	130	140	150	160	170	180	190	200	F_c^{18}	F_s^{18}
	16	206.7	205.6	204.4	203.1	201.7	200.2	198.4	196.3	193.9	190.9	187.0	12.30	13.25
30.79	18	164.4	163.3	162.1	160.9	159.4	157.9	156.1	154.0	151.6	148.6	144.8	8.78	9.58
	20	134.3	133.2	132.1	130.8	129.4	127.8	126.0	124.0	121.5	118.5	114.7	6.53	7.38
	22	114.8	113.7	112.5	111.2	109.8	108.3	106.5	104.4	102.0	99.0	95.1	5.06	5.89
	16	211.3	210.1	208.9	207.5	206.0	204.4	202.5	200.3	197.7	194.6	190.5	12.30	13.27
32.60	18	166.3	165.2	163.9	162.6	161.1	159.4	157.5	155.3	152.8	149.6	145.5	8.77	9.57
	20	136.8	135.6	134.4	133.1	131.6	129.9	128.0	125.8	123.3	120.1	116.0	6.53	7.37
	22	117.1	116.0	114.8	113.4	111.9	110.2	108.4	106.2	103.6	100.4	96.4	5.05	5.86
	16	215.4	214.3	212.9	211.5	210.0	208.2	206.2	203.9	201.2	197.8	103.5	12.31	13.28
34.41	18	168.1	166.9	165.6	164.1	162.6	160.8	158.8	156.5	153.8	150.4	146.1	8.74	9.61
	20	138.9	137.7	136.4	135.0	133.4	131.7	129.7	127.4	124.6	121.3	117.0	6.49	7.38
	22	119.4	118.2	116.9	115.5	113.9	112.1	110.2	107.8	105.1	101.8	97.5	4.99	5.88
	16	219.2	218.0	216.6	215.1	213.5	211.6	209.5	207.1	204.2	200.7	196.2	12.31	13.29
36.22	18	169.4	168.1	166.8	165.3	163.6	161.8	159.7	157.2	154.4	150.9	146.3	8.57	9.59
	20	141.4	140.2	138.8	137.3	135.7	133.8	131.7	129.3	126.4	122.9	118.4	6.44	7.43
	22	122.0	120.8	119.4	117.9	116.2	114.4	112.3	109.9	107.0	103.5	99.0	4.97	5.90
	16	222.7	221.4	219.9	218.3	216.6	214.7	212.5	209.9	206.9	203.2	198.5	12.31	13.31
38.03	18	172.1	170.8	169.4	167.8	166.1	164.1	161.9	159.4	156.3	152.7	147.9	8.54	9.56
	20	143.5	142.1	140.7	139.1	137.4	135.4	133.2	130.7	127.7	124.0	119.2	6.38	7.35
	22	124.2	122.9	121.4	119.8	118.1	116.2	114.0	111.4	108.4	104.7	100.0	4.94	5.85

TABLE 366

Process Times (B) at Retort Temperature of 240°F for Conduction-Heating Foods in 211 x 304 Can

f_h	z	INITIAL FOOD TEMPERATURE (T_{ih})											Equivalent	
		100	110	120	130	140	150	160	170	180	190	200	F_c^{18}	F_s^{18}
30.79	16	84.9	83.9	82.8	81.7	80.4	79.0	77.4	75.6	73.5	71.1	68.1	9.88	11.45
	18	78.1	77.1	76.0	74.9	73.6	72.2	70.6	68.8	66.8	64.3	61.4	7.99	9.60
	20	73.0	72.0	71.0	69.8	68.5	67.1	65.6	63.8	61.7	59.3	56.3	6.53	8.14
	22	68.8	67.8	66.7	65.6	64.3	62.9	61.3	59.5	57.4	55.0	52.0	5.50	7.02
32.60	16	87.6	86.6	85.4	84.2	82.9	81.4	79.7	77.8	75.6	73.0	69.9	9.87	11.48
	18	81.1	80.0	78.9	77.7	76.3	74.8	73.2	71.3	69.1	66.5	63.3	7.96	9.63
	20	75.7	74.7	73.5	72.3	71.0	69.5	67.8	65.9	63.7	61.1	58.0	6.50	8.12
	22	71.3	70.2	69.1	67.9	66.5	65.0	63.3	61.5	59.3	56.7	53.5	5.50	7.01
34.41	16	90.6	89.5	88.3	87.0	85.6	84.0	82.2	80.2	77.9	75.2	71.9	9.92	11.55
	18	83.9	82.8	81.6	80.3	78.9	77.3	75.6	73.6	71.3	68.5	65.2	7.92	9.64
	20	78.3	77.2	76.0	74.7	73.3	71.7	70.0	68.0	65.7	62.9	59.6	6.48	8.10
	22	73.7	72.6	71.4	70.1	68.7	67.1	65.4	63.4	61.1	58.3	55.0	5.50	7.01
36.22	16	93.7	92.5	91.3	89.9	88.4	86.8	84.9	82.8	80.4	77.5	74.0	10.00	11.67
	18	86.7	85.5	84.3	82.9	81.4	79.8	77.9	75.8	73.4	70.5	67.0	7.88	9.62
	20	80.9	79.7	78.5	77.1	75.6	74.0	72.1	70.1	67.6	64.7	61.2	6.47	8.09
	22	76.1	75.0	73.7	72.3	70.8	69.2	67.3	65.2	62.8	59.9	56.4	5.50	7.02
38.03	16	96.8	95.6	94.2	92.8	91.2	89.5	87.5	85.3	82.8	79.8	76.1	9.97	11.71
	18	89.4	88.2	86.9	85.4	83.9	82.1	80.2	78.0	75.4	72.4	68.7	7.86	9.60
	20	83.4	82.2	80.9	79.5	77.9	76.1	74.2	72.0	69.5	66.4	62.8	6.47	8.09
	22	78.4	77.2	75.9	74.4	72.9	71.1	69.2	67.0	64.4	61.4	57.7	5.50	7.02

TABLE 367

Process Times (B) at Retort Temperature of 250°F for Conduction-Heating Foods in 211 x 304 Can

f_h	z	INITIAL FOOD TEMPERATURE (T_{ih})											Equivalent	
		100	110	120	130	140	150	160	170	180	190	200	F_c^{18}	F_s^{18}
	16	54.0	53.1	52.1	51.0	49.9	48.6	47.2	45.6	43.8	41.8	39.3	8.38	10.60
30.79	18	52.4	51.5	50.5	49.4	48.2	47.0	45.6	44.0	42.2	40.1	37.7	7.37	9.57
	20	50.7	49.8	48.8	47.8	46.6	45.3	43.9	42.3	40.6	38.5	36.1	6.41	8.59
	22	49.3	48.4	47.4	46.3	45.1	43.9	42.5	40.9	39.1	37.0	34.6	5.61	7.76
	16	56.4	55.5	54.4	53.3	52.1	50.7	49.2	47.5	45.7	43.5	40.9	8.41	10.66
32.60	18	54.7	53.7	52.7	51.6	50.3	49.0	47.5	45.8	43.9	41.8	39.2	7.35	9.59
	20	53.0	52.0	51.0	49.8	48.6	47.2	45.8	44.1	42.2	40.0	37.4	6.38	8.58
	22	51.4	50.5	49.4	48.3	47.0	45.7	44.2	42.5	40.6	38.5	35.9	5.56	7.73
	16	58.8	57.8	56.7	55.5	54.2	52.8	51.2	49.4	47.4	45.1	42.4	8.42	10.70
34.41	18	57.0	56.0	54.9	53.7	52.4	51.0	49.4	47.6	45.6	43.3	40.6	7.33	9.60
	20	55.2	54.1	53.0	51.8	50.5	49.1	47.5	45.8	43.8	41.5	38.8	6.32	8.54
	22	53.5	52.5	51.4	50.2	48.9	47.5	45.9	44.1	42.2	39.8	37.1	5.49	7.68
	16	61.2	60.1	58.9	57.7	56.3	54.8	53.1	51.3	49.2	46.8	43.9	8.39	10.70
36.22	18	59.3	58.2	57.0	55.8	54.4	52.9	51.2	49.4	47.3	44.9	42.0	7.31	9.59
	20	57.3	56.2	55.1	53.8	52.4	50.9	49.3	47.4	45.3	42.9	40.0	6.26	8.51
	22	55.6	54.5	53.4	52.1	50.7	49.2	47.6	45.7	43.6	41.2	38.3	5.41	7.63
	16	63.5	62.4	61.2	59.8	58.4	56.8	55.1	53.1	50.9	48.4	45.4	8.39	10.73
38.03	18	61.5	60.4	59.2	57.9	56.4	54.8	53.1	51.2	48.9	46.4	43.4	7.28	9.58
	20	59.5	58.4	57.1	55.8	54.4	52.8	51.1	49.1	46.9	44.4	41.3	6.23	8.49
	22	57.7	56.5	55.3	54.0	52.5	51.0	49.2	47.3	45.1	42.5	39.5	5.36	7.59

TABLE 368

Process Times (B) at Retort Temperature of 260°F for Conduction-Heating Foods in 211 x 304 Can

f_h	z	INITIAL FOOD TEMPERATURE (T_{ih})											Equivalent	
		100	110	120	130	140	150	160	170	180	190	200	F_c^{18}	F_s^{18}
30.79	16	41.7	40.8	39.9	38.9	37.8	36.7	35.4	34.0	32.4	30.6	28.6	7.63	10.34
	18	41.0	40.1	39.2	38.2	37.1	36.0	34.7	33.3	31.7	29.9	27.9	6.91	9.58
	20	40.4	39.5	38.6	37.6	36.6	35.4	34.1	32.7	31.1	29.3	27.3	6.33	8.97
	22	39.8	39.0	38.0	37.0	36.0	34.8	33.5	32.1	30.6	28.8	26.7	5.81	8.41
32.60	16	43.7	42.8	41.8	40.8	39.6	38.4	37.1	35.6	33.9	32.0	29.8	7.67	10.39
	18	43.0	42.1	41.1	40.0	38.9	37.7	36.3	34.8	33.2	31.3	29.1	6.89	9.58
	20	42.3	41.4	40.4	39.4	38.2	37.0	35.7	34.2	32.5	30.6	28.4	6.27	8.92
	22	41.7	40.8	39.8	38.8	37.6	36.4	35.0	33.6	31.9	30.0	27.8	5.75	8.36
34.41	16	45.8	44.8	43.8	42.7	41.5	40.2	38.8	37.2	35.4	33.4	31.1	7.70	10.44
	18	44.9	44.0	42.9	41.8	40.6	39.3	37.9	36.3	34.6	32.6	30.3	6.88	9.58
	20	44.2	43.3	42.2	41.1	39.9	38.6	37.2	35.6	33.9	31.9	29.6	6.25	8.91
	22	43.6	42.6	41.6	40.5	39.3	38.0	36.5	35.0	33.2	31.2	28.9	5.67	8.29
36.22	16	47.8	46.8	45.7	44.5	43.3	41.9	40.4	38.8	36.9	34.8	32.4	7.73	10.49
	18	46.9	45.9	44.8	43.6	42.4	41.0	39.5	37.8	36.0	33.9	31.5	6.87	9.58
	20	46.1	45.1	44.0	42.9	41.6	40.2	38.7	37.1	35.2	33.1	30.7	6.21	8.89
	22	45.4	44.4	43.3	42.1	40.9	39.5	38.0	36.3	34.5	32.4	30.0	5.59	8.22
38.03	16	49.8	48.8	47.6	46.4	45.1	43.6	42.1	40.3	38.4	36.2	33.6	7.76	10.53
	18	48.8	47.8	46.6	45.4	44.1	42.6	41.1	39.3	37.4	35.2	32.6	6.86	9.58
	20	48.0	47.0	45.8	44.6	43.3	41.8	40.3	38.5	36.6	34.4	31.8	6.17	8.86
	22	47.2	46.2	45.0	43.8	42.5	41.0	39.5	37.7	35.8	33.6	31.0	5.54	8.17

TABLE 369

Process Times (B) at Retort Temperature of 230°F for Conduction-Heating Foods in 211 x 306 Can

f_h	z	INITIAL FOOD TEMPERATURE (T_{ih})											Equivalent	
		100	110	120	130	140	150	160	170	180	190	200	F_c^{18}	F_s^{18}
31.44	16	208.7	207.6	206.4	205.1	203.7	202.1	200.3	198.2	195.7	192.6	188.7	12.34	13.30
	18	165.5	164.4	163.2	161.9	160.5	158.9	157.0	154.9	152.4	149.4	145.5	8.81	9.60
	20	135.5	134.4	133.2	131.9	130.5	128.9	127.0	124.9	122.4	119.4	115.5	6.55	7.40
	22	115.8	114.7	113.5	112.2	110.8	109.2	107.4	105.3	102.8	99.7	95.8	5.07	5.89
33.29	16	213.3	212.1	210.9	209.5	208.0	206.3	204.3	202.1	199.5	196.2	192.1	12.34	13.31
	18	167.3	166.2	164.9	163.5	162.0	160.3	158.4	156.1	153.5	150.3	146.1	8.80	9.60
	20	137.9	136.8	135.5	134.1	132.6	130.9	129.0	126.7	124.1	120.9	116.7	6.55	7.39
	22	118.2	117.0	115.8	114.4	112.9	111.2	109.3	107.0	104.4	101.2	97.0	5.04	5.89
35.14	16	217.4	216.2	214.9	213.4	211.8	210.0	208.0	205.6	202.9	199.4	105.1	12.34	13.32
	18	169.0	167.8	166.4	165.0	163.4	161.6	159.6	157.2	154.4	151.0	146.6	8.70	9.66
	20	140.4	139.2	137.9	136.4	134.8	133.0	131.0	128.6	125.8	122.4	118.0	6.51	7.43
	22	120.7	119.5	118.2	116.7	115.1	113.3	111.3	108.9	106.1	102.7	98.4	5.00	5.92
36.99	16	221.2	219.9	218.5	217.0	215.3	213.4	211.2	208.8	205.8	202.2	197.6	12.35	13.34
	18	170.7	169.4	168.0	166.5	164.8	162.9	160.7	158.3	155.3	151.8	147.1	8.56	9.59
	20	142.6	141.3	139.9	138.4	136.7	134.8	136.7	130.2	127.3	123.7	119.0	6.44	7.42
	22	123.2	121.9	120.5	119.0	117.3	115.4	113.3	110.8	107.8	104.3	99.6	4.98	5.90
38.84	16	224.6	223.2	221.7	220.1	218.4	216.4	214.1	211.5	208.4	204.7	1-9.8	12.35	13.35
	18	173.8	172.4	170.9	169.3	167.6	165.6	163.3	160.7	157.6	153.9	149.0	8.57	9.59
	20	144.8	143.5	142.0	140.4	138.6	136.6	134.4	131.8	128.7	125.0	120.1	6.39	7.37
	22	125.3	124.0	122.5	120.9	119.1	117.1	114.9	112.3	109.2	105.5	100.6	4.93	5.85

TABLE 370

Process Times (B) at Retort Temperature of 240°F for Conduction-Heating Foods in 211 x 306 Can

f_h	z	INITIAL FOOD TEMPERATURE (T_{ih})											Equivalent	
		100	110	120	130	140	150	160	170	180	190	200	F_c^{18}	F_s^{18}
31.44	16	86.0	85.0	83.9	82.7	81.4	80.0	78.4	76.5	74.4	71.9	68.9	9.91	11.50
	18	79.3	78.3	77.2	76.0	74.7	73.3	71.7	69.8	67.7	65.2	62.2	8.02	9.65
	20	74.1	73.1	72.0	70.8	69.5	68.1	66.5	64.6	62.5	60.0	57.0	6.54	8.16
	22	69.8	68.7	67.7	66.5	65.2	63.7	62.1	60.3	58.2	55.7	52.7	5.52	7.03
33.29	16	88.8	87.7	86.5	85.3	83.9	82.4	80.7	78.7	76.5	73.9	70.7	9.89	11.51
	18	82.3	81.2	80.0	78.8	77.4	75.9	74.2	72.2	70.0	67.4	64.1	7.97	9.66
	20	76.8	75.7	74.6	73.3	71.9	70.4	68.7	66.8	64.6	61.9	58.7	6.52	8.13
	22	72.3	71.2	70.1	68.8	67.4	65.9	64.2	62.3	60.1	57.4	54.2	5.52	7.03
35.14	16	91.9	90.8	89.6	88.3	86.8	85.2	83.3	81.4	79.0	76.2	72.8	9.98	11.63
	18	85.1	84.0	82.8	81.5	80.0	78.4	76.6	74.6	72.2	69.4	66.0	7.93	9.67
	20	79.4	78.3	77.1	75.8	74.3	72.7	70.9	68.9	66.5	63.7	60.3	6.50	8.11
	22	74.8	73.7	72.4	71.1	69.7	68.1	66.3	64.2	61.9	59.1	55.7	5.52	7.04
36.99	16	95.1	93.9	92.7	91.3	89.7	88.0	86.1	84.0	81.5	78.6	75.0	10.03	11.73
	18	88.0	86.8	85.5	84.1	82.6	80.9	79.0	76.8	74.4	71.4	67.8	7.90	9.64
	20	82.1	80.9	79.6	78.2	76.7	75.0	73.1	71.0	68.5	65.5	62.0	6.50	8.12
	22	77.2	76.0	74.7	73.3	71.8	70.1	68.2	66.1	63.6	60.7	57.1	5.52	7.04
38.84	16	98.2	97.0	95.6	94.2	92.5	90.8	88.8	86.5	83.9	80.9	77.1	9.99	11.75
	18	90.7	89.5	88.1	86.7	85.0	83.3	81.3	79.0	76.4	73.4	69.6	7.87	9.62
	20	84.7	83.4	82.1	80.6	79.0	77.2	75.2	73.0	70.4	67.3	63.5	6.50	8.12
	22	79.5	78.2	76.9	75.4	73.8	72.0	70.0	67.8	65.2	62.1	58.4	5.51	7.03

TABLE 371

Process Times (B) at Retort Temperature of 250°F for Conduction-Heating Foods in 211 x 306 Can

f_h	z	INITIAL FOOD TEMPERATURE (T_{ih}) 100	110	120	130	140	150	160	170	180	190	200	Equivalent F_c^{18}	F_s^{18}
31.44	16	54.9	54.0	53.0	51.9	50.7	49.4	48.0	46.4	44.5	42.4	39.9	8.42	10.65
	18	53.3	52.3	51.3	50.2	49.0	47.7	46.3	44.7	42.9	40.8	38.3	7.39	9.61
	20	51.6	50.7	49.6	48.5	47.4	46.1	44.6	43.0	41.2	39.1	36.6	6.43	8.62
	22	50.1	49.2	48.2	47.1	45.9	44.6	43.1	41.5	39.7	37.6	35.1	5.61	7.77
33.29	16	57.4	56.4	55.3	54.2	52.9	51.5	50.0	48.3	46.4	44.2	41.5	8.45	10.71
	18	55.6	54.6	53.6	52.4	51.2	49.8	48.3	46.6	44.6	42.4	39.8	7.37	9.62
	20	53.9	52.9	51.8	50.6	49.4	48.0	46.5	44.8	42.9	40.6	38.0	6.38	8.59
	22	52.3	51.3	50.2	49.1	47.8	46.4	44.9	43.2	41.3	39.0	36.4	5.56	7.74
35.14	16	59.8	58.8	57.6	56.4	55.1	53.6	52.0	50.2	48.2	45.8	43.1	8.44	10.73
	18	58.0	56.9	55.8	54.6	53.2	51.8	50.2	48.4	46.3	44.0	41.2	7.35	9.62
	20	56.1	55.0	53.9	52.7	51.4	49.9	48.3	46.5	44.5	42.1	39.3	6.32	8.55
	22	54.4	53.4	52.2	51.0	49.7	48.2	46.6	44.8	42.8	40.4	37.7	5.48	7.69
36.99	16	62.2	61.1	59.9	58.6	57.2	55.7	54.0	52.1	50.0	47.5	44.6	8.42	10.73
	18	60.3	59.2	58.0	56.7	55.3	53.8	52.1	50.2	48.0	45.6	42.6	7.32	9.61
	20	58.3	57.2	56.0	54.7	53.3	51.8	50.1	48.2	46.0	43.6	40.6	6.27	8.52
	22	56.5	55.4	54.2	52.9	51.5	50.0	48.3	46.4	44.3	41.8	38.9	5.40	7.63
38.84	16	64.6	63.5	62.2	60.9	59.4	57.8	56.0	54.0	51.8	49.2	46.1	8.43	10.78
	18	62.6	61.4	60.2	58.8	57.4	55.7	54.0	52.0	49.7	47.1	44.1	7.30	9.61
	20	60.5	59.3	58.1	56.7	55.3	53.7	51.9	49.9	47.6	45.0	42.0	6.23	8.51
	22	58.6	57.5	56.2	54.9	53.4	51.8	50.0	48.0	45.8	43.2	40.1	5.36	7.59

TABLE 372

Process Times (B) at Retort Temperature of 260°F for Conduction-Heating Foods in 211 x 306 Can

f_h	z	INITIAL FOOD TEMPERATURE (T_{ih})											Equivalent	
		100	110	120	130	140	150	160	170	180	190	200	F_c^{18}	F_s^{18}
	16	42.4	41.6	40.6	39.6	38.5	37.3	36.0	34.6	33.0	31.2	29.0	7.68	10.39
31.44	18	41.7	40.8	39.9	38.9	37.8	36.6	35.3	33.9	32.3	30.4	28.3	6.93	9.61
	20	41.1	40.2	39.3	38.3	37.2	36.0	34.7	33.3	31.7	29.8	27.7	6.34	8.98
	22	40.5	39.6	38.7	37.7	36.6	35.4	34.1	32.7	31.1	29.2	27.1	5.81	8.42
	16	44.5	43.6	42.6	41.5	40.4	39.1	37.7	36.2	34.5	32.6	30.3	7.70	10.43
33.29	18	43.8	42.8	41.8	40.7	39.6	38.3	37.0	35.4	33.7	31.8	29.6	6.92	9.61
	20	43.1	42.1	41.1	40.1	38.9	37.6	36.3	34.7	33.0	31.1	28.9	6.28	8.93
	22	42.4	41.5	40.5	39.4	38.3	37.0	35.6	34.1	32.4	30.5	28.3	5.74	8.36
	16	46.6	45.6	44.6	43.5	42.2	40.9	39.4	37.8	36.0	34.0	31.7	7.74	10.48
35.14	18	45.8	44.8	43.7	42.6	41.4	40.0	38.6	37.0	35.2	33.1	30.8	6.90	9.61
	20	45.0	44.0	43.0	41.9	40.6	39.3	37.9	36.2	34.4	32.4	30.1	6.26	8.93
	22	44.3	43.3	42.3	41.2	39.9	38.6	37.2	35.5	33.7	31.7	29.4	5.66	8.29
	16	48.7	47.7	46.6	45.4	44.1	42.7	41.1	39.5	37.6	35.4	32.9	7.77	10.53
36.99	18	47.7	46.7	45.6	44.4	43.1	41.7	40.2	38.5	36.6	34.5	32.0	6.89	9.61
	20	47.0	45.9	44.8	43.6	42.4	41.0	39.4	37.7	35.8	33.7	31.2	6.22	8.90
	22	46.2	45.1	44.0	42.8	41.6	40.2	38.6	36.9	35.1	32.9	30.4	5.58	8.21
	16	50.8	49.7	48.5	47.3	45.9	44.4	42.8	41.1	39.1	36.8	34.2	7.80	10.58
38.84	18	49.7	48.6	47.5	46.2	44.9	43.4	41.8	40.0	38.0	35.8	33.2	6.88	9.61
	20	48.9	47.8	46.7	45.4	44.1	42.6	41.0	39.2	37.2	35.0	32.4	6.18	8.87
	22	48.1	47.0	45.8	44.6	43.2	41.8	40.1	38.4	36.4	34.1	31.5	5.54	8.18

TABLE 373

Process Times (B) at Retort Temperature of 230°F for Conduction-Heating Foods in 211 x 400 Can

f_h	z	INITIAL FOOD TEMPERATURE (T_{ih})											Equivalent	
		100	110	120	130	140	150	160	170	180	190	200	F_c^{18}	F_s^{18}
	16	216.7	215.5	214.2	212.8	211.2	209.5	207.5	205.3	202.6	199.3	195.0	12.50	13.48
33.98	18	169.7	168.5	167.2	165.8	164.3	162.5	160.6	158.3	155.6	152.3	148.1	8.91	9.72
	20	140.0	138.9	137.6	136.2	134.6	132.9	130.9	128.6	125.9	122.7	118.4	6.64	7.48
	22	120.1	118.9	117.6	116.2	114.7	112.9	111.0	108.7	106.0	102.7	98.5	5.10	5.96
	16	221.1	219.8	218.5	217.0	215.3	213.5	211.4	209.0	206.1	202.7	198.2	12.51	13.50
35.98	18	171.5	170.3	168.9	167.4	165.8	164.0	161.9	159.5	156.6	153.1	148.6	8.78	9.79
	20	142.9	141.6	140.3	138.8	137.1	135.3	133.2	130.8	127.9	124.4	120.0	6.59	7.54
	22	122.9	121.7	120.3	118.8	117.2	115.3	113.2	110.8	108.0	104.5	100.0	5.07	6.00
	16	225.0	223.7	222.2	220.7	218.9	217.0	214.8	212.3	209.2	205.6	200.8	12.51	13.51
37.98	18	173.8	172.5	171.1	169.5	167.7	165.8	163.6	161.1	158.0	154.4	149.6	8.68	9.71
	20	145.1	143.8	142.3	140.7	139.0	137.1	134.9	132.3	129.3	125.6	120.9	6.51	7.50
	22	125.5	124.1	122.7	121.1	119.4	117.5	115.3	112.7	109.7	106.0	101.3	5.04	5.96
	16	228.5	227.2	225.6	224.0	222.2	220.1	217.8	215.1	212.0	208.1	203.1	12.51	13.52
39.98	18	177.1	175.7	174.2	172.5	170.7	168.6	166.3	163.6	160.5	156.6	151.6	8.68	9.71
	20	147.7	146.3	144.8	143.1	141.3	139.3	136.9	134.3	131.1	127.2	122.2	6.48	7.46
	22	127.7	126.3	124.8	123.2	121.3	119.3	117.0	114.3	111.1	107.3	102.3	4.97	5.92
	16	231.7	230.2	228.6	226.9	225.0	222.8	220.4	217.6	214.3	210.2	204.9	12.52	13.53
41.98	18	180.0	178.6	177.0	175.3	173.3	171.2	168.7	165.9	162.6	158.5	153.3	8.68	9.71
	20	150.4	148.9	147.3	145.6	143.7	141.5	139.1	136.3	133.0	128.9	123.6	6.47	7.45
	22	130.5	129.0	127.4	125.7	123.8	121.6	119.2	116.4	113.1	109.0	103.8	4.94	5.94

TABLE 374

Process Times (B) at Retort Temperature of 240°F for Conduction-Heating Foods in 211 x 400 Can

f_h	z	INITIAL FOOD TEMPERATURE (T_{ih})											Equivalent	
		100	110	120	130	140	150	160	170	180	190	200	F_c^{18}	F_s^{18}
	16	90.4	89.3	88.1	86.8	85.4	83.9	82.1	80.2	77.9	75.2	71.9	10.04	11.67
33.98	18	83.8	82.7	81.5	80.2	78.8	77.2	75.5	73.5	71.3	68.6	65.3	8.08	9.79
	20	78.2	77.1	75.9	74.7	73.3	71.7	70.0	68.0	65.7	63.0	59.7	6.61	8.23
	22	73.6	72.6	71.4	70.1	68.7	67.1	65.4	63.4	61.1	58.4	55.2	5.60	7.12
	16	93.8	92.7	91.4	90.1	88.6	86.9	85.1	83.0	80.6	77.8	74.3	10.15	11.81
35.98	18	86.9	85.7	84.5	83.1	81.6	80.0	78.1	76.1	73.6	70.8	67.3	8.04	9.79
	20	81.1	79.9	78.7	77.3	75.8	74.2	72.3	70.3	67.8	65.0	61.5	6.59	8.22
	22	76.3	75.2	73.9	72.6	71.1	69.4	67.6	65.5	63.1	60.2	56.7	5.60	7.13
	16	97.3	96.1	94.7	93.3	91.7	90.0	88.1	85.9	83.3	80.3	76.6	10.17	11.89
37.98	18	89.9	88.7	87.4	85.9	84.4	82.6	80.7	78.5	75.9	72.9	69.3	8.01	9.76
	20	83.9	82.7	81.4	79.9	78.4	76.6	74.7	72.5	69.9	66.9	63.3	6.59	8.22
	22	78.9	77.7	76.4	74.9	73.4	71.6	69.7	67.5	64.9	61.9	58.2	5.60	7.13
	16	100.6	99.3	97.9	96.4	94.8	92.9	90.9	88.6	85.9	82.7	78.8	10.12	11.91
39.98	18	92.9	91.6	90.2	88.7	87.1	85.2	83.2	80.9	78.2	75.0	71.2	7.99	9.74
	20	86.7	85.4	84.0	82.5	80.8	79.0	77.0	74.6	72.0	68.8	64.9	6.59	8.22
	22	81.3	80.0	78.7	77.1	75.5	73.7	71.6	69.3	66.6	63.5	59.6	5.59	7.12
	16	103.8	102.5	101.0	99.4	97.7	95.8	93.6	91.2	88.4	85.1	81.0	10.08	11.92
41.98	18	95.9	94.5	93.1	91.5	89.7	87.8	85.7	83.2	80.4	77.1	73.0	7.98	9.74
	20	89.3	88.0	86.5	84.9	83.2	81.3	79.1	76.7	73.9	70.6	66.5	6.59	8.22
	22	83.7	82.3	80.8	79.3	77.5	75.6	73.5	71.0	68.2	64.9	60.8	5.45	7.04

TABLE 375

Process Times (B) at Retort Temperature of 250°F for Conduction-Heating Foods in 211 x 400 Can

f_h	z	INITIAL FOOD TEMPERATURE (T_{ih})											Equivalent	
		100	110	120	130	140	150	160	170	180	190	200	F_c^{18}	F_s^{18}
	16	58.5	57.5	56.4	55.2	54.0	52.5	51.0	49.3	47.3	45.0	42.3	8.59	10.85
33.98	18	56.7	55.7	54.6	53.4	52.2	50.7	49.2	47.5	45.5	43.2	40.5	7.48	9.75
	20	54.9	53.9	52.8	51.6	50.3	48.9	47.4	45.6	43.7	41.4	38.7	6.47	8.70
	22	53.3	52.3	51.2	50.0	48.7	47.3	45.8	44.0	42.1	39.8	37.1	5.64	7.83
	16	61.1	60.1	58.9	57.6	56.3	54.8	53.2	51.3	49.2	46.8	44.0	8.57	10.87
35.98	18	59.2	58.2	57.0	55.8	54.4	52.9	51.3	49.4	47.3	44.9	42.1	7.46	9.74
	20	57.3	56.2	55.1	53.8	52.5	51.0	49.3	47.5	45.4	43.0	40.2	6.41	8.66
	22	55.6	54.5	53.4	52.1	50.8	49.3	47.6	45.8	43.7	41.3	38.4	5.55	7.77
	16	63.7	62.6	61.4	60.0	58.6	57.0	55.3	53.4	51.2	48.6	45.6	8.55	10.88
37.98	18	61.7	60.6	59.4	58.1	56.6	55.0	53.3	51.4	49.2	46.6	43.6	7.43	9.73
	20	59.7	58.6	57.3	56.0	54.6	53.0	51.3	49.3	47.1	44.6	41.6	6.36	8.63
	22	57.9	56.7	55.5	54.2	52.8	51.2	49.4	47.5	45.3	42.8	39.7	5.48	7.71
	16	66.3	65.1	63.8	62.4	60.9	59.3	57.5	55.4	53.1	50.4	47.2	8.56	10.93
39.98	18	64.2	63.0	61.7	60.4	58.8	57.2	55.4	53.3	51.0	48.3	45.2	7.41	9.73
	20	62.1	60.9	59.6	58.2	56.7	55.0	53.2	51.2	48.8	46.2	43.0	6.32	8.61
	22	60.2	59.0	57.7	56.3	54.8	53.1	51.3	49.3	46.9	44.3	41.1	5.42	7.67
	16	68.9	67.6	66.3	64.8	63.2	61.5	59.6	57.4	55.0	52.2	48.9	8.57	10.95
41.98	18	66.7	65.4	64.1	62.6	61.0	59.3	57.4	55.2	52.8	50.0	46.7	7.39	9.73
	20	64.4	63.2	61.8	60.4	58.8	57.0	55.1	53.0	50.5	47.7	44.4	6.27	8.58
	22	62.4	61.2	59.8	58.4	56.8	55.0	53.1	51.0	48.5	45.7	42.4	5.37	7.64

TABLE 376

Process Times (B) at Retort Temperature of 260°F for Conduction-Heating Foods in 211 x 400 Can

f_h	z	INITIAL FOOD TEMPERATURE (T_{ih})											Equivalent	
		100	110	120	130	140	150	160	170	180	190	200	F_c^{18}	F_s^{18}
	16	45.4	44.5	43.5	42.4	41.2	39.9	38.5	36.9	35.2	33.2	31.0	7.83	10.57
33.98	18	44.6	43.7	42.7	41.6	40.4	39.1	37.7	36.1	34.4	32.4	30.2	7.03	9.73
	20	43.9	43.0	41.9	40.9	39.7	38.4	37.0	35.4	33.7	31.7	29.4	6.38	9.04
	22	43.3	42.3	41.3	40.2	39.0	37.8	36.3	34.8	33.1	31.1	28.8	5.83	8.46
	16	47.7	46.7	45.6	44.4	43.2	41.8	40.3	38.7	36.9	34.8	32.4	7.87	10.63
35.98	18	46.8	45.8	44.7	43.5	42.3	40.9	39.4	37.8	36.0	33.9	31.5	7.01	9.73
	20	46.0	45.0	44.0	42.8	41.5	40.2	38.7	37.1	35.2	33.1	30.7	6.36	9.04
	22	45.3	44.3	43.2	42.1	40.8	39.5	38.0	36.3	34.5	32.4	30.0	5.74	8.38
	16	49.9	48.9	47.7	46.5	45.2	43.7	42.2	40.4	38.5	36.3	33.7	7.90	10.68
37.98	18	48.9	47.9	46.7	45.5	44.2	42.8	41.2	39.4	37.5	35.3	32.8	7.00	9.73
	20	48.1	47.1	45.9	44.7	43.4	42.0	40.4	38.7	36.7	34.5	32.0	6.31	9.01
	22	47.3	46.3	45.1	43.9	42.6	41.2	39.6	37.8	35.9	33.7	31.2	5.66	8.31
	16	52.1	51.0	49.8	48.5	47.2	45.6	44.0	42.2	40.1	37.8	35.1	7.93	10.73
39.98	18	51.1	50.0	48.8	47.5	46.1	44.6	42.9	41.1	39.0	36.7	34.0	6.99	9.73
	20	50.2	49.1	47.9	46.6	45.2	43.7	42.1	40.2	38.2	35.9	33.2	6.27	8.98
	22	49.4	48.3	47.1	45.8	44.4	42.9	41.2	39.4	37.3	35.0	32.3	5.62	8.27
	16	54.4	53.2	51.9	50.6	49.1	47.5	45.8	43.9	41.7	39.3	36.5	7.97	10.78
41.98	18	53.2	52.0	50.8	49.4	48.0	46.4	44.6	42.7	40.6	38.1	35.3	6.97	9.73
	20	52.3	51.1	49.9	48.5	47.0	45.5	43.7	41.8	39.7	37.2	34.4	6.24	8.95
	22	51.4	50.2	49.0	47.6	46.1	44.6	42.8	40.9	38.7	36.3	33.5	5.56	8.21

TABLE 377

Process Times (B) at Retort Temperature of 230°F for Conduction-Heating Foods in 211 x 413 Can

f_h	z	INITIAL FOOD TEMPERATURE (T_{ih}) 100	110	120	130	140	150	160	170	180	190	200	Equivalent F_c^{18}	F_s^{18}
	16	223.3	222.1	220.7	219.2	217.5	215.7	213.6	211.2	208.3	204.8	200.3	12.68	13.67
36.09	18	173.7	172.4	171.1	169.6	167.9	166.1	164.0	161.5	158.7	155.2	150.7	8.94	9.92
	20	144.2	143.0	141.6	140.1	138.5	136.6	134.5	132.1	129.3	125.8	121.3	6.69	7.63
	22	124.1	122.8	121.5	120.0	118.3	116.5	114.4	112.0	109.1	105.6	101.1	5.14	6.07
	16	227.5	226.2	224.8	223.2	221.4	219.5	217.3	214.7	211.7	208.0	203.2	12.68	12.68
38.22	18	175.8	174.4	173.0	171.4	169.7	167.7	165.5	162.9	159.9	156.2	151.4	8.80	9.84
	20	146.8	145.5	144.0	142.4	140.7	138.7	136.5	134.0	130.9	127.2	122.5	6.61	7.61
	22	126.9	125.6	124.1	122.5	120.8	118.8	116.6	114.1	111.0	107.3	102.6	5.11	6.05
	16	231.3	229.9	228.4	226.7	224.9	222.8	220.5	217.8	214.6	210.7	205.7	12.68	13.70
40.34	18	179.2	177.8	176.3	174.6	172.8	170.7	168.4	165.7	162.5	158.6	153.5	8.80	9.84
	20	149.5	148.1	146.6	144.9	143.0	141.0	138.6	135.9	132.8	128.8	123.8	6.57	7.56
	22	129.3	127.9	126.4	124.7	122.9	120.8	118.5	115.8	112.6	108.7	103.7	5.05	6.01
	16	234.7	233.2	231.6	229.9	227.9	225.7	223.3	220.4	217.1	213.0	207.7	12.69	13.71
42.46	18	182.4	180.9	179.3	177.6	175.6	173.5	171.0	168.2	164.8	160.7	155.4	8.81	9.84
	20	152.4	150.9	149.3	147.5	145.6	143.4	141.0	138.1	134.8	130.6	125.3	6.56	7.55
	22	132.2	130.7	129.1	127.4	125.4	123.2	120.8	117.9	114.6	110.5	105.2	5.02	6.01
	16	237.6	236.1	234.4	232.5	230.5	228.2	225.6	222.7	219.1	214.8	209.2	12.69	13.72
44.59	18	185.3	183.7	182.0	180.2	178.1	175.9	173.3	170.3	166.8	162.4	156.9	8.81	9.84
	20	155.5	153.9	152.3	150.4	148.4	146.1	143.5	140.5	137.0	132.7	127.1	6.53	7.58
	22	135.3	133.7	132.0	130.2	128.1	125.9	123.3	120.3	116.8	112.4	106.9	5.01	6.02

TABLE 378

Process Times (B) at Retort Temperature of 240°F for Conduction-Heating Foods in 211 x 413 Can

f_h	z	INITIAL FOOD TEMPERATURE (T_{ih})											Equivalent	
		100	110	120	130	140	150	160	170	180	190	200	F_c^{18}	F_s^{18}
	16	94.5	93.4	92.1	90.7	89.3	87.6	85.8	83.7	81.2	78.4	74.9	10.28	11.94
36.09	18	87.5	86.4	85.1	83.7	82.3	80.6	78.8	76.7	74.2	71.4	67.9	8.17	9.93
	20	81.7	80.5	79.3	77.9	76.4	74.8	72.9	70.8	68.4	65.6	62.1	6.69	8.33
	22	76.9	75.7	74.5	73.1	71.6	70.0	68.1	66.0	63.6	60.8	57.3	5.68	7.22
	16	98.2	97.0	95.6	94.2	92.6	90.8	88.9	86.7	84.1	81.1	77.4	10.32	12.05
38.22	18	90.8	89.5	88.2	86.8	85.2	83.4	81.5	79.3	76.7	73.7	70.0	8.13	9.89
	20	84.7	83.5	82.2	80.7	79.1	77.4	75.4	73.2	70.7	67.6	63.9	6.69	8.33
	22	79.7	78.4	77.1	75.7	74.1	72.3	70.4	68.2	65.6	62.6	58.9	5.69	7.23
	16	101.7	100.4	99.0	97.5	95.8	94.0	91.9	89.6	86.9	83.7	79.8	10.28	12.07
40.34	18	93.9	92.6	91.2	89.7	88.0	86.2	84.1	81.8	79.1	75.9	72.0	8.11	9.87
	20	87.7	86.4	85.0	83.4	81.8	79.9	77.9	75.5	72.8	69.6	65.7	6.69	8.33
	22	82.3	81.0	79.6	78.1	76.4	74.5	72.5	70.1	67.4	64.3	60.3	5.68	7.22
	16	105.2	103.8	102.3	100.7	99.0	97.0	94.8	92.4	89.5	86.2	82.1	10.24	12.09
42.46	18	97.1	95.7	94.3	92.7	90.9	89.0	86.8	84.3	78.1	74.0	74.0	8.11	9.87
	20	90.5	89.1	87.7	86.1	84.3	82.4	80.2	77.7	74.9	71.5	67.4	6.69	8.33
	22	84.8	83.4	81.9	80.3	78.6	76.6	74.4	72.0	69.1	65.8	61.7	5.55	7.14
	16	108.5	107.1	105.6	103.9	102.0	100.0	97.7	95.1	92.1	88.6	84.3	10.21	12.11
44.59	18	100.2	98.8	97.2	95.5	93.7	91.6	89.4	86.8	83.8	80.3	75.9	8.10	9.87
	20	93.2	91.8	90.2	88.5	86.7	84.6	82.4	79.8	76.8	73.3	68.9	6.68	8.32
	22	87.2	85.7	84.2	82.5	80.6	78.6	76.3	73.7	70.7	67.2	62.9	5.39	7.05

TABLE 379

Process Times (B) at Retort Temperature of 250°F for Conduction-Heating Foods in 211 x 413 Can

f_h	z	INITIAL FOOD TEMPERATURE (T_{ih}) 100	110	120	130	140	150	160	170	180	190	200	Equivalent F_c^{18}	F_s^{18}
	16	61.5	60.4	59.3	58.0	56.7	55.2	53.5	51.7	49.6	47.2	44.3	8.71	11.02
36.09	18	59.6	58.5	57.4	56.1	54.8	53.3	51.6	49.8	47.7	45.3	42.4	7.58	9.88
	20	57.7	56.6	55.4	54.2	52.8	51.3	49.7	47.8	45.7	43.3	40.5	6.53	8.78
	22	56.0	54.9	53.7	52.5	51.1	49.6	48.0	46.1	44.0	41.6	38.7	5.66	7.88
	16	64.3	63.1	61.9	60.6	59.1	57.5	55.8	53.8	51.6	49.1	46.0	8.68	11.02
38.22	18	62.3	61.1	59.9	58.6	57.1	55.5	53.8	51.8	49.6	47.0	44.0	7.56	9.87
	20	60.2	59.1	57.8	56.5	55.1	53.5	51.7	49.8	47.6	45.0	42.0	6.47	8.74
	22	58.4	57.2	56.0	54.7	53.2	51.6	49.9	47.9	45.7	43.2	40.1	5.57	7.82
	16	67.0	65.8	64.5	63.1	61.6	59.9	58.1	56.0	53.7	51.0	47.8	8.70	11.07
40.34	18	64.9	63.7	62.4	61.0	59.5	57.8	56.0	53.9	51.6	48.9	45.7	7.53	9.86
	20	62.7	61.5	60.2	58.8	57.3	55.6	53.8	51.7	49.4	46.7	43.5	6.43	8.72
	22	60.8	59.6	58.3	56.9	55.4	53.7	51.9	49.8	47.5	44.8	41.6	5.52	7.78
	16	69.8	68.5	67.1	65.6	64.0	62.3	60.3	58.2	55.7	52.9	49.5	8.71	11.10
42.46	18	67.5	66.3	64.9	63.4	61.8	60.1	58.1	55.9	53.5	50.6	47.3	7.51	9.86
	20	65.3	64.0	62.6	61.1	59.5	57.8	55.8	53.7	51.2	48.4	45.0	6.38	8.70
	22	63.2	62.0	60.6	59.1	57.5	55.7	53.8	51.6	49.2	46.3	43.0	5.46	7.74
	16	72.4	71.1	69.7	68.1	66.4	64.6	62.6	60.3	57.7	54.7	51.2	8.71	11.12
44.59	18	70.1	68.8	67.3	65.8	64.1	62.3	60.2	57.9	55.4	52.4	48.8	7.49	9.86
	20	67.7	66.4	65.0	63.4	61.7	59.9	57.8	55.6	53.0	50.0	46.5	6.34	8.67
	22	65.6	64.3	62.8	61.3	59.6	57.8	55.7	53.4	50.8	47.9	44.3	5.40	7.69

TABLE 380

Process Times (B) at Retort Temperature of 260°F for Conduction-Heating Foods in 211 x 413 Can

f_h	z	INITIAL FOOD TEMPERATURE (T_{ih}) 100	110	120	130	140	150	160	170	180	190	200	Equivalent F_c^{18}	F_s^{18}
36.09	16	47.9	46.9	45.8	44.7	43.4	42.1	40.6	38.9	37.1	35.0	32.6	7.99	10.76
	18	47.1	46.0	45.0	43.8	42.5	41.2	39.7	38.0	36.2	34.1	31.7	7.14	9.86
	20	46.3	45.3	44.2	43.0	41.8	40.4	38.9	37.3	35.4	33.3	30.9	6.48	9.17
	22	45.6	44.6	43.5	42.3	41.1	39.7	38.2	36.6	34.7	32.6	30.2	5.86	8.51
38.22	16	50.3	49.3	48.1	46.9	45.5	44.1	42.5	40.8	38.8	36.6	34.0	8.03	10.82
	18	49.3	48.3	47.1	45.9	44.6	43.1	41.5	39.8	37.8	35.6	33.1	7.12	9.87
	20	48.5	47.5	46.3	45.1	43.8	42.3	40.7	39.0	37.0	34.8	32.3	6.43	9.13
	22	47.7	46.6	45.5	44.3	42.9	41.5	39.9	38.2	36.2	34.0	31.4	5.77	8.42
40.34	16	52.7	51.6	50.3	49.0	47.6	46.1	44.4	42.6	40.5	38.2	35.5	8.06	10.87
	18	51.6	50.5	49.3	48.0	46.6	45.0	43.3	41.5	39.5	37.1	34.4	7.11	9.86
	20	50.8	49.6	48.4	47.1	45.7	44.2	42.5	40.7	38.6	36.3	33.6	6.39	9.10
	22	49.9	48.8	47.5	46.3	44.8	43.3	41.7	39.8	37.7	35.4	32.7	5.72	8.38
42.46	16	55.0	53.8	52.6	51.2	49.7	48.1	46.4	44.4	42.2	39.8	36.9	8.10	10.92
	18	53.9	52.7	51.4	50.0	48.6	47.0	45.2	43.3	41.1	38.6	35.8	7.09	9.86
	20	52.9	51.8	50.5	49.1	47.6	46.0	44.3	42.3	40.2	37.7	34.9	6.35	9.07
	22	52.0	50.8	49.6	48.2	46.7	45.1	43.4	41.4	39.2	36.8	33.9	5.66	8.33
44.59	16	57.4	56.1	54.8	53.3	51.8	50.1	48.3	46.2	43.9	41.4	38.4	8.15	10.99
	18	56.1	54.9	53.5	52.1	50.6	48.9	47.0	45.0	42.7	40.1	37.1	7.09	9.87
	20	55.1	53.9	52.5	51.1	49.5	47.9	46.0	44.0	41.7	39.1	36.1	6.30	9.03
	22	54.1	52.9	51.6	50.1	48.6	46.9	45.0	43.0	40.7	38.1	35.2	5.60	8.27

TABLE 381

Process Times (B) at Retort Temperature of 230°F for Conduction-Heating Foods in 211 x 414 Can

f_h	z	INITIAL FOOD TEMPERATURE (T_{ih}) 100	110	120	130	140	150	160	170	180	190	200	Equivalent F_c^{18}	F_s^{18}
36.22	16	223.7	222.5	221.1	219.6	217.9	216.1	214.0	211.5	208.7	205.2	200.6	12.69	13.69
	18	173.9	172.6	171.3	169.8	168.1	166.3	164.2	161.7	159.8	155.4	150.8	8.94	9.93
	20	144.5	143.3	141.9	140.4	138.8	136.9	134.8	132.4	129.5	126.0	121.5	6.69	7.64
	22	124.3	123.1	121.7	120.2	118.5	116.7	114.6	112.2	109.3	105.8	101.3	5.15	6.08
38.35	16	227.9	226.6	225.2	223.6	221.8	219.9	217.6	215.1	212.0	208.3	203.5	12.69	13.70
	18	176.1	174.8	173.3	171.1	170.0	168.0	165.8	163.2	160.2	156.5	151.7	8.81	9.85
	20	147.0	145.7	144.3	142.7	140.9	139.0	136.7	134.2	131.1	127.4	122.6	6.61	7.62
	22	127.1	125.8	124.3	122.8	121.0	119.0	116.8	114.3	111.2	107.5	102.7	5.12	6.05
40.48	16	231.7	230.3	228.8	227.1	225.3	223.2	220.8	218.1	214.9	211.0	206.0	12.69	13.71
	18	179.6	178.2	176.6	175.0	173.1	171.0	168.7	166.0	162.8	158.8	153.8	8.81	9.85
	20	149.8	148.4	146.8	145.2	143.3	141.2	138.9	136.2	133.0	129.1	124.0	6.58	7.57
	22	129.6	128.2	126.6	125.0	123.1	121.0	118.7	116.0	112.8	108.9	103.8	5.05	6.01
42.61	16	235.1	233.6	232.2	230.2	228.3	226.1	223.6	220.8	217.4	213.3	207.9	12.70	13.72
	18	182.7	181.3	179.6	177.9	175.9	173.8	171.3	168.4	165.1	160.9	155.6	8.82	9.85
	20	152.7	151.2	149.6	147.8	145.9	143.7	141.2	138.4	135.0	130.9	125.5	6.57	7.56
	22	132.5	131.0	129.4	127.6	125.7	123.5	121.0	118.2	114.8	110.7	105.4	5.02	6.02
44.74	16	238.0	236.4	234.7	232.9	230.8	228.6	226.0	223.0	219.4	215.1	209.5	12.70	13.74
	18	185.6	184.0	182.3	180.5	178.4	176.1	173.6	170.6	167.0	162.7	157.1	8.82	9.85
	20	155.8	154.3	152.6	150.7	148.7	146.4	143.8	140.8	137.2	132.9	127.3	6.53	7.59
	22	135.5	134.0	132.3	130.4	128.4	126.1	123.5	120.5	117.0	112.6	107.1	5.01	6.03

TABLE 382

Process Times (B) at Retort Temperature of 240°F for Conduction-Heating Foods in 211 x 414 Can

f_h	z	INITIAL FOOD TEMPERATURE (T_{ih})											Equivalent	
		100	110	120	130	140	150	160	170	180	190	200	F_c^{18}	F_s^{18}
36.22	16	94.8	93.6	92.3	91.0	89.5	87.8	86.0	83.9	81.4	78.6	75.1	10.29	11.96
	18	87.8	86.6	85.3	84.0	82.5	80.8	79.0	76.9	74.4	71.6	68.0	8.17	9.94
	20	81.9	80.7	79.5	78.1	76.6	75.0	73.1	71.0	68.6	65.7	62.2	6.70	8.34
	22	77.1	75.9	74.7	73.3	71.8	70.2	68.3	66.2	63.8	60.9	57.4	5.69	7.23
38.35	16	98.4	97.2	95.9	94.4	92.8	91.1	89.1	86.9	84.3	81.3	77.6	10.33	12.06
	18	91.0	89.8	88.4	87.0	85.4	83.7	81.7	79.5	76.9	73.9	70.1	8.14	9.90
	20	84.9	83.7	82.4	80.9	79.3	77.6	75.6	73.4	70.8	67.8	64.1	6.70	8.34
	22	79.9	78.6	77.3	75.9	74.3	72.5	70.6	68.3	65.8	62.7	59.0	5.69	7.23
40.48	16	102.0	100.7	99.3	97.7	96.1	94.2	92.1	89.8	87.1	83.9	80.0	10.29	12.08
	18	94.2	92.9	91.5	89.9	88.3	86.4	84.4	82.0	79.3	76.1	72.2	8.12	9.88
	20	87.9	86.6	85.2	83.6	82.0	80.1	78.0	75.7	73.0	69.8	65.9	6.70	8.34
	22	82.5	81.2	79.8	78.3	76.6	74.7	72.7	70.3	67.6	64.4	60.5	5.69	7.23
42.61	16	105.4	104.1	102.6	101.0	99.2	97.3	95.1	92.6	89.8	86.4	82.3	10.25	12.12
	18	97.4	96.0	94.5	92.9	91.1	89.2	87.0	84.5	81.7	78.3	74.2	8.11	9.88
	20	90.7	89.4	87.9	86.3	84.5	82.6	80.4	77.9	75.0	71.7	67.5	6.70	8.34
	22	85.0	83.6	82.1	80.5	78.7	76.8	74.6	72.1	69.3	65.9	61.8	5.54	7.14
44.74	16	108.8	107.4	105.8	104.1	102.3	100.2	98.0	95.4	92.4	88.8	84.5	10.22	12.12
	18	100.5	99.0	97.5	95.8	93.9	91.9	89.6	87.0	84.0	80.4	76.1	8.11	9.88
	20	93.4	92.0	90.4	88.7	86.9	84.9	82.6	80.0	77.0	73.4	69.1	6.69	8.33
	22	87.4	85.9	84.4	82.7	80.8	78.8	76.5	73.9	70.9	67.4	63.0	5.39	7.05

TABLE 383

Process Times (B) at Retort Temperature of 250°F for Conduction-Heating Foods in 211 x 414 Can

f_h	z	INITIAL FOOD TEMPERATURE (T_{ih}) 100	110	120	130	140	150	160	170	180	190	200	Equivalent F_c^{18}	F_s^{18}
36.22	16	61.7	60.6	59.4	58.2	56.8	55.3	53.7	51.8	49.7	47.3	44.4	8.72	11.03
	18	59.8	58.7	57.5	56.3	54.9	53.4	51.8	49.9	47.8	45.4	42.5	7.59	9.88
	20	57.8	56.8	55.6	54.3	53.0	51.5	49.8	48.0	45.9	43.4	40.6	6.53	8.79
	22	56.1	55.0	53.9	52.6	51.2	49.7	48.1	46.2	44.1	41.7	38.8	5.66	7.89
38.35	16	64.4	63.3	62.1	60.7	59.3	57.7	55.9	54.0	51.8	49.2	46.2	8.69	11.04
	18	62.4	61.3	60.1	58.7	57.3	55.7	53.9	52.0	49.7	47.2	44.1	7.57	9.88
	20	60.4	59.2	58.0	56.7	55.2	53.6	51.9	49.9	47.7	45.1	42.1	6.47	8.75
	22	58.5	57.4	56.2	54.8	53.4	51.8	50.0	48.1	45.8	43.3	40.2	5.58	7.82
40.48	16	67.2	66.0	64.7	63.3	61.8	60.1	58.2	56.2	53.8	51.1	47.9	8.71	11.08
	18	65.1	63.9	62.6	61.2	59.7	58.0	56.1	54.1	51.7	49.0	45.8	7.54	9.87
	20	62.9	61.7	60.4	59.0	57.5	55.8	53.9	51.9	49.5	46.8	43.6	6.43	8.73
	22	61.0	59.8	58.5	57.1	55.5	53.9	52.0	49.9	47.6	44.9	41.7	5.52	7.78
42.61	16	70.0	68.7	67.3	65.8	64.2	62.5	60.5	58.3	55.9	53.0	49.6	8.72	11.11
	18	67.7	66.5	65.1	63.6	62.0	60.2	58.3	56.1	53.6	50.8	47.4	7.52	9.87
	20	65.4	64.2	62.8	61.3	59.7	57.9	56.0	53.8	51.3	48.5	45.1	6.38	8.71
	22	63.4	62.1	60.8	59.3	57.7	55.9	54.0	51.8	49.3	46.5	43.1	5.47	7.74
44.74	16	72.7	71.3	69.9	68.3	66.6	64.8	62.7	60.4	57.8	54.9	51.3	8.72	11.13
	18	70.3	69.0	67.5	66.0	64.3	62.4	60.4	58.1	55.5	52.5	49.0	7.50	9.87
	20	67.9	66.6	65.1	63.6	61.9	60.0	58.0	55.7	53.1	50.1	46.6	6.34	8.68
	22	65.8	64.5	63.0	61.5	59.8	57.9	55.9	53.6	51.0	48.0	44.4	5.41	7.70

TABLE 384

Process Times (B) at Retort Temperature of 260°F for Conduction-Heating Foods in 211 x 414 Can

f_h	z	INITIAL FOOD TEMPERATURE (T_{ih}) 100	110	120	130	140	150	160	170	180	190	200	Equivalent F_c^{18}	F_s^{18}
36.22	16	48.1	47.1	46.0	44.8	43.6	42.2	40.7	39.0	37.2	35.1	32.7	8.00	10.77
	18	47.2	46.2	45.1	43.9	42.7	41.3	39.8	38.1	36.3	34.2	31.8	7.14	9.87
	20	46.4	45.4	44.3	43.2	41.9	40.5	39.0	37.4	35.5	33.4	31.0	6.48	9.17
	22	45.7	44.7	43.6	42.5	41.2	39.8	38.3	36.7	34.8	32.7	30.3	5.86	8.51
38.35	16	50.5	49.4	48.3	47.0	45.7	44.2	42.7	40.9	38.9	36.7	34.1	8.04	10.83
	18	49.5	48.4	47.3	46.0	44.7	43.2	41.7	39.9	37.9	35.7	33.1	7.13	9.87
	20	48.7	47.6	46.5	45.2	43.9	42.4	40.9	39.1	37.1	34.9	32.4	6.44	9.14
	22	47.9	46.8	45.6	44.4	43.1	41.6	40.0	38.3	36.3	34.1	31.5	5.77	8.43
40.48	16	52.8	51.7	50.5	49.2	47.8	46.3	44.6	42.7	40.7	38.3	35.6	8.08	10.88
	18	51.8	50.6	49.4	48.1	46.7	45.2	43.5	41.6	39.6	37.2	34.5	7.12	9.87
	20	50.9	49.8	48.6	47.3	45.8	44.3	42.6	40.8	38.7	36.4	33.7	6.39	9.11
	22	50.0	48.9	47.7	46.4	45.0	43.5	41.8	39.9	37.9	35.5	32.8	5.72	8.39
42.61	16	55.2	54.0	52.7	51.4	49.9	48.3	46.5	44.6	42.4	39.9	37.0	8.11	10.93
	18	54.0	52.8	51.6	50.2	48.7	47.1	45.3	43.4	41.2	38.7	35.9	7.10	9.87
	20	53.1	51.9	50.6	49.3	47.8	46.2	44.4	42.5	40.3	37.8	35.0	6.35	9.07
	22	52.2	51.0	49.7	48.3	46.9	45.6	43.5	41.5	39.4	38.9	34.0	5.66	8.33
44.74	16	57.5	56.3	55.0	53.5	52.0	50.3	48.4	46.4	44.1	41.5	38.5	8.17	11.00
	18	56.3	55.0	53.7	52.3	50.7	49.0	47.2	45.1	42.8	40.2	37.2	7.09	9.87
	20	55.3	54.0	52.7	51.2	49.7	48.0	46.1	44.1	41.8	39.2	36.2	6.31	9.03
	22	54.3	53.1	51.7	50.3	48.7	47.0	45.2	43.1	40.8	38.3	35.3	5.60	8.28

TABLE 385

Process Times (B) at Retort Temperature of 230°F for Conduction-Heating Foods in 211 x 600 Can

f_h	z	INITIAL FOOD TEMPERATURE (T_{ih})											Equivalent	
		100	110	120	130	140	150	160	170	180	190	200	F_c^{18}	F_s^{18}
	16	229.3	228.0	226.6	225.0	223.3	221.4	219.2	216.6	213.6	209.9	205.2	12.88	13.89
37.88	18	177.5	176.2	174.7	173.2	171.4	169.5	167.3	164.8	161.8	158.1	153.4	8.99	10.05
	20	148.1	146.8	145.4	143.8	142.1	140.2	138.0	135.4	132.4	128.8	124.0	6.76	7.77
	22	127.8	126.5	125.1	123.5	121.8	119.8	117.6	115.1	112.1	108.4	103.7	5.22	6.17
	16	233.5	232.1	230.6	228.9	227.1	225.0	222.7	220.0	216.8	213.0	207.9	12.88	13.90
40.10	18	180.7	179.3	177.8	176.2	174.3	172.3	169.9	167.3	164.1	160.2	155.2	8.94	9.99
	20	150.6	149.2	147.7	146.1	144.2	142.2	139.8	137.2	134.0	130.1	125.1	6.68	7.68
	22	130.5	129.1	127.6	125.9	124.1	122.0	119.7	117.0	113.9	110.0	105.0	5.18	6.12
	16	237.2	235.7	234.1	232.4	230.4	228.3	225.8	223.0	219.6	215.5	210.2	12.89	13.92
42.33	18	184.2	182.7	181.1	179.4	177.4	175.3	172.8	170.0	166.6	162.5	157.2	8.95	10.00
	20	153.8	152.3	150.7	149.0	147.1	144.9	142.4	139.6	136.3	132.2	126.9	6.68	7.68
	22	133.1	131.7	130.1	128.3	126.4	124.2	121.8	118.9	115.6	111.5	106.2	5.10	6.10
	16	240.4	238.9	237.2	235.3	233.3	231.0	228.4	225.4	221.9	217.6	212.0	12.89	13.93
44.56	18	187.3	185.8	184.1	182.2	180.2	177.9	175.3	172.4	168.8	164.5	158.9	8.95	10.00
	20	156.8	155.3	153.6	151.8	149.7	147.4	144.8	141.9	138.3	134.0	128.5	6.64	7.68
	22	136.5	134.9	133.2	131.4	129.4	127.1	124.5	121.5	118.0	113.7	108.1	5.10	6.13
	16	243.2	241.6	239.8	237.9	235.7	233.3	230.6	227.5	223.8	219.2	213.4	12.90	13.94
46.79	18	190.4	188.8	187.0	185.0	182.9	180.5	177.8	174.7	171.0	166.4	160.6	8.95	10.02
	20	160.2	158.6	156.8	154.9	152.8	150.4	147.7	144.5	140.8	136.3	130.4	6.62	7.73
	22	139.4	137.8	136.0	134.1	131.9	129.5	126.8	123.7	120.0	115.4	109.6	5.06	6.10

TABLE 386

Process Times (B) at Retort Temperature of 240°F for Conduction-Heating Foods in 211 x 600 Can

f_h	z	INITIAL FOOD TEMPERATURE (T_{ih})											Equivalent	
		100	110	120	130	140	150	160	170	180	190	200	F^{18}_c	F^{18}_s
	16	98.2	96.9	95.6	94.2	92.6	90.9	89.0	86.8	84.2	81.2	77.6	10.52	12.21
37.88	18	90.8	89.6	88.3	86.9	85.3	83.6	81.6	79.4	76.9	73.9	70.2	8.29	10.06
	20	84.8	83.6	82.2	80.8	79.2	77.5	75.6	73.4	70.8	67.8	64.2	6.81	8.46
	22	79.8	78.6	77.2	75.8	74.2	72.5	70.6	68.4	65.8	62.8	59.2	5.79	7.34
	16	101.9	100.7	99.3	97.7	96.1	94.2	92.2	89.9	87.2	84.0	80.1	10.48	12.26
40.10	18	94.2	92.9	91.5	90.0	88.3	86.5	84.4	82.1	79.4	76.3	72.4	8.26	10.03
	20	87.9	86.6	85.2	83.7	82.0	80.2	78.2	75.8	73.2	70.0	66.1	6.81	8.46
	22	82.6	81.3	79.9	78.4	76.8	74.9	72.9	70.5	67.9	64.7	60.8	5.79	7.34
	16	105.6	104.2	102.8	101.2	99.4	97.5	95.3	92.9	90.0	86.7	82.6	10.43	12.27
42.33	18	97.5	96.2	94.7	93.1	91.3	89.4	87.2	84.8	81.9	78.6	74.5	8.25	10.02
	20	90.9	89.6	88.1	86.5	84.7	82.8	80.6	78.2	75.4	72.0	67.9	6.81	8.46
	22	85.3	83.9	82.4	80.8	79.1	77.1	75.0	72.5	69.7	66.3	62.2	5.72	7.29
	16	109.2	107.7	106.2	104.5	102.7	100.6	98.3	95.8	92.8	89.3	84.9	10.40	12.29
44.56	18	100.8	99.4	97.8	96.1	94.3	92.2	90.0	87.4	84.4	80.9	76.6	8.25	10.02
	20	93.9	92.4	90.9	89.2	87.3	85.3	83.0	80.4	77.5	73.9	69.6	6.81	8.46
	22	87.8	86.4	84.8	83.1	81.3	79.2	77.0	74.4	71.4	67.9	63.6	5.55	7.19
	16	112.7	111.2	109.6	107.8	105.9	103.7	101.3	98.6	95.5	91.8	87.2	10.37	12.29
46.79	18	104.0	102.5	100.8	99.1	97.1	95.0	92.6	89.9	86.8	83.1	78.5	8.25	10.02
	20	96.6	95.1	93.4	91.7	89.7	87.6	85.2	82.5	79.4	75.7	71.1	6.79	8.44
	22	90.4	88.9	87.2	85.5	83.5	81.4	79.0	76.3	73.2	69.4	64.9	5.42	7.12

TABLE 387

Process Times (B) at Retort Temperature of 250°F for Conduction-Heating Foods in 211 x 600 Can

f_h	z	INITIAL FOOD TEMPERATURE (T_{ih})											Equivalent	
		100	110	120	130	140	150	160	170	180	190	200	F_c^{18}	F_s^{18}
	16	64.1	63.0	61.7	60.4	59.0	57.4	55.7	53.8	51.6	49.0	46.0	8.86	11.19
37.88	18	62.1	61.0	59.8	58.4	57.0	55.4	53.7	51.8	49.6	47.0	44.0	7.71	10.02
	20	60.1	58.9	57.7	56.4	55.0	53.4	51.7	49.7	47.5	45.0	42.0	6.62	8.89
	22	58.3	57.1	55.9	54.6	53.2	51.6	49.9	47.9	45.7	43.2	40.2	5.72	7.97
	16	67.0	65.8	64.5	63.1	61.6	59.9	58.1	56.0	53.7	51.0	47.9	8.86	11.23
40.10	18	64.9	63.7	62.4	61.0	59.5	57.8	56.0	53.9	51.6	48.9	45.8	7.69	10.02
	20	62.7	61.5	60.2	58.9	57.3	55.7	53.8	51.8	49.5	46.8	43.6	6.57	8.87
	22	60.8	59.6	58.3	56.9	55.4	53.8	51.9	49.9	47.5	44.9	41.7	5.65	7.91
	16	69.9	68.6	67.2	65.8	64.2	62.4	60.5	58.3	55.9	53.0	49.7	8.87	11.27
42.33	18	67.7	66.4	65.0	63.6	62.0	60.2	58.3	56.1	53.7	50.8	47.5	7.66	10.02
	20	65.4	64.1	62.8	61.3	59.7	57.9	56.0	53.8	51.4	48.5	45.2	6.52	8.84
	22	63.4	62.1	60.7	59.3	57.7	55.9	54.0	51.8	49.4	46.5	43.2	5.59	7.87
	16	72.7	71.4	69.9	68.4	66.7	64.9	62.8	60.6	58.0	55.0	51.5	8.89	11.30
44.56	18	70.4	69.1	67.6	66.1	64.4	62.5	60.5	58.2	55.6	52.7	49.1	7.64	10.01
	20	68.0	66.7	65.2	62.7	62.0	60.2	58.1	55.8	53.3	50.3	46.7	6.47	8.82
	22	65.9	64.5	63.1	61.6	59.9	58.0	56.0	53.7	51.1	48.1	44.6	5.53	7.83
	16	75.6	74.1	72.6	71.0	69.2	67.3	65.2	62.8	60.1	56.9	53.2	8.88	11.31
46.79	18	73.1	71.7	70.2	68.6	66.8	64.9	62.7	60.3	57.6	54.5	50.8	7.62	10.01
	20	70.6	69.2	67.7	66.1	64.3	62.4	60.2	57.8	55.1	52.0	48.3	6.43	8.79
	22	68.4	67.0	65.5	63.8	62.1	60.1	58.0	55.6	52.9	49.7	46.0	5.47	7.78

TABLE 388

Process Times (B) at Retort Temperature of 260°F for Conduction-Heating Foods in 211 x 600 Can

f_h	z	INITIAL FOOD TEMPERATURE (T_{ih})											Equivalent	
		100	110	120	130	140	150	160	170	180	190	200	F_c^{18}	F_s^{18}
	16	50.1	49.0	47.9	46.7	45.4	43.9	42.4	40.6	38.7	36.5	34.0	8.17	10.96
37.88	18	49.1	48.1	46.9	45.7	44.4	43.0	41.4	39.7	37.7	35.5	33.0	7.27	10.02
	20	48.3	47.3	46.1	44.9	43.6	42.2	40.6	38.9	36.9	34.7	32.2	6.58	9.29
	22	47.6	46.5	45.4	44.1	42.8	41.4	39.8	38.1	36.2	34.0	31.4	5.92	8.59
	16	52.6	51.5	50.3	49.0	47.6	46.1	44.4	42.6	40.5	38.2	35.5	8.21	11.02
40.10	18	51.5	50.4	49.2	47.9	46.5	45.0	43.3	41.5	39.4	37.1	34.4	7.26	10.02
	20	50.7	49.6	48.4	47.1	45.7	44.2	42.5	40.7	38.6	36.3	33.6	6.53	9.26
	22	49.8	48.7	47.5	46.2	44.8	43.3	41.6	39.8	37.7	35.4	32.7	5.86	8.53
	16	55.0	53.9	52.6	51.2	49.8	48.2	46.4	44.5	42.3	39.8	37.0	8.24	11.07
42.33	18	53.9	52.7	51.4	50.1	48.6	47.0	45.3	43.3	41.2	38.7	35.9	7.24	10.02
	20	53.0	51.8	50.5	49.2	47.7	46.1	44.4	42.4	40.2	37.8	35.0	6.49	9.22
	22	52.1	50.9	49.6	48.3	46.8	45.2	43.4	41.5	39.3	36.9	34.0	5.80	8.47
	16	57.5	56.3	54.9	53.5	51.9	50.3	48.4	46.4	44.1	41.5	38.5	8.29	11.14
44.56	18	56.3	55.0	53.7	52.3	50.7	49.0	47.2	45.1	42.9	40.3	37.3	7.23	10.02
	20	55.3	54.0	52.7	51.3	49.7	48.0	46.2	44.1	41.9	39.3	36.3	6.45	9.19
	22	54.3	53.1	51.7	50.3	48.7	47.1	45.2	43.2	40.9	38.3	35.3	5.73	8.42
	16	60.0	58.6	57.2	55.7	54.1	52.3	50.4	48.3	45.9	43.2	40.0	8.34	11.20
46.79	18	58.6	57.3	55.9	54.4	52.8	51.0	49.1	46.9	44.5	41.8	38.7	7.22	10.02
	20	57.5	56.2	54.8	53.3	51.7	49.9	48.0	45.9	43.5	40.8	37.6	6.40	9.14
	22	56.5	55.2	53.8	52.3	50.7	48.9	47.0	44.8	42.4	39.7	36.6	5.67	8.37

TABLE 389

Process Times (B) at Retort Temperature of 230°F for Conduction-Heating Foods in 300 x 206 Can

f_h	z	INITIAL FOOD TEMPERATURE (T_{ih}) 100	110	120	130	140	150	160	170	180	190	200	Equivalent F_c^{18}	F_s^{18}
	16	196.4	195.4	194.4	193.2	192.0	190.8	189.0	187.1	184.9	182.3	178.8	12.18	13.11
27.58	18	158.8	157.8	156.8	155.7	154.4	153.0	151.4	149.5	147.4	144.7	141.2	8.72	9.49
	20	128.7	127.7	126.7	125.6	124.3	122.9	121.3	119.4	117.3	114.6	111.1	6.50	7.35
	22	110.3	109.4	108.3	107.2	105.9	104.5	102.9	101.1	98.9	96.2	92.8	5.12	5.88
	16	201.2	200.2	199.1	197.8	196.5	195.0	193.3	191.4	189.1	186.2	182.6	12.18	13.12
29.20	18	161.2	160.2	159.1	157.9	156.5	155.0	153.3	151.4	149.1	146.3	142.6	8.71	9.49
	20	131.1	130.1	129.0	127.7	126.4	124.9	123.2	121.3	119.0	116.1	112.5	6.47	7.31
	22	112.4	111.3	110.2	109.0	107.7	106.2	104.5	102.5	100.2	97.4	93.8	5.06	5.90
	16	205.6	204.5	203.4	202.1	200.7	199.1	197.3	195.2	192.8	189.8	186.0	12.19	13.14
30.82	18	163.2	162.2	161.0	159.7	158.3	156.7	154.9	152.9	150.4	147.4	143.6	8.70	9.49
	20	133.5	132.4	131.3	130.0	128.6	127.0	125.2	123.2	120.7	117.7	113.9	6.47	7.31
	22	114.1	113.0	111.8	110.5	109.1	107.6	105.8	103.7	101.3	98.3	94.4	5.01	5.82
	16	209.7	208.5	207.3	206.0	204.5	202.8	200.9	198.8	196.2	193.1	189.0	12.19	13.15
32.44	18	164.9	163.8	162.5	161.2	159.7	158.1	156.2	154.0	151.4	148.3	144.2	8.69	9.49
	20	135.7	134.6	133.3	132.0	130.5	128.9	127.0	124.8	122.2	119.1	115.0	6.47	7.30
	22	116.2	115.1	113.8	112.5	111.0	109.4	107.5	105.3	102.7	99.6	95.5	5.00	5.81
	16	213.4	212.2	210.9	209.5	208.0	206.2	204.2	202.0	199.3	196.0	191.7	12.19	13.16
34.06	18	166.5	165.3	164.0	162.6	161.0	159.3	157.3	155.0	152.3	149.0	144.8	8.66	9.52
	20	137.6	136.4	135.1	133.7	132.1	130.4	128.4	126.1	123.4	120.1	115.9	6.43	7.31
	22	118.2	117.1	115.8	114.4	112.8	111.1	109.1	106.8	104.1	100.8	96.5	4.94	5.83

TABLE 390

Process Times (B) at Retort Temperature of 240°F for Conduction-Heating Foods in 300 x 206 Can

f_h	z	INITIAL FOOD TEMPERATURE (T_{ih})											Equivalent	
		100	110	120	130	140	150	160	170	180	190	200	F_c^{18}	F_s^{18}
	16	79.7	78.8	77.9	76.8	75.7	74.4	73.0	71.4	69.6	67.4	64.7	9.83	11.36
27.58	18	72.7	71.8	70.8	69.8	68.6	67.4	66.0	64.4	62.5	60.3	57.7	7.96	9.46
	20	67.9	67.0	66.0	65.0	63.8	62.6	61.2	59.6	57.7	55.5	52.9	6.52	8.10
	22	64.0	63.1	62.1	61.1	59.9	58.7	57.3	55.7	53.8	51.6	49.0	5.48	6.98
	16	82.1	81.2	80.2	79.1	77.9	76.5	75.0	73.3	71.4	69.1	66.3	9.81	11.35
29.20	18	75.1	74.2	73.2	72.1	70.9	69.5	68.0	66.3	64.4	62.1	59.2	7.93	9.47
	20	70.4	69.4	68.4	67.3	66.1	64.8	63.3	61.6	59.6	57.3	54.5	6.49	8.10
	22	66.3	65.3	64.3	63.2	62.0	60.7	59.2	57.5	55.5	53.2	50.4	5.46	6.96
	16	84.5	83.5	82.5	81.3	80.0	78.6	77.1	75.3	73.2	70.8	67.8	9.78	11.35
30.82	18	77.9	76.9	75.8	74.7	73.4	72.0	70.4	68.6	66.6	64.1	61.1	7.91	9.53
	20	72.8	71.8	70.7	69.6	68.3	66.9	65.3	63.5	61.5	59.0	56.0	6.46	8.07
	22	68.5	67.6	66.5	65.3	64.0	62.6	61.1	59.3	57.2	54.8	51.8	5.44	6.95
	16	87.0	85.9	84.8	83.6	82.2	80.8	79.1	77.2	75.0	72.5	69.3	9.77	11.38
32.44	18	80.5	79.5	78.4	77.1	75.8	74.3	72.6	70.8	68.6	66.0	62.9	7.88	9.55
	20	75.2	74.2	73.0	71.8	70.5	69.0	67.3	65.4	63.3	60.7	57.5	6.43	8.04
	22	70.8	69.7	68.6	67.4	66.0	64.6	62.9	61.0	58.8	56.3	53.1	5.44	6.95
	16	89.7	88.6	87.4	86.1	84.7	83.1	81.4	79.4	77.1	74.4	71.1	9.82	11.45
34.06	18	83.1	82.0	80.8	79.5	78.1	76.5	74.8	72.8	70.5	67.8	64.5	7.84	9.56
	20	77.5	76.4	75.2	74.0	72.5	71.0	69.2	67.3	65.0	62.3	59.0	6.41	8.02
	22	73.0	71.9	70.7	69.4	68.0	66.5	64.7	62.7	60.5	57.8	54.5	5.44	6.95

TABLE 391

Process Times (B) at Retort Temperature of 250°F for Conduction-Heating Foods in 300 x 206 Can

f_h	z	INITIAL FOOD TEMPERATURE (T_{ih})											Equivalent	
		100	110	120	130	140	150	160	170	180	190	200	F_c^{18}	F_s^{18}
27.58	16	49.6	48.8	47.9	46.9	45.9	44.7	43.5	42.1	40.5	38.6	36.4	8.31	10.47
	18	48.1	47.3	46.4	45.5	44.4	43.3	42.0	40.6	39.0	37.2	35.0	7.35	9.49
	20	46.7	45.8	45.0	44.0	43.0	41.8	40.6	39.1	37.5	35.7	33.5	6.45	8.58
	22	45.4	44.6	43.7	42.7	41.7	40.5	39.3	37.8	36.3	34.4	32.2	5.70	7.81
29.20	16	51.7	50.9	49.9	48.9	47.8	46.6	45.3	43.8	42.1	40.1	37.8	8.27	10.46
	18	50.2	49.3	48.4	47.4	46.2	45.0	43.7	42.2	40.5	38.6	36.2	7.32	9.48
	20	48.6	47.8	46.8	45.8	44.7	43.5	42.1	40.7	39.0	37.0	34.7	6.36	8.52
	22	47.3	46.4	45.4	44.4	43.3	42.1	40.8	39.3	37.6	35.6	33.3	5.60	7.73
30.82	16	53.9	53.0	52.0	50.9	49.8	48.5	47.1	45.5	43.7	41.7	39.2	8.30	10.51
	18	52.3	51.4	50.4	49.3	48.1	46.9	45.5	43.9	42.1	40.0	37.6	7.29	9.49
	20	50.6	49.7	48.7	47.7	46.5	45.2	43.8	42.2	40.4	38.4	35.9	6.34	8.52
	22	49.2	48.3	47.3	46.2	45.0	43.8	42.4	40.8	39.0	36.9	34.5	5.54	7.69
32.44	16	56.1	55.1	54.1	53.0	51.7	50.4	48.9	47.2	45.4	43.2	40.6	8.33	10.57
	18	54.4	53.4	52.4	51.2	50.0	48.7	47.2	45.5	43.6	41.5	38.9	7.27	9.51
	20	52.7	51.7	50.6	49.5	48.3	46.9	45.5	43.8	41.9	39.7	3-.2	6.30	8.50
	22	51.1	50.1	49.1	48.0	46.7	45.4	43.9	42.3	40.4	38.2	35.6	5.49	7.66
34.06	16	58.2	57.2	56.1	54.9	53.6	52.2	50.7	48.9	47.0	44.7	42.0	8.33	10.60
	18	56.4	55.4	54.3	53.1	51.8	50.4	48.9	47.1	45.2	42.9	40.2	7.25	9.51
	20	54.6	53.6	52.5	51.3	50.0	48.6	47.1	45.3	43.3	41.1	38.4	6.25	8.47
	22	53.0	52.0	50.9	49.7	48.4	47.0	45.4	43.7	41.7	39.4	36.7	5.43	7.62

TABLE 392

Process Times (B) at Retort Temperature of 260°F for Conduction-Heating Foods in 300 x 206 Can

f_h	z	INITIAL FOOD TEMPERATURE (T_{ih}) 100	110	120	130	140	150	160	170	180	190	200	Equivalent F^{18}_c	F^{18}_s
27.58	16	37.9	37.1	36.3	35.4	34.5	33.4	32.3	31.0	29.6	28.0	26.2	7.46	10.13
	18	37.4	36.6	35.8	34.9	33.9	32.9	31.7	30.5	29.1	27.5	25.6	6.86	9.50
	20	36.9	36.1	35.3	34.4	33.4	32.4	31.2	30.0	28.6	27.0	25.1	6.36	8.97
	22	36.3	35.6	34.7	33.9	32.9	31.9	30.7	29.5	28.0	26.4	24.6	5.83	8.41
29.20	16	39.8	39.0	38.1	37.2	36.1	35.0	33.8	32.5	31.0	29.3	27.4	7.51	10.20
	18	39.1	38.3	37.4	36.5	35.5	34.4	33.2	31.8	30.3	28.7	26.7	6.84	9.49
	20	38.6	37.8	36.9	36.0	35.0	33.9	32.7	31.3	29.8	28.1	26.2	6.30	8.93
	22	38.1	37.2	36.4	35.4	34.4	33.3	32.1	30.8	29.3	27.6	25.6	5.78	8.37
30.82	16	41.6	40.8	39.8	38.9	37.8	36.6	35.3	33.9	32.4	30.6	28.5	7.56	10.26
	18	40.9	40.1	39.1	38.2	37.1	35.9	34.6	33.2	31.7	29.9	27.8	6.83	9.49
	20	40.3	39.5	38.6	37.6	36.5	35.3	34.1	32.6	31.1	29.3	27.2	6.25	8.88
	22	39.8	38.9	38.0	37.0	35.9	34.8	33.5	32.1	30.5	28.7	26.6	5.73	8.33
32.44	16	43.5	42.6	41.6	40.5	39.4	38.2	36.8	35.4	33.7	31.8	29.6	7.58	10.30
	18	42.7	41.8	40.8	39.8	38.7	37.4	36.1	34.6	32.9	31.1	28.9	6.81	9.50
	20	42.0	41.1	40.2	39.1	38.0	36.8	35.4	33.9	32.3	30.4	28.2	6.19	8.84
	22	41.4	40.5	39.6	38.5	37.4	36.2	34.8	33.3	31.7	29.8	27.6	5.67	8.28
34.06	16	45.3	44.3	43.3	42.2	41.0	39.8	38.4	36.8	35.1	33.1	30.8	7.61	10.34
	18	44.5	43.5	42.5	41.4	40.2	38.9	37.5	36.0	34.2	32.2	30.0	6.80	9.50
	20	43.8	42.8	41.8	40.7	39.5	38.2	36.8	35.3	33.5	31.5	29.3	6.18	8.83
	22	43.1	42.2	41.1	40.0	38.9	37.6	36.2	34.6	32.9	30.9	28.6	5.60	8.22

TABLE 393

Process Times (B) at Retort Temperature of 230°F for Conduction-Heating Foods in 300 x 308 Can

f_h	z	INITIAL FOOD TEMPERATURE (T_{ih})											Equivalent	
		100	110	120	130	140	150	160	170	180	190	200	F_c^{18}	F_s^{18}
38.12	16	226.1	224.8	223.4	221.8	220.0	218.1	215.9	213.3	210.3	206.6	201.8	12.58	13.58
	18	174.7	173.3	171.9	170.3	168.6	166.6	164.4	161.9	158.9	155.2	150.4	8.73	9.76
	20	145.8	144.5	143.1	141.5	139.7	137.8	135.6	133.0	130.0	126.3	121.5	6.55	7.54
	22	126.1	124.8	123.3	121.8	120.0	118.1	115.9	113.3	110.3	106.6	101.8	5.07	6.00
40.37	16	230.1	228.7	227.1	225.5	223.6	221.6	219.2	216.5	213.3	209.4	204.4	12.58	13.59
	18	178.3	176.9	175.4	173.7	171.9	169.8	167.5	164.8	161.6	157.7	152.6	8.73	9.76
	20	148.8	147.4	145.8	144.2	142.3	140.3	137.9	135.2	132.0	128.1	123.1	6.52	7.50
	22	128.6	127.2	125.7	124.0	122.2	120.1	117.8	115.1	111.9	108.0	102.9	5.00	5.95
42.61	16	233.5	232.1	230.4	228.7	226.7	224.5	222.1	219.2	215.9	211.7	206.4	12.59	13.61
	18	181.6	180.1	178.5	176.8	174.8	172.6	170.2	167.3	163.9	159.8	154.5	8.73	9.76
	20	151.7	150.3	148.7	146.9	144.9	142.8	140.3	137.4	134.1	129.9	124.6	6.49	7.49
	22	131.8	130.3	128.7	127.0	125.0	122.8	120.4	117.5	114.1	110.0	104.7	4.97	5.98
44.85	16	236.5	235.0	233.3	231.4	229.3	227.1	224.5	221.5	217.9	213.6	207.9	12.59	13.62
	18	184.5	182.9	181.2	179.4	177.3	175.0	172.4	169.4	165.9	161.5	155.9	8.73	9.76
	20	155.2	153.6	151.9	150.1	148.0	145.7	143.1	140.1	136.6	132.2	126.6	6.47	7.54
	22	134.9	133.4	131.7	129.8	127.8	125.5	122.9	119.9	116.3	112.0	106.4	4.96	5.96
47.10	16	239.0	237.4	235.6	233.7	231.5	229.1	226.4	223.2	219.5	214.9	209.1	12.60	13.63
	18	188.1	186.4	184.6	182.7	180.5	178.1	175.4	172.2	168.5	164.0	158.1	8.71	9.83
	20	158.2	156.5	154.8	152.8	150.7	148.2	145.5	142.4	138.6	134.1	128.2	6.43	7.52
	22	137.7	136.1	134.3	132.3	130.2	127.8	125.0	121.9	118.2	113.6	107.7	4.90	5.94

TABLE 394

Process Times (B) at Retort Temperature of 240°F for Conduction-Heating Foods in 300 x 308 Can

f_h	z	INITIAL FOOD TEMPERATURE (T_{ih})											Equivalent	
		100	110	120	130	140	150	160	170	180	190	200	F_c^{18}	F_s^{18}
	16	97.7	96.5	95.2	93.7	92.2	90.4	88.5	86.3	83.7	80.7	77.0	10.23	11.96
38.12	18	90.3	89.1	87.8	86.4	84.8	83.0	81.1	78.9	76.3	73.3	69.6	8.06	9.81
	20	84.3	83.1	81.8	80.3	78.7	77.0	75.0	72.8	70.3	67.3	63.6	6.63	8.27
	22	79.3	78.1	76.7	75.3	73.7	72.0	70.0	67.8	65.3	62.2	58.5	5.64	7.17
	16	101.4	100.1	98.7	97.2	95.5	93.7	91.6	89.3	86.6	83.4	79.5	10.18	11.98
40.37	18	93.7	92.4	91.0	89.5	87.8	85.9	83.9	81.5	78.8	75.6	71.7	8.03	9.79
	20	87.4	86.1	84.7	83.2	81.5	79.7	77.6	75.2	72.5	69.3	65.4	6.63	8.27
	22	82.0	80.7	79.3	77.8	76.1	74.3	72.2	69.9	67.2	64.0	60.0	5.63	7.16
	16	105.1	103.7	102.2	100.6	98.8	96.9	94.7	92.2	89.4	86.0	81.9	10.14	11.99
42.61	18	97.0	95.6	94.2	92.6	90.8	88.8	86.7	84.2	81.3	78.0	73.8	8.03	9.79
	20	90.4	89.0	87.5	85.9	84.2	82.2	80.0	77.6	74.7	71.3	67.2	6.63	8.27
	22	84.6	83.2	81.7	80.1	78.4	76.4	74.2	71.8	68.9	65.5	61.4	5.45	7.06
	16	108.6	107.2	105.6	103.9	102.1	100.0	97.7	95.1	92.1	88.6	84.2	10.11	11.01
44.85	18	100.2	98.8	97.2	95.6	93.7	91.6	89.3	86.7	83.7	80.2	75.8	8.03	9.79
	20	93.2	91.7	90.2	88.5	86.6	84.6	82.3	79.7	76.7	73.1	68.8	6.61	8.25
	22	87.1	85.7	84.1	82.4	80.5	78.5	76.2	73.6	70.6	67.0	62.7	5.29	6.96
	16	112.1	110.6	108.9	107.2	105.2	103.1	100.6	97.9	94.8	91.0	86.5	10.08	11.98
47.10	18	103.4	101.9	100.2	98.5	96.5	94.4	91.9	89.2	86.1	82.3	77.8	8.03	9.79
	20	95.9	94.3	92.7	90.9	89.0	86.8	84.4	81.7	78.5	74.8	70.2	6.59	8.23
	22	90.1	88.5	86.9	85.1	83.2	81.0	78.6	75.9	72.7	69.0	64.4	5.26	6.98

TABLE 395

Process Times (B) at Retort Temperature of 250°F for Conduction-Heating Foods in 300 x 308 Can

f_h	z	INITIAL FOOD TEMPERATURE (T_{ih})											Equivalent	
		100	110	120	130	140	150	160	170	180	190	200	F_c^{18}	F_s^{18}
38.12	16	64.0	62.9	61.6	60.3	58.9	57.3	55.5	53.6	51.4	48.8	45.8	8.60	10.94
	18	62.0	60.9	59.6	58.3	56.9	55.3	53.5	51.6	49.4	46.8	43.8	7.48	9.79
	20	60.0	58.8	57.6	56.3	54.8	53.2	51.5	49.5	47.3	44.8	41.8	6.40	8.67
	22	58.1	57.0	55.8	54.4	53.0	51.4	49.7	47.7	45.5	43.0	39.9	5.52	7.76
40.37	16	66.9	65.7	64.4	63.0	61.5	59.8	58.0	55.9	53.6	50.9	47.7	8.62	10.99
	18	64.8	63.6	62.3	60.9	59.4	57.7	55.9	53.8	51.4	48.7	45.5	7.46	9.78
	20	62.6	61.4	60.1	58.7	57.2	55.5	53.7	51.6	49.3	46.6	43.4	6.35	8.65
	22	60.7	59.5	58.2	56.8	55.3	53.6	51.8	49.7	47.3	44.6	41.4	5.46	7.71
42.61	16	69.8	68.5	67.1	65.7	64.1	62.3	60.3	58.2	55.7	52.8	49.5	8.63	11.02
	18	67.6	66.3	64.9	63.4	61.8	60.1	58.1	55.9	53.5	50.6	47.2	7.43	9.78
	20	65.3	64.0	62.6	61.1	59.5	57.8	55.8	53.6	51.2	48.3	44.9	6.31	8.63
	22	63.2	62.0	60.6	59.1	57.5	55.7	53.8	51.6	49.1	46.3	42.9	5.40	7.67
44.85	16	72.6	71.3	69.8	68.3	66.6	64.7	62.7	60.4	57.8	54.8	51.2	8.62	11.03
	18	70.3	68.9	67.5	65.9	64.2	62.4	60.3	58.0	55.4	52.4	48.9	7.41	9.78
	20	67.9	66.5	65.1	63.5	61.8	60.0	57.9	55.6	53.0	50.0	46.5	6.26	8.59
	22	65.7	64.4	63.0	61.4	59.7	57.8	55.8	53.5	50.9	47.9	44.3	5.33	7.62
47.10	16	75.5	74.1	72.6	70.9	69.2	67.2	65.1	62.6	59.9	56.8	53.0	8.64	11.07
	18	73.0	71.6	70.1	68.5	66.7	64.7	62.6	60.2	57.4	54.3	50.6	7.39	9.79
	20	70.5	69.1	67.6	66.0	64.2	62.2	60.1	57.7	54.9	51.8	48.0	6.23	8.58
	22	68.3	66.9	65.3	63.7	61.9	60.0	57.8	55.4	52.7	49.5	45.8	5.29	7.60

TABLE 396

Process Times (B) at Retort Temperature of 260°F for Conduction-Heating Foods in 300 x 308 Can

f_h	z	INITIAL FOOD TEMPERATURE (T_{ih})											Equivalent	
		100	110	120	130	140	150	160	170	180	190	200	F_c^{18}	F_s^{18}
	16	50.1	49.1	47.9	46.7	45.4	43.9	42.4	40.6	38.7	36.5	33.9	7.95	10.74
38.12	18	49.1	48.1	46.9	45.7	44.4	42.9	41.4	39.6	37.7	35.5	32.9	7.05	9.79
	20	48.4	47.3	46.1	44.9	43.6	42.2	40.6	38.8	36.9	34.7	32.1	6.36	9.06
	22	47.5	46.5	45.3	44.1	42.8	41.3	39.8	38.0	36.1	33.9	31.3	5.70	8.35
	16	52.6	51.5	50.3	49.0	47.6	46.1	44.4	42.5	40.5	38.1	35.4	7.99	10.79
40.37	18	51.5	50.4	49.2	47.9	46.5	45.0	43.3	41.5	39.4	37.1	34.4	7.03	9.78
	20	50.7	49.6	48.4	47.1	45.6	44.1	42.5	40.6	38.5	36.2	33.5	6.31	9.02
	22	49.8	48.7	47.5	46.2	44.8	43.3	41.6	39.7	37.7	35.3	32.6	5.65	8.31
	16	55.1	53.9	52.6	51.3	49.8	48.2	46.4	44.5	42.3	39.8	37.0	8.03	10.85
42.61	18	53.9	52.7	51.5	50.1	48.6	47.0	45.2	43.3	41.1	38.6	35.8	7.02	9.78
	20	53.0	51.8	50.5	49.2	47.7	46.1	44.3	42.4	40.2	37.7	34.9	6.27	8.99
	22	52.1	50.9	49.6	48.2	46.8	45.1	43.4	41.4	39.3	36.8	33.9	5.58	8.25
	16	57.6	56.3	55.0	53.5	52.0	50.3	48.4	46.4	44.1	41.5	38.5	8.09	10.92
44.85	18	56.3	55.1	53.7	52.3	50.7	49.0	47.2	45.1	42.8	40.2	37.2	7.01	9.79
	20	55.3	54.0	52.7	51.2	49.7	48.0	46.1	44.1	41.8	39.2	36.2	6.22	8.94
	22	54.3	53.1	51.7	50.3	48.7	47.0	45.2	43.1	40.8	38.2	35.2	5.52	8.19
	16	60.0	58.7	57.3	55.8	54.1	52.4	50.4	48.3	45.8	43.1	40.0	8.11	10.95
47.10	18	58.7	57.4	55.9	54.4	52.8	51.0	49.1	46.9	44.5	41.8	38.6	7.00	9.79
	20	57.6	56.3	54.9	53.3	51.7	49.9	48.0	45.8	43.4	40.7	37.5	6.18	8.91
	22	56.5	55.2	53.8	52.3	50.6	48.9	46.9	44.8	42.3	39.6	36.5	5.46	8.14

TABLE 397

Process Times (B) at Retort Temperature of 230°F for Conduction-Heating Foods in 300 x 400 Can

f_h	z	INITIAL FOOD TEMPERATURE (T_{ih})											Equivalent	
		100	110	120	130	140	150	160	170	180	190	200	F_c^{18}	F_s^{18}
	16	232.6	231.2	229.6	227.9	226.1	224.0	221.6	218.9	215.6	211.7	206.5	12.71	13.73
40.91	18	180.4	178.9	117.4	175.7	173.8	171.7	169.4	166.6	163.4	159.4	154.3	8.82	9.86
	20	150.5	149.1	147.5	145.8	144.0	141.9	139.5	136.8	133.5	129.6	124.4	6.58	7.57
	22	130.1	128.7	127.2	125.5	123.6	121.5	119.1	116.4	113.2	109.2	104.1	5.04	6.01
	16	236.3	234.8	233.1	231.3	229.3	227.1	224.6	221.7	218.3	214.1	208.7	12.71	13.74
43.32	18	183.8	182.3	180.7	178.9	176.9	174.7	172.2	169.3	165.9	161.7	156.3	8.82	9.86
	20	153.7	152.2	150.5	148.7	146.7	144.5	142.0	139.1	135.7	131.5	126.1	6.55	7.56
	22	133.6	132.1	130.5	128.7	126.7	124.5	122.0	119.1	115.6	111.4	106.0	5.02	6.04
	16	239.4	237.8	236.1	234.2	232.1	229.7	227.1	224.0	220.4	216.0	210.3	12.72	13.76
45.73	18	187.0	185.4	183.6	181.8	179.7	177.3	174.7	171.6	168.0	163.6	157.8	8.82	9.86
	20	157.4	155.8	154.1	152.2	150.1	147.8	145.1	142.1	138.5	134.0	128.3	6.53	7.62
	22	136.9	135.3	133.6	131.7	129.6	127.2	124.6	121.5	117.9	113.5	107.8	5.00	6.02
	16	242.0	240.3	238.5	236.5	234.3	231.8	229.0	225.8	222.0	217.3	211.3	12.72	13.77
48.13	18	190.7	189.0	187.2	185.2	183.0	180.5	177.7	174.5	170.7	166.0	160.0	8.78	9.93
	20	160.5	158.9	157.0	155.0	152.8	150.4	147.6	144.4	140.6	135.9	129.9	6.49	7.59
	22	139.9	138.2	136.4	134.4	132.2	129.7	126.9	123.7	119.9	115.2	109.2	4.94	5.99
	16	243.8	242.0	240.1	238.0	235.7	233.1	230.2	226.8	222.8	217.9	211.6	12.58	13.76
50.54	18	193.6	191.8	189.9	187.8	185.5	182.9	180.0	176.6	172.6	167.7	161.4	8.70	9.88
	20	163.4	161.7	159.8	157.7	155.4	152.8	149.8	146.5	142.5	137.6	131.2	6.44	7.54
	22	143.2	141.4	139.5	137.4	135.1	132.5	129.6	126.2	122.2	117.3	111.0	4.92	6.00

TABLE 398

Process Times (B) at Retort Temperature of 240°F for Conduction-Heating Foods in 300 x 400 Can

f_h	z	INITIAL FOOD TEMPERATURE (T_{ih})											Equivalent	
		100	110	120	130	140	150	160	170	180	190	200	F_c^{18}	F_s^{18}
40.91	16	102.7	101.4	100.0	98.4	96.8	94.9	92.8	90.4	87.7	84.4	80.5	10.29	12.10
	18	94.9	93.6	92.1	90.6	88.9	87.0	84.9	82.6	79.8	76.6	72.6	8.12	9.89
	20	88.5	87.2	85.8	84.2	82.5	80.7	78.6	76.2	73.4	70.2	66.2	6.71	8.35
	22	83.0	81.7	80.3	78.8	77.1	75.2	73.1	70.7	68.0	64.7	60.8	5.69	7.23
43.32	16	106.6	105.2	103.7	102.1	100.3	98.3	96.1	93.6	90.7	87.2	83.0	10.25	12.11
	18	98.4	97.0	95.5	93.9	92.1	90.1	87.9	85.4	82.5	79.1	74.9	8.12	9.89
	20	91.7	90.3	88.8	87.2	85.4	83.4	81.2	78.7	75.8	72.3	68.1	6.70	8.35
	22	85.8	84.4	82.9	81.3	79.5	77.5	75.3	72.8	69.9	66.4	62.2	5.50	7.12
45.73	16	110.4	109.0	107.4	105.6	103.7	101.6	99.3	96.7	93.6	90.0	85.5	10.22	12.12
	18	101.9	100.4	98.8	97.1	95.2	93.1	90.8	88.1	85.1	81.5	77.0	8.12	9.89
	20	94.7	93.2	91.6	89.9	88.0	85.9	83.6	80.9	77.8	74.2	69.8	6.69	8.33
	22	88.5	87.0	85.5	83.7	81.8	79.7	77.4	74.7	71.7	68.1	63.6	5.34	7.02
48.13	16	114.1	112.6	110.9	109.1	107.1	104.9	102.4	99.6	96.4	92.6	87.9	10.19	12.10
	18	105.2	103.7	102.0	100.2	98.2	96.0	93.5	90.8	87.5	83.7	79.1	8.12	9.89
	20	97.5	96.0	94.3	92.5	90.5	88.3	85.8	83.0	79.8	76.0	71.4	6.65	8.30
	22	91.7	90.2	88.5	86.7	84.7	82.5	80.0	77.3	74.0	70.2	65.6	5.31	7.05
50.54	16	117.8	116.1	114.4	112.5	110.4	108.1	105.5	102.6	99.2	95.2	90.3	10.17	12.08
	18	108.4	106.8	105.1	103.2	101.1	98.7	96.2	93.2	89.8	85.8	81.0	8.11	9.87
	20	100.3	98.7	96.9	95.0	92.9	90.6	88.0	85.1	81.7	77.7	72.8	6.46	8.18
	22	94.9	93.3	91.5	89.6	87.5	85.2	82.6	79.7	76.3	72.3	67.4	5.30	7.07

TABLE 399

Process Times (B) at Retort Temperature of 250°F for Conduction-Heating Foods in 300 x 400 Can

f_h	z	INITIAL FOOD TEMPERATURE (T_{ih})											Equivalent	
		100	110	120	130	140	150	160	170	180	190	200	F_c^{18}	F_s^{18}
40.91	16	67.8	66.6	65.3	63.8	62.3	60.6	58.7	56.6	54.3	51.5	48.3	8.72	11.10
	18	65.7	64.4	63.1	61.7	60.2	58.5	56.6	54.5	52.1	49.4	46.1	7.54	9.88
	20	63.5	62.2	60.9	59.5	58.0	56.3	54.4	52.3	49.9	47.2	43.9	6.43	8.73
	22	61.5	60.3	59.0	57.5	56.0	54.3	52.4	50.3	48.0	45.2	42.0	5.52	7.78
43.32	16	70.9	69.6	68.2	66.7	65.0	63.3	61.3	59.1	56.5	53.6	50.2	8.74	11.13
	18	68.6	67.3	65.9	64.4	62.8	61.0	59.0	56.8	54.3	51.4	47.9	7.52	9.88
	20	66.3	65.0	63.6	62.1	60.5	58.7	56.7	54.5	52.0	49.1	45.6	6.38	8.71
	22	64.2	62.9	61.5	60.0	58.4	56.6	54.6	52.4	49.9	47.0	43.6	5.46	7.74
45.73	16	73.9	72.6	71.1	69.5	67.8	65.9	63.8	61.5	58.8	55.7	52.1	8.73	11.15
	18	71.5	70.2	68.7	67.1	65.4	63.5	61.4	59.1	56.4	53.4	49.7	7.49	9.88
	20	69.1	67.7	66.3	64.7	62.9	61.0	58.9	56.6	54.0	50.9	47.3	6.33	8.67
	22	66.9	65.5	64.1	62.5	60.8	58.9	56.8	54.4	51.8	48.7	45.1	5.39	7.69
48.13	16	77.0	75.6	74.0	72.3	70.5	68.5	66.3	63.9	61.1	57.9	54.0	8.75	11.19
	18	74.5	73.0	71.5	69.8	68.0	66.0	63.8	61.3	58.6	55.3	51.5	7.48	9.88
	20	71.9	70.5	68.9	67.2	65.4	63.4	61.2	58.8	56.0	52.8	48.9	6.30	8.66
	22	69.6	68.2	66.6	65.0	63.1	61.1	58.9	56.5	53.7	50.5	46.7	5.35	7.66
50.54	16	80.0	78.5	76.9	75.1	73.2	71.1	68.8	66.2	63.3	59.9	55.9	8.76	11.22
	18	77.4	75.9	74.2	72.5	70.6	68.5	66.2	63.6	60.6	57.3	53.3	7.46	9.89
	20	74.7	73.2	71.5	69.8	67.9	65.8	63.5	60.9	58.0	54.6	50.6	6.26	8.64
	22	72.3	70.8	69.1	67.4	65.5	63.4	61.1	58.5	55.6	52.2	48.2	5.29	7.62

TABLE 400

Process Times (B) at Retort Temperature of 260°F for Conduction-Heating Foods in 300 x 400 Can

f_h	z	INITIAL FOOD TEMPERATURE (T_{ih})											Equivalent	
		100	110	120	130	140	150	160	170	180	190	200	F_c^{18}	F_s^{18}
	16	53.3	52.2	51.0	49.6	48.2	46.7	45.0	43.1	41.0	38.6	35.9	8.09	10.90
40.91	18	52.2	51.1	49.9	48.5	47.1	45.6	43.9	42.0	39.9	37.5	34.8	7.12	9.88
	20	51.4	50.2	49.0	47.7	46.3	44.7	43.0	41.1	39.1	36.7	33.9	6.39	9.11
	22	50.5	49.3	48.1	46.8	45.4	43.8	42.1	40.3	38.2	35.8	33.1	5.72	8.38
	16	56.0	54.8	53.5	52.1	50.6	48.9	47.2	45.2	43.0	40.4	37.5	8.14	10.97
43.32	18	54.8	53.6	52.3	50.9	49.4	47.8	46.0	44.0	41.8	39.3	36.4	7.11	9.88
	20	53.8	52.6	51.3	49.9	48.4	46.8	45.0	43.0	40.8	38.3	35.4	6.35	9.07
	22	52.9	51.7	50.4	49.0	47.5	45.9	44.1	42.1	39.9	37.4	34.5	5.65	8.32
	16	58.6	57.4	56.0	54.5	52.9	51.2	49.3	47.2	44.9	42.2	39.2	8.19	11.04
45.73	18	57.4	56.1	54.7	53.2	51.6	49.9	48.0	45.9	43.6	40.9	37.9	7.10	9.88
	20	56.3	55.0	53.6	52.2	50.6	48.9	47.0	44.9	42.5	39.9	36.8	6.29	9.02
	22	55.3	54.0	52.7	51.2	49.6	47.9	46.0	43.9	41.5	38.9	35.8	5.58	8.26
	16	61.3	59.9	58.5	56.9	55.2	53.4	51.4	49.2	46.8	44.0	40.8	8.21	11.07
48.13	18	59.9	58.5	57.1	55.5	53.9	52.0	50.1	47.8	45.4	42.6	39.4	7.09	9.88
	20	58.8	57.4	56.0	54.4	52.7	50.9	48.9	46.7	44.3	41.5	38.3	6.26	9.00
	22	57.7	56.3	54.9	53.3	51.7	49.8	47.8	45.6	43.2	40.4	37.2	5.51	8.20
	16	63.9	62.4	60.9	59.3	57.6	55.6	53.5	51.2	48.7	45.7	42.3	8.23	11.10
50.54	18	62.4	61.0	59.5	57.8	56.1	54.2	52.1	49.8	47.2	44.2	40.9	7.08	9.88
	20	61.2	59.8	58.3	56.6	54.9	53.0	50.9	48.6	46.0	43.1	39.7	6.23	8.97
	22	60.0	58.6	57.1	55.5	53.7	51.8	49.7	47.4	44.8	41.9	38.5	5.44	8.13

TABLE 401

Process Times (B) at Retort Temperature of 230°F for Conduction-Heating Foods in 300 x 407 Can

f_h	z	INITIAL FOOD TEMPERATURE (T_{ih})											Equivalent	
		100	110	120	130	140	150	160	170	180	190	200	F_c^{18}	F_s^{18}
42.76	16	236.8	235.3	233.7	231.9	229.9	227.7	225.3	222.4	219.0	214.9	209.5	12.81	13.84
	18	184.0	182.5	180.9	179.1	177.2	175.0	172.5	169.7	166.3	162.1	156.8	8.89	9.93
	20	153.7	152.2	150.6	148.9	146.9	144.7	142.2	139.4	136.0	131.8	126.5	6.63	7.62
	22	133.3	131.8	130.2	128.5	126.5	124.3	121.8	119.0	115.6	111.4	106.1	5.07	6.07
45.27	16	240.2	238.6	236.9	235.0	233.0	230.7	228.0	225.0	221.4	217.0	211.4	12.81	12.85
	18	187.4	185.8	184.1	182.2	180.2	177.8	175.2	172.2	168.6	164.2	158.6	8.89	9.93
	20	157.4	155.8	154.1	152.3	150.2	147.9	145.2	142.2	138.6	134.2	128.6	6.59	7.66
	22	136.9	135.4	133.7	131.8	129.7	127.4	124.8	121.7	118.2	113.8	108.1	5.06	6.08
47.79	16	243.1	241.4	239.6	237.6	235.5	233.0	230.2	227.0	223.3	218.6	212.7	12.82	13.87
	18	191.3	189.6	187.8	185.9	183.7	181.2	178.5	175.3	171.5	166.8	160.9	8.88	10.00
	20	160.9	159.2	157.4	155.4	153.2	150.8	148.0	144.8	141.0	136.4	130.4	6.55	7.66
	22	140.1	138.4	136.6	134.6	132.4	130.0	127.2	124.0	120.2	115.6	109.6	5.00	6.05
50.30	16	245.2	243.5	241.6	239.5	237.2	234.6	231.7	228.3	224.3	219.5	213.2	12.74	13.86
	18	194.4	192.6	190.7	188.6	186.3	183.8	180.8	177.5	173.5	168.6	162.3	8.79	9.98
	20	164.0	162.2	160.3	158.2	155.9	153.3	150.4	147.1	143.1	138.2	131.9	6.51	7.60
	22	143.5	141.7	139.8	137.7	135.4	132.9	129.9	126.6	122.6	117.7	111.4	4.97	6.05
52.82	16	247.9	246.1	244.1	241.9	239.5	236.8	233.7	230.2	226.0	220.9	214.3	12.57	13.84
	18	197.8	195.9	193.9	191.7	189.3	186.6	183.6	180.0	175.8	170.7	164.1	8.75	9.93
	20	167.5	165.6	163.7	161.5	159.0	156.3	153.3	149.7	145.6	140.4	133.8	6.47	7.60
	22	146.9	145.1	143.1	140.9	138.5	135.8	132.7	129.2	125.0	119.9	113.3	4.94	6.04

TABLE 402

Process Times (B) at Retort Temperature of 240°F for Conduction-Heating Foods in 300 x 407 Can

f_h	z	INITIAL FOOD TEMPERATURE (T_{ih}) 100	110	120	130	140	150	160	170	180	190	200	Equivalent F_c^{18}	F_s^{18}
	16	106.0	104.7	103.2	101.6	99.8	97.8	95.6	93.2	90.3	86.9	82.8	10.35	12.20
42.76	18	97.9	96.5	95.1	93.4	91.7	89.7	87.5	85.0	82.2	78.8	74.7	8.19	9.96
	20	91.3	89.9	88.4	86.8	85.0	83.1	80.9	78.4	75.5	72.1	68.0	6.76	8.41
	22	85.5	84.1	82.6	81.0	79.2	77.3	75.1	72.6	69.8	66.4	62.2	5.62	7.22
	16	110.0	108.6	107.0	105.3	103.4	101.4	99.0	96.4	93.4	89.8	85.4	10.31	12.22
45.27	18	101.6	100.1	98.5	96.8	94.9	92.9	90.6	87.9	84.9	81.3	76.9	8.19	9.96
	20	94.5	93.0	91.4	89.7	87.8	85.8	83.5	80.8	77.8	74.2	69.8	6.75	8.40
	22	88.3	86.9	85.3	83.6	81.7	79.6	77.3	74.7	71.7	68.1	63.7	5.43	7.10
	16	114.0	112.4	110.8	108.9	107.0	104.8	102.3	99.6	96.4	92.6	88.0	10.28	12.20
47.79	18	105.1	103.6	101.9	100.1	98.1	95.9	93.5	90.7	87.5	83.7	79.1	8.19	9.96
	20	97.5	95.9	94.3	92.5	90.5	88.3	85.9	83.1	79.9	76.1	71.5	6.73	8.38
	22	91.5	90.0	88.3	86.5	84.5	82.4	79.9	77.1	73.9	70.2	65.5	5.37	7.09
	16	117.8	116.1	114.4	112.5	110.4	108.1	105.5	102.6	99.2	95.3	90.4	10.26	12.17
50.30	18	108.5	106.9	105.1	103.2	101.2	98.9	96.3	93.4	90.0	86.0	81.1	8.18	9.96
	20	100.4	98.8	97.0	95.1	93.1	90.8	88.2	85.3	81.9	77.9	73.0	6.57	8.27
	22	94.9	93.2	91.5	89.6	87.5	85.2	82.6	79.7	76.3	72.4	67.5	5.35	7.12
	16	121.6	119.9	118.0	116.0	113.8	111.4	108.7	105.7	102.1	97.9	92.8	10.26	12.18
52.82	18	111.7	110.0	108.2	106.2	104.0	101.6	98.9	95.8	92.3	88.1	83.0	8.16	9.93
	20	103.7	102.0	100.2	98.2	96.0	93.6	90.9	87.8	84.3	80.1	75.0	6.49	8.25
	22	98.1	96.4	94.6	92.6	90.4	88.0	85.3	82.2	78.7	74.5	69.4	5.32	7.14

TABLE 403

Process Times (B) at Retort Temperature of 250°F for Conduction-Heating Foods in 300 x 407 Can

f_h	z	INITIAL FOOD TEMPERATURE (T_{ih})											Equivalent	
		100	110	120	130	140	150	160	170	180	190	200	F_c^{18}	F_s^{18}
42.76	16	70.3	69.0	67.7	66.2	64.5	62.8	60.8	58.6	56.2	53.3	49.9	8.81	11.21
	18	68.1	66.8	65.4	63.9	62.3	60.5	58.6	56.4	53.9	51.1	47.7	7.60	9.95
	20	65.8	64.5	63.1	61.6	60.0	58.2	56.3	54.1	51.6	48.8	45.4	6.46	8.78
	22	63.7	62.5	61.1	59.6	58.0	56.2	54.2	52.1	49.6	46.7	43.3	5.53	7.81
45.27	16	73.5	72.1	70.7	69.1	67.4	65.5	63.5	61.1	58.5	55.5	51.9	8.81	11.22
	18	71.1	69.8	68.3	66.7	65.0	63.2	61.1	58.8	56.1	53.1	49.5	7.57	9.95
	20	68.7	67.3	65.9	64.3	62.6	60.7	58.7	56.3	53.7	50.7	47.1	6.40	8.75
	22	66.5	65.2	63.7	62.2	60.5	58.6	56.5	54.2	51.6	48.5	44.9	5.46	7.76
47.79	16	76.7	75.3	73.7	72.1	70.3	68.3	66.1	63.7	60.9	57.7	53.9	8.82	11.26
	18	74.2	72.8	71.2	69.6	67.8	65.8	63.6	61.2	58.4	55.2	51.4	7.55	9.96
	20	71.7	70.2	68.7	67.0	65.2	63.2	61.1	58.6	55.8	52.6	48.9	6.36	8.73
	22	69.4	67.9	66.4	64.7	62.9	61.0	58.8	56.3	53.6	50.4	46.6	5.41	7.73
50.30	16	79.9	78.4	76.8	75.0	73.1	71.0	68.7	66.2	63.2	59.9	55.9	8.84	11.30
	18	77.2	75.7	74.1	72.4	70.5	68.4	66.1	63.5	60.6	57.2	53.2	7.53	9.96
	20	74.6	73.1	71.4	69.7	67.8	65.7	63.4	60.8	57.9	54.5	50.6	6.33	8.71
	22	72.2	70.7	69.1	67.3	65.4	63.3	61.0	58.4	55.5	52.2	48.2	5.36	7.69
52.82	16	83.0	81.4	79.7	77.9	75.9	73.7	71.3	68.6	65.5	62.0	57.8	8.85	11.33
	18	80.2	78.7	77.0	75.1	73.1	70.9	68.5	65.8	62.8	59.2	55.0	7.51	9.96
	20	77.4	75.9	74.2	72.3	70.3	68.1	65.7	63.0	60.0	56.4	52.2	6.28	8.68
	22	74.9	73.4	71.7	69.8	67.8	65.6	63.2	60.5	57.5	53.9	49.7	5.30	7.65

TABLE 404

Process Times (B) at Retort Temperature of 260°F for Conduction-Heating Foods in 300 x 407 Can

f_h	z	INITIAL FOOD TEMPERATURE (T_{ih})											Equivalent	
		100	110	120	130	140	150	160	170	180	190	200	F_c^{18}	F_s^{18}
42.76	16	55.5	54.3	53.0	51.6	50.1	48.5	46.7	44.8	42.6	40.1	37.2	8.19	11.02
	18	54.3	53.1	51.8	50.4	48.9	47.3	45.6	43.6	41.4	38.9	36.1	7.18	9.95
	20	53.4	52.2	50.9	49.5	48.0	46.4	44.6	42.7	40.5	38.0	35.1	6.43	9.15
	22	52.4	51.2	50.0	48.6	47.1	45.5	43.7	41.8	39.6	37.1	34.2	5.73	8.40
45.27	16	58.2	57.0	55.6	54.1	52.6	50.9	49.0	46.9	44.6	42.0	38.9	8.25	11.10
	18	57.0	55.7	54.3	52.9	51.3	49.6	47.7	45.6	43.3	40.7	37.7	7.17	9.96
	20	55.9	54.7	53.3	51.8	50.3	48.6	46.7	44.6	42.3	39.7	36.6	6.37	9.10
	22	54.9	53.7	52.3	50.9	49.3	47.6	45.7	43.6	41.3	38.7	35.7	5.66	8.34
47.79	16	61.0	59.6	58.2	56.7	55.0	53.2	51.2	49.0	46.6	43.8	40.6	8.29	11.14
	18	59.6	58.3	56.8	55.3	53.6	51.8	49.9	47.7	45.2	42.5	39.3	7.16	9.96
	20	58.5	57.2	55.7	54.2	52.5	50.7	48.7	46.6	44.1	41.3	38.1	6.33	9.07
	22	57.4	56.1	54.7	53.1	51.5	49.7	47.7	45.5	43.0	40.3	37.1	5.59	8.28
50.30	16	63.7	62.3	60.8	59.2	57.4	55.5	53.4	51.1	48.6	45.6	42.3	8.30	11.18
	18	62.2	60.8	59.3	57.7	55.9	54.0	52.0	49.7	47.1	44.2	40.8	7.15	9.96
	20	61.1	59.7	58.1	56.5	54.8	52.9	50.8	48.5	45.9	43.0	39.6	6.29	9.05
	22	59.9	58.5	57.0	55.3	53.6	51.7	49.6	47.3	44.7	41.8	38.5	5.51	8.21
52.82	16	66.4	64.9	63.4	61.7	59.8	57.8	55.6	53.2	50.5	47.5	43.9	8.33	11.22
	18	64.9	63.4	61.8	60.1	58.3	56.3	54.1	51.7	49.0	45.9	42.4	7.14	9.95
	20	63.6	62.1	60.5	58.8	57.0	55.0	52.8	50.4	47.7	44.6	41.1	6.26	9.02
	22	62.3	60.9	59.3	57.6	55.7	53.7	51.6	49.1	46.4	43.4	39.8	5.45	8.16

TABLE 405

Process Times (B) at Retort Temperature of 230°F for Conduction-Heating Foods in 301 x 411 Can

f_h	z	INITIAL FOOD TEMPERATURE (T_{ih}) 100	110	120	130	140	150	160	170	180	190	200	Equivalent F_c^{18}	F_s^{18}
45.22	16	241.4	239.8	238.1	236.2	234.2	231.8	229.2	226.2	222.6	218.2	212.6	12.90	13.94
	18	188.2	186.7	185.0	183.1	181.0	178.7	176.1	173.1	169.5	165.1	159.4	8.96	10.00
	20	157.9	156.4	154.7	152.8	150.7	148.4	145.8	142.8	139.2	134.8	129.1	6.64	7.70
	22	137.4	135.9	134.2	132.3	130.2	127.9	125.3	122.3	118.7	114.3	108.6	5.10	6.12
47.88	16	244.5	242.8	241.0	239.0	236.8	234.4	231.6	228.4	224.6	220.0	214.0	12.90	13.96
	18	192.4	190.7	188.9	186.9	184.7	182.3	179.5	176.3	172.5	167.8	161.9	8.95	10.07
	20	161.7	160.0	158.2	156.2	154.1	151.6	148.8	145.6	141.8	137.2	131.2	6.60	7.71
	22	140.8	139.1	137.3	135.3	133.1	130.7	127.9	124.7	120.9	116.3	110.3	5.04	6.09
50.54	16	246.8	245.1	243.2	241.1	238.8	236.2	233.3	229.9	225.9	221.0	214.7	12.84	13.96
	18	195.6	193.8	191.9	189.8	187.5	184.9	182.0	178.6	174.6	169.7	163.4	8.85	10.05
	20	165.0	163.2	161.3	159.2	156.9	154.3	151.4	148.0	144.0	139.1	132.8	6.56	7.66
	22	144.3	142.6	140.7	138.6	136.3	133.7	130.8	127.4	123.4	118.5	112.2	5.00	6.09
53.20	16	249.7	247.8	245.8	243.6	241.2	238.4	235.4	231.8	227.6	222.4	215.8	12.65	13.93
	18	199.2	197.3	195.3	193.1	190.7	188.0	184.9	181.3	177.1	171.9	165.3	8.81	10.00
	20	168.7	166.9	164.8	162.6	160.2	157.5	154.4	150.8	146.6	141.5	134.8	6.52	7.66
	22	148.0	146.2	144.1	141.9	139.5	136.8	133.7	130.1	125.9	120.8	114.1	4.98	6.08
55.86	16	254.1	252.2	250.1	247.7	245.2	242.3	239.1	235.4	230.9	225.5	218.5	12.64	13.92
	18	203.0	201.1	198.9	196.6	194.1	191.2	188.0	184.2	179.8	174.4	167.4	8.81	9.99
	20	172.7	170.8	168.7	166.4	163.8	160.9	157.7	154.0	149.5	144.1	137.1	6.51	7.69
	22	151.5	149.6	147.5	145.2	142.6	139.7	136.5	132.8	128.3	122.9	115.9	4.94	6.07

TABLE 406

Process Times (B) at Retort Temperature of 240°F for Conduction-Heating Foods in 301 x 411 Can

f_h	z	INITIAL FOOD TEMPERATURE (T_{ih})											Equivalent	
		100	110	120	130	140	150	160	170	180	190	200	F_c^{18}	F_s^{18}
	16	110.3	108.8	107.2	105.5	103.6	101.6	99.3	96.6	93.6	90.0	85.6	10.40	12.30
45.22	18	101.8	100.3	98.7	97.0	95.2	93.1	90.8	88.2	85.1	81.5	77.2	8.25	10.03
	20	94.7	93.2	91.7	90.0	88.1	86.0	83.7	81.8	78.1	74.5	70.1	6.81	8.46
	22	88.6	87.1	85.5	83.8	82.0	79.9	77.6	74.9	71.9	68.3	64.0	5.50	7.17
	16	114.4	112.9	111.2	109.4	107.4	105.2	102.8	100.0	96.8	93.0	88.4	10.37	12.28
47.88	18	105.5	104.0	102.3	100.5	98.5	96.3	93.9	91.1	87.9	84.1	79.5	8.25	10.03
	20	97.9	96.4	94.7	92.9	90.9	88.7	86.3	83.5	80.3	76.5	71.9	6.78	8.44
	22	91.9	90.3	88.7	86.8	84.9	82.7	80.2	77.4	74.2	70.5	65.8	5.41	7.14
	16	118.4	116.8	115.1	113.1	111.1	108.7	106.2	103.2	99.8	95.8	90.9	10.34	12.26
50.54	18	109.2	107.5	105.8	103.9	101.8	99.5	96.9	93.9	90.6	86.6	81.7	8.25	10.03
	20	101.0	99.4	97.6	95.7	93.6	91.3	88.7	85.8	82.4	78.4	73.5	6.63	8.34
	22	95.4	93.8	92.0	90.1	88.0	85.7	83.1	80.2	76.8	72.8	67.9	5.39	7.16
	16	122.5	120.7	118.9	116.9	114.7	112.2	109.5	106.4	102.9	98.7	93.5	10.34	12.26
53.20	18	112.5	110.8	109.0	107.0	104.8	102.3	99.6	96.5	93.0	88.8	83.6	8.22	10.00
	20	104.5	102.8	100.9	98.9	96.7	94.3	91.5	88.5	84.9	80.7	75.5	6.54	8.31
	22	98.8	97.1	95.3	93.3	91.0	88.6	85.9	82.8	79.2	75.0	69.9	5.37	7.18
	16	126.4	124.6	122.6	120.5	118.2	115.7	112.8	109.6	105.8	101.4	96.0	10.34	12.26
55.86	18	115.8	114.0	112.1	110.0	110.0	107.7	105.1	102.3	99.0	95.3	90.8	85.4	8.20
	20	108.1	106.3	104.4	102.3	100.0	97.4	94.6	91.3	87.6	83.1	77.7	6.52	8.33
	22	102.1	100.3	98.4	96.3	94.0	91.4	88.6	85.3	81.6	77.2	71.7	5.34	7.15

TABLE 407

Process Times (B) at Retort Temperature of 250°F for Conduction-Heating Foods in 301 x 411 Can

f_h	z	INITIAL FOOD TEMPERATURE (T_{ih})											Equivalent	
		100	110	120	130	140	150	160	170	180	190	200	F_c^{18}	F_s^{18}
45.22	16	73.6	72.2	70.8	69.2	67.5	65.6	63.5	61.2	58.6	55.6	52.0	8.88	11.30
	18	71.2	69.9	68.4	66.8	65.1	63.2	61.2	58.9	56.2	53.2	49.6	7.64	10.02
	20	68.8	67.4	66.0	64.4	62.7	60.8	58.7	56.4	53.8	50.8	47.2	6.47	8.81
	22	66.6	65.3	63.8	62.2	60.5	58.7	56.6	54.3	51.7	48.6	45.0	5.51	7.82
47.88	16	77.0	75.5	74.0	72.3	70.5	68.5	66.3	63.9	61.1	57.9	54.1	8.89	11.33
	18	74.5	73.0	71.5	69.8	68.0	66.0	63.8	61.4	58.6	55.4	51.6	7.61	10.02
	20	71.9	70.5	68.9	67.3	65.4	63.5	61.3	58.8	56.0	52.8	49.0	6.42	8.78
	22	69.6	68.2	66.6	65.0	63.2	61.2	59.0	56.5	53.8	50.6	46.8	5.46	7.78
50.54	16	80.3	78.8	77.2	75.4	73.5	71.4	69.1	66.5	63.6	60.2	56.2	8.91	11.37
	18	77.7	76.2	74.5	72.8	70.9	68.8	66.5	63.9	60.9	57.6	53.6	7.59	10.03
	20	75.0	73.5	71.8	70.1	68.2	66.1	63.8	61.2	58.2	54.9	50.9	6.38	8.77
	22	72.6	71.1	69.4	67.7	65.8	63.7	61.4	58.8	55.8	52.5	48.5	5.40	7.74
53.20	16	83.6	82.0	80.3	78.5	76.5	74.3	71.8	69.1	66.0	62.5	58.3	8.92	11.41
	18	80.8	79.3	77.5	75.7	73.7	71.5	69.0	66.3	63.2	59.7	55.5	7.58	10.03
	20	78.0	76.4	74.7	72.9	70.8	68.6	66.2	63.5	60.4	56.8	52.6	6.33	8.73
	22	75.5	73.9	72.2	70.3	68.3	66.1	63.7	61.0	57.9	54.3	50.1	5.35	7.70
55.86	16	87.0	85.3	83.5	81.6	79.4	77.1	74.6	71.7	68.5	64.7	60.3	8.94	11.45
	18	84.0	82.4	80.6	78.6	76.5	74.2	71.6	68.8	65.5	61.8	57.4	7.56	10.03
	20	81.1	79.4	77.6	75.6	73.5	71.2	68.7	65.8	62.6	58.8	54.4	6.31	8.73
	22	78.4	76.8	75.0	73.0	70.9	68.6	66.0	63.2	59.9	56.2	51.8	5.28	7.65

TABLE 408

Process Times (B) at Retort Temperature of 260°F for Conduction-Heating Foods in 301 x 411 Can

f_h	z	INITIAL FOOD TEMPERATURE (T_{ih})											Equivalent	
		100	110	120	130	140	150	160	170	180	190	200	F_c^{18}	F_s^{18}
	16	58.2	57.0	55.6	54.2	52.6	50.9	49.0	46.9	44.6	42.0	39.0	8.31	11.16
45.22	18	57.0	55.7	54.4	52.9	51.3	49.6	47.8	45.7	43.4	40.7	37.7	7.23	10.02
	20	56.0	54.7	53.3	51.9	50.3	48.6	46.7	44.7	42.3	39.7	36.7	6.44	9.17
	22	55.0	53.7	52.4	50.9	49.3	47.6	45.8	43.7	41.4	38.7	35.7	5.72	8.41
	16	61.2	59.8	58.4	56.8	55.2	53.4	51.4	49.2	46.7	44.0	40.8	8.35	11.22
47.88	18	59.8	58.4	57.0	55.5	53.8	52.0	50.0	47.8	45.4	42.6	39.4	7.22	10.02
	20	58.7	57.3	55.9	54.4	52.7	50.9	48.9	46.7	44.3	41.5	38.3	6.38	9.13
	22	57.6	56.3	54.8	53.3	51.6	49.8	47.8	45.7	43.2	40.4	37.2	5.65	8.34
	16	64.0	62.6	61.1	59.5	57.7	55.8	53.7	51.4	48.8	45.9	42.5	8.37	11.25
50.54	18	62.6	61.1	59.6	58.0	56.2	54.3	52.2	49.9	47.3	44.4	41.0	7.21	10.02
	20	61.4	60.0	58.5	56.8	55.1	53.2	51.1	48.8	46.2	43.2	39.9	6.35	9.11
	22	60.2	58.8	57.3	55.7	53.9	52.0	49.9	47.6	45.0	42.1	38.7	5.56	8.27
	16	66.9	65.4	63.8	62.1	60.3	58.3	56.1	53.6	50.9	47.8	44.3	8.40	11.30
53.20	18	65.3	63.9	62.3	60.5	58.7	56.7	54.5	52.1	49.3	46.2	42.7	7.20	10.02
	20	64.1	62.6	61.0	59.3	57.4	55.4	53.2	50.8	48.1	45.0	41.4	6.31	9.08
	22	62.8	61.3	59.7	58.0	56.2	54.1	51.9	49.5	46.8	43.7	40.1	5.50	8.21
	16	69.8	68.2	66.5	64.7	62.8	60.7	58.4	55.8	53.0	49.7	46.0	8.44	11.34
55.86	18	68.1	66.5	64.9	63.1	61.1	59.0	56.7	54.1	51.3	48.0	44.3	7.19	10.02
	20	66.7	65.2	63.5	61.7	59.8	57.6	55.3	52.8	49.9	46.7	42.9	6.26	9.04
	22	65.4	63.8	62.2	60.4	58.4	56.3	54.0	51.4	48.6	45.3	41.6	5.44	8.16

TABLE 409

Process Times (B) at Retort Temperature of 230°F for Conduction-Heating Foods in 303 x 406 Can

f_h	z	INITIAL FOOD TEMPERATURE (T_{ih})											Equivalent	
		100	110	120	130	140	150	160	170	180	190	200	F_c^{18}	F_s^{18}
	16	243.7	242.1	240.3	238.4	236.2	233.8	231.1	227.9	224.2	219.6	213.7	12.91	13.96
47.10	18	191.1	189.4	187.6	185.7	183.5	181.1	178.4	175.2	171.5	166.9	161.1	8.96	10.04
	20	160.8	159.1	157.3	155.4	153.2	150.8	148.1	144.9	141.2	136.6	130.8	6.62	7.73
	22	139.9	138.2	136.5	134.5	132.4	129.9	127.2	124.1	120.3	115.8	109.9	5.06	6.10
	16	246.5	244.8	242.9	240.8	238.5	236.0	233.1	229.7	225.8	221.0	214.7	12.91	13.97
49.87	18	194.8	193.1	191.2	189.2	186.9	184.3	181.4	178.1	174.1	169.3	163.1	8.88	10.08
	20	164.3	162.5	160.6	158.6	156.3	153.7	150.8	147.5	143.6	138.7	132.5	6.58	7.68
	22	143.5	141.7	139.8	137.8	135.5	132.9	130.1	126.7	122.8	117.9	111.7	5.01	6.09
	16	248.8	247.0	245.0	242.8	240.4	237.7	234.6	231.1	226.9	221.8	215.3	12.66	13.95
52.64	18	198.4	196.6	194.6	192.4	190.0	187.3	184.2	180.7	176.5	171.4	164.9	8.82	10.00
	20	167.9	166.0	164.0	161.9	159.5	156.8	153.7	150.2	146.0	140.9	134.3	6.52	7.65
	22	147.3	145.5	143.5	141.3	138.9	136.2	133.2	129.6	125.5	120.4	113.8	4.99	6.09
	16	253.5	251.5	249.4	247.2	244.6	241.8	238.6	234.9	230.5	225.1	218.2	12.65	13.93
55.42	18	202.5	200.5	198.4	196.1	193.6	190.8	187.6	183.8	179.5	174.1	167.2	8.82	10.00
	20	172.1	170.2	168.1	165.8	163.3	160.5	157.2	153.5	149.1	143.8	136.8	6.52	7.69
	22	150.9	149.0	146.9	144.6	142.1	139.2	136.0	132.3	127.9	122.6	115.6	4.94	6.07
	16	257.8	255.8	253.6	251.2	248.5	245.6	242.2	238.3	233.7	228.0	220.8	12.64	13.92
58.19	18	206.6	204.6	202.4	200.0	197.3	194.4	191.0	187.1	182.5	176.8	169.6	8.81	10.02
	20	175.9	173.8	171.6	169.2	166.6	163.6	160.2	156.3	151.7	146.1	138.8	6.49	7.67
	22	154.7	152.7	150.5	148.1	145.4	142.5	139.1	135.2	130.6	124.9	117.7	4.92	6.07

TABLE 410

Process Times (B) at Retort Temperature of 240°F for Conduction-Heating Foods in 303 x 406 Can

f_h	z	INITIAL FOOD TEMPERATURE (T_{ih})											Equivalent	
		100	110	120	130	140	150	160	170	180	190	200	F_c^{18}	F_s^{18}
	16	113.2	111.7	110.1	108.3	106.3	104.2	101.8	99.0	95.9	92.2	87.6	10.38	12.30
47.10	18	104.5	102.9	101.3	99.5	97.6	95.4	93.0	90.3	87.1	83.4	78.8	8.26	10.03
	20	97.0	95.5	93.9	92.1	90.1	88.0	85.6	82.8	79.7	75.9	71.4	6.79	8.45
	22	90.8	89.3	87.7	85.9	83.9	81.8	79.4	76.7	73.5	69.8	65.2	5.42	7.13
	16	117.5	115.9	114.1	112.2	110.2	107.9	105.3	102.4	99.1	95.2	90.3	10.35	12.27
49.87	18	108.3	106.7	104.9	103.1	101.0	98.7	96.2	93.3	89.9	86.0	81.1	8.25	10.03
	20	100.3	98.7	96.9	95.0	93.0	90.7	88.1	85.3	81.9	78.0	73.1	6.69	8.38
	22	94.5	92.9	91.2	89.3	87.2	85.0	82.4	79.5	76.2	72.2	67.4	5.40	7.16
	16	121.6	120.0	118.1	116.1	114.0	111.5	108.9	105.8	102.3	98.1	93.0	10.35	12.27
52.64	18	111.9	110.2	108.3	106.4	104.2	101.8	99.1	96.0	92.5	88.3	83.2	8.23	10.01
	20	103.7	102.0	100.2	98.2	96.0	93.6	90.9	87.9	84.3	80.2	75.1	6.55	8.31
	22	98.1	96.4	94.6	92.6	90.4	88.0	85.3	82.3	78.8	74.6	69.5	5.38	7.19
	16	125.7	124.0	122.0	119.9	117.6	115.1	112.3	109.1	105.4	101.0	95.6	10.35	12.27
55.42	18	115.3	113.5	111.6	109.5	107.2	104.7	101.8	98.6	94.9	90.5	85.2	8.21	9.98
	20	107.5	105.8	103.8	101.7	99.4	96.9	94.1	90.9	87.1	82.8	77.4	6.52	8.33
	22	101.6	99.8	97.9	95.8	93.5	91.0	88.1	84.9	81.2	76.8	71.4	5.34	7.16
	16	129.7	127.9	125.8	123.6	121.2	118.6	115.6	112.2	108.3	103.7	98.1	10.35	12.27
58.19	18	118.6	116.8	114.7	112.5	110.1	107.5	104.5	101.1	97.2	92.6	87.0	8.18	9.96
	20	111.3	109.4	107.4	105.2	102.8	100.1	97.1	93.8	89.9	85.3	79.6	6.50	8.36
	22	105.0	103.2	101.1	98.9	96.5	93.9	90.9	87.5	83.6	79.0	73.4	5.31	7.13

TABLE 411

Process Times (B) at Retort Temperature of 250°F for Conduction-Heating Foods in 303 x 406 Can

f_h	z	INITIAL FOOD TEMPERATURE (T_{ih})											Equivalent	
		100	110	120	130	140	150	160	170	180	190	200	F_c^{18}	F_s^{18}
	16	76.0	74.6	73.0	71.4	69.6	67.7	65.5	63.1	60.4	57.2	53.5	8.89	11.32
47.10	18	73.5	72.1	70.6	68.9	67.2	65.2	63.1	60.7	57.9	54.8	51.0	7.62	10.02
	20	71.0	69.6	68.1	66.4	64.6	62.7	60.5	58.1	55.4	52.2	48.5	6.43	8.79
	22	68.7	67.3	65.8	64.2	62.4	60.4	58.3	55.9	53.1	50.0	46.3	5.47	7.79
	16	79.5	78.0	76.4	74.7	72.8	70.7	68.4	65.9	63.0	59.6	55.7	8.91	11.37
49.87	18	76.9	75.4	73.8	72.0	70.2	68.1	65.8	63.3	60.4	57.0	53.1	7.60	10.03
	20	74.2	72.7	71.1	69.4	67.5	65.4	63.2	60.6	57.7	54.4	50.4	6.40	8.78
	22	71.8	70.4	68.7	67.0	65.1	63.1	60.8	58.2	55.3	52.0	48.1	5.42	7.76
	16	83.0	81.4	79.7	77.9	75.9	73.7	71.3	68.6	65.5	62.0	57.8	8.92	11.41
52.64	18	80.2	78.6	76.9	75.1	73.1	70.9	68.5	65.8	62.8	59.2	55.1	7.58	10.03
	20	77.4	75.8	74.1	72.3	70.3	68.1	65.7	63.0	60.0	56.4	52.3	6.35	8.75
	22	74.9	73.3	71.6	69.8	67.8	65.6	63.2	60.5	57.5	53.9	49.8	5.36	7.71
	16	86.4	84.8	83.0	81.1	79.0	76.7	74.1	71.3	68.1	64.4	60.0	8.94	11.45
55.42	18	83.5	81.8	80.1	78.1	76.0	73.7	71.2	68.4	65.2	61.5	57.1	7.57	10.03
	20	80.6	78.9	77.1	75.2	73.1	70.8	68.3	65.4	62.2	58.5	54.1	6.32	8.73
	22	77.9	76.3	74.5	72.6	70.5	68.2	65.6	62.8	59.6	55.9	51.5	5.30	7.66
	16	89.9	88.1	86.2	84.2	82.0	79.6	76.9	74.0	70.6	66.7	62.1	8.95	11.48
58.19	18	86.8	85.0	83.2	81.1	78.9	76.5	73.9	70.9	67.5	63.6	59.0	7.55	10.03
	20	83.7	82.0	80.1	78.1	75.9	73.5	70.8	67.8	64.4	60.5	55.9	6.28	8.71
	22	81.0	79.2	77.3	75.3	73.1	70.7	68.1	65.1	61.7	57.8	53.2	5.23	7.61

TABLE 412

Process Times (B) at Retort Temperature of 260°F for Conduction-Heating Foods in 303 x 406 Can

f_h	z	INITIAL FOOD TEMPERATURE (T_{ih}) 100	110	120	130	140	150	160	170	180	190	200	Equivalent F_c^{18}	F_s^{18}
47.10	16	60.3	59.0	57.6	56.1	54.4	52.6	50.7	48.5	46.1	43.4	40.2	8.35	11.21
	18	59.0	57.7	56.2	54.7	53.1	51.3	49.4	47.2	44.8	42.1	38.9	7.23	10.03
	20	57.9	56.6	55.2	53.6	52.0	50.2	48.3	46.1	43.7	41.0	37.8	6.40	9.14
	22	56.9	55.5	54.1	52.6	51.0	49.2	47.2	45.1	42.7	39.9	36.8	5.68	8.37
49.87	16	63.3	61.9	60.4	58.8	57.1	55.2	53.1	50.9	48.3	45.4	42.1	8.37	11.25
	18	61.9	60.5	59.0	57.4	55.6	53.8	51.7	49.4	46.9	44.0	40.6	7.22	10.03
	20	60.7	59.3	57.8	56.2	54.5	52.6	50.5	48.3	45.7	42.8	39.5	6.36	9.12
	22	59.6	58.2	56.7	55.1	53.3	51.5	49.4	47.1	44.6	41.7	38.3	5.59	8.29
52.64	16	66.3	64.8	63.3	61.6	59.7	57.8	55.6	53.2	50.5	47.4	43.9	8.40	11.29
	18	64.8	63.3	61.7	60.0	58.2	56.2	54.0	51.6	48.9	45.9	42.3	7.21	10.03
	20	63.5	62.0	60.5	58.8	56.9	55.0	52.8	50.4	47.7	44.6	41.1	6.33	9.09
	22	62.3	60.8	59.2	57.5	55.7	53.7	51.5	49.1	46.4	43.4	39.8	5.51	8.23
55.42	16	69.3	67.7	66.1	64.3	62.4	60.3	58.0	55.4	52.6	49.4	45.7	8.44	11.34
	18	67.6	66.1	64.4	62.6	60.7	58.6	56.3	53.8	51.0	47.7	44.0	7.20	10.03
	20	66.3	64.7	63.1	61.3	59.4	57.3	55.0	52.4	49.6	46.4	42.7	6.28	9.05
	22	65.0	63.4	61.8	60.0	58.0	55.9	53.7	51.1	48.3	45.1	41.4	5.45	8.17
58.19	16	72.3	70.6	68.9	67.0	65.0	62.8	60.4	57.7	54.7	51.4	47.5	8.47	11.38
	18	70.5	68.9	67.1	65.2	63.2	61.0	58.6	56.0	53.0	49.6	45.7	7.19	10.03
	20	69.0	67.4	65.7	63.8	61.8	59.6	57.2	54.5	51.5	48.2	44.3	6.23	9.02
	22	67.6	66.0	64.3	62.4	60.4	58.2	55.8	53.1	50.1	46.7	42.8	5.39	8.12

TABLE 413

Process Times (B) at Retort Temperature of 230°F for Conduction-Heating Foods in 303 x 509 Can

f_h	z	INITIAL FOOD TEMPERATURE (T_{ih}) 100	110	120	130	140	150	160	170	180	190	200	Equivalent F_c^{18}	F_s^{18}
	16	251.2	249.4	247.4	245.3	243.0	240.4	237.4	234.0	229.9	224.9	218.5	13.09	14.20
51.26	18	198.9	197.1	195.2	193.1	190.7	188.1	185.1	181.7	177.6	172.7	166.3	9.02	10.23
	20	167.8	166.0	164.1	162.0	159.6	157.0	154.0	150.6	146.5	141.6	135.2	6.69	7.80
	22	146.8	145.0	143.0	140.9	138.6	135.9	133.0	129.5	125.5	120.5	114.1	5.10	6.19
	16	254.4	252.5	250.4	248.2	245.7	242.9	239.8	236.1	231.9	226.6	219.8	12.88	14.17
54.28	18	203.0	201.1	199.1	196.8	194.3	191.5	188.4	184.8	180.5	175.2	168.4	8.97	10.17
	20	172.0	170.1	168.0	165.8	163.3	160.5	157.4	153.8	149.5	144.2	137.4	6.64	7.79
	22	150.9	149.0	147.0	144.7	142.2	139.5	136.3	132.7	128.4	123.1	116.3	5.07	6.19
	16	259.4	257.4	255.2	252.8	250.2	247.3	244.0	240.1	235.6	230.0	222.9	12.87	14.16
57.29	18	207.3	205.3	203.1	200.8	198.1	195.2	191.9	188.0	183.5	178.0	170.8	8.98	10.17
	20	176.5	174.5	172.3	169.9	167.3	164.4	161.1	157.2	152.7	147.1	140.0	6.63	7.83
	22	154.9	152.9	150.8	148.4	145.8	142.8	139.5	135.7	131.2	125.6	118.4	5.03	6.17
	16	264.0	261.9	259.6	257.1	254.3	251.2	247.7	243.7	238.9	233.1	225.6	12.86	14.15
60.31	18	212.1	210.0	207.7	205.3	202.5	199.4	195.9	191.9	187.1	181.3	173.7	8.97	10.21
	20	180.4	178.3	176.0	173.5	170.8	167.7	164.2	160.2	155.4	149.6	142.0	6.59	7.79
	22	159.0	156.9	154.6	152.1	149.3	146.3	142.8	138.7	133.9	128.1	120.6	4.99	6.17
	16	268.1	265.9	263.5	260.9	258.0	254.8	251.1	246.9	241.8	235.7	227.8	12.86	14.14
63.33	18	216.4	214.2	211.8	209.2	206.3	203.1	199.4	195.2	190.2	184.0	176.1	8.93	10.23
	20	184.6	182.4	180.0	177.3	174.4	171.2	167.5	163.3	158.3	152.1	144.2	6.54	7.77
	22	162.9	160.7	158.3	155.6	152.7	149.5	145.8	141.6	136.6	130.4	122.5	4.95	6.14

TABLE 414

Process Times (B) at Retort Temperature of 240°F for Conduction-Heating Foods in 303 x 509 Can

f_h	z	INITIAL FOOD TEMPERATURE (T_{ih}) 100	110	120	130	140	150	160	170	180	190	200	Equivalent F_c^{18}	F_s^{18}
51.28	16	120.4	118.7	116.9	115.0	112.9	110.5	107.9	104.9	101.5	97.4	92.5	10.55	12.48
	18	110.9	109.3	107.5	105.6	103.4	101.1	98.5	95.5	92.1	88.0	83.0	8.41	10.20
	20	102.7	101.0	99.3	97.3	95.2	92.9	90.2	87.3	83.8	79.8	74.8	6.78	8.50
	22	96.9	95.3	93.5	91.5	89.4	87.1	84.5	81.5	78.1	74.0	69.0	5.50	7.28
54.28	16	124.9	123.2	121.3	119.2	117.0	114.5	111.7	108.6	104.9	100.6	95.4	10.55	12.48
	18	114.8	113.1	111.2	109.1	106.9	104.4	101.6	98.5	94.8	90.5	85.3	8.38	10.18
	20	106.6	104.8	102.9	100.9	98.6	96.2	93.4	90.2	86.6	82.3	77.0	6.67	8.45
	22	100.8	99.1	97.2	95.1	92.9	90.4	87.6	84.5	80.8	76.5	71.3	5.47	7.30
57.29	16	129.3	127.5	125.5	123.3	121.0	118.4	115.4	112.1	108.3	103.7	98.2	10.55	12.48
	18	118.5	116.7	114.7	112.5	110.1	107.5	104.6	101.3	97.4	92.9	87.3	8.36	10.15
	20	110.7	108.9	106.9	104.7	102.3	99.7	96.8	93.5	89.6	85.1	79.5	6.64	8.48
	22	104.6	102.7	100.7	98.6	96.2	93.6	90.6	87.3	83.5	78.9	73.4	5.44	7.27
60.31	16	133.6	131.7	129.6	127.3	124.8	122.1	119.0	115.5	111.5	106.7	100.8	10.55	12.48
	18	122.2	120.3	118.2	115.9	113.4	110.6	107.6	104.1	100.0	95.2	89.4	8.33	10.13
	20	114.7	112.8	110.7	108.4	105.9	103.2	100.1	96.6	92.6	87.8	81.9	6.62	8.50
	22	108.3	106.3	104.2	102.0	99.5	96.7	93.6	90.1	86.1	81.3	75.5	5.38	7.22
63.33	16	137.7	135.7	133.5	131.1	128.5	125.6	122.3	118.6	114.4	109.4	103.3	10.52	12.46
	18	126.6	124.5	122.3	119.9	117.3	114.4	111.2	107.5	103.3	98.2	92.1	8.31	10.16
	20	118.6	116.6	114.4	112.0	109.4	106.5	103.2	99.6	95.3	90.3	84.2	6.58	8.50
	22	111.9	109.8	107.6	105.3	102.6	99.7	96.5	92.8	88.6	83.6	77.4	5.29	7.16

TABLE 415

Process Times (B) at Retort Temperature of 250 °F for Conduction-Heating Foods in 303 x 509 Can

f_h	z	INITIAL FOOD TEMPERATURE (T_{ih}) 100	110	120	130	140	150	160	170	180	190	200	Equivalent F_c^{18}	F_s^{18}
51.26	16	81.6	80.1	78.4	76.6	74.7	72.6	70.2	67.6	64.6	61.2	57.1	9.09	11.57
	18	78.9	77.4	75.7	73.9	72.0	69.9	67.5	64.9	61.9	58.5	54.4	7.76	10.20
	20	76.2	74.6	73.0	71.2	69.3	67.1	64.8	62.2	59.2	55.8	51.7	6.52	8.92
	22	73.7	72.2	70.5	68.8	66.8	64.7	62.4	59.7	56.8	53.3	49.3	5.52	7.87
54.28	16	85.3	83.7	82.0	80.1	78.0	75.8	73.3	70.5	67.4	63.7	59.5	9.11	11.61
	18	82.5	80.9	79.1	77.2	75.2	72.9	70.5	67.7	64.5	60.9	56.6	7.74	10.20
	20	79.6	78.0	76.2	74.3	72.3	70.0	67.6	64.8	61.6	58.0	53.7	6.47	8.88
	22	77.0	75.4	73.7	71.8	69.7	67.5	65.0	62.2	59.1	55.4	51.1	5.46	7.82
57.29	16	89.1	87.4	85.6	83.6	81.4	79.0	76.4	73.5	70.2	66.3	61.8	9.13	11.65
	18	86.1	84.4	82.5	80.6	78.4	76.0	73.4	70.5	67.1	63.3	58.8	7.72	10.20
	20	83.1	81.3	79.5	77.5	75.3	73.0	70.3	67.4	64.1	60.3	55.7	6.44	8.87
	22	80.4	78.6	76.8	74.8	72.6	70.3	67.6	64.7	61.4	57.6	53.0	5.39	7.77
60.31	16	92.8	91.0	89.1	87.0	84.7	82.2	79.5	76.4	72.9	68.8	64.1	9.14	11.69
	18	89.7	87.8	85.9	83.8	81.5	79.0	76.3	73.2	69.7	65.7	60.9	7.70	10.20
	20	86.5	84.7	82.7	80.6	78.3	75.8	73.1	70.0	66.5	62.5	57.7	6.39	8.84
	22	83.6	81.8	79.9	77.8	75.5	73.0	70.2	67.2	63.7	59.6	54.9	5.32	7.72
63.33	16	96.5	94.7	92.6	90.4	88.0	85.4	82.5	79.3	75.6	71.3	66.3	9.16	11.73
	18	93.2	91.3	89.2	87.0	84.7	82.0	79.1	75.9	72.2	68.0	63.0	7.68	10.20
	20	89.8	87.9	85.9	83.7	81.3	78.7	75.8	72.6	68.9	64.6	59.6	6.36	8.82
	22	86.9	85.0	83.0	80.7	78.4	75.7	72.8	69.6	65.9	61.7	56.7	5.27	7.68

TABLE 416

Process Times (B) at Retort Temperature of 260°F for Conduction-Heating Foods in 303 x 509 Can

f_h	z	INITIAL FOOD TEMPERATURE (T_{ih})											Equivalent	
		100	110	120	130	140	150	160	170	180	190	200	F_c^{18}	F_s^{18}
51.26	16	65.0	63.6	62.1	60.4	58.6	56.7	54.6	52.2	49.6	46.6	43.2	8.56	11.45
	18	63.5	62.1	60.6	58.9	57.1	55.2	53.1	50.7	48.1	45.1	41.7	7.37	10.20
	20	62.3	60.9	59.4	57.7	55.9	54.0	51.9	49.5	46.9	43.9	40.5	6.49	9.26
	22	61.2	59.7	58.2	56.5	54.8	52.8	50.7	48.3	45.7	42.8	39.3	5.70	8.41
54.28	16	68.3	66.8	65.1	63.4	61.5	59.5	57.2	54.7	51.9	48.8	45.2	8.59	11.50
	18	66.7	65.2	63.5	61.8	59.9	57.9	55.6	53.1	50.3	47.2	43.6	7.36	10.20
	20	65.4	63.9	62.2	60.5	58.6	56.6	54.3	51.8	49.0	45.9	42.3	6.45	9.24
	22	64.1	62.6	60.9	59.2	57.3	55.3	53.0	50.5	47.8	44.6	41.0	5.62	8.35
57.29	16	71.5	69.9	68.2	66.4	64.4	62.2	59.8	57.2	54.3	51.0	47.1	8.63	11.55
	18	69.8	68.2	66.5	64.6	62.6	60.5	58.1	55.5	52.6	49.2	45.4	7.35	10.20
	20	68.4	66.8	65.1	63.2	61.2	59.1	56.7	54.1	51.2	47.8	44.0	6.40	9.19
	22	67.0	65.4	63.7	61.9	59.9	57.7	55.3	52.7	49.8	46.5	42.6	5.55	8.29
60.31	16	74.7	73.0	71.2	69.3	67.2	64.9	62.4	59.7	56.6	53.1	49.0	8.67	11.60
	18	72.9	71.2	69.4	67.5	65.4	63.1	60.6	57.8	54.7	51.2	47.2	7.34	10.20
	20	71.4	69.7	67.9	66.0	63.9	61.6	59.1	56.3	53.2	49.7	45.7	6.36	9.16
	22	69.9	68.2	66.4	64.5	62.4	60.1	57.6	54.9	51.8	48.3	44.2	5.48	8.23
63.33	16	77.9	76.2	74.3	72.2	70.0	67.6	65.0	62.1	58.9	55.2	51.0	8.69	11.63
	18	76.0	74.2	72.3	70.3	68.1	65.7	63.1	60.2	56.9	53.2	49.0	7.32	10.20
	20	74.4	72.6	70.7	68.7	66.5	64.1	61.5	58.6	55.3	51.7	47.4	6.32	9.13
	22	72.8	71.0	69.1	67.1	64.9	62.5	59.9	57.0	53.7	50.1	45.8	5.41	8.16

TABLE 417

Process Times (B) at Retort Temperature of 230°F for Conduction-Heating Foods in 307 x 113 Can

f_h	z	INITIAL FOOD TEMPERATURE (T_{ih}) 100	110	120	130	140	150	160	170	180	190	200	Equivalent F_c^{18}	F_s^{18}
21.09	16	172.9	172.1	171.3	170.5	169.5	168.4	167.2	165.8	164.1	162.1	159.4	12.12	13.00
	18	144.7	144.0	143.2	142.3	141.3	140.2	139.0	137.6	135.9	133.9	131.3	8.74	9.46
	20	121.5	120.8	120.0	119.1	118.1	117.1	115.8	114.4	112.8	110.7	108.1	6.67	7.27
	22	102.9	102.2	101.4	100.5	99.5	98.5	97.2	95.8	94.2	92.1	89.5	5.35	5.90
22.33	16	177.9	177.1	176.2	175.3	174.3	173.1	171.9	170.4	168.6	166.4	163.6	12.12	13.01
	18	147.9	147.1	146.3	145.3	144.3	143.2	141.9	140.4	138.6	136.5	133.7	8.73	9.46
	20	123.4	122.6	121.8	120.9	119.9	118.7	117.4	115.9	114.2	112.0	109.2	6.67	7.28
	22	103.3	102.5	101.6	100.7	99.7	98.6	97.3	95.8	94.0	91.8	89.0	5.19	5.89
23.57	16	182.6	181.7	180.9	179.9	178.8	177.6	176.2	174.6	172.8	170.5	167.6	12.13	13.03
	18	150.8	150.0	149.1	148.1	147.0	145.8	144.5	142.9	141.0	138.7	135.8	8.72	9.46
	20	125.0	124.2	123.3	122.4	121.3	120.1	118.7	117.1	115.3	113.0	110.0	6.67	7.28
	22	105.1	104.3	103.4	102.4	101.3	100.1	98.8	97.2	95.3	93.0	90.1	5.17	5.86
24.81	16	187.0	186.1	185.2	184.2	183.0	181.8	180.3	178.7	176.7	174.3	171.2	12.13	13.04
	18	153.5	152.6	151.7	150.6	149.5	148.2	146.8	145.1	143.2	140.8	137.7	8.71	9.46
	20	126.4	125.5	124.6	123.6	122.4	121.2	119.7	118.1	116.1	113.7	110.6	6.67	7.29
	22	106.9	106.0	105.1	104.0	102.9	101.6	100.2	98.5	96.6	94.2	91.1	5.17	5.85
26.05	16	191.2	190.3	189.3	188.2	187.0	185.7	184.2	182.5	180.4	177.9	174.6	12.13	13.05
	18	155.8	154.9	153.9	152.9	151.7	150.3	148.8	147.1	145.0	142.5	139.2	8.70	9.46
	20	127.5	126.6	125.6	124.5	123.4	122.0	120.5	118.8	116.7	114.2	110.9	6.64	7.32
	22	108.4	107.5	106.5	105.5	104.3	102.9	101.4	99.7	97.6	95.1	91.8	5.16	5.84

TABLE 418

Process Times (B) at Retort Temperature of 240°F for Conduction-Heating Foods in 307 x 113 Can

f_h	z	INITIAL FOOD TEMPERATURE (T_{ih})											Equivalent	
		100	110	120	130	140	150	160	170	180	190	200	F_c^{18}	F_s^{18}
	16	69.7	69.0	68.3	67.5	66.6	65.7	64.6	63.4	62.0	60.3	58.2	9.89	11.25
21.09	18	63.1	62.5	61.7	60.9	60.1	59.1	58.0	56.8	55.4	53.7	51.7	8.10	9.45
	20	58.1	57.5	56.7	55.9	55.1	54.1	53.0	51.8	50.4	48.7	46.7	6.77	8.10
	22	54.2	53.5	52.7	51.9	51.1	50.1	49.0	47.8	46.4	44.7	42.7	5.69	7.02
	16	71.7	71.0	70.2	69.4	68.4	67.4	66.3	65.0	63.5	61.7	59.6	9.88	11.29
22.33	18	65.0	64.3	63.5	62.7	61.8	60.7	59.6	58.3	56.8	55.0	52.9	8.08	9.47
	20	59.8	59.1	58.3	57.5	56.6	55.5	54.4	53.1	51.6	49.8	47.7	6.71	8.07
	22	55.8	55.1	54.3	53.5	52.6	51.5	50.4	49.1	47.6	45.8	43.7	5.54	6.96
	16	73.5	72.7	71.9	71.0	70.0	68.9	67.7	66.4	64.8	62.9	60.6	9.83	11.28
23.57	18	66.8	66.0	65.2	64.3	63.3	62.3	61.1	59.7	58.1	56.3	54.0	8.05	9.46
	20	61.6	60.8	60.0	59.1	58.1	57.1	55.8	54.5	52.9	51.0	48.8	6.67	8.06
	22	57.8	57.0	56.2	55.3	54.4	53.3	52.1	50.7	49.1	47.3	45.0	5.51	6.99
	16	75.4	74.6	73.7	72.8	71.7	70.6	69.3	67.9	66.2	64.3	61.9	9.84	11.29
24.81	18	68.6	67.8	66.9	66.0	64.9	63.8	62.5	61.1	59.4	57.5	55.1	8.00	9.44
	20	63.3	62.5	61.6	60.7	59.7	58.5	57.2	55.8	54.1	52.2	49.8	6.55	8.01
	22	59.8	59.0	58.1	57.2	56.2	55.0	53.7	52.3	50.6	48.7	46.3	5.51	7.01
	16	77.3	76.4	75.5	74.6	73.5	72.3	71.0	69.4	67.7	65.6	63.1	9.81	11.30
26.05	18	70.3	69.5	68.6	67.6	66.5	65.3	64.0	62.5	60.7	58.7	56.2	7.97	9.44
	20	65.3	64.5	63.6	62.6	61.5	60.3	59.0	57.5	55.7	53.6	51.1	6.51	8.03
	22	61.6	60.8	59.9	58.9	57.8	56.6	55.3	53.8	52.1	50.0	47.5	5.48	6.98

TABLE 419

Process Times (B) at Retort Temperature of 250°F for Conduction-Heating Foods in 307 x 113 Can

f_h	z	INITIAL FOOD TEMPERATURE (T_{ih})											Equivalent	
		100	110	120	130	140	150	160	170	180	190	200	F_c^{18}	F_s^{18}
21.09	16	40.7	40.1	39.4	38.6	37.8	37.0	36.0	34.9	33.7	32.3	30.6	8.26	10.30
	18	39.5	38.9	38.2	37.5	36.7	35.8	34.9	33.8	32.5	31.1	29.5	7.46	9.49
	20	38.4	37.8	37.1	36.4	35.6	34.7	33.8	32.7	31.5	30.0	28.4	6.72	8.71
	22	37.5	36.8	36.2	35.4	34.6	33.8	32.8	31.7	30.5	29.1	27.4	6.04	8.02
22.33	16	42.4	41.7	41.0	40.2	39.3	38.4	37.4	36.3	35.0	33.5	31.7	8.24	10.32
	18	41.1	40.4	39.7	39.0	38.1	37.2	36.2	35.0	33.7	32.2	30.5	7.42	9.46
	20	40.0	39.3	38.6	37.8	36.9	36.0	35.0	33.9	32.6	31.1	29.3	6.58	8.60
	22	38.9	38.3	37.5	36.8	35.9	35.0	34.0	32.8	31.5	30.0	28.3	5.92	7.92
23.57	16	44.1	43.4	42.6	41.8	40.9	40.0	38.9	37.7	36.3	34.7	32.9	8.29	10.39
	18	42.8	42.1	41.3	40.5	39.6	38.6	37.6	36.4	35.0	33.4	31.6	7.39	9.45
	20	41.6	40.9	40.1	39.3	38.4	37.4	36.3	35.1	33.8	32.2	30.3	6.55	8.60
	22	40.5	39.8	39.0	38.2	37.3	36.3	35.2	34.0	32.7	31.1	29.2	5.88	7.91
24.81	16	45.8	45.1	44.3	43.4	42.5	41.4	40.3	39.0	37.6	35.9	34.0	8.33	10.44
	18	44.5	43.7	42.9	42.1	41.1	40.1	39.0	37.7	36.3	34.6	32.6	7.37	9.46
	20	43.2	42.4	41.6	40.8	39.8	38.8	37.7	36.4	35.0	33.3	31.3	6.53	8.60
	22	42.0	41.3	40.5	39.6	38.7	37.6	36.5	35.2	33.8	32.1	30.2	5.82	7.88
26.05	16	47.5	46.7	45.9	45.0	44.0	42.9	41.7	40.4	38.9	37.2	35.1	8.32	10.45
	18	46.1	45.3	44.5	43.6	42.6	41.5	40.3	39.0	37.5	35.8	33.7	7.35	9.46
	20	44.7	44.0	43.1	42.2	41.2	40.2	39.0	37.6	36.1	34.4	32.3	6.51	8.60
	22	43.5	42.8	41.9	41.0	40.0	38.9	37.8	36.4	34.9	33.2	31.1	5.76	7.85

TABLE 420

Process Times (B) at Retort Temperature of 260°F for Conduction-Heating Foods in 307 x 113 Can

f_h	z	INITIAL FOOD TEMPERATURE (T_{ih})											Equivalent	
		100	110	120	130	140	150	160	170	180	190	200	F_c^{18}	F_s^{18}
21.09	16	30.3	29.7	29.1	28.4	27.7	26.9	26.0	25.1	24.0	22.7	21.3	7.34	9.91
	18	30.0	29.4	28.8	28.1	27.4	26.6	25.7	24.7	23.7	22.4	21.0	6.91	9.46
	20	29.6	29.1	28.4	27.7	27.0	26.2	25.3	24.4	23.3	22.1	20.7	6.44	8.98
	22	29.3	28.7	28.1	27.4	26.7	25.9	25.0	24.0	22.9	21.7	20.3	6.03	8.55
22.33	16	31.8	31.2	30.5	29.8	29.0	28.2	27.2	26.2	25.1	23.8	22.3	7.34	9.93
	18	31.4	30.8	30.1	29.4	28.6	27.8	26.9	25.9	24.7	23.4	21.9	6.89	9.47
	20	31.0	30.4	29.7	29.0	28.2	27.4	26.5	25.4	24.3	23.0	21.5	6.40	8.95
	22	30.7	30.0	29.4	28.6	27.9	27.0	26.1	25.1	23.9	22.6	21.1	5.98	8.50
23.57	16	33.2	32.6	31.9	31.1	30.3	29.4	28.4	27.3	26.1	24.8	23.2	7.33	9.95
	18	32.9	32.2	31.5	30.7	29.9	29.0	28.0	27.0	25.8	24.4	22.8	6.87	9.47
	20	32.4	31.8	31.1	30.3	29.5	28.6	27.6	26.5	25.3	24.0	22.4	6.39	8.96
	22	32.0	31.3	30.6	29.9	29.1	28.2	27.2	26.1	24.9	23.5	22.0	5.94	8.48
24.81	16	34.7	34.0	33.2	32.4	31.6	30.6	29.6	28.5	27.2	25.8	24.1	7.34	9.97
	18	34.3	33.6	32.8	32.0	31.2	30.2	29.2	28.1	26.8	25.3	23.7	6.86	9.47
	20	33.8	33.1	32.4	31.6	30.7	29.8	28.7	27.6	26.3	24.9	23.2	6.38	8.96
	22	33.3	32.6	31.9	31.1	30.2	29.3	28.3	27.1	25.9	24.4	22.8	5.90	8.45
26.05	16	36.1	35.4	34.6	33.8	32.9	31.9	30.8	29.6	28.3	26.8	25.0	7.38	10.03
	18	35.6	34.9	34.1	33.3	32.4	31.4	30.3	29.1	27.8	26.3	24.5	6.85	9.47
	20	35.2	34.5	33.7	32.8	31.9	30.9	29.9	28.7	27.3	25.8	24.1	6.38	8.97
	22	34.7	34.0	33.2	32.3	31.4	30.4	29.4	28.2	26.8	25.3	23.6	5.85	8.42

TABLE 421

Process Times (B) at Retort Temperature of 230°F for Conduction-Heating Foods in 307 x 203 Can

f_h	z	INITIAL FOOD TEMPERATURE (T_{ih}) 100	110	120	130	140	150	160	170	180	190	200	Equivalent F_c^{18}	F_s^{18}
	16	200.3	199.4	198.3	197.1	195.8	194.4	192.7	190.8	188.6	185.8	182.3	12.34	13.28
28.40	18	161.6	160.6	159.5	158.3	157.0	155.6	153.9	152.0	149.8	147.0	143.5	8.83	9.61
	20	130.9	129.9	128.8	127.6	126.3	124.9	123.2	121.3	119.1	116.3	112.8	6.56	7.41
	22	112.5	111.5	110.4	109.2	107.9	106.5	104.8	102.9	100.7	97.9	94.4	5.18	5.98
	16	205.2	204.1	203.0	201.7	200.4	198.8	197.1	195.1	192.7	189.8	186.0	12.34	13.29
30.07	18	163.9	162.9	161.7	160.5	159.1	157.6	155.8	153.8	151.4	148.5	144.8	8.82	9.61
	20	133.6	132.5	131.4	130.1	128.7	127.2	125.5	123.5	121.1	118.2	114.4	6.56	7.40
	22	114.3	113.3	112.2	110.9	109.5	108.0	106.3	104.2	101.9	98.9	95.2	5.11	5.95
	16	209.6	208.5	207.3	206.0	204.5	202.9	201.1	198.9	196.4	193.3	189.4	12.34	13.31
31.74	18	165.9	164.8	163.6	162.3	160.8	159.2	157.4	155.2	152.7	149.7	145.7	8.81	9.61
	20	136.0	134.9	133.7	132.4	130.9	129.3	127.4	125.3	122.8	119.7	115.8	6.56	7.40
	22	116.3	115.2	114.0	112.7	111.2	109.6	107.7	105.6	103.1	100.0	96.1	5.07	5.89
	16	213.7	212.5	211.2	209.9	208.3	206.6	204.7	202.5	199.8	196.6	192.4	12.35	13.32
33.41	18	167.5	166.4	165.1	163.7	162.2	160.5	158.5	156.3	153.6	150.4	146.2	8.80	9.61
	20	138.1	137.0	135.7	134.3	132.8	131.1	129.2	126.9	124.3	121.0	116.9	6.55	7.39
	22	118.4	117.2	116.0	114.6	113.1	111.4	109.4	107.2	104.5	101.3	97.1	5.04	5.89
	16	217.4	216.2	214.9	213.4	211.8	210.0	208.0	205.6	202.9	199.5	195.1	12.35	13.33
35.08	18	169.1	167.8	166.5	165.1	163.5	161.7	159.6	157.3	154.5	151.1	146.7	8.71	9.66
	20	140.4	139.1	137.8	136.4	134.8	133.0	130.9	128.6	125.8	122.4	118.0	6.51	7.43
	22	120.7	119.5	118.1	116.7	115.1	113.3	111.3	108.9	106.1	102.7	98.3	5.01	5.92

TABLE 422

Process Times (B) at Retort Temperature of 240°F for Conduction-Heating Foods in 307 x 203 Can

f_h	z	INITIAL FOOD TEMPERATURE (T_{ih})											Equivalent	
		100	110	120	130	140	150	160	170	180	190	200	F_c^{18}	F_s^{18}
28.40	16	81.5	80.6	79.6	78.5	77.4	76.1	74.6	73.0	71.1	68.8	66.1	9.98	11.52
	18	74.3	73.4	72.4	71.3	70.1	68.8	67.4	65.7	63.8	61.6	58.8	8.07	9.57
	20	69.5	68.6	67.6	66.5	65.4	64.1	62.6	61.0	59.1	56.8	54.1	6.61	8.21
	22	65.5	64.6	63.6	62.5	61.3	60.0	58.6	56.9	55.0	52.8	50.0	5.55	7.06
30.07	16	84.0	83.0	81.9	80.8	79.6	78.2	76.7	74.9	72.9	70.5	67.6	9.93	11.49
	18	77.0	76.0	75.0	73.8	72.6	71.2	69.7	67.9	65.9	63.5	60.6	8.03	9.61
	20	72.1	71.1	70.0	68.9	67.7	66.3	64.8	63.0	61.0	58.6	55.7	6.57	8.19
	22	67.9	66.9	65.9	64.7	63.5	62.1	60.6	58.8	56.8	54.4	51.5	5.53	7.05
31.74	16	86.5	85.5	84.4	83.2	81.8	80.4	78.8	76.9	74.8	72.3	69.2	9.92	11.51
	18	79.8	78.8	77.7	76.5	75.2	73.7	72.1	70.3	68.1	65.6	62.6	8.02	9.66
	20	74.6	73.5	72.4	71.2	69.9	68.5	66.9	65.0	62.9	60.4	57.3	6.54	8.16
	22	70.2	69.2	68.1	66.9	65.6	64.1	62.5	60.6	58.5	56.0	52.9	5.52	7.03
33.41	16	89.0	87.9	86.7	85.5	84.1	82.6	80.9	78.9	76.7	74.0	70.8	9.90	11.52
	18	82.5	81.4	80.2	79.0	77.6	76.1	74.4	72.4	70.2	67.5	64.3	7.97	9.67
	20	77.0	75.9	74.8	73.5	72.1	70.6	68.9	67.0	64.7	62.1	58.8	6.52	8.14
	22	72.5	71.4	70.3	69.0	67.6	66.1	64.4	62.4	60.2	57.6	54.3	5.52	7.04
35.08	16	91.9	90.7	89.5	88.2	86.7	85.1	83.3	81.3	79.0	76.2	72.8	9.99	11.63
	18	85.1	84.0	82.7	81.4	80.0	78.3	76.6	74.5	72.2	69.4	66.0	7.94	9.68
	20	79.4	78.3	77.0	75.7	74.3	72.7	70.9	68.8	66.5	63.7	60.3	6.50	8.12
	22	74.7	73.6	72.4	71.1	69.6	68.0	66.2	64.2	61.8	59.1	55.7	5.52	7.04

TABLE 423

Process Times (B) at Retort Temperature of 250°F for Conduction-Heating Foods in 307 x 203 Can

f_h	z	INITIAL FOOD TEMPERATURE (T_{ih})											Equivalent	
		100	110	120	130	140	150	160	170	180	190	200	F_c^{18}	F_s^{18}
28.40	16	50.9	50.0	49.1	48.1	47.1	45.9	44.6	43.1	41.5	39.6	37.3	8.43	10.61
	18	49.4	48.5	47.6	46.6	45.6	44.4	43.1	41.6	40.0	38.1	35.8	7.45	9.61
	20	47.9	47.0	46.1	45.1	44.0	42.9	41.6	40.1	38.5	36.6	34.3	6.52	8.67
	22	46.5	45.7	44.8	43.8	42.7	41.5	40.2	38.8	37.1	35.2	33.0	5.77	7.89
30.07	16	53.1	52.2	51.2	50.2	49.1	47.8	46.4	44.9	43.1	41.1	38.8	8.40	10.61
	18	51.5	50.6	49.6	48.6	47.5	46.2	44.8	43.3	41.5	39.5	37.2	7.42	9.60
	20	49.9	49.0	48.0	47.0	45.8	44.6	43.2	41.7	39.9	37.9	35.5	6.45	8.62
	22	48.5	47.6	46.6	45.6	44.4	43.2	41.8	40.3	38.5	36.5	34.1	5.66	7.80
31.74	16	55.4	54.4	53.4	52.3	51.1	49.8	48.3	46.7	44.9	42.7	40.2	8.43	10.66
	18	53.7	52.7	51.7	50.6	49.4	48.1	46.6	45.0	43.2	41.0	38.5	7.40	9.62
	20	52.0	51.0	50.0	48.9	47.7	46.4	44.9	43.3	41.5	39.4	36.8	6.43	8.62
	22	50.5	49.5	48.5	47.4	46.2	44.9	43.4	41.8	40.0	37.8	35.3	5.61	7.77
33.41	16	57.6	56.6	55.5	54.3	53.1	51.7	50.2	48.5	46.5	44.3	41.6	8.46	10.72
	18	55.8	54.8	53.7	52.6	51.3	49.9	48.4	46.7	44.8	42.5	39.9	7.38	9.63
	20	54.0	53.0	52.0	50.8	49.5	48.1	46.6	44.9	43.0	40.7	38.1	6.38	8.60
	22	52.4	51.4	50.4	49.2	47.9	46.6	45.0	43.3	41.4	39.2	36.5	5.56	7.74
35.08	16	59.8	58.7	57.6	56.4	55.0	53.6	52.0	50.2	48.2	45.8	43.0	8.45	10.73
	18	57.9	56.9	55.7	54.5	53.2	51.7	50.1	48.3	46.3	44.0	41.2	7.36	9.63
	20	56.0	55.0	53.9	52.6	51.3	49.9	48.3	46.5	44.4	42.1	39.3	6.33	8.56
	22	54.4	53.3	52.2	51.0	49.6	48.2	46.6	44.8	42.8	40.4	37.6	5.49	7.69

TABLE 424

Process Times (B) at Retort Temperature of 260°F for Conduction-Heating Foods in 307 x 203 Can

f_h	z	INITIAL FOOD TEMPERATURE (T_{ih})											Equivalent	
		100	110	120	130	140	150	160	170	180	190	200	F_c^{18}	F_s^{18}
28.40	16	39.0	38.2	37.3	36.4	35.4	34.4	33.2	31.9	30.4	28.8	26.9	7.59	10.27
	18	38.4	37.6	36.7	35.8	34.8	33.7	32.6	31.3	29.8	28.2	26.3	6.97	9.62
	20	37.9	37.1	36.2	35.3	34.3	33.3	32.1	30.8	29.3	27.7	25.8	6.45	9.07
	22	37.3	36.5	35.7	34.8	33.8	32.7	31.5	30.2	28.8	27.1	25.2	5.91	8.50
30.07	16	40.9	40.0	39.1	38.2	37.1	36.0	34.8	33.4	31.8	30.1	28.1	7.64	10.34
	18	40.2	39.4	38.5	37.5	36.5	35.3	34.1	32.7	31.2	29.4	27.4	6.95	9.61
	20	39.7	38.8	37.9	37.0	35.9	34.8	33.5	32.2	30.6	28.9	26.9	6.39	9.03
	22	39.1	38.3	37.4	36.4	35.3	34.2	33.0	31.6	30.1	28.3	26.3	5.86	8.46
31.74	16	42.8	41.9	40.9	39.9	38.8	37.6	36.3	34.9	33.2	31.4	29.3	7.69	10.41
	18	42.1	41.2	40.2	39.2	38.1	36.9	35.6	34.1	32.5	30.7	28.5	6.93	9.61
	20	41.4	40.6	39.6	38.6	37.5	36.3	35.0	33.5	31.9	30.0	27.9	6.33	8.98
	22	40.8	40.0	39.0	38.0	36.9	35.7	34.4	32.9	31.3	29.5	27.3	5.81	8.42
33.41	16	44.7	43.7	42.7	41.7	40.5	39.2	37.9	36.3	34.6	32.7	30.4	7.71	10.44
	18	43.9	43.0	42.0	40.9	39.7	38.5	37.1	35.5	33.8	31.9	29.7	6.92	9.62
	20	43.2	42.3	41.3	40.2	39.0	37.8	36.4	34.8	33.1	31.2	29.0	6.28	8.94
	22	42.6	41.6	40.6	39.6	38.4	37.1	35.8	34.2	32.5	30.6	28.3	5.74	8.36
35.08	16	46.6	45.6	44.5	43.4	42.2	40.9	39.4	37.8	36.0	34.0	31.6	7.74	10.49
	18	45.7	44.7	43.7	42.5	41.3	40.0	38.5	36.9	35.1	33.1	30.8	6.91	9.62
	20	45.0	44.0	42.9	41.8	40.6	39.3	37.8	36.2	34.4	32.4	30.0	6.27	8.94
	22	44.3	43.3	42.2	41.1	39.9	38.6	37.1	35.5	33.7	31.7	29.3	5.67	8.30

TABLE 425

Process Times (B) at Retort Temperature of 260°F for Conduction-Heating Foods in 307 x 214 Cans

f_h	z	INITIAL FOOD TEMPERATURE (T_{ih})											Equivalent	
		100	110	120	130	140	150	160	170	180	190	200	F_c^{18}	F_s^{18}
39.38	16	229.0	227.7	226.2	224.6	222.8	220.7	218.5	215.8	212.7	208.9	204.0	12.63	13.64
	18	177.2	175.9	174.4	172.7	170.9	168.9	166.6	164.0	160.9	157.1	152.2	8.76	9.80
	20	147.7	146.3	144.8	143.2	141.4	139.4	137.1	134.5	131.4	127.5	122.6	6.54	7.53
	22	127.9	126.5	125.1	123.4	121.6	119.6	117.3	114.7	111.6	107.8	102.8	5.07	6.00
41.70	16	232.9	231.4	229.8	228.1	226.2	224.1	221.7	218.9	215.6	211.5	206.3	12.64	13.65
	18	180.8	179.4	177.8	176.1	174.2	172.0	169.6	166.8	163.5	159.5	154.3	8.77	9.80
	20	151.0	149.5	148.0	146.2	144.3	142.2	139.8	137.0	133.7	129.6	124.4	6.54	7.52
	22	130.7	129.3	127.7	126.0	124.1	122.0	119.5	116.7	113.4	109.4	104.2	5.00	5.98
44.01	16	236.2	234.6	233.0	231.2	229.1	226.9	224.3	221.4	217.9	213.6	208.1	12.64	13.67
	18	184.0	182.5	180.8	179.0	177.0	174.7	172.2	169.2	165.8	161.5	156.0	8.77	9.80
	20	154.2	152.7	151.0	149.2	147.2	144.9	142.4	139.4	136.0	131.7	126.2	6.50	7.54
	22	134.2	132.7	131.0	129.2	127.2	124.9	122.3	119.4	115.9	111.6	106.2	4.99	6.00
46.33	16	239.0	237.4	235.6	233.7	231.6	229.2	226.5	223.4	219.8	215.3	209.5	12.65	13.68
	18	187.4	185.8	184.0	182.1	180.0	177.6	174.9	171.8	168.2	163.7	157.9	8.77	9.84
	20	157.6	156.0	154.2	152.3	150.2	147.8	145.2	142.0	138.4	133.9	128.1	6.48	7.57
	22	137.1	135.5	133.8	131.8	129.7	127.4	124.7	121.6	117.9	113.4	107.6	4.94	5.97
48.65	16	241.2	239.5	237.7	235.7	233.4	230.9	228.1	224.9	221.0	216.3	210.2	12.64	13.69
	18	190.5	188.8	186.9	184.9	182.7	180.2	177.4	174.1	170.3	165.6	159.5	8.69	9.87
	20	160.5	158.8	157.0	155.0	152.7	150.3	147.4	144.2	140.3	135.6	129.5	6.44	7.52
	22	140.1	138.4	136.6	134.6	132.4	129.9	127.0	123.8	119.9	115.2	109.1	4.90	5.96

TABLE 426

Process Times (B) at Retort Temperature of 260°F for Conduction-Heating Foods in 307 x 214 Cans

f_h	z	INITIAL FOOD TEMPERATURE (T_{ih}) 100	110	120	130	140	150	160	170	180	190	200	Equivalent F_c^{18}	F_s^{18}
39.38	16	100.0	98.7	97.3	95.9	94.2	92.4	90.4	88.1	85.5	82.4	78.6	10.25	12.02
	18	92.4	91.1	89.7	88.2	86.6	84.8	92.8	80.5	77.9	74.8	70.9	8.08	9.84
	20	86.2	84.9	83.6	82.1	80.4	78.6	76.6	74.3	71.7	68.6	64.8	6.66	8.30
	22	81.0	79.7	78.4	76.9	75.2	73.4	71.4	69.1	66.5	63.4	59.6	5.66	7.20
41.70	16	103.8	102.4	101.0	99.4	97.7	95.8	93.6	91.2	88.4	85.1	81.1	10.20	12.03
	18	95.8	94.5	93.0	91.5	89.7	87.8	85.7	83.3	80.5	77.2	73.1	8.07	9.83
	20	89.3	88.0	86.5	85.0	83.2	81.3	79.2	76.8	74.0	70.7	66.6	6.66	8.30
	22	83.7	82.4	80.9	79.4	77.6	75.7	73.6	71.2	68.4	65.1	61.0	5.56	7.14
44.01	16	107.5	106.1	104.5	102.9	101.0	99.0	96.8	94.2	91.3	87.8	83.5	10.17	12.05
	18	99.2	97.8	96.3	94.6	92.8	90.8	88.5	86.0	83.0	79.5	75.3	8.08	9.83
	20	92.3	90.9	89.4	87.7	85.9	83.9	81.6	79.1	76.1	72.6	68.4	6.65	8.29
	22	86.3	84.9	83.4	81.7	79.9	77.9	75.6	73.1	70.2	66.7	62.4	5.39	7.04
46.33	16	111.1	109.6	108.0	106.2	104.3	102.2	99.8	97.2	94.1	90.4	85.9	10.14	12.04
	18	102.5	101.0	99.4	97.6	95.7	93.6	91.2	88.6	85.5	81.8	77.3	8.07	9.83
	20	95.1	93.6	92.0	90.3	88.4	86.2	83.9	81.2	78.1	74.4	69.9	6.63	8.27
	22	89.2	87.7	86.1	84.3	82.4	80.3	77.9	75.2	72.1	68.4	63.9	5.29	6.99
48.65	16	114.6	113.1	111.4	109.5	107.5	105.3	102.8	100.0	96.7	92.9	88.2	10.11	12.02
	18	105.7	104.1	102.4	100.6	98.6	96.4	93.9	91.0	87.8	83.9	79.2	8.07	9.83
	20	97.9	96.3	94.6	92.8	90.7	88.5	86.0	83.2	80.0	76.1	71.4	6.54	8.21
	22	92.2	90.7	89.0	87.1	85.1	82.9	80.4	77.6	74.3	70.5	65.8	5.27	7.02

TABLE 427

Process Times (B) at Retort Temperature of 250°F for Conduction-Heating Foods in 307 x 214 Can

f_h	z	INITIAL FOOD TEMPERATURE (T_{ih})											Equivalent	
		100	110	120	130	140	150	160	170	180	190	200	F_c^{18}	F_s^{18}
	16	65.7	64.5	63.3	61.9	60.4	58.8	57.0	55.0	52.7	50.0	46.9	8.65	11.01
39.38	18	63.7	62.5	61.2	59.8	58.3	56.7	54.9	52.9	50.6	48.0	44.9	7.51	9.83
	20	61.5	60.4	59.1	57.7	56.2	54.8	52.8	50.8	48.6	45.9	42.7	6.41	8.70
	22	59.6	58.5	57.2	55.8	54.3	52.7	50.9	48.9	46.6	44.0	40.9	5.51	7.76
	16	68.7	67.5	66.1	64.7	63.1	61.4	59.5	57.3	54.9	52.1	48.8	8.67	11.05
41.70	18	66.5	65.3	63.9	62.5	60.9	59.2	57.3	55.1	52.7	49.9	46.6	7.48	9.82
	20	64.3	63.0	61.7	60.2	58.7	56.9	55.0	52.9	50.5	47.7	44.4	6.36	8.67
	22	62.3	61.0	59.7	58.2	56.7	54.9	53.0	50.9	48.5	45.7	42.4	5.45	7.72
	16	71.6	70.3	68.9	67.4	65.7	63.9	61.9	59.6	57.1	54.1	50.6	8.67	11.07
44.01	18	69.3	68.0	66.6	65.1	63.4	61.6	59.6	57.3	54.8	51.8	48.3	7.45	9.82
	20	67.0	65.7	64.3	62.7	61.1	59.2	57.2	55.0	52.4	49.5	46.0	6.31	8.64
	22	64.9	63.6	62.2	60.6	59.0	57.1	55.1	52.9	50.3	47.4	43.9	5.39	7.67
	16	74.6	73.2	71.7	70.1	68.4	66.4	64.3	62.0	59.3	56.2	52.5	8.67	11.10
46.33	18	72.2	70.8	69.3	67.7	65.9	64.0	61.9	59.5	56.8	53.7	50.1	7.43	9.82
	20	69.7	68.3	66.8	65.2	63.5	61.5	59.4	57.0	54.4	51.3	47.6	6.27	8.62
	22	67.5	66.1	64.6	63.0	61.2	59.3	57.2	54.8	52.2	49.1	45.4	5.33	7.64
	16	77.5	76.1	74.5	72.8	71.0	69.0	66.7	64.3	61.4	58.2	54.3	8.69	11.13
48.65	18	75.0	73.5	72.0	70.3	68.4	66.4	64.2	61.7	58.9	55.6	51.8	7.42	9.83
	20	72.4	70.9	69.4	67.7	65.8	63.8	61.6	59.1	56.3	53.0	49.2	6.24	8.60
	22	70.1	68.6	67.1	65.4	63.5	61.5	59.3	56.8	54.0	50.7	46.9	5.29	7.61

TABLE 428

Process Times (B) at Retort Temperature of 260°F for Conduction- Heating Foods in 307 x 214 Can

f_h	z	INITIAL FOOD TEMPERATURE (T_{ih})											Equivalent	
		100	110	120	130	140	150	160	170	180	190	200	F_c^{18}	F_s^{18}
39.38	16	51.6	50.5	49.3	48.0	46.7	45.2	43.5	41.7	39.7	37.4	34.8	8.01	10.81
	18	50.5	49.4	48.2	47.0	45.6	44.1	42.5	40.7	38.7	36.4	33.8	7.08	9.82
	20	49.7	48.6	47.4	46.2	44.8	43.3	41.7	39.9	37.9	35.6	32.9	6.37	9.08
	22	48.9	47.8	46.6	45.3	43.9	42.5	40.8	39.0	37.0	34.7	32.1	5.71	8.37
41.70	16	54.1	53.0	51.7	50.4	48.9	47.4	45.6	43.7	41.6	39.2	36.4	8.05	10.86
	18	53.0	51.8	50.6	49.3	47.8	46.2	44.5	42.6	40.5	38.0	35.3	7.06	9.82
	20	52.1	50.9	49.7	48.4	46.9	45.3	43.6	41.7	39.6	37.1	34.4	6.33	9.04
	22	51.2	50.0	48.8	47.5	46.0	44.4	42.7	40.8	38.7	36.2	33.5	5.64	8.31
44.01	16	56.7	55.5	54.1	52.7	51.2	49.5	47.7	45.7	43.5	40.9	38.0	8.10	10.93
	18	55.5	54.2	52.9	51.5	50.0	48.3	46.5	44.5	42.2	39.7	36.7	7.05	9.83
	20	54.5	53.2	51.9	50.5	49.0	47.3	45.5	43.5	41.2	38.7	35.7	6.28	9.00
	22	53.5	52.3	51.0	49.6	48.0	46.4	44.5	42.5	40.3	37.7	34.8	5.58	8.25
46.33	16	59.2	57.9	56.5	55.1	53.4	51.7	49.8	47.7	45.3	42.6	39.5	8.14	10.98
	18	57.9	56.6	55.2	53.7	52.1	50.4	48.5	46.3	44.0	41.3	38.2	7.04	9.83
	20	56.8	55.5	54.2	52.7	51.1	49.3	47.4	45.3	42.9	40.2	37.1	6.23	8.96
	22	55.8	54.5	53.1	51.6	50.0	48.3	46.4	44.3	41.9	39.2	36.1	5.52	8.20
48.65	16	61.8	60.4	58.9	57.4	55.7	53.8	51.8	49.6	47.1	44.3	41.0	8.16	11.01
	18	60.3	59.0	57.5	56.0	54.3	52.4	50.4	48.2	45.7	42.9	39.6	7.03	9.82
	20	59.2	57.9	56.4	54.8	53.1	51.3	49.3	47.1	44.6	41.7	38.5	6.20	8.94
	22	58.1	56.7	55.3	53.7	52.0	50.2	48.2	45.9	43.4	40.6	37.4	5.44	8.13

TABLE 429

Process Times (B) at Retort Temperature of 230°F for Conduction-Heating Foods in 307 x 306 Can

f_h	z	INITIAL FOOD TEMPERATURE (T_{ih})											Equivalent	
		100	110	120	130	140	150	160	170	180	190	200	F_c^{18}	F_s^{18}
45.31	16	240.0	238.4	236.7	234.9	232.8	230.5	227.8	224.8	221.2	216.8	211.2	12.80	13.83
	18	187.3	185.7	184.0	182.1	180.0	177.7	175.1	172.0	168.4	164.1	158.4	8.88	9.92
	20	157.4	155.8	154.1	152.2	150.1	147.8	145.2	142.1	138.6	134.2	128.5	6.58	7.65
	22	136.9	135.3	133.6	131.7	129.6	127.3	124.7	121.7	118.1	113.7	108.0	5.05	6.07
47.98	16	243.0	241.4	239.6	237.6	235.4	232.9	230.1	226.9	223.1	218.5	212.5	12.80	13.85
	18	191.4	189.7	187.9	185.9	183.7	181.2	178.5	175.2	171.4	166.8	160.8	8.86	9.99
	20	161.0	159.3	157.5	155.5	153.3	150.9	148.1	144.9	141.1	136.4	130.4	6.54	7.64
	22	140.2	138.5	136.7	134.7	132.5	130.1	127.3	124.1	120.3	115.6	109.6	4.98	6.03
50.64	16	245.2	243.4	241.5	239.4	237.1	234.5	231.6	228.2	224.2	219.3	212.9	12.68	13.84
	18	194.6	192.8	190.9	188.8	186.5	183.9	181.0	177.6	173.6	168.7	162.3	8.76	9.95
	20	164.2	162.4	160.5	158.4	156.1	153.5	150.6	147.2	143.2	138.3	132.0	6.49	7.59
	22	143.8	142.1	140.1	138.1	135.7	133.1	130.2	126.8	122.8	117.9	111.6	4.96	6.04
53.31	16	248.5	246.7	244.6	242.4	240.0	237.3	234.2	230.6	226.4	221.2	214.6	12.54	13.82
	18	198.3	196.5	194.5	192.3	189.8	187.1	184.0	180.4	176.2	171.1	164.4	8.74	9.92
	20	168.1	166.3	164.3	162.1	159.6	156.9	153.8	150.2	146.0	140.8	134.2	6.46	7.60
	22	147.4	145.6	143.6	141.4	138.9	136.2	133.1	129.5	125.3	120.2	113.5	4.92	6.03
55.97	16	252.9	251.0	248.9	246.6	244.0	241.1	237.9	234.1	229.7	224.3	217.3	12.54	13.81
	18	202.1	200.1	198.0	195.7	193.1	190.3	187.0	183.3	178.8	173.4	166.4	8.74	9.91
	20	172.0	170.1	168.0	165.7	163.1	160.2	157.0	153.2	148.8	143.4	136.4	6.45	7.63
	22	151.0	149.1	147.0	144.7	142.1	139.2	136.0	132.2	127.8	122.4	115.4	4.89	6.02

TABLE 430

Process Times (B) at Retort Temperature of 240°F for Conduction-Heating Foods in 307 x 306 Can

f_h	z	INITIAL FOOD TEMPERATURE (T_{ih})											Equivalent	
		100	110	120	130	140	150	160	170	180	190	200	F_c^{18}	F_s^{18}
	16	110.0	108.6	107.0	105.3	103.4	101.4	99.0	96.4	93.4	89.8	85.4	10.30	12.21
45.31	18	101.6	100.1	98.5	96.8	94.9	92.9	90.6	87.9	84.9	81.3	76.9	8.18	9.95
	20	94.4	93.0	91.4	89.7	87.8	85.8	83.4	80.8	77.8	74.2	69.8	6.74	8.39
	22	88.3	86.8	85.3	83.6	81.7	79.6	77.3	74.7	71.6	68.0	63.7	5.42	7.09
	16	114.2	112.6	111.0	109.2	107.2	105.0	102.5	99.7	96.5	92.7	88.1	10.27	12.18
47.98	18	105.3	103.8	102.1	100.3	98.3	96.1	93.6	90.9	87.7	83.9	79.2	8.18	9.95
	20	97.6	96.1	94.4	92.6	90.6	88.4	86.0	83.2	80.0	76.2	71.5	6.72	8.37
	22	91.7	90.2	88.5	86.7	84.7	82.5	80.1	77.3	74.1	70.3	65.6	5.36	7.09
	16	118.2	116.6	114.8	112.9	110.8	108.5	105.9	103.0	99.6	95.6	90.7	10.25	12.16
50.64	18	108.9	107.3	105.5	103.6	101.5	99.2	96.6	93.6	90.3	86.2	81.3	8.17	9.94
	20	100.7	99.1	97.3	95.4	93.3	91.0	88.4	85.5	82.1	78.1	73.2	6.52	8.24
	22	95.3	93.6	91.9	89.9	87.9	85.5	82.9	80.0	76.6	72.6	67.7	5.34	7.11
	16	122.2	120.5	118.7	116.6	114.4	112.0	109.3	106.2	102.6	98.4	93.2	10.25	12.16
53.31	18	112.3	110.5	108.7	106.7	104.5	102.0	99.3	96.2	92.6	88.4	83.3	8.14	9.91
	20	104.3	102.6	100.8	98.8	96.5	94.1	91.4	88.3	84.7	80.5	75.3	6.47	8.25
	22	98.7	96.9	95.1	93.1	90.9	88.4	85.7	82.6	79.0	74.8	69.7	5.31	7.12
	16	126.1	124.3	122.4	120.3	117.9	115.4	112.5	109.3	105.5	101.1	95.7	10.25	12.16
55.97	18	115.5	113.7	111.8	109.7	107.3	104.8	101.9	98.7	94.9	90.5	85.1	8.12	9.89
	20	108.0	106.2	104.2	102.1	99.8	97.2	94.4	91.1	87.4	83.0	77.5	6.45	8.27
	22	102.0	100.2	98.2	96.1	93.8	91.2	88.4	85.1	81.4	76.9	71.5	5.28	7.10

TABLE 431

Process Times (B) at Retort Temperature of 250°F for Conduction-Heating Foods in 307 x 306 Can

f_h	z	INITIAL FOOD TEMPERATURE (T_{ih})											Equivalent	
		100	110	120	130	140	150	160	170	180	190	200	F_c^{18}	F_s^{18}
45.31	16	73.5	72.2	70.7	69.1	67.4	65.5	63.5	61.1	58.5	55.5	51.9	8.79	11.21
	18	71.2	69.8	68.3	66.8	65.1	63.2	61.1	58.8	56.2	53.1	49.5	7.56	9.94
	20	68.7	67.4	65.9	64.3	62.6	60.7	58.7	56.4	53.7	50.7	47.1	6.39	8.73
	22	66.6	65.2	63.8	62.2	60.5	58.6	56.5	54.2	51.6	48.5	44.9	5.45	7.74
47.98	16	76.9	75.5	73.9	72.3	70.5	68.5	66.3	63.8	61.0	57.8	54.0	8.81	11.25
	18	74.4	73.0	71.4	69.8	68.0	66.0	63.8	61.3	58.5	55.3	51.5	7.54	9.94
	20	71.9	70.4	68.9	67.2	65.4	63.4	61.2	58.8	56.0	52.8	49.0	6.35	8.71
	22	69.6	68.1	66.6	64.9	63.1	61.1	58.9	56.5	53.7	50.5	46.7	5.40	7.71
50.64	16	80.3	78.8	77.1	75.4	73.5	71.4	69.1	66.5	63.5	60.1	56.1	8.82	11.29
	18	77.6	76.1	74.5	72.7	70.8	68.7	66.4	63.8	60.9	57.5	53.5	7.52	9.95
	20	74.9	73.4	71.8	70.0	68.1	66.0	63.7	61.1	58.2	54.8	50.8	6.31	8.69
	22	72.5	71.0	69.4	67.6	65.7	63.6	61.3	58.7	55.8	52.4	48.4	5.34	7.67
53.31	16	83.6	82.0	80.3	78.4	76.4	74.2	71.8	69.1	66.0	62.4	58.2	8.84	11.33
	18	80.8	79.2	77.5	75.6	73.6	71.4	69.0	66.3	63.2	59.6	55.4	7.50	9.95
	20	78.0	76.4	74.7	72.8	70.8	68.6	66.1	63.4	60.3	56.8	52.5	6.27	8.66
	22	75.4	73.8	72.1	70.3	68.3	66.1	63.6	60.9	57.8	54.2	50.0	5.28	7.63
55.97	16	86.9	85.3	83.5	81.5	79.4	77.1	74.5	71.7	68.4	64.7	60.2	8.85	11.36
	18	84.0	82.3	80.5	78.6	76.4	74.1	71.6	68.7	65.5	61.7	57.3	7.48	9.95
	20	81.0	79.3	77.5	75.6	73.5	71.2	68.6	65.7	62.5	58.7	54.3	6.24	8.66
	22	78.4	76.7	74.9	73.0	70.8	68.5	66.0	63.1	59.8	56.1	51.7	5.22	7.58

TABLE 432

Process Times (B) at Retort Temperature of 260°F for Conduction-Heating Foods in 307 x 306 Can

f_h	z	INITIAL FOOD TEMPERATURE (T_{ih})											Equivalent	
		100	110	120	130	140	150	160	170	180	190	200	F_c^{18}	F_s^{18}
45.31	16	58.3	57.0	55.6	54.2	52.6	50.9	49.0	46.9	44.6	42.0	39.0	8.24	11.09
	18	57.0	55.7	54.4	52.9	51.3	49.6	47.7	45.7	43.3	40.7	37.7	7.16	9.94
	20	55.9	54.7	53.3	51.9	50.3	48.6	46.7	44.6	42.3	39.7	36.6	6.36	9.09
	22	55.0	53.7	52.3	50.9	49.3	47.6	45.7	43.6	41.3	38.7	35.7	5.65	8.33
47.98	16	61.2	59.8	58.4	56.8	55.2	53.4	51.4	49.2	46.7	43.9	40.7	8.27	11.13
	18	59.8	58.4	57.0	55.5	53.8	52.0	50.0	47.8	45.3	42.6	39.4	7.15	9.94
	20	58.7	57.3	55.9	54.4	52.7	50.9	48.9	46.7	44.2	41.5	38.2	6.31	9.05
	22	57.6	56.3	54.8	53.3	51.6	49.8	47.8	45.6	43.2	40.4	37.2	5.57	8.26
50.64	16	64.0	62.6	61.1	59.5	57.7	55.8	53.7	51.4	48.8	45.9	42.5	8.29	11.17
	18	62.6	61.2	59.6	58.0	56.2	54.3	52.2	49.9	47.3	44.4	41.0	7.14	9.94
	20	61.4	60.0	58.5	56.8	55.1	53.1	51.1	48.7	46.1	43.2	39.8	6.28	9.03
	22	60.2	58.8	57.3	55.6	53.9	52.0	49.9	47.5	45.0	42.0	38.6	5.49	8.19
53.31	16	66.9	65.4	63.8	62.1	60.3	58.3	56.0	53.6	50.9	47.8	44.2	8.33	11.22
	18	65.4	63.9	62.3	60.5	58.7	56.7	54.5	52.0	49.3	46.2	42.6	7.12	9.94
	20	64.1	62.6	61.0	59.3	57.4	55.4	53.2	50.8	48.0	44.9	41.4	6.24	9.00
	22	62.8	61.3	59.7	58.0	56.1	54.1	51.9	49.5	46.8	43.7	40.1	5.43	8.14
55.97	16	69.8	68.2	66.5	64.7	62.8	60.7	58.4	55.8	52.9	49.7	45.9	8.36	11.26
	18	68.1	66.5	64.9	63.1	61.1	59.0	56.7	54.1	51.3	48.0	44.3	7.11	9.94
	20	66.7	65.2	63.5	61.7	59.7	57.6	55.3	52.7	49.9	46.6	42.9	6.19	8.96
	22	65.4	63.8	62.1	60.3	58.4	56.3	54.0	51.4	48.5	45.3	41.5	5.36	8.09

TABLE 433

Process Times (B) at Retort Temperature of 230°F for Conduction-Heating Foods in 307 x 400 Can

f_h	z	INITIAL FOOD TEMPERATURE (T_{ih}) 100	110	120	130	140	150	160	170	180	190	200	Equivalent F_c^{18}	Equivalent F_s^{18}
50.79	16	248.0	246.2	244.3	242.2	239.9	237.3	234.3	230.9	226.9	222.0	215.6	12.90	14.02
	18	196.5	194.7	192.8	190.7	188.4	185.8	182.8	179.4	175.4	170.5	164.2	8.89	10.09
	20	165.8	164.0	162.1	160.0	157.7	155.1	152.1	148.7	144.7	139.8	133.4	6.59	7.69
	22	145.0	143.3	141.3	139.2	136.9	134.3	131.4	128.0	124.0	119.0	112.7	5.03	6.11
53.78	16	251.4	249.5	247.5	245.2	242.8	240.0	236.9	233.3	229.0	223.8	217.1	12.71	13.99
	18	200.6	198.7	196.7	194.5	192.0	189.3	186.1	182.5	178.3	173.1	166.3	8.85	10.04
	20	170.0	168.1	166.1	163.9	161.4	158.7	155.5	151.9	147.7	142.5	135.7	6.55	7.69
	22	149.1	147.3	145.2	143.0	140.5	137.8	134.7	131.1	126.8	121.6	114.9	4.99	6.10
56.77	16	256.3	254.3	252.2	249.8	247.2	244.3	241.0	237.2	232.7	227.2	220.1	12.70	13.98
	18	204.8	202.8	200.7	198.3	195.7	192.8	189.5	185.7	181.2	175.7	168.6	8.85	10.03
	20	174.4	172.4	170.3	167.9	165.3	162.4	159.1	155.3	150.8	145.3	138.2	6.53	7.72
	22	153.1	151.2	149.0	146.7	144.1	141.2	137.9	134.1	129.6	124.1	117.0	4.96	6.10
59.75	16	260.8	258.7	256.5	254.0	251.3	248.2	244.7	240.7	236.0	230.2	222.8	12.69	13.97
	18	209.7	207.6	205.3	202.9	200.1	197.1	193.6	189.6	184.9	179.1	171.6	8.85	10.09
	20	178.3	176.2	173.9	171.5	168.7	165.7	162.2	158.2	153.5	147.7	140.2	6.49	7.68
	22	157.1	155.0	152.8	150.3	147.6	144.5	141.0	137.0	132.3	126.5	119.0	4.92	6.08
62.74	16	264.9	262.7	260.3	257.7	254.9	251.7	248.0	243.8	238.9	232.8	224.9	12.68	13.96
	18	213.9	211.7	209.3	206.7	203.8	200.6	197.0	192.8	187.8	181.7	173.9	8.80	10.10
	20	182.4	180.2	177.9	175.3	172.4	169.2	165.5	161.3	156.4	150.3	142.5	6.45	7.67
	22	161.0	158.8	156.4	153.8	150.9	147.7	144.1	139.9	134.9	128.8	121.0	4.88	6.06

TABLE 434

Process Times (B) at Retort Temperature of 240°F for Conduction-Heating Foods in 307 x 400 Can

f_h	z	INITIAL FOOD TEMPERATURE (T_{ih}) 100	110	120	130	140	150	160	170	180	190	200	Equivalent F_c^{18}	F_s^{18}
50.79	16	119.0	117.4	115.6	113.7	111.6	109.3	106.7	103.7	100.3	96.3	91.4	10.39	12.31
	18	109.7	108.1	106.3	104.4	102.3	99.9	97.4	94.4	91.0	87.0	82.1	8.29	10.07
	20	101.5	99.9	98.1	96.2	94.1	91.8	89.2	86.2	82.8	78.8	73.9	6.66	8.37
	22	95.9	94.2	92.5	90.5	88.4	86.1	83.5	80.6	77.2	73.1	68.2	5.42	7.19
53.78	16	123.5	121.8	119.9	117.9	115.7	113.2	110.5	107.3	103.7	99.5	94.3	10.39	12.32
	18	113.5	111.8	109.9	107.9	105.6	103.2	100.4	97.3	93.7	89.4	84.2	8.26	10.04
	20	105.4	103.7	101.8	99.8	97.6	85.1	92.4	89.2	85.6	81.4	76.2	6.57	8.35
	22	99.7	98.0	96.1	94.1	91.8	89.4	86.6	83.5	79.9	75.7	70.4	5.39	7.21
56.77	16	127.9	126.1	124.1	122.0	119.6	117.0	114.1	110.8	107.0	102.5	97.0	10.39	12.32
	18	117.2	115.3	113.4	111.2	108.9	106.3	103.4	100.1	96.3	91.8	86.3	8.23	10.01
	20	109.5	107.7	105.7	103.6	101.2	98.6	95.7	92.4	88.6	84.1	78.6	6.54	8.37
	22	103.4	101.6	99.6	97.5	95.1	92.5	89.6	86.3	82.5	78.0	72.5	5.36	7.18
59.75	16	132.1	130.2	218.1	125.9	123.4	120.7	117.6	114.2	110.2	105.4	99.6	10.39	12.32
	18	120.9	119.0	116.9	114.6	112.2	109.4	106.4	102.9	98.9	94.2	88.4	8.21	10.00
	20	113.5	111.6	109.5	107.2	104.8	102.0	99.0	95.5	91.5	86.8	81.0	6.51	8.39
	22	107.1	105.2	103.1	100.8	98.4	95.6	92.6	89.1	85.1	80.4	74.6	5.29	7.13
62.74	16	136.1	134.1	131.9	129.6	127.0	124.1	120.9	117.2	113.0	108.1	102.0	10.36	12.29
	18	125.2	123.2	121.0	118.6	116.0	113.2	110.0	106.3	102.1	97.1	91.1	8.18	10.03
	20	117.3	115.3	113.1	110.8	108.2	105.3	102.1	98.4	94.2	89.3	83.2	6.48	8.40
	22	110.6	108.6	106.4	104.1	101.5	98.6	95.4	91.8	87.6	82.6	76.5	5.20	7.06

TABLE 435

Process Times (B) at Retort Temperature of 250°F for Conduction-Heating Foods in 307 x 400 Can

f_h	z	INITIAL FOOD TEMPERATURE (T_{ih})											Equivalent	
		100	110	120	130	140	150	160	170	180	190	200	F_c^{18}	F_s^{18}
	16	80.7	79.2	77.6	75.8	73.9	71.8	69.5	66.9	63.9	60.5	56.5	8.95	11.42
50.79	18	78.1	76.5	74.9	73.1	71.2	69.1	66.8	64.2	61.3	57.8	53.8	7.63	10.07
	20	75.4	73.8	72.2	70.4	68.5	66.4	64.1	61.5	58.5	55.1	51.1	6.42	8.80
	22	72.9	71.4	69.8	68.0	66.1	64.0	61.7	59.1	56.1	52.7	48.7	5.43	7.77
	16	84.5	82.8	81.1	79.2	77.2	75.0	72.5	69.8	66.7	63.1	58.8	8.97	11.46
53.78	18	81.6	80.0	78.3	76.4	74.4	72.2	69.7	66.9	63.8	60.2	56.0	7.61	10.07
	20	78.8	77.1	75.4	73.5	71.5	69.3	66.8	64.1	61.0	57.4	53.1	6.36	8.77
	22	76.2	74.6	72.9	71.0	69.0	66.7	64.3	61.5	58.4	54.8	50.6	5.37	7.72
	16	88.2	86.5	84.7	82.7	80.5	78.2	75.6	72.7	69.4	65.6	61.1	8.99	11.50
56.77	18	85.2	83.5	81.7	79.7	77.5	75.2	72.6	69.7	66.4	62.6	58.1	7.59	10.07
	20	82.2	80.5	78.7	76.7	74.5	72.2	69.6	66.7	63.4	59.6	55.1	6.33	8.76
	22	79.5	77.8	76.0	74.0	71.9	69.5	66.9	64.0	60.7	56.9	52.4	5.30	7.67
	16	91.9	90.1	88.2	86.1	83.8	81.3	78.6	75.6	72.1	68.1	63.4	9.00	11.54
59.75	18	88.7	86.9	85.0	82.9	80.7	78.2	75.4	72.4	68.9	64.9	60.2	7.57	10.07
	20	85.5	83.8	81.8	79.8	77.5	75.0	72.3	69.2	65.8	61.8	57.0	6.29	8.73
	22	82.7	80.9	79.0	76.9	74.7	72.2	69.5	66.4	63.0	59.0	54.2	5.23	7.62
	16	95.5	93.7	91.6	89.5	87.1	84.5	81.6	78.4	74.8	70.6	65.6	9.02	11.58
62.74	18	92.2	90.3	88.3	86.1	83.7	81.2	78.3	75.1	71.4	67.2	62.3	7.55	10.06
	20	88.9	87.0	85.0	82.8	80.4	77.9	75.0	71.8	68.1	63.9	59.0	6.26	8.71
	22	86.0	84.1	82.1	79.9	77.5	74.9	72.1	68.8	65.2	61.0	56.0	5.18	7.59

TABLE 436

Process Times (B) at Retort Temperature of 260°F for Conduction-Heating Foods in 307 x 400 Can

f_h	z	INITIAL FOOD TEMPERATURE (T_{ih})											Equivalent	
		100	110	120	130	140	150	160	170	180	190	200	F_c^{18}	F_s^{18}
	16	64.4	62.9	61.4	59.8	58.0	56.1	54.0	51.7	49.1	46.1	42.7	8.42	11.30
50.79	18	62.9	61.5	59.9	58.3	56.5	54.6	52.5	50.2	47.6	44.6	41.2	7.25	10.07
	20	61.7	60.3	58.8	57.1	55.4	53.4	51.3	49.0	46.4	43.5	40.1	6.38	9.14
	22	60.5	59.1	57.6	55.9	54.2	52.2	50.1	47.8	45.2	42.3	38.9	5.59	8.30
	16	67.6	66.1	64.5	62.7	60.9	58.8	56.6	54.1	51.4	48.3	44.7	8.46	11.35
53.78	18	66.0	64.5	62.9	61.1	59.3	57.2	55.0	52.6	49.8	46.7	43.1	7.24	10.07
	20	64.7	63.2	61.6	59.9	58.0	56.0	53.7	51.3	48.5	45.4	41.8	6.34	9.11
	22	63.4	61.9	60.3	58.6	56.7	54.7	52.5	50.0	47.2	44.1	40.5	5.52	8.24
	16	70.8	69.2	67.5	65.7	63.7	61.6	59.2	56.6	53.7	50.4	46.6	8.49	11.40
56.77	18	69.1	67.5	65.8	64.0	62.0	59.8	57.5	54.9	52.0	48.7	44.9	7.23	10.06
	20	67.7	66.1	64.4	62.6	60.6	58.5	56.1	53.5	50.6	47.3	43.5	6.29	9.07
	22	66.3	64.7	63.0	61.2	59.2	57.1	54.7	52.1	49.2	45.9	42.1	5.45	8.18
	16	74.0	72.3	70.5	68.6	66.5	64.2	61.8	59.0	56.0	52.5	48.5	8.53	11.45
59.75	18	72.1	70.5	68.7	66.8	64.7	62.4	59.9	57.2	54.2	50.7	46.7	7.21	10.06
	20	70.7	69.0	67.2	65.3	63.2	60.9	58.5	55.7	52.7	49.2	45.2	6.25	9.04
	22	69.2	67.5	65.7	63.8	61.7	59.5	57.0	54.3	51.2	27.7	43.7	5.38	8.12
	16	77.1	75.4	73.5	71.5	69.3	66.9	64.3	61.4	58.2	54.6	50.4	8.55	11.48
62.74	18	75.2	73.4	71.6	69.5	67.4	65.0	62.4	59.5	56.3	52.7	48.5	7.20	10.06
	20	73.6	71.9	70.0	68.0	65.8	63.4	60.8	57.9	54.7	51.1	46.9	6.21	9.02
	22	72.0	70.3	68.4	66.4	64.2	61.8	59.2	56.3	53.1	49.5	45.3	5.31	8.05

TABLE 437

Process Times (B) at Retort Temperature of 230°F for Conduction-Heating Foods in 307 x 409 Can

f_h	z	INITIAL FOOD TEMPERATURE (T_{ih})											Equivalent	
		100	110	120	130	140	150	160	170	180	190	200	F_c^{18}	F_s^{18}
54.37	16	253.9	252.0	250.0	247.7	245.2	242.4	239.3	235.7	231.4	226.1	219.3	12.83	14.12
	18	202.7	200.8	198.7	196.5	194.0	191.2	188.0	184.4	180.1	174.8	168.0	8.94	10.13
	20	171.8	169.9	167.8	165.6	163.1	160.3	157.2	153.5	149.2	144.0	137.2	6.61	7.77
	22	150.7	148.8	146.8	144.5	142.0	139.2	136.1	132.4	128.1	122.9	116.1	5.04	6.16
57.57	16	259.2	257.2	255.0	252.6	250.0	247.0	243.7	239.8	235.3	229.7	222.5	12.82	14.10
	18	207.1	205.1	203.0	200.6	198.0	195.0	191.7	187.8	183.3	177.7	170.5	8.94	10.13
	20	176.5	174.5	172.3	169.9	167.3	164.3	161.0	157.1	152.6	147.0	139.8	6.60	7.79
	22	155.0	153.0	150.8	148.5	145.8	142.9	139.5	135.7	131.1	125.5	118.4	5.01	6.15
60.77	16	263.9	261.8	259.5	257.0	254.2	251.1	247.6	243.5	238.8	232.8	225.3	12.81	14.09
	18	212.4	210.3	208.0	205.5	202.7	199.6	196.1	192.0	187.2	181.3	173.7	8.94	10.19
	20	180.6	178.5	176.2	173.7	170.9	167.8	164.3	160.2	155.4	149.5	141.9	6.54	7.75
	22	159.2	157.1	154.8	152.3	149.5	146.4	142.9	138.8	134.0	128.1	120.5	4.96	6.14
63.97	16	268.2	266.0	263.6	260.9	258.0	254.7	251.0	246.7	241.7	235.5	227.5	12.80	14.08
	18	216.8	214.6	212.2	209.5	206.6	203.3	199.6	195.3	190.2	184.1	176.1	8.88	10.18
	20	185.1	182.9	180.5	177.9	174.9	171.7	167.9	163.7	158.6	152.4	144.4	6.51	7.75
	22	163.4	161.2	158.8	156.1	153.2	149.9	146.2	141.9	136.9	130.7	122.7	4.91	6.12
67.17	16	273.2	270.9	268.3	265.6	262.5	259.0	255.2	250.7	245.3	238.8	230.4	12.84	14.14
	18	220.9	218.6	216.0	213.2	210.2	206.7	202.8	198.3	193.0	186.5	178.1	8.83	10.13
	20	189.7	187.3	184.8	182.0	178.9	175.5	171.6	167.1	161.8	155.3	146.9	6.50	7.76
	22	167.7	165.3	162.8	160.0	157.0	153.5	149.6	145.1	139.8	133.3	124.9	4.80	6.09

TABLE 438

Process Times (B) at Retort Temperature of 240°F for Conduction-Heating Foods in 307 x 409 Can

f_h	z	INITIAL FOOD TEMPERATURE (T_{ih}) 100	110	120	130	140	150	160	170	180	190	200	Equivalent F_c^{18}	F_s^{18}
54.37	16	124.9	123.1	121.2	119.2	116.9	114.4	111.7	108.5	104.9	100.6	95.3	10.50	12.43
	18	114.7	113.0	111.1	109.0	106.8	104.3	101.5	98.4	94.7	90.4	85.1	8.35	10.13
	20	106.6	104.8	102.9	100.9	98.6	96.1	93.4	90.2	86.6	82.3	77.0	6.64	8.42
	22	100.8	99.0	97.1	95.1	92.8	90.4	87.6	84.4	80.8	76.5	71.2	5.45	7.27
57.57	16	129.6	127.7	125.7	123.5	121.1	118.5	115.6	112.2	108.4	103.8	98.2	10.50	12.44
	18	118.6	116.8	114.8	112.6	110.2	107.6	104.7	101.3	97.5	92.9	87.3	8.32	10.11
	20	111.0	109.1	107.1	104.9	102.5	99.9	97.0	93.6	89.8	85.2	79.6	6.61	8.45
	22	104.8	102.9	100.9	98.7	96.4	93.7	90.8	87.4	83.6	79.0	73.4	5.41	7.24
60.77	16	134.1	132.1	130.0	127.7	125.2	122.4	119.3	115.8	111.7	106.9	101.0	10.50	12.43
	18	122.7	120.8	118.7	116.4	113.9	111.1	108.0	104.4	100.4	95.6	89.7	8.29	10.10
	20	115.2	113.2	111.1	108.8	106.3	103.5	100.4	96.9	92.8	88.0	82.1	6.58	8.47
	22	108.7	106.7	104.6	102.3	99.8	97.0	93.9	90.4	86.3	81.5	75.6	5.33	7.18
63.97	16	138.3	136.3	134.0	131.6	129.0	126.0	122.8	119.1	114.8	109.7	103.5	10.47	12.41
	18	127.3	125.3	123.0	120.6	118.0	115.1	111.8	108.1	103.8	98.7	92.5	8.27	10.13
	20	119.3	117.2	115.0	112.6	109.9	107.0	103.7	100.0	95.8	90.7	84.5	6.54	8.48
	22	112.5	110.4	108.2	105.8	103.1	100.2	96.9	93.2	88.9	83.9	77.7	5.24	7.11
67.17	16	142.4	140.3	137.9	135.4	132.6	129.5	126.1	122.2	117.7	112.4	105.9	10.45	12.38
	18	131.8	129.7	127.3	124.8	122.0	118.9	115.5	111.6	107.1	101.8	95.3	8.24	10.16
	20	123.4	121.2	118.9	116.3	113.6	110.5	107.1	103.2	98.7	93.3	86.8	6.52	8.47
	22	116.2	114.0	111.7	109.1	106.4	103.3	99.8	95.9	91.5	86.1	79.6	5.15	7.04

TABLE 439

Process Times (B) at Retort Temperature of 250°F for Conduction-Heating Foods in 307 x 409 Can

f_h	z	INITIAL FOOD TEMPERATURE (T_{ih}) 100	110	120	130	140	150	160	170	180	190	200	Equivalent F_c^{18}	F_s^{18}
54.37	16	85.4	83.8	82.0	80.1	78.1	75.8	73.3	70.5	67.4	63.8	59.4	9.07	11.57
	18	82.5	80.9	79.2	77.3	75.2	73.0	70.5	67.7	64.5	60.9	56.6	7.70	10.16
	20	79.6	78.0	76.3	74.4	72.3	70.1	67.6	64.8	61.6	58.0	53.7	6.43	8.85
	22	77.1	75.4	73.7	71.8	69.7	67.5	65.0	62.2	59.1	55.4	51.1	5.43	7.79
57.57	16	89.4	87.7	85.8	83.8	81.6	79.2	76.6	73.7	70.3	66.5	61.9	9.09	11.62
	18	86.4	84.6	82.8	80.8	78.6	76.2	73.6	70.6	67.3	63.4	58.9	7.68	10.16
	20	83.3	81.6	79.7	77.7	75.5	73.2	70.5	67.6	64.2	60.4	55.8	6.40	8.84
	22	80.6	78.9	77.0	75.0	72.9	70.4	67.8	64.9	61.5	57.7	53.1	5.35	7.74
60.77	16	93.3	91.5	89.5	87.4	85.1	82.6	79.8	76.7	73.2	69.1	64.3	9.10	11.65
	18	90.1	88.3	86.3	84.2	81.9	79.4	76.6	73.5	70.0	65.9	61.1	7.66	10.16
	20	86.9	85.1	83.1	81.0	78.7	76.2	73.4	70.3	66.8	62.7	57.9	6.35	8.80
	22	84.0	82.2	80.3	78.1	75.9	73.3	70.6	67.4	63.9	59.9	55.0	5.28	7.68
63.97	16	97.3	95.3	93.3	91.1	88.6	86.0	83.1	79.8	76.1	71.8	66.7	9.13	11.70
	18	93.8	91.9	89.9	87.6	85.2	82.6	79.7	76.4	72.7	68.4	63.3	7.64	10.16
	20	90.5	88.6	86.5	84.3	81.9	79.2	76.3	73.0	69.3	65.0	60.0	6.32	8.78
	22	87.5	85.6	83.5	81.3	78.9	76.2	73.3	70.0	66.3	62.0	57.0	5.23	7.65
67.17	16	101.2	99.2	97.0	94.7	92.1	89.3	86.3	82.8	78.9	74.4	69.1	9.15	11.74
	18	97.6	95.5	93.4	91.1	88.5	85.7	82.7	79.2	75.3	70.8	65.5	7.62	10.16
	20	94.1	92.0	89.9	87.5	85.0	82.2	79.2	75.7	71.8	67.3	62.0	6.26	8.75
	22	90.9	88.9	86.8	84.4	81.9	79.1	76.0	72.6	68.7	64.2	58.9	5.19	7.62

TABLE 440

Process Times (B) at Retort Temperature of 260°F for Conduction-Heating Foods in 307 x 409 Can

f_h	z	INITIAL FOOD TEMPERATURE (T_{ih})											Equivalent	
		100	110	120	130	140	150	160	170	180	190	200	F_c^{18}	F_s^{18}
54.37	16	68.3	66.8	65.2	63.4	61.5	59.5	57.2	54.8	52.0	48.8	45.2	8.56	11.46
	18	66.7	65.2	63.6	61.8	59.9	57.9	55.6	53.1	50.4	47.2	43.6	7.33	10.16
	20	65.4	63.9	62.3	60.5	58.6	56.6	54.3	51.8	49.1	45.9	42.3	6.42	9.20
	22	64.1	62.6	61.0	59.2	57.3	55.3	53.0	50.5	47.8	44.6	41.0	5.59	8.32
57.57	16	71.8	70.2	68.4	66.6	64.6	62.4	60.0	57.4	54.4	51.1	47.2	8.60	11.51
	18	70.0	68.4	66.7	64.9	62.8	60.7	58.3	55.7	52.7	49.4	45.5	7.31	10.16
	20	68.6	67.0	65.3	63.4	61.4	59.3	56.9	54.2	51.3	48.0	44.1	6.36	9.15
	22	67.2	65.6	63.9	62.0	60.0	57.9	55.5	52.9	49.9	46.6	42.7	5.51	8.25
60.77	16	75.2	73.5	71.6	69.7	67.6	65.3	62.8	60.0	56.9	53.4	49.3	8.63	11.56
	18	73.3	71.6	69.8	67.8	65.7	63.4	60.9	58.1	55.0	51.5	47.4	7.30	10.16
	20	71.8	70.1	68.3	66.3	64.2	61.9	59.4	56.6	53.5	50.0	45.9	6.32	9.12
	22	70.3	68.6	66.8	64.8	62.7	60.4	57.9	55.1	52.0	48.5	44.4	5.44	8.18
63.97	16	78.6	76.8	74.8	72.8	70.6	68.1	65.5	62.6	59.3	55.6	51.3	8.65	11.59
	18	76.6	74.8	72.9	70.8	68.6	66.2	63.5	60.6	57.3	53.6	49.3	7.29	10.16
	20	75.0	73.2	71.3	69.2	67.0	64.6	61.9	59.0	55.7	52.0	47.7	6.28	9.09
	22	73.3	71.5	69.6	67.6	65.3	62.9	60.3	57.3	54.1	50.4	46.1	5.36	8.11
67.17	16	81.9	80.0	78.0	75.9	73.5	71.0	68.2	65.1	61.7	57.8	53.3	8.67	11.63
	18	79.8	77.9	75.9	73.8	71.4	68.9	66.1	63.0	59.6	55.7	51.2	7.27	10.16
	20	78.1	76.2	74.2	72.0	69.7	67.2	64.4	61.3	57.9	54.0	49.5	6.23	9.06
	22	76.4	74.5	72.5	70.3	68.0	65.4	62.6	59.6	56.1	52.2	47.7	5.30	8.05

TABLE 441

Process Times (B) at Retort Temperature of 230°F for Conduction-Heating Foods in 307 x 510 Can

f_h	z	INITIAL FOOD TEMPERATURE (T_{ih})											Equivalent	
		100	110	120	130	140	150	160	170	180	190	200	F_c^{18}	F_s^{18}
	16	263.8	261.7	259.5	257.0	254.4	251.3	247.9	244.0	239.3	233.6	226.3	13.01	14.30
58.89	18	211.0	209.0	206.7	204.3	201.6	198.6	195.2	191.2	186.6	180.9	173.5	9.08	10.28
	20	179.8	177.7	175.5	173.1	170.4	167.3	163.9	160.0	155.3	149.6	142.3	6.69	7.90
	22	158.0	156.0	153.8	151.3	148.6	145.6	142.2	138.3	133.6	127.9	120.5	5.09	6.25
	16	268.8	266.7	264.3	261.7	258.9	255.7	252.1	247.9	243.0	236.9	229.1	13.00	14.29
62.35	18	216.6	214.4	212.1	209.5	206.6	203.4	199.8	195.7	190.7	184.7	176.9	9.06	10.34
	20	184.3	182.1	179.7	177.1	174.3	171.1	167.5	163.3	158.4	152.3	144.5	6.63	7.85
	22	162.6	160.4	158.0	155.4	152.6	149.4	145.8	141.6	136.7	130.6	122.8	5.03	6.22
	16	273.3	271.0	268.5	265.8	262.8	259.4	255.6	251.2	246.0	239.6	231.4	12.99	14.28
65.82	18	221.3	219.0	216.5	213.8	210.8	207.4	203.6	199.2	194.0	187.6	179.4	9.01	10.32
	20	189.3	187.0	184.5	181.8	178.8	175.4	171.6	167.2	162.0	155.6	147.4	6.61	7.87
	22	167.2	164.9	162.4	159.7	156.6	153.3	149.5	145.1	139.8	133.5	125.2	4.96	6.20
	16	278.7	276.3	273.7	270.8	267.6	264.1	260.1	255.4	249.9	243.2	234.6	12.98	14.33
69.28	18	225.8	223.4	220.8	217.9	214.8	211.2	207.2	202.6	197.1	190.4	181.7	8.97	10.27
	20	194.1	191.7	189.0	186.2	183.0	179.5	175.4	170.8	165.3	158.6	150.0	6.58	7.86
	22	171.7	169.3	166.7	163.8	160.7	157.1	153.1	148.5	143.0	136.3	127.6	4.85	6.17
	16	282.9	280.3	277.6	274.6	271.3	267.5	263.3	258.5	252.7	245.6	236.6	12.85	14.29
72.75	18	231.4	228.9	226.1	223.1	219.8	216.1	211.8	207.0	201.2	194.2	185.1	8.97	10.31
	20	198.9	196.4	193.6	190.6	187.3	183.6	179.4	174.5	168.7	161.7	152.6	6.55	7.85
	22	177.0	174.4	171.7	168.7	165.4	161.6	157.4	152.5	146.8	139.7	130.7	4.81	6.18

TABLE 442

Process Times (B) at Retort Temperature of 240°F for Conduction-Heating Foods in 307 x 510 Can

f_h	z	INITIAL FOOD TEMPERATURE (T_{ih})											Equivalent	
		100	110	120	130	140	150	160	170	180	190	200	F_c^{18}	F_s^{18}
	16	132.2	130.3	128.3	126.1	123.6	120.9	117.9	114.5	110.6	105.9	100.2	10.68	12.62
58.89	18	121.0	119.2	117.1	114.9	112.4	109.7	106.7	103.3	99.4	94.7	89.0	8.45	10.25
	20	113.3	111.4	109.3	107.1	104.7	102.0	99.0	95.6	91.6	87.0	81.2	6.72	8.58
	22	107.0	105.1	103.0	100.8	98.3	95.7	92.6	89.2	85.3	80.6	74.9	5.50	7.34
	16	137.1	135.1	132.9	130.5	128.0	125.1	121.9	118.3	114.1	109.2	103.2	10.67	12.62
62.35	18	125.6	123.6	121.4	119.1	116.5	113.6	110.5	106.8	102.7	97.7	91.7	8.42	10.25
	20	117.8	115.8	113.7	111.3	108.7	105.9	102.7	99.1	94.9	90.0	83.9	6.68	8.59
	22	111.2	109.2	107.0	104.7	102.1	99.2	96.0	92.4	88.2	83.3	77.3	5.41	7.27
	16	141.6	139.5	137.2	134.8	132.0	129.0	125.7	121.8	117.4	112.2	105.8	10.64	12.59
65.82	18	130.6	128.4	126.2	123.7	120.9	117.9	114.6	110.7	106.3	101.1	94.8	8.40	10.29
	20	122.3	120.2	117.9	115.4	112.7	109.7	106.3	102.5	98.1	92.9	86.5	6.64	8.60
	22	115.3	113.1	110.9	108.4	105.7	102.6	99.3	95.5	91.0	85.8	79.5	5.30	7.19
	16	146.1	143.8	141.4	138.8	135.9	132.8	129.2	125.2	120.6	115.1	108.4	10.61	12.56
69.28	18	135.4	133.2	130.8	128.1	125.3	122.1	118.6	114.5	109.9	104.4	97.7	8.37	10.31
	20	126.7	124.5	122.0	119.4	116.6	113.4	109.8	105.8	101.2	95.7	89.0	6.62	8.58
	22	119.2	117.0	114.6	112.0	109.1	105.9	102.4	98.4	93.7	88.3	81.5	5.21	7.12
	16	151.1	148.7	146.2	143.4	140.4	137.1	133.4	129.2	124.3	118.5	111.5	10.71	12.67
72.75	18	140.0	137.7	135.2	132.4	129.4	126.1	122.4	118.1	113.3	107.5	100.5	8.32	10.32
	20	130.9	128.6	126.1	123.3	120.3	117.0	113.3	109.0	104.2	98.4	91.4	6.55	8.52
	22	123.4	121.1	118.5	115.8	112.8	109.4	105.7	101.5	96.6	90.9	83.8	5.16	7.09

TABLE 443

Process Times (B) at Retort Temperature of 250°F for Conduction-Heating Foods in 307 x 510 Can

f_h	z	INITIAL FOOD TEMPERATURE (T_{ih})											Equivalent	
		100	110	120	130	140	150	160	170	180	190	200	F^{18}	F^{18}
	16	91.3	89.6	87.7	85.6	83.4	81.0	78.3	75.3	71.8	67.9	63.2	9.25	11.79
58.89	18	88.2	86.5	84.6	82.5	80.3	77.9	75.2	72.2	68.7	64.8	60.1	7.81	10.31
	20	85.1	83.3	81.4	79.4	77.2	74.7	72.0	69.0	65.6	61.7	57.0	6.51	8.96
	22	82.3	80.6	78.7	76.6	74.4	72.0	69.3	66.2	62.8	58.9	54.2	5.44	7.83
	16	95.6	93.7	91.7	89.6	87.2	84.6	81.8	78.6	75.0	70.8	65.8	9.26	11.83
62.35	18	92.3	90.4	88.4	86.2	83.9	81.3	78.5	75.3	71.7	67.5	62.5	7.79	10.31
	20	89.0	87.1	85.1	83.0	80.6	78.0	75.2	72.0	68.4	64.2	59.2	6.46	8.92
	22	86.1	84.2	82.2	80.0	77.7	75.1	72.2	69.0	65.4	61.3	56.3	5.37	7.78
	16	99.9	97.9	95.8	93.5	91.0	88.3	85.3	81.9	78.1	73.7	68.5	9.30	11.88
65.82	18	96.3	94.4	92.3	90.0	87.5	84.8	81.7	78.4	74.6	70.2	64.9	7.77	10.31
	20	92.9	90.9	88.8	86.5	84.0	81.3	78.3	74.9	71.1	66.7	61.5	6.42	8.90
	22	89.8	87.9	85.7	83.4	81.0	78.2	75.2	71.9	68.0	63.6	58.4	5.32	7.74
	16	104.1	102.0	99.8	97.4	94.7	91.9	88.7	85.2	81.1	76.5	71.0	9.31	11.92
69.28	18	100.4	98.3	96.1	93.6	91.0	88.2	85.0	81.4	77.4	72.8	67.3	7.75	10.31
	20	96.7	94.7	92.4	90.0	87.4	84.5	81.4	77.8	73.8	69.2	63.7	6.36	8.86
	22	93.5	91.4	89.2	86.8	84.2	81.3	78.2	74.6	70.6	66.0	60.5	5.27	7.71
	16	108.3	106.1	103.8	101.2	98.5	95.5	92.1	88.4	84.2	79.3	73.6	9.34	11.97
72.75	18	104.4	102.2	99.8	97.3	94.6	91.5	88.2	84.5	80.3	75.4	69.6	7.74	10.31
	20	100.6	98.4	96.0	93.5	90.8	87.8	84.4	80.7	76.5	71.6	65.9	6.31	8.83
	22	97.2	95.0	92.7	90.2	87.4	84.4	81.1	77.4	73.1	68.3	62.5	5.24	7.69

TABLE 444

Process Times (B) at Retort Temperature of 260°F for Conduction-Heating Foods in 307 x 510 Can

f_h	z	INITIAL FOOD TEMPERATURE (T_{ih})											Equivalent	
		100	110	120	130	140	150	160	170	180	190	200	F_c^{18}	F_s^{18}
58.89	16	73.4	71.7	70.0	68.1	66.0	63.8	61.3	58.7	55.6	52.2	48.3	8.76	11.69
	18	71.6	69.9	68.2	66.3	64.2	62.0	59.6	56.9	53.9	50.5	46.5	7.45	10.31
	20	70.1	68.5	66.7	64.8	62.8	60.6	58.1	55.4	52.4	49.0	45.1	6.47	9.27
	22	68.7	67.1	65.3	63.4	61.4	59.1	56.7	54.0	51.0	47.6	43.6	5.61	8.36
62.35	16	77.1	75.3	73.4	71.4	69.3	66.9	64.3	61.5	58.3	54.7	50.5	8.79	11.74
	18	75.1	73.4	71.5	69.5	67.4	65.0	62.4	59.6	56.4	52.8	48.6	7.43	10.31
	20	73.6	71.8	70.0	68.0	65.8	63.4	60.9	58.0	54.8	51.2	47.0	6.43	9.25
	22	72.0	70.3	68.4	66.4	64.2	61.9	59.3	56.5	53.3	49.7	45.5	5.53	8.28
65.82	16	80.7	78.9	76.9	74.8	72.5	70.0	67.3	64.3	60.9	57.1	52.7	8.82	11.77
	18	78.7	76.8	74.9	72.7	70.5	68.0	65.2	62.2	58.9	55.1	50.6	7.42	10.31
	20	77.0	75.2	73.2	71.1	68.8	66.3	63.6	60.6	57.2	53.4	49.0	6.38	9.21
	22	75.3	73.5	71.5	69.4	67.1	64.6	61.9	58.9	55.5	51.7	47.3	5.44	8.20
69.28	16	84.4	82.4	80.3	78.1	75.7	73.1	70.2	67.0	63.5	59.5	54.8	8.84	11.81
	18	82.2	80.2	78.2	75.9	73.5	70.9	68.0	64.9	61.3	57.3	52.7	7.41	10.31
	20	80.4	78.4	76.4	74.1	71.7	69.1	66.2	63.1	59.5	55.5	50.9	6.33	9.17
	22	78.6	76.6	74.6	72.3	69.9	67.3	64.4	61.3	57.7	53.7	49.1	5.38	8.14
72.75	16	88.0	85.9	83.8	81.4	78.9	76.1	73.1	69.8	66.1	61.9	57.0	8.88	11.86
	18	85.7	83.6	81.5	79.1	76.6	73.8	70.8	67.5	63.8	59.6	54.7	7.39	10.31
	20	83.8	81.7	79.5	77.2	74.7	71.9	68.9	65.6	61.9	57.6	52.8	6.29	9.13
	22	81.8	79.8	77.6	75.3	72.7	70.0	67.0	63.7	59.9	55.7	50.9	5.31	8.09

TABLE 445

Process Times (B) at Retort Temperature of 230°F for Conduction-Heating Foods in 307 x 512 Can

f_h	z	INITIAL FOOD TEMPERATURE (T_{ih})											Equivalent	
		100	110	120	130	140	150	160	170	180	190	200	F^{18}_c	F^{18}_s
	16	264.6	262.6	260.3	257.9	255.2	252.1	248.7	244.7	240.0	234.3	226.9	13.03	14.32
59.29	18	211.9	209.8	207.6	205.1	202.4	199.4	195.9	192.0	187.3	181.5	174.1	9.09	10.30
	20	180.5	178.4	176.2	173.7	171.0	168.0	164.5	160.5	155.9	150.1	142.7	6.70	7.91
	22	158.7	156.7	154.4	152.0	149.2	146.2	142.8	138.8	134.1	128.4	121.0	5.09	6.26
	16	269.7	267.5	265.1	262.5	259.7	256.5	252.8	248.6	243.7	237.6	229.7	13.02	14.31
62.77	18	217.4	215.2	212.8	210.2	207.3	204.1	200.5	196.3	191.3	185.2	117.4	9.07	10.35
	20	185.0	182.8	180.5	177.9	175.0	171.8	168.1	163.9	159.0	152.9	145.0	6.64	7.87
	22	163.2	161.0	158.7	156.1	153.2	150.0	146.3	142.1	137.2	131.1	123.2	5.03	6.23
	16	274.3	272.0	269.4	266.7	263.7	260.3	256.4	252.0	246.8	240.3	232.1	13.02	14.31
66.26	18	222.1	219.8	217.3	214.5	211.5	208.1	204.3	199.8	194.6	188.2	179.9	9.02	10.33
	20	190.1	187.8	185.3	182.6	179.5	176.1	172.3	167.9	162.6	156.2	147.9	6.62	7.88
	22	167.9	165.6	163.1	160.3	157.3	153.9	150.1	145.6	140.4	134.0	125.7	4.96	6.21
	16	279.6	277.1	274.5	271.6	268.4	264.9	260.8	256.1	250.6	243.9	235.1	12.99	14.35
69.75	18	226.7	224.3	221.7	218.8	215.6	212.0	208.0	203.3	197.8	191.0	182.3	8.98	10.29
	20	194.9	192.4	189.8	186.9	183.7	180.1	176.1	171.4	165.9	159.2	150.4	6.59	7.87
	22	172.5	170.0	167.4	164.5	161.3	157.8	153.7	149.0	143.5	136.8	128.1	4.84	6.17
	16	283.8	281.2	278.5	275.4	272.1	268.3	264.1	259.2	253.4	246.3	237.1	12.86	14.29
73.23	18	232.4	229.8	227.0	224.0	220.7	216.9	212.7	207.8	202.0	194.9	185.7	8.98	10.33
	20	199.8	197.2	194.5	191.4	188.1	184.3	180.1	175.2	169.4	162.3	153.1	6.56	7.86
	22	177.8	175.3	172.5	169.5	166.1	162.4	158.1	153.2	147.4	140.3	131.2	4.82	6.19

TABLE 446

Process Times (B) at Retort Temperature of 240°F for Conduction-Heating Foods in 307 x 512 Can

f_h	z	INITIAL FOOD TEMPERATURE (T_{ih}) 100	110	120	130	140	150	160	170	180	190	200	Equivalent F_c^{18}	F_s^{18}
	16	132.9	131.0	128.9	126.7	124.2	121.5	118.5	115.0	111.1	106.4	100.6	10.70	12.64
59.29	18	121.6	119.7	117.6	115.4	112.9	110.2	107.2	103.8	99.8	95.1	89.4	8.46	10.26
	20	113.9	112.0	109.9	107.7	105.2	102.5	99.5	96.0	92.1	87.4	81.6	6.73	8.59
	22	107.5	105.6	103.5	101.3	98.8	96.1	93.1	89.7	85.7	81.0	75.2	5.51	7.35
	16	137.7	135.7	133.5	131.5	128.6	125.7	122.5	118.8	114.6	109.7	103.6	10.69	12.63
62.77	18	126.3	124.3	122.1	119.7	117.1	114.2	111.0	107.4	103.2	98.2	92.1	8.44	10.27
	20	118.4	116.4	114.2	111.9	109.3	106.4	103.2	99.5	95.3	90.4	84.3	6.69	8.60
	22	111.8	109.7	107.6	105.2	102.6	99.7	96.5	92.9	88.7	83.7	77.6	5.41	7.27
	16	142.3	140.2	137.9	135.4	132.6	129.6	126.2	122.4	117.9	112.7	106.3	10.66	12.60
66.26	18	131.2	129.1	126.8	124.3	121.6	118.5	115.1	111.3	106.9	101.6	95.2	8.41	10.31
	20	122.9	120.8	118.5	116.0	113.2	110.2	106.8	103.0	98.5	93.3	86.9	6.65	8.61
	22	115.8	113.7	111.4	108.9	106.2	103.1	99.7	95.9	91.5	86.2	79.8	5.30	7.19
	16	146.8	144.5	142.1	139.4	136.6	133.4	129.8	125.8	121.1	115.6	108.8	10.63	12.57
69.75	18	136.1	133.8	131.4	128.8	125.9	122.7	119.1	115.1	110.4	104.9	98.1	8.38	10.33
	20	127.3	125.1	122.7	120.0	117.1	113.9	110.4	106.3	101.7	96.1	89.4	6.63	8.59
	22	119.8	117.6	115.2	112.5	109.6	106.5	102.9	98.8	94.2	88.7	81.9	5.21	7.12
	16	151.9	149.5	147.0	144.2	141.2	137.8	134.1	129.8	124.9	119.1	112.0	10.75	12.70
73.23	18	140.8	138.4	135.9	133.1	130.1	126.7	123.0	118.7	113.8	108.0	100.9	8.33	10.33
	20	131.6	129.2	126.7	123.9	120.9	117.5	113.8	109.6	104.7	98.9	91.8	6.55	8.53
	22	124.1	121.7	119.2	116.4	113.4	110.0	106.3	102.0	97.1	91.3	84.2	5.17	7.10

TABLE 447

Process Times (B) at Retort Temperature of 250°F for Conduction-Heating Foods in 307 x 512 Can

f_h	z	INITIAL FOOD TEMPERATURE (T_{ih})											Equivalent	
		100	110	120	130	140	150	160	170	180	190	200	F_c^{18}	F_s^{18}
59.29	16	91.9	90.1	88.2	86.1	83.9	81.4	78.7	75.7	72.2	68.3	63.6	9.27	11.81
	18	88.7	87.0	85.0	83.0	80.7	78.3	75.6	72.5	69.1	65.1	60.4	7.82	10.32
	20	85.6	83.8	81.9	79.8	77.6	75.1	72.4	69.4	66.0	62.0	57.3	6.52	8.97
	22	82.8	81.0	79.1	77.0	74.8	72.3	69.6	66.6	63.2	59.2	54.5	5.44	7.84
62.77	16	96.1	94.3	92.2	90.1	87.7	85.1	82.2	79.0	75.4	71.2	66.2	9.28	11.85
	18	92.8	90.9	88.9	86.7	84.4	81.8	78.9	75.7	72.0	67.8	62.9	7.80	10.32
	20	89.5	87.6	85.6	83.4	81.0	78.4	75.6	72.4	68.7	64.5	59.5	6.47	8.93
	22	86.6	84.7	82.7	80.5	78.1	75.5	72.6	69.4	65.8	61.6	56.6	5.37	7.79
66.26	16	100.4	98.5	96.3	94.0	91.5	88.8	85.7	82.3	78.5	74.1	68.8	9.32	11.91
	18	96.9	94.9	92.8	90.5	88.0	85.2	82.2	78.8	75.0	70.5	65.3	7.78	10.32
	20	93.4	91.4	89.3	87.0	84.5	81.8	78.7	75.3	71.5	67.1	61.8	6.42	8.91
	22	90.3	88.3	86.2	83.9	81.4	78.7	75.6	72.2	68.4	64.0	58.7	5.32	7.75
69.75	16	104.7	102.6	100.3	97.9	95.3	92.4	89.2	85.6	81.6	76.9	71.4	9.33	11.94
	18	100.9	98.8	96.6	94.2	91.5	88.6	85.5	81.9	77.8	73.2	67.7	7.76	10.32
	20	97.3	95.2	93.0	90.5	87.9	85.0	81.8	78.2	74.2	69.5	64.0	6.36	8.87
	22	94.1	92.0	89.7	87.3	84.7	81.8	78.6	75.0	71.0	66.3	60.8	5.28	7.72
73.23	16	108.9	106.7	104.4	101.8	99.0	96.0	92.7	88.9	84.7	79.8	74.0	9.36	11.99
	18	105.0	102.8	100.4	97.9	95.1	92.1	88.7	85.0	80.7	75.8	70.0	7.75	10.33
	20	101.1	99.0	96.6	94.0	91.3	88.3	84.9	81.2	76.9	72.0	66.2	6.32	8.84
	22	97.8	95.6	93.2	90.7	87.9	84.9	81.5	77.8	73.5	68.6	62.8	5.25	7.70

TABLE 448

Process Times (B) at Retort Temperature of 260°F for Conduction-Heating Foods in 307 x 512 Can

f_h	z	INITIAL FOOD TEMPERATURE (T_{ih}) 100	110	120	130	140	150	160	170	180	190	200	Equivalent F_c^{18}	F_s^{18}
	16	73.8	72.2	70.4	68.5	66.4	64.2	61.7	59.0	56.0	52.5	48.6	8.78	11.71
59.29	18	72.0	70.4	68.6	66.7	64.6	62.4	59.9	57.2	54.2	50.7	46.8	7.46	10.32
	20	70.6	68.9	67.1	65.2	63.1	60.9	58.5	55.7	52.7	49.3	45.3	6.48	9.28
	22	69.1	67.5	65.7	63.8	61.7	59.5	57.0	54.3	51.3	47.8	43.9	5.61	8.36
	16	77.5	75.8	73.9	71.9	69.7	67.3	64.7	61.8	58.6	55.0	50.8	8.81	11.76
62.77	18	75.6	73.8	72.0	69.9	67.8	65.4	62.8	59.9	56.7	53.1	48.9	7.45	10.32
	20	74.0	72.3	70.4	68.4	66.2	63.8	61.2	58.3	55.1	51.5	47.3	6.44	9.26
	22	72.5	70.7	68.8	66.8	64.6	62.2	59.6	56.8	53.6	49.9	45.7	5.53	8.29
	16	81.2	79.3	77.4	75.2	72.9	70.4	67.7	64.6	61.3	57.4	53.0	8.84	11.79
66.26	18	79.2	77.3	75.3	73.2	70.9	68.4	65.6	62.6	59.2	55.4	50.9	7.43	10.32
	20	77.5	75.6	73.6	71.5	69.2	66.7	63.9	60.9	57.5	53.7	49.2	6.39	9.22
	22	75.8	73.9	71.9	69.8	67.5	65.0	62.2	59.2	55.8	52.0	47.5	5.45	8.21
	16	84.9	82.9	80.8	78.6	76.1	73.5	70.6	67.4	63.9	59.8	55.2	8.86	11.83
69.75	18	82.7	80.7	78.6	76.4	74.0	71.3	68.4	65.3	61.7	57.6	53.0	7.42	10.32
	20	80.9	78.9	76.8	74.6	72.2	69.5	66.6	63.4	59.9	55.8	51.2	6.34	9.18
	22	79.1	77.1	75.0	72.8	70.3	67.7	64.8	61.6	58.1	54.0	49.3	5.38	8.15
	16	88.5	86.5	84.3	81.9	79.4	76.6	73.6	70.2	66.5	62.2	57.3	8.90	11.89
73.23	18	86.2	84.1	81.9	79.6	77.0	74.3	71.2	67.9	64.1	59.9	55.0	7.41	10.32
	20	84.3	82.2	80.0	77.6	75.1	72.3	69.3	66.0	62.2	58.0	53.1	6.30	9.14
	22	82.3	80.3	78.1	75.7	73.2	70.4	67.4	64.0	60.3	56.0	51.1	5.32	8.09

TABLE 449

Process Times (B) at Retort Temperature of 230°F for Conduction-Heating Foods in 307 x 704 Can

f_h	z	INITIAL FOOD TEMPERATURE (T_{ih})											Equivalent	
		100	110	120	130	140	150	160	170	180	190	200	F_c^{18}	F_s^{18}
	16	272.5	270.3	268.0	265.4	262.5	259.3	255.6	251.5	246.5	240.4	232.6	13.23	14.53
62.69	18	219.4	217.2	214.8	212.2	209.4	206.2	202.5	198.3	193.4	187.3	179.5	9.24	10.51
	20	186.6	184.4	182.0	179.4	176.6	173.4	169.7	165.5	160.6	154.5	146.7	6.77	8.00
	22	164.6	162.4	160.0	157.4	154.6	151.3	147.7	143.5	138.5	132.5	124.6	5.14	6.34
	16	277.4	275.1	272.6	269.9	266.8	263.4	259.6	255.1	249.9	243.5	235.2	13.23	14.52
66.37	18	224.4	222.1	219.6	216.9	213.8	210.5	206.6	202.2	196.9	190.5	182.2	9.18	10.50
	20	191.8	189.5	187.0	184.3	181.2	177.8	174.0	169.5	164.3	157.9	149.6	6.74	8.00
	22	169.4	167.1	164.6	161.8	158.8	155.4	151.5	147.1	141.9	135.4	127.1	5.08	6.31
	16	283.1	280.7	278.0	275.1	271.9	268.3	264.3	259.6	254.0	247.3	238.5	13.24	14.58
70.06	18	229.3	226.9	224.2	221.3	218.1	214.5	210.5	205.8	200.2	193.4	184.7	9.14	10.45
	20	197.0	194.6	191.9	189.0	185.8	182.2	178.2	173.5	167.9	161.1	152.4	6.71	8.00
	22	174.3	171.9	169.2	166.3	163.1	159.5	155.5	150.8	145.2	138.4	129.7	4.96	6.28
	16	287.6	285.0	282.2	279.2	275.8	272.0	267.8	262.8	257.0	249.8	240.6	13.09	14.54
73.75	18	235.1	232.5	229.8	226.7	223.3	219.6	215.3	210.3	204.5	197.4	188.1	9.13	10.48
	20	202.1	199.6	196.8	193.7	109.3	186.6	182.3	177.4	171.5	164.4	155.2	6.67	7.98
	22	179.8	177.2	174.4	171.4	168.0	164.2	159.9	155.0	149.2	142.0	132.8	4.90	6.28
	16	292.9	290.2	287.3	284.1	280.5	276.6	272.1	266.9	260.8	253.3	243.6	13.05	14.49
77.44	18	240.6	237.9	235.0	231.8	228.2	224.3	219.8	214.6	208.5	201.0	191.3	9.11	10.50
	20	207.2	204.5	201.5	198.3	194.8	190.8	186.3	181.2	175.0	167.5	157.8	6.64	7.98
	22	185.5	182.8	179.9	176.7	173.1	169.1	164.7	159.5	153.3	145.8	136.2	4.89	6.32

TABLE 450

Process Times (B) at Retort Temperature of 240°F for Conduction-Heating Foods in 307 x 704 Can

f_h	z	INITIAL FOOD TEMPERATURE (T_{ih})											Equivalent	
		100	110	120	130	140	150	160	170	180	190	200	F_c^{18}	F_s^{18}
	16	138.6	136.5	134.4	132.0	129.4	126.5	123.3	119.7	115.5	110.5	104.4	10.89	12.84
62.69	18	126.8	124.8	122.6	120.2	117.6	114.7	111.5	107.9	103.7	98.7	92.7	8.60	10.42
	20	119.0	117.0	114.8	112.4	109.8	107.0	103.8	100.1	95.9	91.0	84.9	6.82	8.73
	22	112.3	110.3	108.1	105.7	103.1	100.3	97.1	93.4	89.2	84.3	78.2	5.54	7.41
	16	143.5	141.3	139.0	136.5	133.8	130.7	127.3	123.5	119.1	113.8	107.4	10.86	12.81
66.37	18	132.1	129.9	127.6	125.1	122.4	119.3	115.9	112.1	107.6	102.4	96.0	8.57	10.46
	20	123.7	121.6	119.3	116.8	114.0	111.0	107.6	103.7	99.3	94.0	87.6	6.78	8.74
	22	116.7	114.5	112.2	109.7	107.0	103.9	100.5	96.7	92.3	87.0	80.6	5.43	7.32
	16	148.2	146.0	143.5	140.9	138.0	134.8	131.2	127.1	122.4	116.9	110.1	10.83	12.78
70.06	18	137.3	135.0	132.6	129.9	127.0	123.8	120.2	116.2	111.5	105.9	99.1	8.54	10.49
	20	128.4	126.2	123.7	121.1	118.2	115.0	111.4	107.3	102.7	97.1	90.3	6.75	8.72
	22	120.9	118.7	116.2	113.6	110.7	107.5	103.9	99.8	95.1	89.6	82.8	5.32	7.24
	16	153.4	151.0	148.4	145.7	142.6	139.2	135.5	131.2	126.2	120.4	113.3	10.91	12.87
73.75	18	142.2	139.8	137.3	134.5	131.4	128.1	124.3	120.0	115.1	109.2	102.1	8.49	10.49
	20	133.0	130.6	128.1	125.3	122.2	118.8	115.1	110.8	105.9	100.0	92.9	6.70	8.68
	22	125.3	122.9	120.4	117.6	114.5	111.2	107.4	103.1	98.2	92.3	85.2	5.27	7.21
	16	158.9	156.4	153.7	150.7	147.5	144.0	140.0	135.5	130.4	124.2	116.7	11.06	13.03
77.44	18	147.2	144.7	142.0	139.0	135.8	132.3	128.3	123.8	118.7	112.5	105.0	8.46	10.51
	20	137.4	134.9	132.2	129.3	126.1	122.6	118.6	114.1	108.9	102.8	95.3	6.58	8.59
	22	129.8	127.3	124.6	121.7	118.5	115.0	111.0	106.5	101.3	95.2	87.7	5.23	7.20

TABLE 451

Process Times (B) at Retort Temperature of 250°F for Conduction-Heating Foods in 307 x 704 Can

f_h	z	INITIAL FOOD TEMPERATURE (T_{ih})											Equivalent	
		100	110	120	130	140	150	160	170	180	190	200	F_c^{18}	F_s^{18}
	16	96.4	94.5	92.5	90.3	88.0	85.4	82.5	79.3	75.7	71.5	66.5	9.45	12.02
62.69	18	93.1	91.2	89.2	87.0	84.6	82.0	79.2	76.0	72.3	68.1	63.2	7.96	10.48
	20	89.8	87.9	85.9	83.7	81.3	78.7	75.9	72.7	69.0	64.8	59.9	6.61	9.08
	22	86.8	84.9	82.9	80.7	78.4	75.8	72.9	69.7	66.1	61.9	56.9	5.50	7.92
	16	100.9	98.9	96.8	94.5	92.0	89.2	86.2	82.8	79.0	74.5	69.3	9.49	12.08
66.37	18	97.4	95.4	93.3	91.0	88.5	85.7	82.7	79.3	75.4	71.0	65.7	7.94	10.48
	20	93.9	91.9	89.8	87.5	85.0	82.2	79.2	75.8	71.9	67.5	62.2	6.56	9.05
	22	90.8	88.8	86.7	84.4	81.9	79.1	76.1	72.7	68.8	64.4	59.1	5.44	7.87
	16	105.4	103.3	101.1	98.6	96.0	93.1	89.9	86.3	82.2	77.6	72.0	9.50	12.12
70.06	18	101.7	99.6	97.3	94.9	92.2	89.3	86.1	82.6	78.5	73.8	68.3	7.92	10.48
	20	98.0	95.9	93.7	91.2	88.6	85.7	82.5	78.9	74.8	70.1	64.6	6.50	9.01
	22	94.8	92.7	90.4	88.0	85.3	82.4	79.2	75.6	71.6	66.9	61.3	5.39	7.84
	16	109.9	107.7	105.3	102.8	100.0	96.9	93.6	89.8	85.5	80.6	74.7	9.53	12.17
73.75	18	105.9	103.7	101.4	98.8	96.0	93.0	89.6	85.8	81.5	76.6	70.8	7.90	10.49
	20	102.1	99.9	97.5	95.0	92.2	89.1	85.7	82.0	77.7	72.8	66.9	6.45	8.98
	22	98.7	96.5	94.1	91.5	88.8	85.7	82.3	78.6	74.3	69.3	63.5	5.35	7.81
	16	114.3	112.0	109.5	106.8	103.9	100.7	97.2	93.2	88.7	83.5	77.4	9.56	12.21
77.44	18	110.2	107.8	105.3	102.7	99.7	96.5	93.0	89.0	84.5	79.3	73.2	7.88	10.48
	20	106.1	103.8	101.3	98.6	95.7	92.5	89.0	85.0	80.5	75.3	69.2	6.41	8.95
	22	102.6	100.3	97.8	95.1	92.1	88.9	85.4	81.4	76.9	71.8	65.6	5.32	7.79

TABLE 452

Process Times (B) at Retort Temperature of 260°F for Conduction-Heating Foods in 307 x 704 Can

f_h	z	INITIAL FOOD TEMPERATURE (T_{ih})											Equivalent	
		100	110	120	130	140	150	160	170	180	190	200	F_c^{18}	F_s^{18}
	16	77.6	75.9	74.0	72.0	69.8	67.4	64.8	62.0	58.8	55.1	50.9	8.98	11.93
62.69	18	75.7	74.0	72.1	70.1	67.9	65.6	62.9	60.1	56.9	53.2	49.0	7.60	10.48
	20	74.2	72.4	70.5	68.5	66.3	64.0	61.4	58.5	55.3	51.7	47.5	6.58	9.41
	22	72.6	70.9	69.0	67.0	64.8	62.4	59.8	57.0	53.8	50.1	45.9	5.67	8.44
	16	81.5	79.7	77.7	75.6	73.3	70.7	68.0	65.0	61.6	57.7	53.3	9.01	11.97
66.37	18	79.5	77.6	75.7	73.5	71.2	68.7	66.0	62.9	59.5	55.7	51.2	7.58	10.48
	20	77.8	76.0	74.0	71.8	69.5	67.0	64.3	61.2	57.8	54.0	49.5	6.53	9.37
	22	76.1	74.3	72.3	70.1	67.8	65.3	62.6	59.5	56.1	52.3	47.9	5.58	8.35
	16	85.4	83.5	81.4	79.1	76.7	74.0	71.1	67.9	64.3	60.3	55.6	9.03	12.01
70.06	18	83.2	81.3	79.2	76.9	74.5	71.8	68.9	65.7	62.2	58.1	53.4	7.57	10.48
	20	81.4	79.5	77.4	75.1	72.7	70.0	67.1	63.9	60.3	56.3	51.6	6.48	9.33
	22	79.6	77.6	75.5	73.3	70.9	68.2	65.3	62.1	58.5	54.5	49.8	5.51	8.29
	16	89.3	87.2	85.0	82.6	80.1	77.3	74.2	70.9	67.1	62.8	57.9	9.07	12.06
73.75	18	87.0	84.9	82.7	80.3	77.7	75.0	71.9	68.5	64.8	60.5	55.5	7.56	10.48
	20	85.0	82.9	80.7	78.4	75.8	73.0	70.0	66.6	62.8	58.5	53.6	6.43	9.29
	22	83.1	81.0	78.8	76.4	73.9	71.1	68.0	64.6	60.9	56.6	51.7	5.44	8.22
	16	93.1	91.0	88.6	86.1	83.5	80.5	77.3	73.8	69.8	65.3	60.1	9.10	12.11
77.44	18	90.7	88.5	86.2	83.7	81.0	78.1	74.8	71.3	67.3	62.9	57.7	7.54	10.48
	20	88.6	86.4	84.1	81.6	78.9	76.0	72.8	69.2	65.3	60.8	55.6	6.39	9.25
	22	86.5	84.3	82.0	79.5	76.8	73.9	70.7	67.2	63.2	58.7	53.5	5.36	8.16

TABLE 453

Process Times (B) at Retort Temperature of 230°F for Conduction-Heating Foods in 401 x 205 Can

f_h	z	INITIAL FOOD TEMPERATURE (T_{ih}) 100	110	120	130	140	150	160	170	180	190	200	Equivalent F_c^{18}	F_s^{18}
35.23	16	221.7	220.5	219.2	217.7	216.1	214.3	212.3	209.9	207.1	203.7	199.3	12.70	13.69
	18	173.2	171.9	170.6	169.2	167.5	165.7	163.7	161.3	158.5	155.1	150.7	9.05	9.90
	20	143.1	141.9	140.5	139.1	137.5	135.7	133.6	131.3	128.5	125.1	120.7	6.72	7.60
	22	122.9	121.7	120.3	118.9	117.3	115.5	113.4	111.1	108.3	104.9	100.5	5.16	6.06
37.30	16	226.1	224.8	223.4	221.8	220.1	218.2	216.1	213.6	210.6	207.0	202.3	12.70	13.71
	18	174.9	173.7	172.2	170.7	169.0	167.1	164.9	162.4	159.5	155.9	151.2	8.86	9.91
	20	146.0	144.7	143.3	141.8	140.0	138.1	136.0	133.5	130.5	126.9	122.3	6.66	7.67
	22	126.0	124.7	123.3	121.7	120.0	118.1	115.9	113.4	110.5	106.9	102.2	5.14	6.09
39.38	16	230.0	228.6	227.1	225.5	223.7	221.7	219.4	216.8	213.7	209.8	204.9	12.71	13.72
	18	177.9	176.6	175.1	173.3	171.6	169.6	167.3	164.7	161.6	157.8	152.9	8.82	9.86
	20	148.3	146.9	145.5	143.8	142.0	140.0	137.7	135.1	132.0	128.2	123.2	6.59	7.59
	22	128.4	127.1	125.6	124.0	122.2	120.1	117.9	115.2	112.1	108.3	103.4	5.10	6.04
41.45	16	233.5	232.1	230.5	228.8	226.9	224.8	222.3	219.6	216.3	212.3	207.1	12.71	13.73
	18	181.2	179.7	178.2	176.5	174.6	172.4	170.0	167.3	164.0	160.0	154.8	8.82	9.86
	20	151.3	149.8	148.2	146.5	144.6	142.5	140.1	137.3	134.1	130.0	124.9	6.58	7.57
	22	130.8	129.4	127.8	126.1	124.2	122.1	119.7	116.9	113.6	109.6	104.4	5.03	6.01
43.52	16	236.6	235.1	233.4	231.6	229.6	227.4	224.9	222.0	218.5	214.3	208.9	12.72	13.74
	18	184.1	182.6	181.0	179.2	177.2	175.0	172.4	169.5	166.1	161.9	156.4	8.83	9.86
	20	153.9	152.4	150.8	149.0	147.0	144.8	142.2	139.3	135.9	131.7	126.2	6.54	7.57
	22	133.9	132.4	130.8	129.0	127.0	124.7	122.2	119.3	115.9	111.6	106.2	5.02	6.04

TABLE 454

Process Times (B) at Retort Temperature of 240°F for Conduction-Heating Foods in 401 x 205 Can

f_h	z	INITIAL FOOD TEMPERATURE (T_{ih}) 100	110	120	130	140	150	160	170	180	190	200	Equivalent F_c^{18}	F_s^{18}
35.23	16	93.1	92.0	90.8	89.4	88.0	86.4	84.5	82.5	80.1	77.4	73.9	10.25	11.90
	18	86.3	85.1	83.9	82.6	81.1	79.5	77.7	75.6	73.3	70.5	67.1	8.20	9.94
	20	80.5	79.4	78.2	76.8	75.4	73.8	72.0	69.9	67.6	64.8	61.4	6.72	8.35
	22	75.8	74.7	73.5	72.1	70.7	69.1	67.3	65.2	62.9	60.1	56.7	5.70	7.23
37.30	16	96.7	95.5	94.2	92.8	91.2	89.5	87.6	85.4	83.0	80.0	76.4	10.36	12.04
	18	89.5	88.3	87.0	85.6	84.0	82.3	80.4	78.2	75.7	72.8	69.2	8.17	9.93
	20	83.5	82.3	81.0	79.6	78.0	76.3	74.4	72.3	69.8	66.8	63.2	6.71	8.35
	22	78.6	77.4	76.1	74.7	73.1	71.4	69.5	67.3	64.8	61.9	58.3	5.70	7.24
39.38	16	100.2	98.9	97.6	96.1	94.5	92.7	90.6	88.4	85.7	82.6	78.8	10.32	12.09
	18	92.6	91.3	90.0	88.5	86.8	85.0	83.0	80.7	78.1	75.0	71.2	8.14	9.90
	20	86.4	85.1	83.8	82.3	80.7	78.9	76.8	74.6	71.9	68.8	65.0	6.71	8.35
	22	81.2	79.9	78.6	77.1	75.5	73.7	71.6	69.4	66.7	63.6	59.8	5.70	7.24
41.45	16	103.6	102.3	100.8	99.3	97.6	95.7	93.5	91.1	88.4	85.1	81.1	10.28	12.10
	18	95.7	94.4	92.9	91.3	89.6	87.7	85.6	83.2	80.4	77.2	73.1	8.12	9.89
	20	89.2	87.9	86.5	84.9	83.2	81.3	79.2	76.8	74.0	70.7	66.7	6.71	8.35
	22	83.7	82.3	80.9	79.3	77.6	75.7	73.6	71.2	68.4	65.1	61.1	5.65	7.21
43.52	16	106.9	105.5	104.0	102.4	100.6	98.6	96.4	93.8	90.9	87.5	83.3	10.24	12.12
	18	98.7	97.3	95.8	94.2	92.4	90.4	88.2	85.6	82.7	79.3	75.1	8.12	9.89
	20	92.0	90.6	89.1	87.4	85.6	83.6	81.4	78.9	76.0	72.5	68.3	6.71	8.35
	22	86.1	84.7	83.1	81.5	79.7	77.7	75.5	73.0	70.0	66.6	62.4	5.49	7.11

TABLE 455

Process Times (B) at Retort Temperature of 250°F for Conduction-Heating Foods in 401 x 205 Can

f_h	z	INITIAL FOOD TEMPERATURE (T_{ih})											Equivalent	
		100	110	120	130	140	150	160	170	180	190	200	F_c^{18}	F_s^{18}
	16	60.4	59.4	58.2	57.0	55.7	54.2	52.6	50.8	48.8	46.4	43.6	8.75	11.04
35.23	18	58.6	57.5	56.4	55.2	53.8	52.4	50.8	49.0	46.9	44.5	41.8	7.61	9.90
	20	56.7	55.6	54.5	53.3	51.9	50.5	48.9	47.1	45.0	42.7	39.9	6.57	8.82
	22	55.0	54.0	52.8	51.6	50.3	48.8	47.2	45.4	43.3	41.0	38.2	5.72	7.93
	16	63.1	62.0	60.8	59.5	58.1	56.5	54.8	52.9	50.8	48.3	45.3	8.71	11.04
37.30	18	61.2	60.0	58.8	57.5	56.1	54.6	52.9	51.0	48.8	46.3	43.4	7.59	9.89
	20	59.2	58.0	56.8	55.5	54.1	52.6	50.9	49.0	46.8	44.3	41.4	6.51	8.77
	22	57.4	56.3	55.1	53.8	52.4	50.8	49.1	47.2	45.0	42.5	39.6	5.63	7.86
	16	65.8	64.6	63.4	62.0	60.5	58.9	57.1	55.1	52.8	50.1	47.0	8.71	11.07
39.38	18	63.8	62.6	61.3	59.9	58.4	56.8	55.0	53.0	50.7	48.1	45.0	7.56	9.88
	20	61.6	60.5	59.2	57.8	56.3	54.7	52.9	50.9	48.6	46.0	42.8	6.46	8.75
	22	59.7	58.6	57.3	55.9	54.4	52.8	51.0	49.0	46.7	44.1	41.0	5.56	7.82
	16	68.5	67.3	65.9	64.5	62.9	61.2	59.3	57.2	54.8	52.0	48.7	8.73	11.11
41.45	18	66.3	65.1	63.8	62.3	60.7	59.0	57.1	55.0	52.6	49.8	46.6	7.54	9.88
	20	64.1	62.9	61.5	60.1	58.5	56.8	54.9	52.8	50.4	47.6	44.3	6.42	8.73
	22	62.1	60.9	59.5	58.1	56.5	54.8	52.9	50.8	48.4	45.6	42.3	5.51	7.77
	16	71.1	69.8	68.4	66.9	65.3	63.5	61.5	59.3	56.7	53.8	50.4	8.74	11.14
43.52	18	68.9	67.6	66.2	64.6	63.0	61.2	59.2	57.0	54.5	51.5	48.1	7.52	9.88
	20	66.5	65.2	63.8	62.3	60.7	58.9	56.9	54.6	52.1	49.2	45.8	6.38	8.71
	22	64.5	63.1	61.7	60.2	58.6	56.8	54.8	52.6	50.0	47.1	43.7	5.45	7.73

TABLE 456

Process Times (B) at Retort Temperature of 260°F for Conduction-Heating Foods in 401 x 205 Can

f_h	z	INITIAL FOOD TEMPERATURE (T_{ih})											Equivalent	
		100	110	120	130	140	150	160	170	180	190	200	F_c^{18}	F_s^{18}
	16	47.0	46.0	44.9	43.8	42.6	41.2	39.8	38.2	36.4	34.3	32.0	8.00	10.76
35.23	18	46.1	45.2	44.1	43.0	41.7	40.4	38.9	37.3	35.5	33.5	31.1	7.16	9.88
	20	45.4	44.4	43.4	42.2	41.0	39.7	38.2	36.6	34.8	32.8	30.4	6.50	9.18
	22	44.7	43.7	42.7	41.6	40.3	39.0	37.5	35.9	34.1	32.1	29.7	5.91	8.56
	16	49.3	48.3	47.2	46.0	44.7	43.2	41.7	40.0	38.1	35.9	33.4	8.03	10.81
37.30	18	48.4	47.3	46.2	45.0	43.7	42.3	40.8	39.1	37.1	35.0	32.5	7.15	9.88
	20	47.6	46.6	45.4	44.2	42.9	41.5	40.0	38.3	36.4	34.2	31.7	6.47	9.17
	22	46.8	45.8	44.7	43.5	42.2	40.8	39.2	37.5	35.6	33.4	30.9	5.82	8.48
	16	51.6	50.5	49.4	48.1	46.7	45.2	43.6	41.8	39.8	37.5	34.9	8.07	10.87
39.38	18	50.6	49.5	48.3	47.0	45.7	44.2	42.6	40.7	38.7	36.5	33.8	7.13	9.88
	20	49.8	48.7	47.5	46.2	44.9	43.4	41.7	39.9	37.9	35.6	33.0	6.42	9.13
	22	48.9	47.8	46.6	45.4	44.0	42.5	40.9	39.1	37.1	34.8	32.2	5.76	8.42
	16	53.9	52.8	51.5	50.2	48.8	47.2	45.5	43.6	41.5	39.0	36.3	8.10	10.91
41.45	18	52.8	51.6	50.4	49.1	47.6	46.1	44.4	42.5	40.3	37.9	35.2	7.12	9.88
	20	51.9	50.8	49.5	48.2	46.7	45.2	43.5	41.6	39.4	37.0	34.3	6.38	9.10
	22	51.0	49.9	48.6	47.3	45.9	44.3	42.6	40.7	38.6	36.2	33.4	5.70	8.37
	16	56.2	55.0	53.7	52.3	50.8	49.1	47.3	45.3	43.1	40.6	37.7	8.15	10.97
43.52	18	55.0	53.8	52.5	51.1	49.6	47.9	46.1	44.1	41.9	39.4	36.5	7.11	9.88
	20	54.1	52.8	51.5	50.1	48.6	47.0	45.2	43.2	41.0	38.4	35.5	6.35	9.07
	22	53.1	51.9	50.6	49.2	47.7	46.0	44.2	42.2	40.0	37.5	34.6	5.64	8.32

TABLE 457

Process Times (B) at Retort Temperature of 230°F for Conduction-Heating Foods in 401 x 205 Can

f_h	z	INITIAL FOOD TEMPERATURE (T_{ih})											Equivalent	
		100	110	120	130	140	150	160	170	180	190	200	F_c^{18}	F_s^{18}
43.50	16	238.6	237.1	235.4	233.6	231.6	229.4	226.9	224.0	220.5	216.3	210.9	12.86	13.90
	18	185.6	184.1	182.5	180.7	178.7	176.4	173.9	171.0	167.6	163.4	157.9	8.93	9.98
	20	155.1	153.6	152.0	150.2	148.2	146.0	143.4	140.5	137.1	132.9	127.4	6.64	7.66
	22	134.8	133.3	131.6	129.8	127.8	125.6	123.1	120.2	116.7	112.5	107.1	5.09	6.11
46.06	16	242.0	140.4	138.6	236.7	234.6	232.3	229.6	226.5	222.9	218.4	212.6	12.87	13.91
	18	188.9	187.3	185.6	183.7	181.6	179.2	176.5	173.5	169.8	165.3	159.6	8.93	9.97
	20	159.1	157.5	155.7	153.8	151.7	149.3	146.7	143.6	139.9	135.5	129.7	6.62	7.70
	22	138.3	136.7	135.0	133.1	131.0	128.6	125.9	122.8	119.2	114.7	109.0	5.07	6.09
48.62	16	244.8	243.1	241.2	239.2	237.0	234.5	231.7	228.4	224.6	219.9	213.8	12.87	12.93
	18	192.9	191.2	189.4	187.4	185.2	182.7	179.9	176.6	172.7	168.0	162.0	8.89	10.04
	20	162.4	160.7	158.9	156.9	154.6	152.1	149.3	146.1	142.2	137.5	131.4	6.57	7.68
	22	141.5	139.8	138.0	135.9	133.7	131.2	128.4	125.2	121.3	116.6	110.5	5.01	6.06
51.18	16	246.8	145.0	243.1	241.0	238.6	236.0	233.1	229.6	225.6	220.6	214.2	12.73	13.92
	18	196.0	194.3	192.3	190.2	187.9	185.2	182.3	178.8	174.8	169.8	163.4	8.81	10.00
	20	165.5	163.7	161.8	159.7	157.3	154.7	151.7	148.3	144.3	139.3	132.9	6.52	7.63
	22	145.0	143.3	141.3	139.2	136.9	134.2	131.3	127.8	123.8	118.8	112.4	4.99	6.08
53.74	16	250.2	248.3	246.3	244.0	241.6	238.8	235.7	232.1	227.9	222.7	215.9	12.62	13.89
	18	199.7	197.8	195.8	193.6	191.1	188.4	185.2	181.6	177.4	172.2	165.5	8.79	9.97
	20	169.3	167.4	165.4	163.2	160.7	158.0	154.9	151.3	147.0	141.8	135.1	6.50	7.65
	22	148.5	146.6	144.6	142.4	139.9	137.2	134.0	130.4	126.2	121.0	114.3	4.95	6.06

TABLE 458

Process Times (B) at Retort Temperature of 240°F for Conduction-Heating Foods in 401 x 205 Can

f_h	z	INITIAL FOOD TEMPERATURE (T_{ih}) 100	110	120	130	140	150	160	170	180	190	200	Equivalent F_c^{18}	F_s^{18}
43.50	16	107.4	106.0	104.5	102.9	101.1	99.1	96.8	94.3	91.4	88.0	83.7	10.39	12.26
	18	99.2	97.8	96.3	94.6	92.8	90.8	88.6	86.1	83.2	79.7	75.5	8.23	10.00
	20	92.4	91.0	89.5	87.9	86.1	84.1	81.8	79.3	76.4	73.0	68.7	6.79	8.45
	22	86.5	85.1	83.6	82.0	80.2	78.2	76.0	73.4	70.5	67.1	62.9	5.60	7.22
46.06	16	111.5	110.0	108.4	106.6	104.7	102.6	100.3	97.6	94.5	90.9	86.4	10.36	12.27
	18	102.9	101.4	99.8	98.0	96.1	94.0	91.7	89.0	85.9	82.3	77.8	8.23	10.00
	20	95.6	94.1	92.5	90.8	88.9	86.8	84.4	81.8	78.7	75.0	70.6	6.78	8.43
	22	89.4	87.9	86.3	84.6	82.6	80.5	78.2	75.5	72.4	68.8	64.3	5.42	7.11
48.62	16	115.4	113.9	112.2	110.3	108.3	106.1	103.6	100.8	97.5	93.7	89.0	10.33	12.25
	18	106.4	104.9	103.2	101.3	99.3	97.1	94.6	91.8	88.5	84.7	80.0	8.23	10.00
	20	98.7	97.1	95.4	93.6	91.6	89.3	86.9	84.0	80.8	76.9	72.2	6.75	8.41
	22	92.8	91.2	89.5	87.7	85.7	83.4	81.0	78.1	74.9	71.0	66.3	5.39	7.13
51.18	16	119.3	117.6	115.9	113.9	111.8	109.5	106.9	103.9	100.5	96.4	91.5	10.31	12.23
	18	109.9	108.2	106.4	104.5	102.4	100.0	97.4	94.5	91.0	87.0	82.0	8.22	9.99
	20	101.6	100.0	98.-	96.3	94.1	91.8	89.2	86.2	82.8	78.7	73.8	6.55	8.28
	22	96.1	94.5	92.7	90.8	88.7	86.3	83.7	80.7	77.3	73.3	68.3	5.37	7.15
53.74	16	123.1	121.4	119.5	117.5	115.3	112.8	110.1	107.0	103.4	99.1	93.9	10.31	12.23
	18	113.1	111.4	109.5	107.5	105.2	102.8	100.0	96.9	93.3	89.1	83.9	8.19	9.97
	20	105.1	103.4	101.5	99.5	97.3	94.8	92.1	89.0	85.4	81.1	75.9	6.52	8.29
	22	99.4	97.7	95.8	93.8	91.5	89.1	86.3	83.2	79.6	75.4	70.2	5.34	7.16

TABLE 459

Process Times (B) at Retort Temperature of 250°F for Conduction-Heating Foods in 401 x 205 Can

f_h	z	INITIAL FOOD TEMPERATURE (T_{ih})											Equivalent	
		100	110	120	130	140	150	160	170	180	190	200	F_c^{18}	F_s^{18}
	16	71.3	70.0	68.6	67.1	65.5	63.7	61.7	59.5	56.9	54.0	50.6	8.86	11.26
43.50	18	69.1	67.8	66.4	64.9	63.2	61.4	59.4	57.2	54.7	51.8	48.3	7.63	10.00
	20	66.7	65.4	64.0	62.5	60.9	59.1	57.1	54.9	52.3	49.4	46.0	6.48	8.81
	22	64.7	63.3	61.9	60.4	58.8	57.0	55.0	52.8	50.3	47.3	43.9	5.54	7.83
	16	74.6	73.2	71.7	70.1	68.4	66.5	64.4	62.0	59.3	56.3	52.6	8.85	11.28
46.06	18	72.2	70.8	69.3	67.7	66.0	64.1	62.0	59.6	56.9	53.9	50.2	7.61	9.99
	20	69.7	68.3	66.8	65.2	63.5	61.6	59.5	57.1	54.5	51.4	47.7	6.42	8.77
	22	67.5	66.1	64.6	63.0	61.3	59.4	57.3	54.9	52.3	49.2	45.5	5.47	7.78
	16	77.9	76.4	74.8	73.1	71.3	69.3	67.1	64.6	61.8	58.5	54.7	8.87	11.32
48.62	18	75.3	73.9	72.3	70.6	68.8	66.7	64.5	62.0	59.2	56.0	52.1	7.58	10.00
	20	72.7	71.3	69.7	68.0	66.2	64.1	61.9	59.4	56.6	53.4	49.5	6.39	8.76
	22	70.4	68.9	67.4	65.7	63.8	61.8	59.6	57.1	54.3	51.0	47.2	5.43	7.75
	16	81.1	79.5	77.9	76.1	74.2	72.1	69.7	67.1	64.1	60.7	56.7	8.88	11.35
51.18	18	78.4	76.9	75.2	73.4	71.5	69.4	67.0	64.4	61.4	58.0	54.0	7.57	10.01
	20	75.7	74.1	72.5	70.7	68.8	68.6	64.3	61.7	58.7	55.3	51.2	6.35	8.74
	22	73.2	71.7	70.1	68.3	66.3	64.2	61.9	59.3	56.3	52.9	48.8	5.37	7.71
	16	84.3	82.7	80.9	79.1	77.0	74.8	72.3	69.6	66.5	62.9	58.6	8.90	11.39
53.74	18	81.4	79.8	78.1	76.2	74.2	72.0	69.5	66.8	63.7	60.1	55.8	7.55	10.00
	20	78.6	77.0	75.2	73.4	71.3	69.1	66.7	63.9	60.8	57.2	52.9	6.31	8.71
	22	76.0	74.4	72.7	70.8	68.8	66.6	64.1	61.4	58.2	54.6	50.4	5.31	7.67

TABLE 460

Process Times (B) at Retort Temperature of 260°F for Conduction-Heating Foods in 401 x 205 Can

f_h	z	INITIAL FOOD TEMPERATURE (T_{ih}) 100	110	120	130	140	150	160	170	180	190	200	Equivalent F_c^{18}	F_s^{18}
43.50	16	56.3	55.1	53.8	52.4	50.9	49.2	47.4	45.5	43.2	40.7	37.8	8.25	11.08
	18	55.1	53.9	52.6	51.2	49.7	48.1	46.3	44.3	42.0	39.5	36.6	7.22	10.00
	20	54.2	53.0	51.7	50.3	48.7	47.1	45.3	43.3	41.1	38.6	35.6	6.45	9.18
	22	53.2	52.0	50.7	49.3	47.8	46.2	44.4	42.4	40.1	37.6	34.7	5.75	8.43
46.06	16	59.1	57.8	56.5	55.0	53.4	51.6	49.7	47.6	45.3	42.6	39.5	8.31	11.16
	18	57.8	56.6	55.2	53.7	52.1	50.4	48.4	46.3	44.0	41.3	38.2	7.21	10.00
	20	56.8	55.5	54.1	52.6	51.1	49.3	47.4	45.3	42.9	40.2	37.2	6.39	9.13
	22	55.8	54.5	53.1	51.6	50.0	48.3	46.4	44.3	41.9	39.2	36.2	5.68	8.36
48.62	16	61.9	60.6	59.1	57.5	55.9	54.0	52.0	49.8	47.3	44.5	41.2	8.33	11.20
	18	60.5	59.2	57.7	56.1	54.5	52.6	50.6	48.4	45.9	43.1	39.8	7.20	10.00
	20	59.4	58.0	56.6	55.0	53.3	51.5	49.5	47.3	44.8	41.9	38.7	6.35	9.10
	22	58.3	56.9	55.5	53.9	52.2	50.4	48.4	46.2	43.7	40.9	37.6	5.60	8.30
51.18	16	64.7	63.3	61.7	60.1	58.3	56.4	54.3	51.9	49.3	46.3	42.9	8.35	11.23
	18	63.2	61.8	60.2	58.6	56.8	54.9	52.8	50.4	47.8	44.8	41.4	7.19	10.00
	20	62.0	60.6	59.0	57.4	55.6	53.7	51.6	49.2	46.6	43.6	40.2	6.32	9.08
	22	60.8	59.4	57.8	56.2	54.4	52.5	50.3	48.0	45.4	42.4	39.0	5.52	8.23
53.74	16	67.5	66.0	64.3	62.6	60.7	58.7	56.5	54.0	51.3	48.2	44.6	8.39	11.28
	18	65.9	64.4	62.8	61.0	59.2	57.1	54.9	52.4	49.7	46.6	43.0	7.17	10.00
	20	64.6	63.1	61.5	59.7	57.9	55.8	53.6	51.2	48.4	45.3	41.7	6.28	9.05
	22	63.3	61.8	60.2	58.5	56.6	54.6	52.3	49.9	47.1	44.0	40.4	5.47	8.18

TABLE 461

Process Times (B) at Retort Temperature of 230°F for Conduction-Heating Foods in 401 x 411 Can

f_h	z	INITIAL FOOD TEMPERATURE (T_{ih})											Equivalent	
		100	110	120	130	140	150	160	170	180	190	200	F_c^{18}	F_s^{18}
	16	283.7	281.2	278.5	275.5	272.2	268.5	264.4	259.6	253.9	246.9	237.9	13.03	14.45
71.80	18	231.0	228.5	225.8	222.9	219.6	215.9	211.7	206.9	201.2	194.3	185.3	9.06	10.39
	20	198.5	196.0	193.3	190.3	187.1	183.4	179.2	174.4	168.7	161.8	152.8	6.62	7.92
	22	176.2	173.7	171.0	168.0	164.7	161.0	156.9	152.1	146.4	139.4	130.5	4.87	6.23
	16	289.4	286.7	283.9	280.7	277.2	273.4	268.9	263.9	257.8	250.5	241.0	12.95	14.39
76.02	18	237.5	234.9	232.0	228.9	225.4	221.5	217.1	212.0	206.0	198.6	189.1	9.04	10.42
	20	204.4	201.8	198.9	195.8	192.3	188.4	184.0	178.9	172.9	165.5	156.0	6.59	7.92
	22	182.7	180.1	177.2	174.1	170.6	166.7	162.3	157.2	151.2	143.8	134.3	4.85	6.26
	16	295.5	292.7	289.7	286.4	282.7	278.6	273.9	268.6	262.2	254.4	244.4	12.94	14.37
80.24	18	243.3	240.5	237.5	234.1	230.5	226.4	221.7	216.3	210.0	202.2	192.2	9.00	10.40
	20	210.1	207.3	204.2	200.9	197.2	193.1	188.5	183.1	176.8	169.0	158.9	6.54	7.89
	22	189.2	186.4	183.4	180.0	176.4	172.3	167.6	162.2	155.9	148.1	138.1	4.84	6.26
	16	302.2	299.3	296.1	292.6	288.8	284.4	279.5	273.9	267.2	259.0	248.5	12.98	14.42
84.47	18	249.5	246.5	243.3	239.8	236.0	231.6	226.7	221.1	214.4	206.2	195.7	8.97	10.39
	20	215.9	213.0	209.8	206.3	202.4	198.1	193.2	187.5	180.8	172.7	162.1	6.50	7.88
	22	195.4	192.4	189.2	185.7	181.9	177.5	172.6	167.0	160.3	152.1	141.6	4.82	6.24
	16	308.5	305.4	302.0	298.4	294.3	289.8	284.6	278.7	271.7	263.1	252.0	12.92	14.42
88.69	18	255.7	252.6	249.3	245.6	241.6	237.0	231.9	226.0	218.9	210.3	199.3	8.96	10.41
	20	221.9	218.8	215.4	211.8	207.7	203.2	198.0	192.1	185.1	176.5	165.4	6.38	7.85
	22	201.4	198.3	195.0	191.3	187.2	182.7	177.6	171.6	164.6	156.0	144.9	4.80	6.23

TABLE 462

Process Times (B) at Retort Temperature of 240°F for Conduction-Heating Foods in 401 x 411 Can

f_h	z	INITIAL FOOD TEMPERATURE (T_{ih}) 100	110	120	130	140	150	160	170	180	190	200	Equivalent F_c^{18}	F_s^{18}
71.80	16	150.1	147.8	145.3	142.6	139.6	136.3	132.6	128.5	123.7	118.0	111.0	10.76	12.71
	18	139.2	136.9	134.4	131.7	128.7	125.4	121.8	117.6	112.8	107.1	100.2	8.43	10.41
	20	130.2	127.9	125.4	122.7	119.7	116.5	112.8	108.6	103.8	98.1	91.2	6.68	8.64
	22	122.6	120.3	117.8	115.1	112.1	108.8	105.2	101.0	96.2	90.5	83.5	5.23	7.16
76.02	16	156.4	153.9	151.3	148.4	145.3	141.8	137.9	133.5	128.4	122.4	115.0	10.93	12.90
	18	144.9	142.4	139.8	136.9	133.8	130.3	126.4	122.0	116.9	110.9	103.5	8.39	10.42
	20	135.3	132.9	130.3	127.4	124.2	120.8	116.9	112.5	107.4	101.4	94.0	6.55	8.54
	22	127.8	125.3	122.7	119.8	116.7	113.2	109.3	104.9	99.8	93.8	86.4	5.19	7.15
80.24	16	162.6	160.0	157.2	154.1	150.8	147.2	143.0	138.4	133.0	126.7	118.9	11.07	13.06
	18	150.5	147.9	145.1	142.1	138.7	135.1	131.0	126.3	120.9	114.6	106.8	8.36	10.44
	20	140.5	137.9	135.1	132.1	128.8	125.1	121.0	116.4	111.0	104.6	96.9	6.46	8.48
	22	132.9	130.3	127.5	124.5	121.2	117.5	113.4	108.7	103.4	97.0	89.2	5.13	7.13
84.47	16	168.5	165.8	162.9	159.7	156.2	152.3	148.0	143.1	137.4	130.7	122.6	11.01	13.05
	18	155.9	153.1	150.2	147.0	143.5	139.7	135.3	130.4	124.8	118.1	109.9	8.33	10.43
	20	145.9	143.2	140.2	137.0	133.5	129.7	125.3	120.4	114.8	108.1	99.9	6.43	8.47
	22	137.9	135.2	132.2	129.0	125.5	121.7	117.3	112.4	106.8	100.1	91.9	5.08	7.10
88.69	16	174.3	171.5	168.4	165.0	161.4	157.3	152.8	147.6	141.7	134.7	126.1	10.94	13.04
	18	161.1	158.3	155.2	151.9	148.2	144.1	139.6	134.4	128.5	121.5	112.9	8.30	10.40
	20	151.2	148.3	145.3	141.9	138.2	134.2	129.6	124.5	118.6	111.5	102.9	6.42	8.48
	22	142.7	139.9	136.8	133.4	129.7	125.7	121.2	116.0	110.1	103.0	94.5	5.02	7.05

TABLE 463

Process Times (B) at Retort Temperature of 250°F for Conduction-Heating Foods in 401 x 411 Can

f_h	z	INITIAL FOOD TEMPERATURE (T_{ih})											Equivalent	
		100	110	120	130	140	150	160	170	180	190	200	F^{18}_c	F^{18}_s
71.80	16	107.4	105.2	102.9	100.4	97.7	94.7	91.4	87.8	83.6	78.8	73.1	9.43	12.05
	18	103.5	101.3	99.0	96.5	93.8	90.9	87.6	83.9	79.7	74.9	69.2	7.83	10.41
	20	99.8	97.6	95.3	92.8	90.1	87.1	83.8	80.2	76.0	71.2	65.5	6.41	8.92
	22	96.4	94.3	92.0	89.5	86.8	83.8	80.5	76.8	72.7	67.9	62.2	5.31	7.77
76.02	16	112.5	110.2	107.7	105.1	102.2	99.1	95.6	91.7	87.3	82.2	76.2	9.47	12.11
	18	108.3	106.1	103.6	101.0	98.1	95.0	91.5	87.6	83.2	78.1	72.1	7.81	10.40
	20	104.4	102.1	99.7	97.0	94.2	91.0	87.5	83.6	79.2	74.1	68.1	6.36	8.89
	22	100.9	98.6	96.2	93.5	90.7	87.5	84.0	80.1	75.7	70.6	64.6	5.28	7.74
80.24	16	117.5	115.1	112.5	109.8	106.7	103.4	99.7	95.6	91.0	85.6	79.2	9.50	12.17
	18	113.2	110.8	108.2	105.4	102.4	99.0	95.4	91.3	86.6	81.2	74.9	7.79	10.40
	20	109.0	106.6	104.0	101.2	98.2	94.9	91.2	87.1	82.5	77.1	70.7	6.32	8.87
	22	105.3	102.9	100.4	97.6	94.5	91.2	87.5	83.4	78.8	73.4	67.1	5.24	7.72
84.47	16	122.6	120.1	117.4	114.4	111.3	107.8	103.9	99.6	94.7	89.0	82.3	9.56	12.25
	18	118.0	115.5	112.8	109.8	106.6	103.1	99.3	94.9	90.0	84.4	77.7	7.77	10.40
	20	113.7	111.1	108.4	105.5	102.3	98.8	94.9	90.6	85.7	80.1	73.4	6.32	8.88
	22	109.8	107.3	104.6	101.6	98.4	94.9	91.1	86.7	81.9	76.2	69.5	5.20	7.69
88.69	16	127.7	125.0	122.2	119.1	115.7	112.1	108.0	103.5	98.3	92.4	85.4	9.61	12.32
	18	122.8	120.1	117.3	114.2	110.8	107.2	103.1	98.6	93.4	87.5	80.5	7.76	10.41
	20	118.3	115.6	112.7	109.7	106.3	102.6	98.6	94.0	88.9	83.0	75.9	6.31	8.89
	22	114.2	111.6	108.7	105.6	102.3	98.6	94.5	90.0	84.9	78.9	71.9	5.16	7.67

TABLE 464

Process Times (B) at Retort Temperature of 260°F for Conduction-Heating Foods in 401 x 411 Can

f_h	z	INITIAL FOOD TEMPERATURE (T_{ih})											Equivalent	
		100	110	120	130	140	150	160	170	180	190	200	F_c^{18}	F_s^{18}
71.80	16	87.1	85.1	83.0	80.7	78.2	75.4	72.5	69.2	65.5	61.4	56.5	8.97	11.95
	18	84.9	82.9	80.7	78.4	75.9	73.2	70.2	66.9	63.3	59.1	54.3	7.49	10.40
	20	83.0	81.0	78.8	76.5	74.0	71.3	68.3	65.0	61.4	57.2	52.4	6.38	9.23
	22	81.1	79.1	77.0	74.6	72.1	69.4	66.5	63.2	59.5	55.3	50.5	5.41	8.19
76.02	16	91.5	89.4	87.1	84.7	82.0	79.2	76.0	72.5	68.7	64.2	59.2	9.01	12.01
	18	89.1	87.0	84.7	82.3	79.6	76.7	73.6	70.1	66.2	61.8	56.7	7.47	10.40
	20	87.1	85.0	82.7	80.2	77.6	74.7	71.6	68.1	64.2	59.8	54.7	6.33	9.19
	22	85.1	82.9	80.6	78.2	75.6	72.7	69.5	66.1	62.2	57.8	52.7	5.33	8.11
80.24	16	95.9	93.7	91.3	88.7	85.9	82.8	79.5	75.9	71.8	67.1	61.7	9.03	12.05
	18	93.3	91.1	88.7	86.1	83.3	80.3	77.0	73.3	69.2	64.5	59.1	7.46	10.40
	20	91.1	88.9	86.5	83.9	81.1	78.1	74.8	71.1	67.0	62.3	57.0	6.28	9.15
	22	88.9	86.7	84.3	81.7	78.9	75.9	72.6	68.9	64.8	60.1	54.8	5.24	8.03
84.47	16	100.3	97.9	95.4	92.6	89.7	86.5	83.0	79.2	74.8	69.9	64.3	9.06	12.09
	18	97.5	95.2	92.6	89.9	87.0	83.8	80.3	76.4	72.1	67.2	61.5	7.45	10.40
	20	95.2	92.8	90.3	87.5	84.6	81.4	77.9	74.1	69.7	64.8	59.2	6.24	9.11
	22	92.8	90.5	87.9	85.2	82.3	79.1	75.6	71.7	67.4	62.5	56.8	5.17	7.97
88.69	16	104.6	102.1	99.4	96.6	93.5	90.1	86.5	82.4	77.9	72.7	66.8	9.09	12.14
	18	101.7	99.2	96.5	93.7	90.6	87.3	83.6	79.5	75.0	69.9	63.9	7.44	10.40
	20	99.2	96.7	94.0	91.2	88.1	84.8	81.1	77.0	72.5	67.3	61.4	6.19	9.08
	22	96.7	94.2	91.5	88.7	85.6	82.2	78.6	74.5	70.0	64.8	58.9	5.10	7.90

TABLE 465

Process Times (B) at Retort Temperature of 230°F for Conduction-Heating Foods in 401 x 602 Can

f_h	z	INITIAL FOOD TEMPERATURE (T_{ih})											Equivalent	
		100	110	120	130	140	150	160	170	180	190	200	F_c^{18}	F_s^{18}
	16	300.3	297.4	294.4	291.0	287.3	283.2	278.4	273.0	266.6	258.7	248.6	13.19	14.63
81.11	18	247.1	244.3	241.2	237.9	234.1	230.0	225.3	219.9	213.4	205.6	195.4	9.18	10.59
	20	213.2	210.4	207.3	204.0	200.3	196.1	191.4	186.0	179.6	171.7	161.6	6.67	8.04
	22	191.9	189.0	186.0	182.6	178.9	174.8	170.1	164.6	158.2	150.3	140.2	4.94	6.37
	16	307.7	304.7	301.5	297.9	294.0	289.6	284.6	278.9	272.1	263.7	253.0	13.23	14.68
85.88	18	254.0	251.0	247.7	244.2	240.2	235.9	230.9	225.1	218.3	210.0	199.3	9.15	10.58
	20	219.8	216.8	213.6	210.0	206.1	201.7	196.7	191.0	184.2	175.9	165.1	6.64	8.03
	22	198.9	195.9	192.6	189.1	185.2	180.8	175.8	170.0	163.2	154.9	144.2	4.92	6.35
	16	314.8	311.6	308.2	304.4	300.3	295.6	290.4	284.3	277.1	268.3	257.0	13.16	14.68
90.65	18	261.0	257.9	254.5	250.7	246.6	241.9	236.7	230.6	223.4	214.6	203.3	9.13	10.60
	20	226.6	223.5	220.0	216.3	212.1	207.5	202.2	196.2	189.0	180.2	168.9	6.51	7.99
	22	205.7	202.6	199.1	195.4	191.2	186.6	181.3	175.3	168.1	159.3	148.0	4.90	6.33
	16	321.2	317.9	314.3	310.3	305.9	301.1	295.5	289.1	281.6	272.3	260.4	13.08	14.64
95.43	18	267.8	264.5	260.9	256.9	252.5	247.7	242.1	235.7	228.2	218.9	207.0	9.10	10.59
	20	234.3	230.9	227.3	223.4	219.0	214.1	208.6	202.2	194.7	185.4	173.5	6.48	8.02
	22	212.4	209.1	205.5	201.5	197.2	192.3	186.7	180.4	172.8	163.6	151.6	4.89	6.32
	16	328.3	324.8	321.1	316.9	312.3	307.2	301.4	294.7	286.7	277.0	264.5	13.09	14.64
100.20	18	274.7	271.2	267.4	263.3	258.7	253.5	247.7	241.0	233.1	223.4	210.9	9.07	10.58
	20	241.8	238.3	234.5	230.4	225.8	220.7	214.8	208.1	200.2	190.5	178.0	6.47	8.06
	22	218.9	215.4	211.6	207.5	202.9	197.8	192.0	185.2	177.3	167.6	155.1	4.88	6.31

TABLE 466

Process Times (B) at Retort Temperature of 240°F for Conduction-Heating Foods in 401 x 602 Can

f_h	z	INITIAL FOOD TEMPERATURE (T_{ih})											Equivalent	
		100	110	120	130	140	150	160	170	180	190	200	F_c^{18}	F_s^{18}
	16	164.8	162.2	159.3	156.3	152.9	149.2	145.1	140.4	134.9	128.5	120.6	11.30	13.29
81.11	18	152.5	149.9	147.1	144.0	140.7	137.0	132.8	128.1	122.7	116.3	108.4	8.54	10.63
	20	142.4	139.8	137.0	133.9	130.6	126.9	122.7	118.0	112.6	106.1	98.3	6.60	8.63
	22	134.7	132.1	129.3	126.2	122.8	119.1	115.0	110.3	104.8	98.4	90.6	5.25	7.25
	16	171.5	168.8	165.8	162.5	159.0	155.1	150.7	145.7	139.9	133.1	124.8	11.24	13.29
85.88	18	158.7	155.9	152.9	149.7	146.1	142.2	137.8	132.8	127.1	120.3	111.9	8.50	10.62
	20	148.5	145.7	142.7	139.5	135.9	132.0	127.6	122.6	116.9	110.1	101.8	6.57	8.62
	22	140.4	137.6	134.6	131.4	127.8	123.9	119.5	114.5	108.7	101.9	93.6	5.19	7.22
	16	178.1	175.2	172.0	168.6	164.9	160.7	156.1	150.8	144.7	137.6	128.8	11.16	13.28
90.65	18	164.7	161.7	158.6	155.2	151.4	147.3	142.6	137.4	131.3	124.1	115.3	8.47	10.59
	20	154.5	151.6	148.4	145-0	141.3	137.1	132.5	127.2	121.1	114.0	105.2	6.55	8.63
	22	145.8	142.9	139.8	136.3	132.6	128.4	123.8	118.5	112.5	105.3	96.5	5.12	7.17
	16	184.6	181.6	178.3	174.6	170.0	166.5	161.4	155.9	149.5	142.0	132.7	11.12	13.28
95.43	18	171.0	167.9	164.6	161.0	157.0	152.7	147.8	142.2	135.9	128.3	119.1	8.44	10.58
	20	160.4	157.3	154.0	150.4	146.4	142.1	137.2	131.7	125.3	117.7	108.5	6.52	8.62
	22	151.2	148.1	144.8	141.2	137.2	132.9	128.0	122.5	116.1	108.5	99.3	5.03	7.09
	16	191.0	187.8	184.3	180.5	176.4	171.8	166.7	160.9	154.1	146.2	136.5	11.07	13.28
100.20	18	177.3	174.1	170.6	166.8	162.6	158.1	152.9	147.1	140.4	132.5	122.8	8.42	10.58
	20	166.1	162.9	159.4	155.6	151.5	146.9	141.8	136.0	129.2	121.3	111.6	6.44	8.58
	22	156.8	153.6	150.1	146.3	142.1	137.6	132.4	126.6	119.9	112.0	102.3	4.99	7.07

TABLE 467

Process Times (B) at Retort Temperature of 250°F for Conduction-Heating Foods in 401 x 602 Can

f_h	z	INITIAL FOOD TEMPERATURE (T_{ih})											Equivalent	
		100	110	120	130	140	150	160	170	180	190	200	F_c^{18}	F_s^{18}
	16	119.0	116.6	114.0	111.2	108.1	104.7	101.0	96.9	92.2	86.8	80.3	9.70	12.37
81.11	18	114.6	112.2	109.6	106.8	103.7	100.4	96.6	92.5	87.8	82.4	75.9	7.97	10.59
	20	110.4	108.0	105.4	102.6	99.5	96.1	92.4	88.3	83.6	78.2	71.7	6.47	9.02
	22	106.7	104.3	101.7	98.8	85.8	92.4	88.7	84.6	79.9	74.4	68.0	5.37	7.85
	16	124.8	122.2	119.5	116.5	113.2	109.7	105.7	101.4	96.4	90.6	83.8	9.77	12.47
85.88	18	120.1	117.5	114.8	111.8	108.5	105.0	101.0	96.7	91.7	85.9	79.1	7.95	10.59
	20	115.7	113.1	110.3	107.4	104.1	100.6	96.6	92.2	87.3	81.5	74.7	6.46	9.03
	22	111.8	109.2	106.4	103.4	100.2	96.6	92.7	88.3	83.3	77.6	70.8	5.32	7.82
	16	130.5	127.8	124.9	121.7	118.3	114.5	110.4	105.8	100.5	94.4	87.3	9.82	12.55
90.65	18	125.5	122.8	119.9	116.7	113.3	109.5	105.4	100.8	95.5	89.4	82.3	7.93	10.59
	20	120.9	118.2	115.2	112.1	108.7	104.9	100.8	96.1	90.9	84.8	77.6	6.45	9.04
	22	116.8	114.0	111.1	108.0	104.5	100.8	96.6	92.0	86.7	80.7	73.5	5.28	7.80
	16	136.2	133.3	130.2	126.9	123.3	119.4	115.0	110.1	104.6	98.2	90.6	9.87	12.61
95.43	18	130.9	128.0	124.9	121.6	118.0	114.1	109.7	104.8	99.3	92.9	85.3	7.92	10.59
	20	126.0	123.1	120.1	116.8	113.2	109.2	104.8	100.0	94.4	88.0	80.5	6.45	9.05
	22	121.7	118.8	115.7	112.4	108.8	104.9	100.5	95.6	90.1	83.7	76.2	5.24	7.77
	16	141.7	138.7	135.5	132.0	128.3	124.1	119.5	114.4	108.6	101.9	93.9	9.90	12.66
100.20	18	136.1	133.1	129.9	126.4	122.6	118.5	113.9	108.8	103.0	96.3	88.3	7.90	10.59
	20	131.1	128.1	124.8	121.4	117.6	113.4	108.8	103.7	97.9	91.2	83.3	6.41	9.02
	22	126.5	123.5	120.3	116.8	113.1	108.9	104.3	99.2	93.4	86.7	78.7	5.20	7.74

TABLE 468

Process Times (B) at Retort Temperature of 260°F for Conduction-Heating Foods in 401 x 602 Can

f_h	z	INITIAL FOOD TEMPERATURE (T_{ih})											Equivalent	
		100	110	120	130	140	150	160	170	180	190	200	F_c^{18}	F_s^{18}
	16	97.1	94.8	92.4	89.8	87.0	83.9	80.5	76.8	72.7	68.0	62.6	9.23	12.26
81.11	18	94.5	92.2	89.8	87.2	84.4	81.3	77.9	74.2	70.1	65.4	60.0	7.64	10.59
	20	92.3	90.0	87.6	85.0	82.2	79.1	75.7	72.0	67.9	63.2	57.7	6.44	9.32
	22	90.1	87.8	85.4	82.8	80.0	76.9	73.5	69.8	65.7	61.0	55.5	5.38	8.18
	16	102.0	99.6	97.0	94.3	91.3	88.1	84.5	80.6	76.2	71.2	65.4	9.27	12.31
85.88	18	99.2	96.8	94.3	91.5	88.5	85.3	81.7	77.8	73.4	68.4	62.7	7.62	10.59
	20	96.9	94.4	91.9	89.1	86.1	82.9	79.3	75.4	71.0	66.0	60.3	6.38	9.27
	22	94.5	92.1	89.5	86.7	83.7	80.5	76.9	73.0	68.6	63.6	57.9	5.30	8.11
	16	106.9	104.4	101.7	98.7	95.6	92.2	88.4	84.3	79.6	74.4	68.3	9.31	12.37
90.65	18	104.0	101.4	98.7	95.8	92.6	89.2	85.5	81.3	76.7	71.4	65.3	7.61	10.59
	20	101.4	98.9	96.1	93.2	90.1	86.6	82.9	78.7	74.1	68.8	62.8	6.34	9.24
	22	98.8	96.3	93.6	90.6	87.5	84.1	80.3	76.2	71.5	66.3	60.2	5.22	8.03
	16	111.8	109.1	106.2	103.2	99.9	96.2	92.3	87.9	83.0	77.5	71.1	9.33	12.40
95.43	18	108.6	106.0	103.1	100.0	96.7	93.1	89.2	84.8	79.9	74.4	68.0	7.60	10.59
	20	105.9	103.2	100.4	97.3	94.0	90.4	86.4	82.1	77.2	71.6	65.3	6.29	9.20
	22	103.1	100.5	97.6	94.5	91.2	87.6	83.6	79.3	74.4	68.9	62.5	5.14	7.96
	16	116.6	113.8	110.8	107.6	104.1	100.3	96.1	91.6	86.4	80.6	73.9	9.35	12.44
100.20	18	113.3	110.5	107.5	104.3	100.8	97.0	92.8	88.3	83.1	77.3	70.6	7.59	10.59
	20	110.4	107.6	104.6	101.3	97.9	94.1	89.9	85.3	80.2	74.4	67.7	6.25	9.16
	22	107.4	104.6	101.6	98.4	94.9	91.1	87.0	82.4	77.3	71.5	64.8	5.08	7.91

TABLE 469

Process Times (B) at Retort Temperature of 230°F for Conduction-Heating Foods in 404 x 200 Can

f_h	z	INITIAL FOOD TEMPERATURE (T_{ih})											Equivalent	
		100	110	120	130	140	150	160	170	180	190	200	F_c^{18}	F_s^{18}
28.48	16	203.2	202.2	201.1	199.9	198.6	197.2	195.5	193.6	191.4	188.6	185.0	12.62	13.57
	18	164.3	163.3	162.3	161.1	159.8	158.3	156.7	154.8	152.5	149.7	146.2	9.03	9.82
	20	133.4	132.4	131.3	130.1	128.8	127.4	125.7	123.8	121.6	118.8	115.2	6.75	7.62
	22	114.3	113.3	112.2	111.0	109.7	108.3	106.6	104.7	102.4	99.7	96.1	5.31	6.09
30.16	16	208.1	207.1	206.0	204.7	203.3	201.8	200.0	198.0	195.6	192.7	188.9	12.62	13.58
	18	166.8	165.8	164.6	163.4	162.0	160.5	158.7	156.7	154.3	151.4	147.6	9.02	9.82
	20	135.7	134.6	133.5	132.2	130.9	129.3	127.6	125.6	123.2	120.2	116.5	6.71	7.57
	22	116.4	115.4	114.2	113.0	111.6	110.0	108.3	106.3	103.9	101.0	97.2	5.26	6.11
31.84	16	212.7	211.6	210.4	209.1	207.6	206.0	204.2	202.0	199.5	196.4	192.5	12.62	13.60
	18	169.0	167.8	166.6	165.3	163.9	162.2	160.4	158.3	155.7	152.7	148.7	9.01	9.82
	20	138.2	137.1	135.9	134.6	133.1	131.5	129.7	127.5	125.0	121.9	117.9	6.71	7.57
	22	118.1	117.0	115.8	114.5	113.0	111.4	109.5	107.4	104.9	101.8	97.8	5.19	6.03
33.51	16	216.9	215.8	214.5	213.1	211.6	209.9	207.9	205.7	203.0	199.8	195.6	12.63	13.61
	18	170.7	169.5	168.3	166.9	165.4	163.6	161.7	159.5	156.8	153.6	149.4	9.00	9.82
	20	140.5	139.3	138.1	136.7	135.1	133.4	131.5	129.2	126.6	123.3	119.1	6.71	7.56
	22	120.4	119.2	117.9	116.5	115.0	113.3	111.4	109.1	106.5	103.2	99.0	5.19	6.02
35.19	16	220.8	219.6	218.3	216.8	215.2	213.4	211.4	209.0	206.2	202.8	198.4	12.63	13.62
	18	172.5	171.3	169.9	168.5	166.9	165.1	163.0	160.7	157.9	154.5	150.1	9.00	9.86
	20	142.5	141.2	139.9	138.5	136.8	135.0	133.0	130.6	127.9	124.5	120.1	6.67	7.56
	22	122.4	121.2	119.9	118.4	116.8	115.0	113.0	110.6	107.8	104.4	100.0	5.13	6.03

TABLE 470

Process Times (B) at Retort Temperature of 240°F for Conduction-Heating Foods in 404 x 200 Can

f_h	z	INITIAL FOOD TEMPERATURE (T_{ih})											Equivalent	
		100	110	120	130	140	150	160	170	180	190	200	F_c^{18}	F_s^{18}
	16	82.6	81.7	80.7	79.6	78.4	77.1	75.6	74.0	72.1	69.8	67.1	10.22	11.76
28.49	18	75.3	74.3	73.3	72.3	71.1	69.8	68.3	66.7	64.8	62.5	59.8	8.28	9.79
	20	70.3	69.3	68.3	67.3	66.1	64.8	63.3	61.7	59.8	57.5	54.8	6.78	8.37
	22	66.2	65.3	64.3	63.2	62.1	60.8	59.3	57.6	55.7	53.5	50.7	5.70	7.23
	16	85.1	84.1	83.1	81.9	80.7	79.3	77.8	76.0	74.0	71.6	68.7	10.20	11.77
30.16	18	77.8	76.8	75.7	74.6	73.3	72.0	70.4	68.7	66.7	64.3	61.3	8.24	9.79
	20	72.9	71.9	70.8	69.7	68.4	67.1	65.5	63.8	61.8	59.4	56.4	6.74	8.38
	22	68.6	67.7	66.6	65.5	64.2	62.9	61.3	59.6	57.5	55.2	52.2	5.68	7.21
	16	87.6	86.6	85.4	84.2	82.9	81.5	79.8	78.0	75.9	73.3	70.3	10.17	11.76
31.84	18	80.6	79.6	78.5	77.3	76.0	74.5	72.9	71.0	68.9	66.4	63.3	8.22	9.85
	20	75.4	74.4	73.3	72.1	70.7	69.3	67.7	65.8	63.7	61.2	58.1	6.71	8.35
	22	71.0	70.0	68.9	67.7	66.3	64.9	63.3	61.4	59.3	56.8	53.7	5.66	7.19
	16	90.1	89.0	87.9	86.6	85.2	83.7	82.0	80.0	77.8	75.1	71.9	10.16	11.79
33.51	18	83.4	82.3	81.1	79.9	78.5	76.9	75.2	73.3	71.0	68.4	65.1	8.19	9.88
	20	77.9	76.8	75.6	74.4	73.0	71.4	69.7	67.8	65.5	62.9	59.6	6.69	8.33
	22	73.3	72.2	71.1	69.8	68.4	66.9	65.2	63.2	61.0	58.3	55.1	5.66	7.19
	16	92.8	91.7	90.5	89.2	87.7	86.1	84.3	82.2	79.9	77.1	73.7	10.20	11.85
35.19	18	86.0	84.9	83.6	82.3	80.9	79.2	77.4	75.4	73.0	70.3	66.9	8.15	9.89
	20	80.3	79.2	77.9	76.6	75.1	73.5	71.7	69.7	67.3	64.6	61.1	6.67	8.31
	22	75.6	74.5	73.2	71.9	70.4	68.8	67.0	65.0	62.6	59.9	56.4	5.66	7.19

TABLE 471

Process Times (B) at Retort Temperature of 250°F for Conduction-Heating Foods in 404 x 200 Can

f_h	z	INITIAL FOOD TEMPERATURE (T_{ih})											Equivalent	
		100	110	120	130	140	150	160	170	180	190	200	F_c^{18}	F_s^{18}
	16	51.4	50.5	49.6	48.6	47.5	46.3	45.0	43.6	41.9	40.0	37.8	8.67	10.86
28.49	18	49.8	49.0	48.1	47.1	46.0	44.8	43.5	42.1	40.4	38.5	36.2	7.66	9.83
	20	48.3	47.5	46.6	45.6	44.5	43.3	42.0	40.5	38.9	37.0	34.7	6.74	8.89
	22	47.0	46.1	45.2	44.2	43.2	42.0	40.7	39.2	37.6	35.7	33.4	5.95	8.09
	16	53.6	52.7	51.7	50.6	49.5	48.3	46.9	45.3	43.6	41.6	39.2	8.62	10.84
30.16	18	52.0	51.1	50.1	49.0	47.9	46.6	45.3	43.7	42.0	40.0	37.6	7.63	9.82
	20	50.4	49.5	48.5	47.4	46.3	45.0	43.7	42.1	40.4	38.4	36.0	6.64	8.83
	22	48.9	48.0	47.1	46.0	44.9	43.6	42.2	40.7	39.0	36.9	34.5	5.85	8.00
	16	55.8	54.9	53.8	52.7	51.5	50.2	48.8	47.1	45.3	43.1	40.6	8.64	10.88
31.84	18	54.1	53.2	52.1	51.0	49.8	48.5	47.1	45.4	43.6	41.5	38.9	7.60	9.82
	20	52.4	51.5	50.5	49.3	48.1	46.8	45.4	43.7	41.9	39.8	37.2	6.61	8.81
	22	50.9	50.0	48.9	47.8	46.6	45.3	43.9	42.2	40.4	38.3	35.7	5.78	7.95
	16	58.1	57.1	56.0	54.8	53.6	52.2	50.6	48.9	47.0	44.7	42.1	8.67	10.94
33.51	18	56.3	55.3	54.2	53.0	51.8	50.4	48.9	47.1	45.2	43.0	40.3	7.58	9.84
	20	54.5	53.5	52.4	51.3	50.0	48.6	47.1	45.4	43.4	41.2	38.5	6.58	8.80
	22	52.9	51.9	50.8	49.7	48.4	47.0	45.5	43.8	41.8	39.6	36.9	5.73	7.92
	16	60.3	59.2	58.1	56.9	55.5	54.1	52.5	50.7	48.6	46.3	43.5	8.69	10.98
35.19	18	58.4	57.4	56.2	55.0	53.7	52.2	50.6	48.8	46.8	44.4	41.6	7.56	9.84
	20	56.5	55.5	54.4	53.1	51.8	50.3	48.7	46.9	44.9	42.5	39.8	6.52	8.76
	22	54.9	53.8	52.7	51.5	50.1	48.7	47.1	45.3	43.2	40.9	38.1	5.67	7.88

TABLE 472

Process Times (B) at Retort Temperature of 260°F for Conduction-Heating Foods in 404 x 200 Can

f_h	z	INITIAL FOOD TEMPERATURE (T_{ih})											Equivalent	
		100	110	120	130	140	150	160	170	180	190	200	F_c^{18}	F_s^{18}
	16	39.2	38.4	37.6	36.7	35.7	34.6	33.4	32.1	30.7	29.0	27.1	7.78	10.47
28.49	18	38.7	37.9	37.0	36.1	35.1	34.0	32.9	31.5	30.1	28.4	26.5	7.17	9.83
	20	38.2	37.4	36.5	35.6	34.6	33.5	32.3	31.0	29.6	27.9	26.0	6.66	9.29
	22	37.6	36.8	36.0	35.1	34.1	33.0	31.8	30.5	29.0	27.4	25.5	6.10	8.70
	16	41.2	40.3	39.4	38.5	37.4	36.3	35.0	33.6	32.1	30.3	28.3	7.83	10.55
30.16	18	40.5	39.7	38.8	37.8	36.7	35.6	34.3	33.0	31.4	29.7	27.7	7.15	9.83
	20	40.0	39.1	38.2	37.3	36.2	35.1	33.8	32.4	30.9	29.1	27.1	6.59	9.24
	22	39.4	38.6	37.7	36.7	35.6	34.5	33.2	31.9	30.3	28.6	26.6	6.04	8.66
	16	43.1	42.2	41.2	40.2	39.1	37.9	36.6	35.1	33.5	31.7	29.5	7.89	10.61
31.84	18	42.4	41.5	40.5	39.5	38.4	37.2	35.9	34.4	32.8	30.9	28.8	7.14	9.83
	20	41.8	40.9	39.9	38.9	37.8	36.6	35.3	33.8	32.2	30.3	28.2	6.54	9.20
	22	41.2	40.3	39.3	38.3	37.2	36.0	34.7	33.2	31.6	29.7	27.6	5.99	8.62
	16	45.0	44.0	43.0	42.0	40.8	39.5	38.1	36.6	34.9	32.9	30.7	7.92	10.66
33.51	18	44.2	43.3	42.3	41.2	40.0	38.8	37.4	35.8	34.1	32.2	29.9	7.12	9.83
	20	43.5	42.6	41.6	40.5	39.3	38.1	36.7	35.2	33.4	31.5	29.3	6.48	9.15
	22	42.9	42.0	41.0	39.9	38.7	37.5	36.1	34.5	32.8	30.9	28.6	5.94	8.57
	16	46.9	45.9	44.8	43.7	42.5	41.2	39.7	38.1	36.3	34.2	31.9	7.94	10.70
35.19	18	46.0	45.1	44.0	42.9	41.6	40.3	38.9	37.2	35.4	33.4	31.0	7.11	9.83
	20	45.3	44.3	43.3	42.1	40.9	39.6	38.1	36.5	34.7	32.7	30.3	6.45	9.14
	22	44.6	43.6	42.6	41.5	40.2	38.9	37.4	35.8	34.0	32.0	29.6	5.86	8.51

TABLE 473

Process Times (B) at Retort Temperature of 230°F for Conduction-Heating Foods in 404 x 211 Can

f_h	z	INITIAL FOOD TEMPERATURE (T_{ih})											Equivalent	
		100	110	120	130	140	150	160	170	180	190	200	F_c^{18}	F_s^{18}
45.30	16	242.1	240.6	238.9	237.0	234.9	232.6	230.0	226.9	223.3	219.0	213.3	12.94	13.99
	18	188.8	187.3	185.6	183.7	181.6	179.3	176.7	173.6	170.0	165.6	160.0	8.99	10.04
	20	158.4	156.8	155.1	153.2	151.2	148.8	146.2	143.2	139.6	135.2	129.6	6.66	7.73
	22	137.9	136.3	134.6	132.7	130.6	128.3	125.7	122.6	119.1	114.7	109.0	5.12	6.15
47.97	16	245.3	243.6	241.8	239.8	237.6	235.2	232.4	229.2	225.4	220.7	214.7	12.95	14.00
	18	192.9	191.2	189.4	187.5	185.3	182.8	180.0	176.8	173.0	168.4	162.4	8.99	10.10
	20	162.2	160.5	158.7	156.7	154.5	152.1	149.3	146.1	142.3	137.6	131.7	6.63	7.74
	22	141.2	139.5	137.7	135.8	133.6	131.1	128.3	125.1	121.3	116.7	110.7	5.06	6.11
50.63	16	247.7	245.9	244.0	241.9	239.6	237.0	234.1	230.7	226.7	221.8	215.5	12.90	14.01
	18	196.2	194.5	192.5	190.4	188.1	185.5	182.6	179.2	175.2	170.3	164.0	8.89	10.09
	20	165.5	163.7	161.8	159.7	157.4	154.8	151.9	148.5	144.5	139.6	133.3	6.59	7.69
	22	144.8	143.0	141.1	139.0	136.7	134.1	131.1	127.8	123.7	118.8	112.5	5.03	6.11
53.30	16	250.4	248.6	246.6	244.3	241.9	239.2	236.1	232.5	228.3	223.1	216.5	12.70	13.99
	18	199.8	197.9	195.9	193.7	191.3	188.5	185.4	181.9	177.7	172.5	165.8	8.85	10.03
	20	169.2	167.3	165.3	163.1	160.7	157.9	154.9	151.3	147.1	141.9	135.2	6.54	7.68
	22	148.4	146.6	144.6	142.4	139.9	137.2	134.1	130.5	126.3	121.2	114.5	5.00	6.10
55.96	16	254.9	252.9	250.8	248.5	245.9	243.1	239.8	236.1	231.7	226.2	219.2	12.69	13.97
	18	203.6	201.7	199.6	197.2	194.7	191.8	188.6	184.8	180.4	175.0	168.0	8.85	10.03
	20	173.2	171.3	169.2	166.9	164.3	161.4	158.2	154.4	150.0	144.6	137.6	6.54	7.72
	22	152.0	150.0	147.9	145.6	143.0	140.2	136.9	133.2	128.7	123.3	116.3	4.96	6.09

TABLE 474

Process Times (B) at Retort Temperature of 240°F for Conduction-Heating Foods in 404 x 211 Can

f_h	z	INITIAL FOOD TEMPERATURE (T_{ih})											Equivalent	
		100	110	120	130	140	150	160	170	180	190	200	F_c^{18}	F_s^{18}
45.30	16	110.5	109.1	107.5	105.8	103.9	101.8	99.5	96.9	93.9	90.3	85.9	10.44	12.35
	18	102.0	100.6	99.0	97.3	95.4	93.3	91.0	88.4	85.4	81.8	77.4	8.29	10.06
	20	95.0	93.5	91.9	90.2	88.3	86.3	83.9	81.3	78.3	74.7	70.3	6.84	8.49
	22	88.8	87.4	85.8	84.1	82.2	80.1	77.8	75.2	72.1	68.6	64.2	5.53	7.20
47.97	16	114.7	113.2	111.5	109.7	107.7	105.5	103.0	100.3	97.1	93.3	88.6	10.41	12.33
	18	105.8	104.3	102.6	100.8	98.8	96.6	94.1	91.4	88.2	84.4	79.7	8.28	10.06
	20	98.2	96.6	95.0	93.2	91.2	89.0	86.5	83.7	80.5	76.7	72.1	6.81	8.47
	22	92.1	90.5	88.9	87.1	85.1	82.9	80.4	77.7	74.4	70.6	66.0	5.43	7.16
50.63	16	118.8	117.1	115.4	113.4	111.4	109.0	106.4	103.5	100.1	96.1	91.2	10.38	12.31
	18	109.5	107.8	106.1	104.1	102.1	99.7	97.1	94.2	90.8	86.8	81.9	8.28	10.06
	20	101.3	99.7	97.9	96.0	93.9	91.6	89.0	86.0	82.7	78.7	73.7	6.67	8.37
	22	95.6	94.0	92.2	90.3	88.2	85.9	83.3	80.4	77.0	73.0	68.1	5.41	7.19
53.30	16	122.8	121.1	119.2	117.2	115.0	112.5	109.8	106.7	103.2	98.9	93.8	10.38	12.31
	18	112.9	111.1	109.3	107.3	105.1	102.6	99.9	96.8	93.2	89.0	83.9	8.26	10.04
	20	104.7	103.0	101.2	99.2	96.9	94.5	91.8	88.7	85.1	80.9	75.7	6.57	8.34
	22	99.1	97.4	95.5	93.5	91.3	88.8	86.1	83.0	79.5	75.2	70.1	5.39	7.21
55.96	16	126.7	124.9	123.0	120.8	118.5	116.0	113.1	109.9	106.1	101.7	96.3	10.38	12.31
	18	116.1	114.3	112.4	110.3	108.0	105.4	102.5	99.3	95.6	91.1	85.7	8.23	10.01
	20	108.4	106.6	104.7	102.5	100.2	97.7	94.8	91.6	87.8	83.4	77.9	6.54	8.36
	22	102.4	100.6	98.6	96.5	94.2	91.7	88.8	85.5	81.8	77.4	71.9	5.36	7.18

TABLE 475

Process Times (B) at Retort Temperature of 250°F for Conduction-Heating Foods in 404 x 211 Can

f_h	z	INITIAL FOOD TEMPERATURE (T_{ih})											Equivalent	
		100	110	120	130	140	150	160	170	180	190	200	F_c^{18}	F_s^{18}
	16	73.7	72.4	70.9	69.4	67.6	65.8	63.7	61.4	58.7	55.7	52.1	8.92	11.34
45.30	18	71.4	70.0	68.6	67.0	65.3	63.4	61.3	59.0	56.4	53.3	49.8	7.67	10.05
	20	68.9	67.6	66.1	64.6	62.8	61.0	58.9	56.6	53.9	50.9	47.3	6.50	8.84
	22	66.8	65.4	64.0	62.4	60.7	58.8	56.7	54.4	51.8	48.8	45.2	5.54	7.84
	16	77.1	75.7	74.2	72.5	70.7	68.7	66.5	64.0	61.3	58.1	54.3	8.93	11.37
47.97	18	74.6	73.2	71.6	70.0	68.2	66.2	64.0	61.5	58.8	55.5	51.7	7.65	10.06
	20	72.1	70.6	69.1	67.4	65.6	63.6	61.4	59.0	56.2	53.0	49.2	6.45	8.82
	22	69.8	68.3	66.8	65.1	63.3	61.3	59.1	56.7	53.9	50.7	46.9	5.48	7.80
	16	80.5	79.0	77.4	75.6	73.7	71.6	69.3	66.7	63.8	60.4	56.4	8.95	11.41
50.63	18	77.9	76.3	74.7	72.9	71.0	68.9	66.6	64.0	61.1	57.7	53.7	7.63	10.06
	20	75.2	73.6	72.0	70.2	68.3	66.2	63.9	61.3	58.4	55.0	51.0	6.41	8.80
	22	72.7	71.2	69.6	67.8	65.9	63.8	61.5	58.9	56.0	52.6	48.6	5.43	7.77
	16	83.8	82.2	80.5	78.7	76.7	74.5	72.0	69.3	66.2	62.6	58.4	8.96	11.45
53.30	18	81.0	79.4	77.7	75.9	73.9	71.7	69.2	66.5	63.4	59.8	55.6	7.61	10.06
	20	78.2	76.6	74.9	73.0	71.0	68.8	66.4	63.6	60.6	57.0	52.8	6.36	8.77
	22	75.7	74.1	72.4	70.5	68.5	66.3	63.9	61.1	58.0	54.5	50.2	5.37	7.73
	16	87.2	85.5	83.7	81.8	79.6	77.3	74.8	71.9	68.7	64.9	60.5	8.98	11.49
55.96	18	84.2	82.5	80.7	78.8	76.7	74.4	71.8	68.9	65.7	62.0	57.5	7.59	10.06
	20	81.3	79.6	77.8	75.8	73.7	71.4	68.8	66.0	62.7	59.0	54.6	6.34	8.76
	22	78.6	76.9	75.1	73.2	71.1	68.8	66.2	63.3	60.1	56.3	51.9	5.31	7.68

TABLE 476

Process Times (B) at Retort Temperature of 260°F for Conduction-Heating Foods in 404 x 211 Can

f_h	z	INITIAL FOOD TEMPERATURE (T_{ih})											Equivalent	
		100	110	120	130	140	150	160	170	180	190	200	F_c^{18}	F_s^{18}
45.30	16	58.4	57.1	55.7	54.3	52.7	51.0	49.1	47.1	44.7	42.1	39.1	8.35	11.20
	18	57.1	55.8	54.5	53.0	51.5	49.7	47.9	45.8	43.5	40.8	37.8	7.27	10.06
	20	56.1	54.8	53.5	52.0	50.4	48.7	46.8	44.8	42.4	39.8	36.8	6.47	9.21
	22	55.1	53.8	52.5	51.0	49.4	47.7	45.9	43.8	41.5	38.8	35.8	5.75	8.44
47.97	16	61.3	59.9	58.5	57.0	55.3	53.5	51.5	49.3	46.8	44.1	40.9	8.39	11.26
	18	59.9	58.6	57.1	55.6	53.9	52.1	50.1	47.9	45.5	42.7	39.5	7.26	10.06
	20	58.8	57.5	56.0	54.5	52.8	51.0	49.0	46.8	44.4	41.6	38.4	6.41	9.16
	22	57.7	56.4	55.0	53.4	51.8	49.9	48.0	45.8	43.3	40.5	37.3	5.68	8.38
50.63	16	64.2	62.8	61.2	59.6	57.9	55.9	53.8	51.5	48.9	46.0	42.6	8.41	11.29
	18	62.7	61.3	59.8	58.1	56.4	54.5	52.4	50.0	47.5	44.5	41.1	7.25	10.06
	20	61.5	60.1	58.6	57.0	55.2	53.3	51.2	48.9	46.3	43.3	40.0	6.38	9.14
	22	60.3	58.9	57.4	55.8	54.0	52.1	50.0	47.7	45.1	42.2	38.8	5.59	8.30
53.30	16	67.1	65.6	64.0	62.3	60.4	58.4	56.2	53.7	51.0	47.9	44.4	8.44	11.34
	18	65.5	64.0	62.4	60.7	58.8	56.8	54.6	52.2	49.4	46.4	42.8	7.23	10.06
	20	64.2	62.7	61.1	59.4	57.6	55.5	53.3	50.9	48.2	45.1	41.5	6.35	9.12
	22	62.9	61.5	59.9	58.1	56.3	54.3	52.1	49.6	46.9	43.8	40.2	5.53	8.24
55.96	16	69.9	68.4	66.7	64.9	62.9	60.8	58.5	55.9	53.1	49.8	46.1	8.48	11.38
	18	68.2	66.7	65.0	63.2	61.3	59.1	56.8	54.3	51.4	48.2	44.4	7.22	10.06
	20	66.9	65.3	63.6	61.8	59.9	57.8	55.5	52.9	50.0	46.8	43.0	6.30	9.08
	22	65.5	64.0	62.3	60.5	58.5	56.4	54.1	51.6	48.7	45.4	41.7	5.46	8.19

TABLE 477

Process Times (B) at Retort Temperature of 230°F for Conduction-Heating Foods in 404 x 307 Can

f_h	z	INITIAL FOOD TEMPERATURE (T_{ih})											Equivalent	
		100	110	120	130	140	150	160	170	180	190	200	F_c^{18}	F_s^{18}
60.21	16	264.6	262.5	260.2	257.7	255.0	251.9	248.4	244.4	239.6	233.8	226.3	12.92	14.21
	18	212.5	210.4	208.1	205.6	202.9	199.8	196.3	192.3	187.5	181.7	174.1	9.01	10.25
	20	180.8	178.7	176.4	173.9	171.2	168.1	164.6	160.6	155.8	150.0	142.4	6.63	7.83
	22	159.2	157.1	154.9	152.4	149.6	146.5	143.0	139.0	134.2	128.4	120.9	5.02	6.20
63.75	16	269.5	267.3	264.9	262.2	259.3	256.1	252.4	248.1	243.1	236.9	228.9	12.91	14.20
	18	217.6	215.4	213.0	210.4	207.4	204.2	200.5	196.2	191.2	185.0	177.0	8.97	10.28
	20	185.6	183.4	181.0	178.3	175.4	172.2	168.5	164.2	159.2	153.0	145.0	6.57	7.81
	22	163.8	161.6	159.2	156.5	153.6	150.4	146.7	142.4	137.4	131.2	123.2	4.97	6.17
67.29	16	274.9	272.5	270.0	267.2	264.1	260.7	256.8	252.3	246.9	240.4	232.0	12.96	14.25
	18	222.2	219.9	217.3	214.6	211.5	208.0	204.1	199.6	194.3	187.8	179.4	8.92	10.22
	20	190.7	188.4	185.8	183.0	180.0	176.5	172.6	168.1	162.8	156.3	147.9	6.56	7.83
	22	168.6	166.2	163.7	160.9	157.8	154.4	150.5	146.0	140.6	134.1	125.7	4.86	6.15
70.83	16	279.3	276.8	274.1	271.2	267.9	264.3	260.2	255.5	249.9	243.0	234.1	12.81	14.22
	18	227.6	225.1	222.4	219.5	216.2	212.6	208.5	203.8	198.2	191.3	182.4	8.91	10.23
	20	195.5	193.1	190.4	187.5	184.2	180.6	176.5	171.7	166.1	159.3	150.4	6.51	7.80
	22	173.6	171.1	168.4	165.5	162.3	158.6	154.5	149.8	144.2	137.3	128.5	4.79	6.13
74.37	16	284.0	281.4	278.6	275.5	272.1	268.3	264.0	259.0	253.2	246.0	236.7	12.73	14.16
	18	233.0	230.5	227.6	224.6	221.2	217.4	213.0	208.1	202.2	195.0	185.7	8.90	10.26
	20	200.4	197.9	195.1	192.0	188.6	184.8	180.5	175.5	169.6	162.4	153.1	6.48	7.80
	22	179.0	176.5	173.6	170.6	167.2	163.4	159.0	154.1	148.2	141.0	131.7	4.77	6.16

TABLE 478

Process Times (B) at Retort Temperature of 240°F for Conduction-Heating Foods in 404 x 307 Can

f_h	z	INITIAL FOOD TEMPERATURE (T_{ih})											Equivalent	
		100	110	120	130	140	150	160	170	180	190	200	F_c^{18}	F_s^{18}
	16	133.7	131.8	129.7	127.4	125.0	122.2	119.1	115.6	111.6	106.8	101.0	10.60	12.54
60.21	18	122.2	120.3	118.2	115.9	113.4	110.7	107.6	104.1	100.1	95.3	89.5	8.38	10.17
	20	114.8	112.9	110.8	108.5	106.0	103.2	100.2	96.7	92.6	87.9	82.0	6.66	8.54
	22	108.3	106.4	104.3	102.0	99.5	96.8	93.7	90.2	86.2	81.4	75.6	5.42	7.26
	16	138.5	136.5	134.3	131.9	129.2	126.3	123.0	119.3	115.1	110.0	103.9	10.58	12.52
63.75	18	127.4	125.3	123.1	120.7	118.0	115.1	111.9	108.2	103.9	98.8	92.7	8.35	10.21
	20	119.3	117.3	115.1	112.7	110.0	107.1	103.9	100.2	95.9	90.8	84.7	6.61	8.54
	22	112.6	110.5	108.3	105.9	103.3	100.3	97.1	93.4	89.1	84.1	77.9	5.31	7.18
	16	143.1	141.0	138.6	136.1	133.3	130.2	126.8	122.9	118.4	113.0	106.5	10.55	12.49
67.29	18	132.4	130.2	127.9	125.3	122.5	119.4	116.0	112.1	107.6	102.3	95.7	8.32	10.24
	20	123.9	121.7	119.4	116.8	114.1	111.0	107.5	103.6	99.1	93.8	87.3	6.58	8.53
	22	116.7	114.5	112.2	109.6	106.8	103.8	100.3	96.4	91.9	86.6	80.1	5.21	7.10
	16	147.9	145.6	143.1	140.5	137.5	134.3	130.7	126.6	121.8	116.2	109.3	10.58	12.52
70.83	18	137.2	134.9	132.4	129.7	126.8	123.6	119.9	115.8	111.1	105.5	98.6	8.28	10.25
	20	128.3	126.0	123.6	120.9	117.9	114.7	111.1	107.0	102.2	96.6	89.8	6.55	8.51
	22	120.8	118.5	116.1	113.4	110.5	107.2	103.6	99.5	94.7	89.1	82.3	5.13	7.05
	16	153.2	150.8	148.2	145.4	142.3	138.9	135.1	130.8	125.8	119.9	112.7	10.73	12.68
74.37	18	141.9	139.5	136.9	134.1	131.1	127.7	123.8	119.5	114.6	108.7	101.5	8.24	10.26
	20	132.6	130.2	127.6	124.8	121.7	118.3	114.5	110.2	105.2	99.3	92.1	6.44	8.42
	22	125.1	122.7	120.1	117.3	114.3	110.9	107.1	102.7	97.8	91.9	84.7	5.10	7.04

TABLE 479

Process Times (B) at Retort Temperature of 250°F for Conduction-Heating Foods in 404 x 307 Can

f_h	z	INITIAL FOOD TEMPERATURE (T_{ih})											Equivalent	
		100	110	120	130	140	150	160	170	180	190	200	F_c^{18}	F_s^{18}
60.21	16	92.8	91.0	89.1	87.0	84.7	82.2	79.5	76.4	72.9	68.9	64.1	9.18	11.73
	18	89.6	87.8	85.9	83.8	81.5	79.0	76.3	73.2	69.7	65.7	60.9	7.74	10.24
	20	86.4	84.6	82.7	80.6	78.3	75.8	73.1	70.0	66.5	62.5	57.7	6.43	8.89
	22	83.6	81.8	79.9	77.8	75.5	73.0	70.3	67.2	63.7	59.7	54.9	5.36	7.76
63.75	16	97.2	95.3	93.2	91.0	88.6	85.9	83.0	79.8	76.1	71.8	66.8	9.21	11.78
	18	93.8	91.9	89.8	87.6	85.2	82.6	79.6	76.4	72.7	68.4	63.4	7.72	10.24
	20	90.4	88.5	86.5	84.2	81.8	79.2	76.3	73.0	69.3	65.1	60.0	6.39	8.86
	22	87.4	85.5	83.5	81.3	78.9	76.2	73.3	70.0	66.3	62.1	57.0	5.30	7.71
67.29	16	101.5	99.5	97.3	95.0	92.4	89.7	86.6	83.1	79.2	74.7	69.4	9.23	11.83
	18	97.9	95.9	93.7	91.4	88.8	86.1	83.0	79.5	75.6	71.1	65.8	7.70	10.24
	20	94.4	92.4	90.2	87.9	85.3	82.5	79.5	76.0	72.1	67.6	62.3	6.33	8.82
	22	91.3	89.2	87.1	84.7	82.2	79.4	76.3	72.9	69.0	64.5	59.1	5.25	7.68
70.83	16	105.8	103.7	101.4	98.9	96.3	93.3	90.1	86.5	82.4	77.6	72.0	9.26	11.87
	18	102.0	99.9	97.6	95.1	92.5	89.5	86.3	82.7	78.5	73.8	68.2	7.68	10.25
	20	98.3	96.2	93.9	91.4	88.8	85.8	82.6	79.0	74.9	70.1	64.5	6.28	8.78
	22	95.0	92.9	90.6	88.2	85.5	82.5	79.3	75.7	71.6	66.8	61.2	5.21	7.65
74.37	16	110.1	107.8	105.5	102.9	100.1	97.0	93.6	89.8	85.5	80.5	74.6	9.29	11.92
	18	106.1	103.8	101.4	98.8	96.0	93.0	89.6	85.7	81.4	76.5	70.6	7.67	10.24
	20	102.2	100.0	97.6	95.0	92.2	89.1	85.7	81.9	77.6	72.6	66.7	6.24	8.76
	22	98.8	96.5	94.1	91.6	88.8	85.7	82.3	78.5	74.2	69.2	63.3	5.18	7.63

TABLE 480

Process Times (B) at Retort Temperature of 260°F for Conduction-Heating Foods in 404 x 307 Can

f_h	z	INITIAL FOOD TEMPERATURE (T_{ih})											Equivalent	
		100	110	120	130	140	150	160	170	180	190	200	F_c^{18}	F_s^{18}
	16	74.7	73.0	71.2	69.3	67.2	64.9	62.4	59.6	56.6	53.1	49.0	8.71	11.64
60.21	18	72.9	71.2	69.4	67.4	65.3	63.1	60.6	57.8	54.7	51.2	47.2	7.38	10.24
	20	71.4	69.7	67.9	65.9	63.8	61.6	59.1	56.3	53.2	49.7	45.7	6.40	9.20
	22	69.9	68.2	66.4	64.5	62.4	60.1	57.6	54.8	51.8	48.3	44.2	5.52	8.27
	16	78.4	76.7	74.7	72.7	70.5	68.1	65.4	62.5	59.3	55.6	51.3	8.74	11.68
63.75	18	76.5	74.7	72.8	70.7	68.5	66.1	63.5	60.6	57.3	53.6	49.3	7.37	10.24
	20	74.9	73.1	71.2	69.1	66.9	64.5	61.9	58.9	55.7	52.0	47.7	6.35	9.17
	22	73.3	71.5	69.6	67.5	65.3	62.9	60.2	57.3	54.1	50.4	46.1	5.44	8.19
	16	82.2	80.3	78.3	76.1	73.8	71.2	68.4	65.4	61.9	58.0	53.5	8.76	11.72
67.29	18	80.1	78.2	76.2	74.0	71.7	69.1	66.3	63.3	59.8	55.9	51.4	7.35	10.24
	20	78.3	76.5	74.4	72.3	69.9	67.4	64.6	61.5	58.1	54.2	49.7	6.30	9.13
	22	76.6	74.7	72.7	70.5	68.2	65.7	62.9	59.8	56.4	52.4	47.9	5.36	8.12
	16	85.9	83.9	81.8	79.5	77.0	74.4	71.4	68.2	64.6	60.5	55.7	8.79	11.77
70.83	18	83.6	81.7	79.5	77.3	74.8	72.1	69.2	65.9	62.3	58.2	53.5	7.34	10.24
	20	81.8	79.8	77.7	75.4	72.9	70.3	67.3	64.1	60.5	56.4	51.6	6.25	9.09
	22	79.9	78.0	75.8	73.6	71.1	68.4	65.5	62.2	58.6	54.5	49.8	5.29	8.06
	16	89.6	87.5	85.3	82.9	80.3	77.5	74.4	71.0	67.2	62.9	57.9	8.83	11.81
74.37	18	87.2	85.1	82.9	80.5	77.9	75.1	72.0	68.6	64.8	60.5	55.5	7.32	10.24
	20	85.2	83.1	80.9	78.5	75.9	73.1	70.0	66.6	62.8	58.5	53.5	6.21	9.06
	22	83.2	81.2	78.9	76.5	73.9	71.1	68.1	64.7	60.8	56.5	51.6	5.22	8.00

TABLE 481

Process Times (B) at Retort Temperature of 230°F for Conduction-Heating Foods in 404 x 309 Can

f_h	z	INITIAL FOOD TEMPERATURE (T_{ih})											Equivalent	
		100	110	120	130	140	150	160	170	180	190	200	F_c^{18}	F_s^{18}
	16	268.0	265.9	263.5	261.0	258.1	254.9	251.3	247.1	242.2	236.2	228.4	12.95	14.24
62.30	18	216.0	213.8	211.5	208.9	206.0	202.8	199.2	195.1	190.1	184.1	176.3	9.02	10.30
	20	183.8	181.6	179.3	176.7	173.8	170.7	167.0	162.9	157.9	151.9	144.1	6.60	7.82
	22	162.1	160.0	157.6	155.0	152.2	149.0	145.4	141.2	136.3	130.2	122.4	5.01	6.19
	16	272.9	270.6	268.1	265.4	262.3	259.0	255.1	250.7	245.5	239.1	230.9	12.95	14.23
65.96	18	220.9	218.6	216.1	213.4	210.4	207.0	203.2	198.8	193.6	187.2	178.9	8.96	10.27
	20	189.1	186.8	184.3	181.6	178.6	175.2	171.4	167.0	161.8	155.4	147.1	6.59	7.84
	22	167.0	164.7	162.2	159.5	156.5	153.1	149.3	144.9	139.7	133.3	125.0	4.93	6.18
	16	278.3	275.9	273.3	270.4	267.2	263.7	259.6	255.0	249.4	242.7	234.0	12.90	14.27
69.63	18	225.9	223.5	220.8	218.0	214.8	211.2	207.2	202.5	197.0	190.2	181.6	8.93	10.24
	20	194.1	191.7	189.1	186.2	183.0	179.4	175.4	170.7	165.2	158.5	149.8	6.54	7.82
	22	171.9	169.4	166.8	163.9	160.7	157.2	153.1	148.5	143.0	136.2	127.5	4.81	6.14
	16	282.8	280.2	277.5	274.4	271.1	267.3	263.1	258.2	252.4	245.3	236.1	12.77	14.20
73.29	18	231.8	229.2	226.5	223.4	220.1	216.3	212.1	207.2	201.4	194.3	185.1	8.93	10.28
	20	199.3	196.7	194.0	190.9	187.6	183.8	179.6	174.7	168.9	161.8	152.6	6.51	7.82
	22	177.5	175.0	172.2	169.2	165.8	162.1	157.8	152.9	147.1	140.0	130.9	4.79	6.17
	16	288.4	285.7	282.8	279.6	276.1	272.1	267.7	262.5	256.4	249.0	239.4	12.76	14.19
76.96	18	237.0	234.3	231.4	228.2	224.7	220.7	216.3	211.1	205.0	197.6	188.0	8.90	10.29
	20	204.1	201.5	198.6	195.4	191.9	187.9	183.5	178.3	172.2	164.8	155.1	6.47	7.81
	22	183.3	180.6	177.7	174.5	171.0	167.0	162.6	157.4	151.3	143.9	134.3	4.78	6.19

TABLE 482

Process Times (B) at Retort Temperature of 240°F for Conduction-Heating Foods in 404 x 309 Can

f_h	z	INITIAL FOOD TEMPERATURE (T_{ih})											Equivalent	
		100	110	120	130	140	150	160	170	180	190	200	F_c^{18}	F_s^{18}
	16	136.8	134.8	132.6	130.2	127.7	124.8	121.6	118.0	113.8	108.9	102.9	10.62	12.56
62.30	18	125.4	123.4	121.2	118.8	116.3	113.4	110.2	106.6	102.4	97.5	91.5	8.39	10.22
	20	117.6	115.6	113.4	111.1	108.5	105.6	102.5	98.8	94.7	89.7	83.7	6.65	8.56
	22	111.0	109.0	106.8	104.4	101.9	99.0	95.8	92.2	88.0	83.1	77.1	5.38	7.24
	16	141.6	139.5	137.2	134.7	132.0	128.9	125.6	121.7	117.3	112.1	105.7	10.59	12.53
65.96	18	130.6	128.5	126.2	123.7	121.0	117.9	114.6	110.7	106.3	101.1	94.7	8.36	10.25
	20	122.3	120.2	117.9	115.4	112.7	109.6	106.3	102.4	98.0	92.8	86.4	6.61	8.56
	22	115.3	113.1	110.8	108.4	105.6	102.6	99.2	95.4	91.0	85.8	79.4	5.27	7.15
	16	146.2	144.0	141.6	138.9	136.1	132.9	129.3	125.3	120.6	115.1	108.4	10.56	12.50
69.63	18	135.7	133.4	131.0	128.4	125.5	122.3	118.8	114.7	110.1	104.5	97.8	8.32	10.27
	20	126.9	124.7	122.3	119.6	116.8	113.6	110.0	106.0	101.3	95.8	89.1	6.59	8.54
	22	119.5	117.2	114.8	112.2	109.3	106.1	102.5	98.5	93.8	88.3	81.6	5.17	7.08
	16	151.7	149.3	146.8	144.0	141.0	137.6	133.9	129.6	124.7	118.9	111.8	10.70	12.65
73.29	18	140.6	138.2	135.7	132.9	129.9	126.5	122.8	118.5	113.6	107.8	100.7	8.28	10.28
	20	131.4	129.0	126.5	123.7	120.7	117.3	113.6	109.3	104.4	98.6	91.5	6.50	8.47
	22	123.9	121.6	119.0	116.2	113.2	109.8	106.1	101.8	96.9	91.1	84.0	5.13	7.07
	16	157.1	154.6	151.9	149.0	145.8	142.3	138.4	133.9	128.8	122.7	115.2	10.85	12.81
76.96	18	145.5	143.0	140.3	137.4	134.2	130.7	126.8	122.3	117.2	111.1	103.6	8.25	10.30
	20	135.8	133.3	130.6	127.7	124.5	121.0	117.1	112.6	107.5	101.4	93.9	6.39	8.38
	22	128.4	125.9	123.2	120.3	117.1	113.6	109.7	105.2	100.1	94.0	86.5	5.08	7.05

TABLE 483

Process Times (B) at Retort Temperature of 250°F for Conduction-Heating Foods in 404 x 309 Can

f_h	z	INITIAL FOOD TEMPERATURE (T_{ih})											Equivalent	
		100	110	120	130	140	150	160	170	180	190	200	F_c^{18}	F_s^{18}
	16	95.4	93.6	91.6	89.4	87.0	84.5	81.6	78.4	74.8	70.6	65.7	9.22	11.79
62.30	18	92.1	90.3	88.3	86.1	83.7	81.2	78.3	75.1	71.5	67.3	62.4	7.75	10.27
	20	88.8	87.0	85.0	82.8	80.5	77.9	75.0	71.8	68.2	64.1	59.1	6.43	8.89
	22	85.9	84.1	82.1	79.9	77.5	75.0	72.1	68.9	65.3	61.1	56.2	5.34	7.75
	16	99.9	98.0	95.8	93.6	91.1	88.3	85.3	81.9	78.1	73.7	68.5	9.26	11.84
65.96	18	96.4	94.4	92.3	90.0	87.5	84.8	81.8	78.4	74.6	70.2	65.0	7.73	10.27
	20	93.0	91.0	88.9	86.6	84.1	81.4	78.3	75.0	71.1	66.7	61.5	6.38	8.86
	22	89.9	87.9	85.8	83.5	81.0	78.3	75.3	71.9	68.1	63.6	58.4	5.29	7.71
	16	104.4	102.3	100.1	97.7	95.0	92.1	89.0	85.4	81.4	76.7	71.2	9.27	11.88
69.63	18	100.7	98.6	96.3	93.9	91.3	88.4	85.2	81.7	77.6	73.0	67.4	7.71	10.27
	20	97.0	94.9	92.7	90.3	87.6	84.8	81.6	78.0	74.0	69.3	63.8	6.32	8.82
	22	93.8	91.7	89.5	87.1	84.4	81.5	78.4	74.8	70.8	66.1	60.6	5.24	7.68
	16	108.8	106.6	104.3	101.7	99.0	95.9	92.6	88.8	84.6	79.7	73.9	9.31	11.93
73.29	18	104.9	102.7	100.3	97.8	95.0	92.0	88.6	84.9	80.6	75.7	69.9	7.70	10.27
	20	101.1	98.9	96.5	94.0	91.2	88.2	84.8	81.1	76.8	71.9	66.1	6.27	8.79
	22	97.7	95.5	93.1	90.6	87.8	84.8	81.4	77.7	73.4	68.5	62.7	5.21	7.66
	16	113.2	110.9	108.4	105.8	102.9	99.7	96.2	92.2	87.8	82.6	76.5	9.32	11.97
76.96	18	109.1	106.7	104.3	101.6	98.7	95.5	92.0	88.0	83.6	78.4	72.3	7.68	10.27
	20	105.1	102.8	100.3	97.6	94.7	91.5	88.0	84.1	79.6	74.4	68.4	6.23	8.76
	22	101.5	99.2	96.8	94.1	91.2	88.0	84.5	80.5	76.1	70.9	64.8	5.18	7.64

TABLE 484

Process Times (B) at Retort Temperature of 260°F for Conduction-Heating Foods in 404 x 309 Can

f_h	z	INITIAL FOOD TEMPERATURE (T_{ih})											Equivalent	
		100	110	120	130	140	150	160	170	180	190	200	F_c^{18}	F_s^{18}
	16	76.9	75.2	73.3	71.3	69.2	66.8	64.2	61.4	58.2	54.6	50.4	8.75	11.69
62.30	18	75.0	73.3	71.4	69.4	67.2	64.9	62.3	59.5	56.3	52.7	48.5	7.40	10.27
	20	73.5	71.7	69.9	67.9	65.7	63.3	60.8	57.9	54.7	61.1	46.9	6.40	9.21
	22	71.9	70.2	68.3	66.3	64.1	61.8	59.2	56.4	53.2	49.6	45.4	5.49	8.25
	16	80.8	79.0	77.0	74.9	72.6	70.1	67.3	64.3	61.0	57.1	52.7	8.78	11.73
65.96	18	78.8	76.9	74.9	72.8	70.5	68.0	65.3	62.3	58.9	55.1	50.7	7.38	10.27
	20	77.1	75.2	73.3	71.1	68.8	66.4	63.6	60.6	57.2	53.4	49.0	6.34	9.17
	22	75.4	73.5	71.6	69.4	67.1	64.7	61.9	58.9	55.5	51.7	47.3	5.41	8.17
	16	84.7	82.7	80.6	78.4	76.0	73.3	70.4	67.3	63.7	59.7	55.0	8.81	11.77
69.63	18	82.5	80.5	78.4	76.2	73.8	71.1	68.3	65.1	61.5	57.5	52.8	7.37	10.27
	20	80.7	78.7	76.6	74.4	72.0	69.3	66.4	63.3	59.7	55.7	51.0	6.29	9.13
	22	78.9	76.9	74.8	72.6	70.2	67.5	64.6	61.5	57.9	53.9	49.2	5.34	8.10
	16	88.5	86.4	84.2	81.9	79.3	76.6	73.5	70.2	66.4	62.2	57.3	8.85	11.83
73.29	18	86.2	84.1	81.9	79.6	77.0	74.2	71.2	67.8	64.1	59.8	54.9	7.35	10.27
	20	84.2	82.2	80.0	77.6	75.1	72.3	69.3	65.9	62.2	57.9	53.0	6.25	9.09
	22	8.23	80.2	78.0	75.7	73.1	70.4	67.3	64.0	60.2	56.0	51.1	5.27	8.04
	16	92.3	90.1	87.8	85.3	82.7	79.8	76.6	73.1	69.1	64.7	59.5	8.87	11.86
76.96	18	89.8	87.7	85.4	82.9	80.2	77.3	74.1	70.6	66.7	62.2	57.0	7.34	10.27
	20	87.8	85.6	83.3	80.8	78.1	75.2	72.0	68.5	64.6	60.1	55.0	6.20	9.06
	22	85.7	83.5	81.2	78.7	76.1	73.1	70.0	66.4	62.5	58.0	52.9	5.19	7.97

TABLE 485

Process Times (B) at Retort Temperature of 230°F for Conduction-Heating Foods in 404 x 700 Can

f_h	z	INITIAL FOOD TEMPERATURE (T_{ih})											Equivalent	
		100	110	120	130	140	150	160	170	180	190	200	F_c^{18}	F_s^{18}
91.67	16	319.1	315.9	312.4	308.6	304.4	299.8	294.4	288.3	281.0	272.2	260.7	13.37	14.90
	18	264.6	261.4	257.9	254.1	249.9	245.2	239.9	233.8	226.5	217.6	206.2	9.28	10.75
	20	229.5	226.4	222.9	219.1	214.9	210.2	204.9	198.8	191.5	182.6	171.2	6.62	8.10
	22	208.4	205.2	201.8	198.0	193.8	189.1	183.8	177.6	170.4	161.5	150.0	4.98	6.43
97.06	16	326.4	323.0	319.3	315.3	310.9	305.9	300.3	293.8	286.1	276.7	264.6	13.28	14.85
	18	272.2	268.8	265.2	261.1	256.7	251.7	246.1	239.6	231.9	222.5	210.4	9.24	10.74
	20	238.2	234.8	231.1	227.1	222.7	217.7	212.1	205.6	197.9	188.5	176.4	6.59	8.14
	22	216.0	212.6	208.9	204.9	200.5	195.5	189.9	183.4	175.7	166.3	154.2	4.97	6.41
102.45	16	334.6	331.0	327.2	322.9	318.2	313.0	307.0	300.2	292.1	282.1	269.3	13.31	14.87
	18	280.0	276.4	272.5	268.3	263.6	258.4	252.4	245.6	237.4	227.5	214.7	9.21	10.73
	20	246.6	243.1	239.2	235.0	230.3	225.0	219.1	212.2	204.1	194.2	181.4	6.57	8.17
	22	223.3	219.7	215.9	211.6	206.9	201.7	195.7	188.9	180.8	170.8	158.0	4.96	6.40
107.85	16	343.1	339.4	335.3	330.8	325.9	320.4	314.1	306.9	298.4	287.9	274.4	13.30	14.90
	18	287.4	283.7	279.6	275.2	270.2	264.7	258.5	251.2	242.7	232.2	218.8	9.17	10.72
	20	254.8	251.0	246.9	242.5	237.5	232.0	225.8	218.5	210.0	199.5	186.1	6.54	8.16
	22	230.6	226.8	222.8	218.3	213.4	207.8	201.6	194.4	185.8	175.4	161.9	4.96	6.41
113.24	16	350.7	346.8	342.5	337.8	332.7	326.9	320.3	312.7	303.7	292.6	278.6	13.24	14.88
	18	295.1	291.2	286.9	282.2	277.1	271.3	254.7	257.1	248.2	237.2	223.0	9.13	10.71
	20	262.7	258.8	254.5	249.8	244.6	238.9	232.3	224.7	215.7	204.8	190.6	6.52	8.14
	22	237.7	233.7	229.4	224.8	219.6	213.8	207.2	199.6	190.7	179.7	165.5	4.96	6.41

TABLE 486

Process Times (B) at Retort Temperature of 240°F for Conduction-Heating Foods in 404 x 700 Can

f_h	z	INITIAL FOOD TEMPERATURE (T_{ih})											Equivalent	
		100	110	120	130	140	150	160	170	180	190	200	F_c^{18}	F_s^{18}
	16	180.4	177.5	174.3	170.8	167.0	162.8	158.1	152.8	146.7	139.4	130.5	11.36	13.48
91.67	18	166.8	163.8	160.7	157.2	153.4	149.2	144.5	139.2	133.1	125.8	116.9	8.61	10.74
	20	156.5	153.5	150.3	146.9	143.1	138.9	134.2	128.9	122.7	115.5	106.6	6.67	8.75
	22	147.7	144.8	141.6	138.1	134.3	130.1	125.4	120.1	114.0	106.7	97.8	5.21	7.27
	16	187.8	184.7	181.3	177.6	173.6	169.2	164.2	158.6	152.1	144.4	135.0	11.30	13.48
97.06	18	173.9	170.8	167.4	163.7	159.7	155.3	150.3	144.7	138.2	130.5	121.1	8.58	10.73
	20	163.1	160.0	156.6	153.0	148.9	144.5	139.5	133.9	127.4	119.7	110.3	6.63	8.74
	22	153.8	150.6	127.3	143.6	139.6	135.1	130.2	124.5	118.0	110.4	101.0	5.11	7.19
	16	195.0	191.7	188.1	184.3	180.0	175.3	170.1	164.1	157.3	149.2	139.2	11.25	13.48
102.45	18	181.0	177.7	174.2	170.3	166.1	161.4	156.1	150.2	143.3	135.2	125.3	8.56	10.74
	20	169.6	166.3	162.7	158.9	154.6	149.9	144.7	138.8	131.9	123.8	113.9	6.54	8.69
	22	160.1	156.8	153.2	149.4	145.1	140.4	135.2	129.2	122.4	114.3	104.3	5.07	7.16
	16	202.0	198.5	194.8	190.7	186.3	181.3	175.8	169.6	162.3	153.8	143.3	11.20	13.47
107.85	18	188.1	184.6	180.8	176.8	172.3	167.4	161.9	155.6	148.4	139.8	129.4	8.54	10.75
	20	176.0	172.5	168.7	164.7	160.2	155.3	149.7	143.5	136.3	127.7	117.3	6.47	8.65
	22	166.3	162.8	159.1	155.0	150.5	145.6	140.1	133.8	126.6	118.1	107.6	5.03	7.14
	16	209.5	205.8	201.9	197.6	192.9	187.7	182.0	175.4	167.8	158.9	147.9	11.26	13.56
113.24	18	194.9	191.3	187.3	183.1	178.4	173.2	167.4	160.8	153.3	144.3	133.3	8.51	10.74
	20	182.5	178.9	174.9	170.7	166.0	160.8	155.0	148.4	140.9	131.9	120.9	6.45	8.64
	22	172.4	168.8	164.8	160.5	155.9	150.7	144.9	138.3	130.7	121.8	110.8	4.97	7.10

TABLE 487

Process Times (B) at Retort Temperature of 250°F for Conduction=Heating Foods in 404 x 700 Can

f_h	z	INITIAL FOOD TEMPERATURE (T_{ih})											Equivalent	
		100	110	120	130	140	150	160	170	180	190	200	F_c^{18}	F_s^{18}
	16	132.1	129.4	126.4	123.2	119.8	116.0	111.8	107.1	101.8	95.6	88.4	9.99	12.72
91.67	18	127.1	124.3	121.4	118.2	114.7	110.9	106.7	102.0	96.7	90.6	83.3	8.07	10.74
	20	122.4	119.6	116.7	113.5	110.0	106.2	102.0	97.4	92.0	85.9	78.6	6.57	9.17
	22	118.2	115.5	112.5	109.3	105.9	102.1	97.9	93.2	87.9	81.7	74.5	5.38	7.90
	16	138.5	135.6	132.5	129.1	125.4	121.4	117.0	112.0	106.4	99.9	92.2	10.04	12.80
97.06	18	133.1	130.2	127.1	123.7	120.0	116.0	111.6	106.6	101.0	94.5	86.8	8.06	10.75
	20	128.2	125.3	122.1	118.8	115.1	111.1	106.6	101.7	96.1	89.6	81.9	6.56	9.17
	22	123.8	120.9	117.7	114.4	110.7	106.7	102.2	97.3	91.7	85.2	77.5	5.33	7.87
	16	144.8	141.8	138.5	134.9	131.0	126.8	122.1	116.9	110.9	104.1	95.9	10.08	12.85
102.45	18	139.1	136.0	132.7	129.2	125.3	121.0	116.4	111.1	105.2	98.3	90.2	8.04	10.75
	20	133.9	130.8	127.5	124.0	120.1	115.9	111.2	105.9	100.0	93.1	85.0	6.52	9.14
	22	129.3	126.2	122.9	119.4	115.5	111.2	106.6	101.3	95.4	88.5	80.4	5.29	7.84
	16	151.1	147.8	144.4	140.6	136.5	132.1	127.1	121.6	115.4	108.2	99.6	10.08	12.87
107.85	18	145.0	141.8	138.3	134.5	130.5	126.0	121.1	115.5	109.3	102.1	93.5	8.03	10.75
	20	139.6	136.3	132.9	129.1	125.0	120.6	115.6	110.1	103.9	96.6	88.1	6.46	9.10
	22	134.7	131.5	128.0	124.3	120.2	115.7	110.8	105.3	99.0	91.8	83.3	5.24	7.79
	16	157.3	153.9	150.2	146.3	142.0	137.3	132.1	126.3	119.8	112.2	103.2	10.08	12.89
113.24	18	150.8	147.4	143.8	139.9	135.6	130.9	125.7	119.9	113.3	105.8	96.8	8.01	10.75
	20	145.2	141.8	138.1	134.2	129.9	125.2	120.0	114.3	107.7	100.1	91.1	6.42	9.07
	22	140.1	136.7	133.1	129.1	124.8	120.2	115.0	109.2	102.6	95.0	86.1	5.17	7.74

TABLE 488

Process Times (B) at Retort Temperature of 260°F for Conduction-Heating Foods in 404 x 700 Can

f_h	z	INITIAL FOOD TEMPERATURE (T_{ih}) 100	110	120	130	140	150	160	170	180	190	200	Equivalent F_c^{18}	F_s^{18}
	16	108.2	105.6	102.9	100.0	96.8	93.3	89.5	85.3	80.6	75.3	69.2	9.47	12.54
91.67	18	105.2	102.7	99.9	97.0	93.8	90.3	86.5	82.3	77.6	72.3	66.2	7.76	10.74
	20	102.6	100.1	97.3	94.4	91.2	87.7	83.9	79.7	75.0	69.7	63.6	6.46	9.37
	22	100.0	97.5	94.7	91.8	88.6	85.1	81.3	77.1	72.5	67.1	61.0	5.32	8.15
	16	113.7	111.0	108.1	105.0	101.6	97.9	93.9	89.5	84.5	78.9	72.4	9.50	12.59
97.06	18	110.5	107.8	104.9	101.8	98.4	94.7	90.7	86.3	81.3	75.7	69.2	7.74	10.74
	20	107.7	105.0	102.1	99.0	95.6	91.9	87.9	83.5	78.5	72.9	66.4	6.40	9.33
	22	104.9	102.2	99.3	96.2	92.8	89.1	85.1	80.7	75.7	70.1	63.6	5.23	8.07
	16	119.2	116.3	113.2	109.9	106.4	102.5	98.3	93.6	88.3	82.4	75.5	9.53	12.63
102.45	18	115.8	112.9	109.8	106.5	103.0	99.1	94.9	90.2	84.9	79.0	72.1	7.73	10.74
	20	112.8	109.9	106.9	103.6	100.0	96.1	91.9	87.2	82.0	76.0	69.2	6.36	9.29
	22	109.8	106.9	103.8	100.5	97.0	93.1	88.9	84.2	78.9	73.0	66.1	5.17	8.01
	16	124.6	121.6	118.3	114.9	111.1	107.0	102.6	97.6	92.1	85.9	78.6	9.55	12.66
107.85	18	121.0	118.0	114.7	111.3	107.5	103.4	99.0	94.1	88.5	82.3	75.1	7.72	10.74
	20	117.8	114.8	111.6	108.1	104.4	100.3	95.8	90.9	85.4	79.1	71.9	6.31	9.25
	22	114.6	111.6	108.4	104.9	101.1	97.1	92.6	87.7	82.1	75.9	68.7	5.10	7.94
	16	130.0	126.8	123.4	119.8	115.8	111.6	106.9	101.7	95.9	89.3	81.7	9.57	12.70
113.24	18	126.2	123.0	119.6	116.0	112.1	107.8	103.1	97.9	92.1	85.6	78.0	7.71	10.74
	20	122.8	119.6	116.3	112.6	108.7	104.4	99.7	94.5	88.7	82.2	74.6	6.27	9.21
	22	119.4	116.2	112.8	109.2	105.3	101.0	96.3	91.1	85.3	78.8	71.2	5.04	7.89

TABLE 489

Process Times (B) at Retort Temperature of 230°F for Conduction-Heating Foods in 603 x 700 Can

f_h	z	INITIAL FOOD TEMPERATURE (T_{ih})											Equivalent	
		100	110	120	130	140	150	160	170	180	190	200	F_c^{18}	F_s^{18}
	16	445.3	439.4	433.0	425.9	418.2	409.5	399.6	388.2	374.8	358.3	337.0	13.87	15.72
170.00	18	388.8	382.9	376.4	369.4	361.6	352.9	343.1	331.7	318.2	301.7	280.5	9.39	11.25
	20	344.5	338.6	332.1	325.1	317.3	308.6	298.8	287.4	273.9	257.4	236.2	6.81	8.47
	22	312.0	306.1	299.6	292.6	284.8	276.1	266.3	254.9	241.4	225.0	203.7	4.86	6.60
	16	462.4	456.1	449.3	441.8	433.6	424.4	414.0	401.9	387.7	370.2	347.7	14.03	15.91
180.00	18	403.3	397.0	390.2	382.7	374.5	365.3	354.9	342.8	328.6	311.1	288.6	9.39	11.25
	20	355.9	349.6	342.8	335.4	327.2	318.0	307.5	295.5	281.2	263.8	241.3	6.70	8.40
	22	324.1	317.9	311.1	303.6	295.4	286.2	275.7	263.7	249.4	232.0	209.5	4.83	6.58
	16	479.0	472.3	465.2	457.3	448.6	438.9	427.9	415.2	400.1	381.7	358.0	14.00	15.95
190.00	18	417.3	410.7	403.5	395.6	386.9	377.2	366.2	353.5	338.4	320.0	296.3	9.39	11.25
	20	368.1	361.5	354.3	346.4	337.7	328.0	317.0	304.3	289.2	270.8	247.1	6.57	8.33
	22	336.2	329.6	322.4	314.5	305.8	296.1	285.1	272.4	257.3	238.9	215.2	4.78	6.54
	16	495.3	488.3	480.8	472.5	463.3	453.1	441.5	428.1	412.3	392.9	367.9	13.95	15.96
200.00	18	430.9	423.9	416.4	408.1	399.0	388.7	377.1	363.7	347.9	328.5	303.5	9.39	11.25
	20	381.6	374.6	367.1	358.8	349.6	339.4	327.8	314.4	298.6	279.2	254.2	6.55	8.36
	22	348.0	341.0	333.5	325.2	316.1	305.8	294.2	280.8	265.0	245.6	220.6	4.70	6.49
	16	511.2	503.9	496.0	487.3	477.7	466.9	454.8	440.7	424.1	403.7	377.5	13.91	15.97
210.00	18	444.1	436.8	428.9	420.2	410.6	399.8	387.6	373.6	356.9	336.6	310.4	9.39	11.25
	20	394.7	387.4	379.5	370.8	361.2	350.5	338.3	324.2	307.6	287.3	261.0	6.52	8.38
	22	359.4	352.1	344.2	335.5	325.9	315.1	302.9	288.9	272.3	251.9	225.7	4.62	6.43

TABLE 490

Process Times (B) at Retort Temperature of 240°F for Conduction-Heating Foods in 603 x 700 Can

f_h	z	INITIAL FOOD TEMPERATURE (T_{ih})											Equivalent	
		100	110	120	130	140	150	160	170	180	190	200	F_c^{18}	F_s^{18}
	16	287.8	282.3	276.4	269.9	262.9	255.1	246.4	236.6	225.2	211.7	195.3	11.96	14.44
170.00	18	268.3	262.9	257.0	250.5	243.5	235.7	227.0	217.2	205.8	192.3	175.8	8.81	11.24
	20	251.4	245.9	240.0	233.6	226.5	218.8	210.1	200.2	188.8	175.4	158.9	6.50	8.86
	22	237.4	231.9	226.0	219.6	212.6	204.8	196.1	186.2	174.9	161.4	144.9	4.89	7.17
	16	300.5	294.7	288.5	281.7	274.2	266.0	256.8	246.4	234.3	220.0	202.6	11.94	14.46
180.00	18	280.4	274.6	268.3	261.5	254.1	245.9	236.7	226.2	214.2	199.9	182.5	8.79	11.24
	20	262.8	257.0	250.7	243.9	236.5	228.2	219.0	208.6	196.5	182.3	164.8	6.46	8.84
	22	248.1	242.3	236.1	229.3	221.8	213.6	204.4	193.9	181.9	167.6	150.2	4.82	7.12
	16	313.2	307.1	300.5	293.3	285.4	276.7	267.0	256.0	243.3	228.2	209.8	11.92	14.47
190.00	18	292.3	286.2	279.6	272.4	264.5	255.8	246.1	235.1	222.4	207.3	188.9	8.76	11.24
	20	274.0	267.9	261.3	254.1	246.2	237.5	227.8	216.8	204.1	189.0	170.6	6.42	8.82
	22	258.7	252.6	246.0	238.9	231.0	222.3	212.6	201.6	188.8	173.8	155.4	4.76	7.08
	16	326.0	319.5	312.6	305.0	296.7	287.6	277.3	265.7	252.4	236.5	217.1	11.94	14.52
200.00	18	304.2	297.8	290.8	283.3	275.0	265.8	255.6	244.0	230.6	214.8	195.4	8.74	11.24
	20	285.1	278.7	271.7	264.2	255.9	246.7	236.5	224.9	211.5	195.7	176.3	6.38	8.80
	22	269.2	262.8	255.9	248.3	240.0	230.9	220.6	209.0	195.7	179.8	160.4	4.71	7.04
	16	338.5	331.8	324.5	316.5	307.8	298.2	287.5	275.3	261.3	244.6	224.3	11.97	14.56
210.00	18	316.0	309.2	301.9	294.0	285.3	275.7	265.0	252.8	238.7	222.1	201.7	8.72	11.25
	20	296.2	289.4	282.1	274.2	265.5	255.9	245.2	233.0	218.9	202.3	181.9	6.35	8.79
	22	279.8	273.0	265.7	257.8	249.1	239.5	228.7	216.6	202.5	185.9	165.5	4.67	7.02

TABLE 491

Process Times (B) at Retort Temperature of 250°F for Conduction-Heating Foods in 603 x 700 Can

f_h	z	INITIAL FOOD TEMPERATURE (T_{ih})											Equivalent	
		100	110	120	130	140	150	160	170	180	190	200	F_c^{18}	F_s^{18}
	16	222.8	217.8	212.3	206.4	200.0	192.9	185.1	176.4	166.6	155.2	141.7	11.01	13.97
170.00	18	212.9	207.8	202.3	196.4	190.0	182.9	175.2	166.5	156.6	145.2	131.8	8.39	11.24
	20	204.5	199.4	194.0	188.1	181.6	174.6	166.8	158.1	148.3	136.9	123.4	6.51	9.26
	22	196.9	191.8	186.4	180.5	174.0	167.0	159.2	150.5	140.7	129.3	115.8	5.06	7.71
	16	233.9	228.5	222.7	216.5	209.7	202.2	194.0	184.8	174.3	162.3	148.0	11.06	14.04
180.00	18	223.3	217.9	212.1	205.9	199.1	191.6	183.4	174.2	163.7	151.7	137.4	8.37	11.24
	20	214.5	209.1	203.3	197.1	190.2	182.8	174.6	165.4	154.9	142.9	128.6	6.47	9.23
	22	206.4	201.0	195.2	189.0	182.2	174.7	166.5	157.3	146.8	134.8	120.5	5.00	7.66
	16	244.9	239.2	233.1	226.5	219.3	211.4	202.7	193.0	182.0	169.3	154.2	11.11	14.11
190.00	18	233.7	228.0	221.9	215.2	208.1	200.2	191.5	181.8	170.8	158.1	143.0	8.36	11.25
	20	224.4	218.7	212.6	205.9	198.8	190.9	182.2	172.5	161.5	148.8	133.7	6.44	9.21
	22	215.8	210.1	204.0	197.4	190.2	182.3	173.6	163.9	152.9	140.2	125.1	4.93	7.61
	16	255.7	249.7	243.3	236.3	228.8	220.5	211.4	201.1	189.5	176.1	160.3	11.16	14.17
200.00	18	243.9	237.9	231.5	224.5	217.0	208.7	199.5	189.3	177.7	164.3	148.5	8.35	11.25
	20	234.1	228.1	221.7	214.7	207.2	198.9	189.8	179.5	167.9	154.5	138.7	6.39	9.17
	22	225.1	219.1	212.6	205.7	198.1	189.8	180.7	170.5	158.9	145.5	129.6	4.87	7.55
	16	266.5	260.2	253.5	246.2	238.2	229.5	219.9	209.2	197.0	182.9	166.3	11.21	14.24
210.00	18	254.1	247.8	241.0	233.7	225.8	217.1	207.5	196.7	184.6	170.5	153.9	8.34	11.24
	20	243.8	237.5	230.7	223.4	215.5	206.8	197.2	186.5	174.3	160.2	143.6	6.34	9.14
	22	234.2	227.9	221.2	213.9	205.9	197.3	187.6	176.9	164.7	150.7	134.0	4.80	7.49

TABLE 492

Process Times (B) at Retort Temperature of 260°F for Conduction-Heating Foods in 603 x 700 Can

f_h	z	INITIAL FOOD TEMPERATURE (T_{ih})											Equivalent	
		100	110	120	130	140	150	160	170	180	190	200	F_c^{18}	F_s^{18}
	16	186.7	181.9	176.8	171.4	165.4	159.0	152.0	144.2	135.5	125.7	114.3	10.35	13.60
170.00	18	180.8	176.1	171.0	165.5	159.6	153.2	146.1	138.4	129.7	119.8	108.4	8.10	11.24
	20	175.4	170.6	165.5	160.1	154.2	147.7	140.7	132.9	124.2	114.4	103.0	6.35	9.39
	22	170.0	165.2	160.1	154.6	148.7	142.3	135.3	127.5	118.8	108.9	97.5	4.87	7.81
	16	196.3	191.2	185.8	180.0	173.8	167.0	159.5	151.3	142.1	131.7	119.6	10.39	13.65
180.00	18	190.0	185.0	179.6	173.8	167.6	160.8	153.3	145.1	135.9	125.4	113.4	8.09	11.24
	20	184.2	179.2	173.8	168.0	161.7	154.9	147.5	139.2	130.0	119.6	107.5	6.29	9.34
	22	178.5	173.4	168.0	162.3	156.0	149.2	141.7	133.5	124.3	113.9	101.8	4.82	7.76
	16	205.8	200.5	194.8	188.7	182.1	174.9	167.0	158.3	148.6	137.6	124.9	10.41	13.69
190.00	18	199.2	193.9	188.2	182.1	175.5	168.3	160.4	151.7	142.0	131.0	118.3	8.07	11.24
	20	193.0	187.7	182.0	175.9	169.3	162.1	154.2	145.5	135.8	124.8	112.1	6.23	9.29
	22	186.9	181.6	175.9	169.8	163.2	156.0	148.2	139.5	129.8	118.7	106.0	4.77	7.72
	16	215.4	209.7	203.8	197.3	190.4	182.8	174.5	165.4	155.1	143.5	130.2	10.47	13.76
200.00	18	208.3	202.7	196.7	190.3	183.3	175.8	167.5	158.3	148.1	136.5	123.1	8.06	11.24
	20	201.7	196.1	190.1	183.7	176.8	169.2	160.9	151.8	141.5	129.9	116.6	6.18	9.25
	22	195.3	189.7	183.7	177.3	170.3	162.8	154.5	145.4	135.1	123.5	110.1	4.72	7.68
	16	224.8	218.9	212.6	205.9	198.6	190.7	182.0	172.4	161.6	149.4	135.4	10.51	13.82
210.00	18	217.4	211.5	205.2	198.4	191.1	183.2	174.5	164.9	154.2	142.0	127.9	8.05	11.24
	20	210.4	204.5	198.3	191.5	184.2	176.3	167.6	158.0	147.2	135.0	121.0	6.13	9.22
	22	203.7	197.8	191.6	184.8	177.5	169.6	160.9	151.3	140.5	128.3	114.3	4.67	7.64

References

REFERENCES

1. **Ball, C. O.**, Thermal process time for canned foods, *Bull. Natl. Res. Counc.*, 7 (Part 1), No. 37, 1923.
2. **Ball, C. O.**, Mathematical solution of problems on thermal processing of canned food, *Univ. Calif. Berkeley Publ. Public Health*, 1, 15, 1928.
3. **Bigelow, W. D., Bohart, G. S., Richardson, A. C., and Ball, C. O.**, Heat penetration in processing canned foods, *Natl. Canners Assoc. Bull.*, No. 16L, 1920.
4. **Esty, J. R. and Mayer, K. F.**, The heat resistance of *B. botulinus* and allied anerobes, *J. Infect. Dis.*, 31, 650, 1922.
5. **Greenberg, R. A., Tompkin, R. B., Bladel, B. O., Kittaka, R. S., and Anellis, A.**, Incidence of mesophilic Clostridium spores in raw pork, beef and chicken in the processing plants in the United States and Canada, *Appl. Microbiol.*, 14, 789, 1966.
6. **Insalata, N. H., Witzeman, J. S., Berman, J. H., and Borker, E.**, A study of the incidence of spores of *Clostridium botulinum* in frozen vacuum pouch-pack vegetables, *Proc. 96th Annu. Meet. Am. Public Health Assoc.*, American Public Health Association, Washington, D.C., 1968, 124.
7. **Jen, Y., Manson, J. E., Stumbo, C. R., and Zahradnik, J. W.**, A procedure for estimating sterilization of and quality factor degradation in thermally processed foods, *J. Food Sci.*, 36, 692, 1971.
8. **Olson, F. C. W. and Jackson, J. M.**, Heating curves — theory and practical applications, *Ind. Eng. Chem.*, 34, 337, 1942.
9. **Purohit, K. S.**, Refinement and extension of f_h/U:g par- for process calculation, *J. Food Sci.*, 38, 726, 1973.
10. **Riemann, H.**, Aerobic toxins, in *Chemical and Biological Hazards in Foods,* Iowa State University Press, Ames, 1962, 279.
11. **Schultz, O. T. and Olson, F. C. W.**, Thermal processing of canned foods in tin containers. I. Variation in heating rate with can size for products heating by convection, *Food Res.*, 3, 647, 1938.
12. **Schultz, O. T. and Olson, F. C. W.**, Thermal processing of foods in tin containers. III. Recent improvements in the general method of thermal process calculations — a special coordinate paper and methods of converting initial and retort temperatures, *Food Res.*, 5, 399, 1940.
13. **Secrist, J. L. and Stumbo, C. R.**, Application of spore resistance in the newer methods of process evaluation, *Food Technol.*, 10, 543, 1956.
14. **Steinkraus, K. H. and Ayers, J. C.**, Incidence of putrefactive anerobic spores in meat, *J. Food Sci.*, 29, 87, 1964.
15. **Stumbo, C. R.**, Bacteriological considerations relating to process evaluation, *Food Technol.*, 2, 115, 1948.
16. **Stumbo, C. R.**, A technique for studying resistance of bacterial spores to temperatures in the higher range, *Food Technol.*, 2, 228, 1948.
17. **Stumbo, C. R.**, Thermobacteriology as applied to food processing, *Adv. Food Res.*, 2, 47, 1949.
18. **Stumbo, C. R.**, Further considerations relating to evaluation of thermal processes for foods, *Food Technol.*, 3, 126, 1949.
19. **Stumbo, C. R.**, New procedures for evaluating thermal processes for foods in cylindrical containers, *Food Technol.*, 7, 309, 1953.
20. **Stumbo, C. R.**, *Thermobacteriology in Food Processing,* 2nd ed., Academic Press, New York, 1973.
21. **Stumbo, C. R. and Longley, R. E.**, New parameters for process calculation, *Food Technol.*, 20, 109, 1966.
22. **Stumbo, C. R., Murphy, J. R., and Cochran, J.**, Nature of thermal death curves for P.A. 3679 and *Clostridium botulinum, Food Technol.*, 4, 321, 1950.
23. **Stumbo, C. R., Purohit, K. S., and Ramakrishnan, T. V.**, Thermal process lethality guide for low-acid foods in metal containers, *J. Food Sci.*, 40, 1316, 1975.
24. **Teixeira, A. A., Dixon, J. R., Zahradnik, J. W., and Zinsmeister, G. E.**, Computer optimization of nutrient retention in the thermal processing of conduction-heated foods, *Food Technol.*, 23, 845, 1969.
25. **Townsend, C. T., Esty, J. R., and Baselt, F. C.**, Heat resistance studies on spores of putrefactive anerobes in relation to determination of safe processes for canned foods, *Food Res.*, 3, 323, 1938.
26. **Xezones, H. and Hutchings, I. J.**, Thermal resistance of *Clostridium botulinum* (62A) spores as affected by fundamental food constituents, *Food Technol.*, 19, 1003, 1965.

Appendix

SYMBOLS AND DEFINITIONS

The following are definitions of the symbols that have appeared in the text. These are arranged in alphabetical order for ease of location.

a The initial population of spores or vegetative cells of an organism per unit volume of an inoculated medium just prior to applying lethal heat.

b The final or surviving population of spores or vegetative cells of an organism per unit volume of a medium after heat treatment at a constant temperature for some designated period of time.

B The thermal processing time without correcting for the time required to bring the retort to processing temperature.

D The time, at any specified lethal temperature, required to inactivate a population of spores or vegetative cells of an organism by one logarithm cycle or 90%. Mathematically, D is equal to the reciprocal of the slope of the survivor curve.

D_r The time required, at some designated reference temperature, to thermally inactivate a population of spores or vegetative cells of an organism by one log cycle or 90%.

F The equivalent, in minutes at some specified temperature, of all lethal heat with respect to its capacity to inactivate spores or vegetative cells of a specific organism.

F_c The F value of all lethal heat received by the geometrical center of a container of food product during processing.

F_λ The F value of all lethal heat received by any point in a container of food product other than the geometrical center of that container.

F_s Integrated lethality of heat received by all points in a container of food product during processing.

F_i The time at any other temperature equivalent to 1 min of processing time at some specific reference process temperature. In most cases the specific reference process temperature employed is 250°F.

f_h The time in minutes, required for the straight line portion of the semilogarithmic heating curve to traverse one logarithmic cycle. Also the f of the first straight line portion of a broken heating curve.

g The difference, in degrees Fahrenheit, between the retort temperature and the maximum food temperature at the point of concern.

g_c The g when the point of concern is the geometrical center or cold point of the food container.

g_λ The g when the point of concern is any point within the container other than the geometrical center or cold point.

g_{bh} The difference between the retort temperature and the food temperature at the time of a break in a heating curve.

I_h The difference between the retort temperature and the food temperature at the time when heating is started.

I_c The difference between cooling water temperature and the food temperature when cooling is started.

j A heating lag factor.

j_{ch} The j of the heating curve for the geometrical center of a container. This factor when multiplied by I_h, locates the intersection of an extension of the straight-line portion of the semilogarithmic heating curve and a vertical line that represents the beginning of heating.

j_{cc} The j of the cooling curve for the geometrical center of a container. This factor, when multiplied by I_c, locates the intersection of an extension of the straight line portion of the cooling curve and a vertical line representing the start of cooling.

$j_{\lambda h}$ The j of the heating curve for an iso-j region enclosing 0.19 of container volume.

$j_{\lambda c}$ The j of the cooling curve for an iso-j region enclosing 0.19 of container volume.

k The thermal diffusivity value.

ℓ The time, in minutes, required to bring the retort to processing temperature.

L The lethal rate value. It is equal to the reciprocal of time, at any lethal temperature, equivalent to 1 min at some designated reference temperature or 1/Fi.

p_t The operators process time, or the time, in minutes, from the instant the retort achieves processing temperature until the instant the steam is turned off and cooling is started.

T_{ih} The initial food temperature at the time heating is started.

T_{ic} The initial food temperature at the time cooling is initiated.

T_{pih} The pseudo-initial temperature when heating is started. This temperature is indicated by the intersection of the extension of the straight line portion of the heating curve and a vertical line that represents the start of heating.

T_{pic} The pseudo-initial temperature of the food when cooling is initiated. This temperature is indicated by the intersection of the extension of the straight line portion of the cooling curve and a vertical line representing the beginning of cooling.

T_r The retort or processing temperature employed.

T_w The temperature of the cooling water.

U The equivalent time, in minutes at retort temperature, of all lethal heat received by some designated point in the container during processing.

U_c The U value of all lethal heat received at the geometrical center of the container.

U_λ The U value of all lethal heat received by any point in the container other than the geometrical center.

z The number of Fahrenheit degrees required for the thermal destruction curve to traverse one logarithmic cycle. Mathematically, z is equal to the reciprocal of the slope of the thermal death curve.

CAN VOLUME AND PROCESS VALUES FOR 41 CAN SIZES

The process value which a thermally processed food should receive depends on the resistance of the organism of importance, the initial population of the organism per container, and the decimal reduction of the organism required to achieve practical sterility.

For safe thermal processes of low-acid canned foods, the organism of concern is spores of *Clostridium botulinum*. The D_{250} value used for these spores is 0.2 min and a 12 log cycle reduction generally is considered minimum. In our computation, the initial load is assumed to be one organism per cubic centimeter of the container capacity. For foods in a 202 × 204 can (approximately 97 cm^3), the process value desired would be determined as follows:

$$\begin{aligned} F\ (\text{Process value}) &= D_{250}\,(\log a - \log b) \\ F &= 0.2\,(\log 97 - \log 10^{-12}) \\ F &= 0.2\,(1.99 + 12) \\ F\ (\text{Process value}) &= 2.80 \text{ min at } 250°F \end{aligned}$$

For commercial sterility the process value determination is based on the elimination of spores of *C. sporogenes* with a D_{250} value of 1.5 min. A reduction by four log cycles is sufficient to achieve a considerable degree of freedom from economic spoilage. For the can size 202 × 204:

$$\begin{aligned} F\ (\text{Process value}) &= D_{250}\,(\log a - \log b) \\ F &= 1.5\,(\log 97 - 10^{-4}) \\ F &= 1.5\,(1.99 + 4) \\ F\ (\text{Process value}) &= 8.99 \text{ or } 9.0 \text{ min at } 250°F \end{aligned}$$

Table 1A shows the process values desired to achieve both safety and commercial sterility for foods processed in 41 different can sizes. The respective process values should be considered as F_c, the process value at the cold point of the container for convection-heating foods and F_s, the integrated lethal capacity for conduction-heating foods. Although the different foods processed in containers of a particular size should receive the same process value, the process time needed would be variable since this would be influenced by the specific processing conditions employed and the heat transfer characteristics of the food.

Table 1A
CAN SIZE, VOLUME, AND PROCESS VALUES FOR THERMALLY PROCESSED FOODS

Can size	Container volume (cc)	Process value for safety	Process value for commercial sterility
202 × 204	96.54	2.80	8.99
202 × 214	128.71	2.82	9.16
202 × 308	160.89	2.84	9.31
202 × 314	180.20	2.85	9.38
211 × 200	137.35	2.83	9.21
211 × 210	190.17	2.86	9.42
211 × 212	200.73	2.86	9.45
211 × 214	211.30	2.87	9.49
211 × 300	221.86	2.87	9.52
211 × 304	242.30	2.88	9.58
211 × 306	253.55	2.88	9.61

Table 1A (continued)
CAN SIZE, VOLUME, AND PROCESS VALUES FOR THERMALLY PROCESSED FOODS

Can size	Container volume (cc)	Process value for safety	Process value for commercial sterility
211 × 400	306.37	2.90	9.73
211 × 413	375.04	2.91	9.86
211 × 414	380.32	2.92	9.87
211 × 600	475.40	2.94	10.02
300 × 206	212.78	2.87	9.49
300 × 308	332.46	2.90	9.78
300 × 400	385.65	2.92	9.88
300 × 407	432.20	2.93	9.95
301 × 411	479.00	2.94	10.02
303 × 406	482.86	2.94	10.03
303 × 509	626.21	2.96	10.20
307 × 113	203.03	2.86	9.46
307 × 203	255.99	2.88	9.61
307 × 214	353.08	2.91	9.82
307 × 306	423.69	2.93	9.94
307 × 400	512.00	2.94	10.06
307 × 409	591.40	2.95	10.16
307 × 510	741.44	2.97	10.31
307 × 512	759.10	2.98	10.32
307 × 704	970.93	3.00	10.48
401 × 205	386.65	2.92	9.88
401 × 211	461.48	2.93	10.00
401 × 411	860.56	2.99	10.40
401 × 602	1147.40	3.01	10.59
404 × 200	355.91	2.91	9.83
404 × 211	506.47	2.94	10.06
404 × 307	670.72	2.97	10.24
404 × 309	698.10	2.97	10.27
404 × 700	1450.90	3.03	10.74
603 × 700	3133.96	3.10	11.24

AN EXAMPLE OF USING THE PROCESS LETHALITY GUIDE TABLES FOR CONDUCTION-HEATING PRODUCTS

Example: Conduction-heating and commercial sterility. Assume the following data for a conduction-heating product in 303 × 406 cans:

Retort temperature — 240°F
Initial food temperature — 155°F
Product f_h — 51 min
The z — 18F°

To obtain the process time that would be the minimum suggested for a commercially sterile product locate the table that contains the required data for the process variables noted above. The corresponding Table is 410 (Figure 3). Now, proceed with the table according to the following sequential steps:

1. Locate the can size of 303 × 406.
2. Note that the retort temperature on the table is 240°F.
3. Find the initial food temperature of 150°F on the table. (Since the actual initial food temperature of 155°F is not in the table, for reasons of safety, the next lower table value of 150°F should be used.)
4. Use the table f_h value of 52.64 for the product. (The table value f_h of 52.64 is used, in the interest of assurance of sterility, as the next higher f_h value since the actual f_h of 51 is not shown in the table.)
5. Locate the z of 18.
6. Then at f_h of 52.64, z of 18 proceed horizontally across the line of figures to the vertical column of figures under the initial temperature of 150°F. At the intersect, located at (6), the processing time is found to be 101.8 min.

For this particular product, processing at approximately 102 min at 240°F should assure a reasonable degree of commercial sterility for the process variables identified.

TABLE 410

Process Times (B) at Retort Temperature of (2) 240°F for Conduction-Heating Foods in (1) 303 x 406 Can

INITIAL FOOD TEMPERATURE (T_{ih})

f_h	z	100	110	120	130	140	(3) 150	160	170	180	190	200	Equivalent F_c^{18}	Equivalent F_s^{18}
	16	113.2	111.7	110.1	108.3	106.3	104.2	101.8	99.0	95.9	92.2	87.6	10.38	12.30
47.10	18	104.5	102.9	101.3	99.5	97.6	95.4	93.0	90.3	87.1	83.4	78.8	8.26	10.03
	20	97.0	95.5	93.9	92.1	90.1	88.0	85.6	82.8	79.7	75.9	71.4	6.79	8.45
	22	90.8	89.3	87.7	85.9	83.9	81.8	79.4	76.7	73.5	69.8	65.2	5.42	7.13
	16	117.5	115.9	114.1	112.2	110.2	107.9	105.3	102.4	99.1	95.2	90.3	10.35	12.27
49.87	18	108.3	106.7	104.9	103.1	101.0	98.7	96.2	93.3	89.9	86.0	81.1	8.25	10.03
	20	100.3	98.7	96.9	95.0	93.0	90.7	88.1	85.3	81.9	78.0	73.1	6.69	8.38
	22	94.5	92.9	91.2	89.3	87.2	85.0	82.4	79.5	76.2	72.2	67.4	5.40	7.16
	16	121.6	120.0	118.1	116.1	114.0	111.5	108.9	105.8	102.3	98.1	93.0	10.35	12.27
(4) 52.64	(5) 18	111.9	110.2	108.3	106.4	104.2	(6) 101.8	99.1	96.0	92.5	88.3	83.2	8.23	10.01
	20	103.7	102.0	100.2	98.2	96.0	93.6	90.9	87.9	84.3	80.2	75.1	6.55	8.31
	22	98.1	96.4	94.6	92.6	90.4	88.0	85.3	82.3	78.8	74.6	69.5	5.38	7.19
	16	125.7	124.0	122.0	119.9	117.6	115.1	112.3	109.1	105.4	101.0	95.6	10.35	12.27
55.42	18	115.3	113.5	111.6	109.5	107.2	104.7	101.8	98.6	94.9	90.5	85.2	8.21	9.98
	20	107.5	105.8	103.8	101.7	99.4	96.9	94.1	90.9	87.1	82.8	77.4	6.52	8.33
	22	101.6	99.8	97.9	95.8	93.5	91.0	88.1	84.9	81.2	76.8	71.4	5.34	7.16
	16	129.7	127.9	125.8	123.6	121.2	118.6	115.6	112.2	108.3	103.7	98.1	10.35	12.27
58.19	18	118.6	116.8	114.7	112.5	110.1	107.5	104.5	101.1	97.2	92.6	87.0	8.18	9.96
	20	111.3	109.4	107.4	105.2	102.8	100.1	97.1	93.8	89.9	85.3	79.6	6.50	8.36
	22	105.0	103.2	101.1	98.9	96.5	93.9	90.9	87.5	83.6	79.0	73.4	5.31	7.13

FIGURE 3. A typical page of data for conduction-heating foods to achieve commercial sterility.